# Assessment
# of
# Athletic Injuries

## ATHLETIC TRAINING EDUCATION SERIES

**SANDRA J. SHULTZ, PhD, ATC**
**PEGGY A. HOUGLUM, MS, ATC, PT**
**DAVID H. PERRIN, PhD, ATC**
UNIVERSITY OF VIRGINIA, CHARLOTTESVILLE


**DAVID H. PERRIN, PhD, ATC**
SERIES EDITOR
UNIVERSITY OF VIRGINIA, CHARLOTTESVILLE

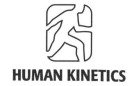

**HUMAN KINETICS**

**Library of Congress Cataloging-in-Publication Data**

Shultz, Sandra J.
    Assessment of athletic injuries / Sandra J. Shultz, Peggy A. Houglum, David H. Perrin.
        p. ; cm. -- (Athletic training education series)
    Includes bibliographical references and index.
    ISBN 0-7360-0158-1
    1. Sports--Accidents and injuries--Diagnosis--Examinations, questions, etc. 2. Sports medicine--Examinations, questions, etc. I. Houglum, Peggy A., 1948- II. Perrin, David H., 1954- III. Title. IV. Series.
    [DNLM: 1. Athletic Injuries--diagnosis--Examination Questions. 2. Physical Education and Training--methods--Examination Questions.  3. Sports Medicine--methods--Examination Questions. QT  18.2 S562a 2000]
    RD97 .S538 2000
    617.1'027'076--dc21                                          00-025395

ISBN: 0-7360-0158-1

**Acquisitions Editor**: Loarn D. Robertson, PhD; **Series Editors**: Kristine Enderle and Elaine Mustain; **Developmental Editor**: Elaine Mustain; **Assistant Editors**: Amanda S. Ewing and Melissa Feld; **Copyeditor**: Joyce Sexton; **Proofreader**: Sarah Wiseman; **Indexer**: Marie Rizzo; **Permission Manager**: Cheri Banks; **Graphic Designer**: Stuart Cartwright; **Graphic Artist**: Yvonne Griffith; **Photo Editor**: Clark Brooks; **Cover Designer**: Stuart Cartwright; **Photographer (interior)**: Tom Roberts, except where otherwise noted; **Art Manager**: Craig Newsom; **Illustrator**: Argosy; **Printer**: United Graphics

Printed in the United States of America       10  9  8  7  6  5  4  3  2

**Human Kinetics**
Web site: www.HumanKinetics.com

*United States:* Human Kinetics, P.O. Box 5076, Champaign, IL 61825-5076
800-747-4457
e-mail: humank@hkusa.com

*Canada:* Human Kinetics, 475 Devonshire Road, Unit 100, Windsor, ON N8Y 2L5
800-465-7301 (in Canada only)
e-mail: orders@hkcanada.com

*Europe:* Human Kinetics, 107 Bradford Road, Stanningley
Leeds LS28  6AT, United Kingdom
+44 (0) 113 255 5665
e-mail: hk@hkeurope.com

*Australia:* Human Kinetics, 57A Price Avenue, Lower Mitcham, South Australia 5062
08  8277 1555
e-mail: liahka@senet.com.au

*New Zealand:* Human Kinetics, P.O. Box 105-231, Auckland Central
09-523-3462
e-mail: hkp@ihug.co.nz

To my cherished family and in loving memory of my sister Patty. Through you, I have come to appreciate even more the magnitude of God's loving grace and his most perfect gift in our lives.

Sandra J. Shultz

*John 3:16*

To Cosette Perry, my first-grade teacher, whose enthusiasm in the classroom was my first exposure to the effectiveness of excellent teaching. Her wonderful ability to instill a desire for knowledge became my foundation for a lifetime of learning.

Peggy A. Houglum

# CONTENTS

# INTRODUCTION TO THE ATHLETIC TRAINING EDUCATION SERIES

The five textbooks of the Athletic Training Education Series—*Introduction to Athletic Training, Assessment of Athletic Injuries, Therapeutic Exercise for Athletic Injuries, Therapeutic Modalities for Athletic Injuries,* and *Management Strategies in Athletic Training,* Second Edition—were written for student athletic trainers and as a reference for practicing certified athletic trainers. Many textbooks have been written that in one way or another address the competencies in athletic training. However, absent from these books has been a coordinated approach to the competencies that serves to optimally prepare student athletic trainers for the National Athletic Trainers' Association (NATA) certification examination. If you are a student athletic trainer, you must master the material included in each of the content areas delineated in the NATA publication *Competencies in Athletic Training.* The philosophy of the Athletic Training Education Series is to address these competencies in a comprehensive and sequential manner while avoiding unnecessary duplication.

The series covers the educational content areas developed by the Education Council of the National Athletic Trainers' Association for accredited curriculum development. These content areas and the text (or in some cases, texts) of the series that primarily addresses each content area is as follows:

- Risk management and injury prevention *(Introduction* and *Management Strategies)*
- Pathology of injury and illnesses *(Introduction, Assessment, Therapeutic Exercise,* and *Therapeutic Modalities)*
- Assessment and evaluation *(Assessment* and *Therapeutic Exercise)*
- Acute care of injury and illness *(Introduction* and *Management Strategies)*
- Pharmacology *(Introduction* and *Therapeutic Modalities)*
- Therapeutic modalities *(Therapeutic Modalities)*
- Therapeutic exercise *(Therapeutic Exercise)*
- General medical conditions and disabilities *(Introduction* and *Assessment)*
- Nutritional aspects of injury and illness *(Introduction)*
- Psychosocial intervention and referral *(Introduction, Therapeutic Modalities,* and *Therapeutic Exercise)*
- Health care administration *(Management Strategies)*
- Professional development and responsibilities *(Introduction* and *Management Strategies)*

The authors for this series—Craig Denegar, Susan Hillman, Peggy Houglum, Richard Ray, Sandy Shultz, and I—are six certified athletic trainers with well over a century of collective experience as clinicians, educators, and leaders in the athletic training profession. The clinical experience of the authors spans virtually every setting in which athletic trainers practice, including the high school, sports medicine clinic, college, professional sport, hospital, and industrial settings. The professional positions of the authors include undergraduate and graduate curriculum director, head athletic trainer, professor, clinic director, and researcher. The authors have chaired or served on the NATA's most important committees, including the Professional Education Committee, the Education Task Force, Education Council, Research Committee of the Research and Education Foundation, Journal Committee, Appropriate Medical Coverage for Intercollegiate Athletics Task Force, Continuing Education Committee, and many others. The six authors of the series have created the most comprehensive and progressive collection of texts and related instructional materials presently available to athletic training students and educators. These materials, designed to accompany an accredited athletic training curriculum, will also serve to optimally prepare you for successful completion of the certification examination.

You will find several elements common to all the books in the series. These include

- chapter objectives and summaries tied to one another so that students can know and achieve their learning goals,
- chapter opening scenarios that illustrate the importance and relevance of the chapter content,
- cross-referencing among texts for a complete education on the subject, and
- thorough reference lists for further reading and research.

To enhance instruction, the series also includes Microsoft® PowerPoint presentations and instructor guides that comprise features such as course syllabuses, lecture and chapter outlines, case studies, and test banks. Where most appropriate, laboratory manuals accompany texts. Other features vary from book to book, depending on the requirements of the subject matter, but all include various aids for assimilation and review of information, extensive illustrations, and material to help the student apply the facts in the text.

Beyond the introductory text by Hillman, the order in which the books should be used is determined by the philosophy of your curriculum director. In any case, each book can stand alone so that an entire curriculum doesn't need to be revamped to use one or more parts of the series.

When I entered the profession of athletic training nearly 25 years ago, one text—*Prevention and Care of Athletic Injuries* by Klafs and Arnheim—covered nearly all the subject matter necessary to pass the NATA Board of Certification examination and practice as an entry-level athletic trainer. Since that time we have witnessed an amazing expansion of the subject matter necessary to practice athletic training and an equally impressive growth of practice settings in which athletic trainers work. I trust you will find the Athletic Training Education Series an invaluable resource as you prepare for a successful career as a certified athletic trainer and a most useful reference in your professional practice.

David H. Perrin, PhD, ATC
Series Editor

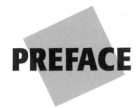

# PREFACE

*Assessment of Athletic Injuries*, one of five texts of the Athletic Training Education Series, addresses several clinical practice content areas you will need to master to pass the NATA BOC certification exam, including Pathology of Injury and Illnesses, Assessment and Evaluation, and General Medical Conditions and Disabilities. According to the 1998 Role Delineation Study conducted by Columbia Assessment Services for the NATA, approximately 23% of the certified athletic trainer's time is devoted to injury recognition and evaluation. Indeed, you will need to master the material in this book in order to properly manage, treat, and rehabilitate athletic injuries.

Each day of your career as a certified athletic trainer will present new challenges, and the ability to recognize, evaluate, and assess athletic injuries is essential to the proper management of the broad spectrum of injuries you will encounter. These injuries will range from acute to chronic, obvious to subtle, and minor to life threatening. The essential components of the injury assessment include obtaining an accurate history of the injury; inspecting the injured area and related structures; active and passive testing of motion; conducting strength and neurological assessment; palpating bony landmarks and soft tissues; and assessing function to determine readiness to return to unrestricted physical activity. In addition, special tests are necessary to isolate relevant structures and identify specific pathologies, including ligament stress testing and fracture assessment. The order and extent to which you address these components of the injury assessment will be determined in part by the injury setting. *Assessment of Athletic Injuries* offers a unique presentation of injury assessment, divided into on-field, sideline, and off-field protocols. These protocols allow you to specifically focus your evaluation skills for emergent, non-emergent, and post-acute conditions. Checklists in the text provide the framework for developing a systematic approach to injury evaluation in each setting.

Each chapter of *Assessment of Athletic Injuries* is designed to optimize your understanding and mastery of the material. You will first find chapter objectives that highlight key learning points for each chapter. A real-life scenario will follow to illustrate the complexity and exciting challenge of athletic injury assessment. Chapters 1 and 2 review injury classifications and present the general principles of injury assessment. Chapters 3 through 12 focus on injury recognition and assessment of specific body regions. Chapter 13 discusses general medical conditions and disabilities that you may encounter in physically active people. In chapters devoted to specific body regions, a brief review of the key anatomical structures (including applied illustrations) is presented immediately after the opening scenario, although your sound understanding of human anatomy from prior courses is assumed for this text. The various classifications of injuries, such as contusions, sprains and strains, impingements, fractures and dislocations, and neurovascular and neuromuscular injuries commonly seen for each body region, are addressed in this section. Next, a plan for on-field, sideline, and off-field assessment is presented, including a detailed review of the techniques for history, observation, range of motion, strength, palpation, special tests, and functional assessment appropriate for the structures examined in that chapter. In all chapters, a summary and list of review and critical thinking questions will help ensure that you have adequately mastered the material. Throughout each chapter, you will find various learning aids in the margins as well: terms that, while they are not defined in the text, may be unfamiliar to some readers, are defined; warnings not to omit procedures that may make the difference between complete recovery or permanent disability or even death are marked with an exclamation point; and statements that occur earlier in the text and are important to recall at certain points are repeated and designated with an icon of an index finger tied with string. Most chapters conclude with lists of both cited references and recommended references.

An instructor guide, including case studies, course projects, chapter worksheets, sample test questions, and a sample course syllabus is available for instructors, as is a Microsoft® PowerPoint graphics package that may be adapted as desired to suit each person's lecture content and style.

We trust you will find *Assessment of Athletic Injuries* an indispensable resource for the development of your confidence in assessing and differentiating the various pathologies that you will encounter over your career as a certified athletic trainer. This book can stand alone, but it should be noted, however, that using the entire Athletic Training Education Series will be especially effective in preparing you for the challenging NATA BOC certification examination and for a gratifying career in athletic training and sports medicine.

Sandra J. Shultz, PhD, ATC, CSCS
Peggy A. Houglum, MS, ATC, PT
David H. Perrin, PhD, ATC

# ACKNOWLEDGMENTS

Throughout the development of this text, there are a number of people who have contributed and whom we wish to recognize. In particular, we extend our sincere appreciation to our colleagues, Ethan Saliba and the University of Virginia Sports Medicine/Athletic Training Staff, for their invaluable support and patient cooperation during two weeks of photo shoots in the athletic treatment facility. To Julie Bernier, EdD, ATC, and John Cottone, ATC, for their thoughtful review of the initial draft and the excellent feedback they provided. To Dr. Theodore E. Keats, Professor of Medicine-Radiology, and the Film Library staff in the Department of Radiology, University of Virginia Health Sciences, for their assistance in obtaining the radiographic and Salter-Harris illustrations of skeletal pathologies. To Dr. Kenneth E. Greer, Professor and Chairman of the Department of Dermatology, University of Virginia Health Sciences for his personal time and contribution in obtaining the photographs of dermatological conditions. And to Dr. Frank C. McCue III, Professor of Orthopedic Surgery, and Dr. Brian C. Hoard, Associate Professor of Medicine-Dentistry, University of Virginia Health Sciences for providing selected hand and dental photographs. This text has been greatly enhanced by the collective contributions of these outstanding professionals.

Finally, we would like to thank our publisher Rainer Martens at Human Kinetics, as well as Loarn Robertson, Joanna Hatzopoulos, and especially Elaine Mustain, our developmental editor, for their support and invaluable contributions. Elaine's tireless efforts and quality suggestions are acknowledged beyond words and positively reflected in the quality and content of this text.

Sandra J. Shultz, PhD, ATC, CSCS
Peggy A. Houglum, MS, ATC, PT
David H. Perrin, PhD, ATC

# CHAPTER ONE

# Classification
# of Injuries

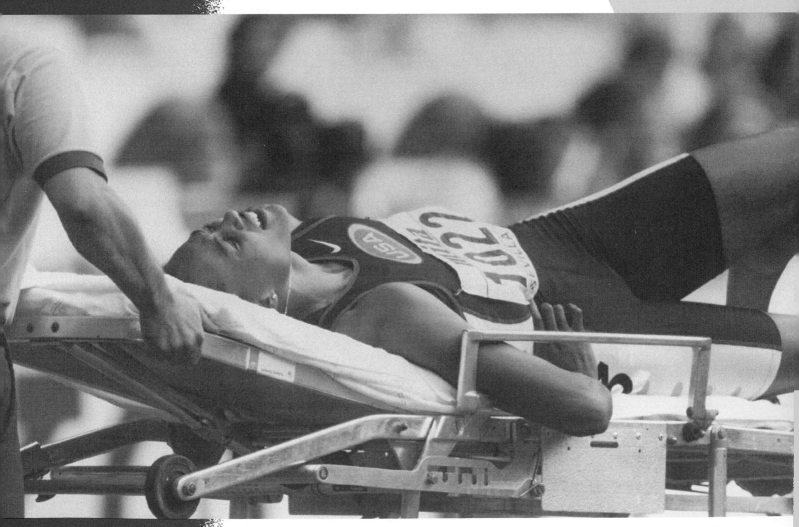

# OBJECTIVES

At the completion of this chapter, the reader will be able to do the following:

1. Classify injuries as either acute or chronic based on the onset and duration of symptoms

2. Define the common chronic inflammatory conditions, including signs and symptoms

3. Define the various classifications of closed soft tissue wounds, including degrees of severity

4. Define and classify closed and open wounds of the bone and joint articulations

5. Classify nerve injuries according to mechanism, severity, and signs and symptoms

6. Identify the classifications of open (exposed) wounds

Diane was looking forward to her new position as the first full-time head athletic trainer at Blue Ridge High School. Before hiring Diane, the school had had no certified athletic trainer; a coach (who had taken a couple of athletic training courses in college) and the school nurse had worked together to take care of the athletes when injury occurred. It wasn't long after the start of spring football that the athletic training room was packed with injured athletes.

"Steve, what can I help you with?" Diane asked the senior starting quarterback.

"Oh, my knee is acting up again. It seems to do this every year since I first injured it as a freshman. It hurts right here in the front below my kneecap. Coach said I strained it, but the nurse said I had tendinitis . . . so I don't really know what it is," Steve said. "What's the difference, anyway?"

"Well," Diane began to explain. "A strain is typically an acute injury caused by stretching or pulling a muscle or tendon. Tendinitis, on the other hand, is more of a chronic inflammation or irritation of the tendon."

"Chronic? Acute?" Steve asked.

"Sorry," Diane said. "Those are terms we use to describe how your symptoms began or how long you have had them. An acute injury is one that you usually know you have right when it occurs, and symptoms start almost immediately. With a chronic injury, the symptoms usually last longer and often appear gradually over time, and the person can't identify exactly when the injury occurred."

"Well, from what you are saying, tendinitis sounds more like it," Steve answered. "Boy, it sure would be nice, and less confusing, if everyone used the same words to describe my injury!"

Diane couldn't help but agree. She would later recall a number of times when it had been difficult to determine an athlete's previous injury based on what the coach called it. Now, more than ever, she appreciated the importance of using consistent terminology both when documenting injuries and when communicating with parents, coaches, and other health professionals.

As you read this text, you will find that the injuries for each joint or body region are classified by type. Proper injury terminology is essential for communicating effectively with other health professionals and accurately documenting the findings of your assessments. This chapter will briefly review the generally accepted scheme of injury classification and the cardinal signs and symptoms typically associated with these injuries. With few exceptions, the injury classifications and descriptors presented here will remain consistent, regardless of the joint or body region involved.

## SIGN VERSUS SYMPTOM

*Crepitus is a crackling, grating, or grinding sensation caused by abnormal movement between two structures.*

When people refer to the "signs and symptoms" that characterize a particular injury, it is important to note that these terms are not synonymous but rather define two separate sets of injury descriptors. A **sign** refers to a finding that is observed or that can be objectively measured as a result of the injury, such as swelling, discoloration, deformity, crepitus, or redness. A **symptom**, on the other hand, denotes a subjective complaint or an abnormal sensation the patient describes that cannot be directly observed. Complaints or perceptions of pain, nausea, altered sensation, **fatigue**, and so on are examples of symptoms that patients commonly report.

# ACUTE VERSUS CHRONIC

Injuries are classified as either acute or chronic. **Acute** injuries are conditions that have a sudden onset and are of short duration. They typically result from a one-time traumatic event or mechanism. Usually, the athlete clearly knows and recalls the mechanism of injury, as the signs and symptoms associated with the injury typically begin to surface immediately.

**Chronic** injuries, on the other hand, usually have a gradual onset and are of prolonged duration. Many times the exact mechanism or time of injury is not known. Chronic injury usually results from an accumulation of minor insults or repetitive stress that would not be sufficient to cause injury if the same stress or insult were applied in an isolated event. Consequently, chronic injuries are primarily inflammatory conditions in which the demands on the tissues exceed the ability to heal and recover before additional stress is applied. Common inflammatory conditions are listed in table 1.1. Chronic injury often occurs following periods of inadequate rest or recovery, overuse of a muscle or body part, overactivity, repetitive overloading of

| Table 1.1 | Common Chronic Inflammatory Conditions | |
|---|---|---|
| **Condition** | **Description** | **Signs and symptoms** |
| Apophysitis | Inflammation of a bony projection or outgrowth that serves as a muscle attachment | Pain, tenderness, swelling, increased bony prominence, pain with muscle tension |
| Bursitis | Inflammation or swelling of a bursa (synovial-filled membrane that lies between adjacent structures to limit friction and ease movement) | Pain, redness, heat, palpable fluid accumulation, crepitus and/or fluid thickening |
| Capsulitis | Inflammation of a joint capsule | Pain, localized joint inflammation and swelling, decreased range of motion |
| Myositis | Inflammatory response in a muscle or its surrounding connective tissue; can lead to ossification | Pain, inflammation, tenderness, decreased range of motion; possible calcium deposit |
| Neuritis | Inflammation or irritation of a nerve or nerve sheath | Local and referred pain, pain with percussion, tenderness, impaired sensation and motor function |
| Periostitis | Inflammation of the membranous lining of a bone | Pain, palpable swelling or "bumpiness" and tenderness along the bone; pain with attaching muscle action |
| Tendinitis | Inflammation of a tendon attaching muscle to bone | Pain, swelling, palpable tenderness and crepitus; pain with active and resistive muscle action |
| Tenosynovitis | Inflammation of the synovial sheath covering a tendon | Pain with palpation and movement of the tendon within the sheath; swelling or thickening, snowball crepitus, and decreased range of motion |

a structure, or repetitive friction between two structures. As such, these injuries may also be referred to as **overuse injuries**. Chronic injuries are often more difficult to treat than acute injuries, as the longer the pathologic or diseased state continues, the longer it takes for healing to occur and symptoms to subside.

# CLOSED (UNEXPOSED) WOUNDS

**Closed wounds** include any injury that does not involve disruption of the skin surface. Although closed wounds are not always visually obvious, most result in visible signs and symptoms (i.e., swelling, discoloration, and deformity) that aid in evaluating and identifying the injury. Common examples of closed wounds include contusions, ligament sprains, muscle and tendon strains, inflammatory conditions, some bony fractures, joint dislocations, and neurovascular injuries.

## CLOSED SOFT TISSUE INJURIES

Closed injuries to soft tissue can occur as contusions, sprains, or strains. These types of soft tissue injury are further classified according to the degree of severity or the extent of injury.

### *Contusion*

*A hematoma is a localized mass or "blood [hema] tumor [toma]" caused by an accumulation of blood in a confined area of a tissue or space.*

A **contusion** or "bruise" refers to the compression of soft tissue by a direct blow or impact sufficient to cause disruption or damage to the small capillaries in the tissue. This trauma will cause local bleeding or hemorrhage, resulting in **ecchymosis**, or discoloration of the tissue. There will also be localized pain and tenderness. Ecchymosis and swelling may occur immediately or may be delayed, depending on the severity of injury. The severity of a contusion can be described as first, second, or third degree, usually according to the extent of tissue damage and functional impairment. A **first-degree** contusion involves only superficial tissue damage, causing minimal swelling and localized tenderness and no limitations in strength or range of motion. A **second-degree** contusion is characterized by increased pain and hemorrhage due to increased area and depth of tissue damage, resulting in mild to moderate limitations in range of motion, muscle function, or both. A **third-degree** contusion is a severe tissue compression, resulting in severe pain, significant hemorrhage, and hematoma formation, as well as severe limitations in range of motion and muscle function. With third-degree contusions, you should have a high index of suspicion that deeper structures (e.g., bone, muscle) may also have been damaged by the offending impact but may be masked by the signs and symptoms associated with the superficial soft tissue damage.

### *Sprain*

A **sprain** is an injury to a ligament or capsular structure. Because ligaments attach one bone to another, sprains are associated with joint injury. Sprains result from forces that cause two or more connecting bones to separate or go beyond their normal range of motion—subsequently stretching and tearing the attaching ligament(s) or capsule. To describe the severity or extent of injury, sprains are further classified as first, second, or third degree.

*Laxity denotes hypermobility or increased joint movement.*

• **First Degree.** A first-degree sprain is characterized by mild overstretching and does not cause any visual disruption in the tissue. Signs and symptoms include mild pain and tenderness over the involved ligament and little or no disability. Active and passive range of motion usually is not limited, but the athlete will typically experience pain at the end of the range as the ligament becomes taut. When the joint is stressed, the athlete will complain of pain but you will not notice any joint laxity.

With first-degree injuries, inflammation and discoloration are usually minor and may be delayed until the next day. However, in some body regions, such as the lateral ankle, a relatively minor sprain can cause considerable and rapid swelling if a major capillary running adjacent to the ligament is disrupted. Therefore, the degree of swelling and discoloration may be a poor indication of injury severity.

*Instability is defined as abnormal joint movement caused by disruption of a ligament or capsular integrity.*

• **Second Degree.** With a second-degree injury, further stretching and partial disruption or macrotearing of the ligament occur. Second-degree injuries represent the broadest range of injury; therefore the severity of signs and symptoms and disability will vary considerably. Signs and symptoms range from moderate to severe pain, point tenderness, ecchymosis, and swelling. Range of motion and normal function are usually limited secondary to pain and swelling. **Stress testing** will show varying degrees of joint instability, but the ligament will still be sufficiently intact to provide an end point to joint motion.

• **Third Degree.** A third-degree sprain is characterized by complete disruption (rupture) or loss of ligament integrity. The athlete may have experienced a "pop" at the time of injury. Signs and symptoms include immediate pain and disability, rapid swelling, ecchymosis, and loss of function. Stress testing of the ligament will reveal moderate to severe joint instability, and there will be no end feel. Third-degree injuries can be initially deceiving in that range of motion and stress testing is typically less painful than with second-degree injuries, since no tension will be placed on the injured structure if it is completely torn.

### Strains

*Dysynchrony is a misfiring or mistiming of a muscle contraction.*

Whereas sprains involve stretching or tearing of a ligament, **strains** involve stretching or tearing of a muscle or tendon. Muscle and tendon strains occur most often as a result of a violent, forceful contraction or overstretching of the myotendon unit. Fatigue, lack of proper warm-up, and muscle imbalance or dysynchrony are common predisposing factors. Similarly to sprains, strains are classified by severity as first-, second-, and third-degree injuries.

• **First Degree.** A first-degree strain is characterized by overstretching and microtearing of the muscle or tendon, but there is no gross fiber disruption. The athlete will complain of mild pain and tenderness but will typically have a full active and passive range of motion and little or no disability. Pain will usually accompany resisted muscle contraction. Following a first-degree strain, it is not uncommon for an athlete to continue to practice or compete, as pain and tenderness are often delayed until the next day.

*Palpable means detectable by touching or feeling.*

• **Second Degree.** Second-degree strains involve further stretching and partial tearing of muscle or tendon fibers. As with sprains, second-degree strains represent the broadest range of injury, and signs and symptoms can vary considerably. These include immediate pain, localized tenderness, and disability. Varying degrees of swelling, ecchymosis, decreased range of motion, and decreased strength will also be noted. The athlete will complain of pain with active muscle contraction and passive muscle stretch. Depending on injury severity, there may or may not be a palpable defect.

• **Third Degree.** In third-degree strains, a muscle or tendon is completely ruptured. Signs and symptoms include an audible pop, immediate pain, and loss of function of the myotendon unit. There will be a palpable defect in superficially lying muscles. Muscle hemorrhage and diffuse swelling will be present. Depending on the function or contribution of the injured muscle or tendon for a given movement, range of motion and strength may or may not be affected and may or may not be painful.

## BONE AND JOINT ARTICULATIONS

The general classifications of closed wounds comprising disruptions in a bone, joint surface, or joint articulation include **fractures**, dislocations, and subluxations.

### *Closed Fractures*

Simple or closed fractures involve disruption in the continuity of a bone without disruption of the skin surface. Traumatic fractures are caused by direct impact or by an indirect force that exceeds the tensile strength of the bone. The direction of force or impact often dictates the type of fracture that results. Repetitive forces or impact at lower applied loads can also cause chronic weakening or failure of bone tissue resulting in a stress fracture. Table 1.2 presents the common classifications of closed fractures.

| Table 1.2 | Classifications of Closed Fractures | |
|---|---|---|
| **Classification** | **Illustration** | **Description** |
| Comminuted | | Fracture resulting in multiple fragments or shattering of the bone at the site of injury. |
| Compression | | Failure of the bone and subsequent compression or impaction of the fracture ends due to axial compression forces. |
| Greenstick | | Incomplete fracture through the bone, most often occuring in young bones. Resembles the breaking of a "green stick." |
| Oblique | | The fracture line extends obliquely or diagonally in relation to the long axis of the bone. |
| Spiral | | An S-shaped fracture line that twists around and through the bone due to rotation or torsional forces. |
| Transverse | | The fracture line runs transverse or horizontal to the long axis of the bone. Usually caused by direct lateral impact or stress failure. |
| Avulsion | | The pulling away of a piece of bone secondary to tensioning of an attaching ligament, tendon, or muscle. |

*(continued)*

| Table 1.2 *(continued)* | | |
|---|---|---|
| **Classification** | **Illustration** | **Description** |
| Osteochondral | | A fracture that extends through the articular cartilage (i.e., joint surface) and into the underlying bone. |
| Stress or "fatigue" | | Complete or incomplete failure of a bone due to repetitive stress or loading. Weakening and failure occur when bone breakdown/absorption exceeds bone production. |

- **Traumatic Fractures.** Signs and symptoms of a traumatic fracture include immediate pain, rapid swelling, bony tenderness, crepitus with movement of the bony fragments, and possible deformity if the fracture is displaced. False joint movement may also occur when the fracture is near a movable joint. With displaced fractures, there is always a danger of secondary injury to the surrounding soft tissue and neurovascular structures. Therefore, the evaluation process should always include assessment of neurovascular status distal to the suspected fracture site.

For details on immediate care and immobilization of suspected fractures, refer to *Introduction to Athletic Training* (Hillman 2000), chapter 8.

- **Stress Fractures.** Signs and symptoms of stress fractures are not usually quite so obvious, and often the athlete initially dismisses them. The onset of pain is often gradual, but may appear suddenly once bone failure occurs. Pain or a deep ache may at first be noticeable only during activity and may subside with rest, progressing to more constant pain if the offending activity continues. Swelling will be minimal, and there will be localized tenderness over the fracture site.

### Epiphyseal Injury

Epiphyseal injury or fracture involves the disruption or separation of the **epiphysis** or epiphyseal plate (growth plate). Epiphyseal injury is a concern in children and in adolescents before the cessation of growth, as disruption can cause premature closing and growth abnormalities in the involved bone. The most widely accepted classification system is the Salter-Harris classification system (Harris 1983) (see table 1.3). Signs and symptoms are consistent with those previously mentioned for closed fractures.

### Dislocation

*Spontaneous reduction is an unassisted relocation of a joint following dislocation or subluxation.*

Joint **dislocation**, or "luxation," is a complete disassociation of two joint surfaces. Joint dislocation most commonly results from forces that cause the joint to exceed its normal range of motion, forcing the bony articulation to separate. Consequently, joint dislocation usually involves severe stretching or complete disruption of one or more of the supporting ligaments (third-degree sprain). Signs and symptoms include immediate pain, rapid swelling, deformity, and loss of function. As with displaced fractures, signs and symptoms associated with neurovascular impairment may also be present and should be monitored. In some instances, joint dislocation may not be obvious if the joint spontaneously reduces immediately following the

## Table 1.3 Salter-Harris Classifications of Epiphyseal Fractures

| Classification | Illustration | Description |
| --- | --- | --- |
| Type I | | Complete separation of the epiphyseal plate (epiphysis from the metaphysis). No associated fracture. |
| Type II | | Separation of the epiphysis with associated fracture of the metaphysis. |
| Type III | | Fracture of the epiphysis extending from the epiphyseal plate through the articular surface. |
| Type IV | | Fracture extending through the epiphysis, epiphyseal plate, and metaphysis. |
| Type V | | Crushing or compression of the epiphyseal plate. This injury has a high incidence of premature closure. |

Reprinted, by permission, from R.B. Salter, 1999, *Textbook of disorders and injuries of the musculoskeletal system*. 3rd ed. (Philadelphia: Lippincott Williams & Wilkins).

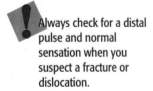

Always check for a distal pulse and normal sensation when you suspect a fracture or dislocation.

injury. In the case of a spontaneous reduction, the athlete may complain of a feeling of the joint slipping or "giving out," or a sensation of the joint "going out and coming back in." Chronic joint instability often follows an acute dislocation, precipitating recurrent episodes of dislocation or subluxation (see the next section) at lower forces and applied loads. This is particularly true of the patellofemoral, glenohumeral, and phalangeal joints.

### Subluxation

**Subluxation** of a joint is an incomplete disassociation of two joint surfaces. Depending on the degree of subluxation, these injuries vary quite a bit in terms of signs and symptoms of pain, disability, swelling, and joint instability. Often, subluxations are difficult to identify, as deformity may be minimal and they often spontaneously reduce. History becomes important in identification of these injuries, and the athlete may complain of a sensation of the joint's slipping or momentarily giving out at the time of injury.

## NERVE INJURIES

*Ischemia is tissue anemia caused by lack of blood flow to an area.*

Nerve injury can result from compression or tensioning of the neural structure. Nervous tissue is very sensitive to compression and ischemia, and injury may occur secondary to a direct blow, acute swelling of tissue within an enclosed space, or any pathology that compromises the space through which the nerve courses. Laceration of the nerve can occur secondary to fracture, dislocation, penetrating trauma, or excessive tensioning or stretch. Signs and symptoms of pain, sensation, and motor function can vary considerably depending on the extent of nerve injury. Sensory impairment can range from **anesthesia** (no sensation) to **paresthesia** (tingling, burning, or numbness) to **hyperesthesia** (hypersensitivity), and motor function can range from no loss in muscle strength or function to weakness to complete loss of muscle function (paralysis).

Classifications for the extent of nerve disruption include neuropraxia, axonotmesis, and neurotmesis.

- The least severe nerve disruption is a **neuropraxia**—a transient and reversible loss in nerve function secondary to trauma or irritation. Neuropraxia entails mechanical deformation of the nerve, but no disruption of the nerve fibers. Signs and symptoms of sensory and motor deficits are short-lived, ranging from a few seconds to two weeks depending on the extent of nerve trauma. A direct blow over the peroneal nerve at the proximal fibular head and the ulnar nerve at the medial elbow is a common mechanism for a neuropraxia.

- **Axonotmesis** denotes a partial disruption in the nerve. With an axonotmesis, sufficient nervous tissue is intact to allow eventual regeneration. However, signs and symptoms of sensory and motor deficits will be prolonged, lasting anywhere from two weeks to up to one year, so that considerable atrophy and weakness may result.

- **Neurotmesis**, the most severe nerve injury, is characterized by complete severance of the nerve resulting in permanent loss of function of the innervated structures distal to the point of injury. With a neurotmesis, no regeneration is evident one year after the injury.

Other terms used to describe nerve pathology include neuralgia and neuroma.

- **Neuralgia** is an achiness or pain along the distribution of a nerve secondary to chronic irritation or inflammation. Neuralgia is a common symptom in nerve compression syndromes such as tarsal tunnel syndrome, ulnar nerve compression, carpal tunnel syndrome, and disc herniation, which will be discussed later in this text.

- A **neuroma** is a thickening of a nerve, or "nerve tumor," secondary to chronic irritation or inflammation.

# OPEN (EXPOSED) WOUNDS

**Open**, or exposed, **wounds** are injuries that involve a disruption in the continuity of the skin, caused by friction or by blunt or sharp trauma. The classifications for open wounds are listed in table 1.4.

- An **abrasion**, or "strawberry," is particularly painful because of the large surface area that is exposed. Abrasions most commonly occur in soccer, baseball, and softball as a result of sliding. "Floor burns" are also abrasions, a consequence of sliding or of friction against a wooden floor as commonly occurs in basketball and volleyball. The use of sliding and knee pads is highly effective in preventing these minor but painful superficial skin wounds. Signs and symptoms include a burning or "stinging" pain and minimal bleeding. It is important to cleanse these wounds thoroughly, making sure to remove all of the dirt and debris to avoid infection.

- A **blister**—common in nonathletes as well as athletes—is an area of skin that is exposed to excessive friction or rubbing. Friction from new or ill-fitting shoes in

| **Table 1.4   Classification of Open (Exposed) Wounds** | |
|---|---|
| **Classification** | **Description** |
| Abrasion | Broad scraping or shearing off of the superficial skin layers with sliding of the skin against a rough or high-friction surface. |
| Blister | Separation and accumulation of fluid or blood between superficial skin layers secondary to repetitive friction or shearing movements. |
| Incision | A cut through all layers of the skin by a sharp object or instrument (e.g., knife), resulting in smooth, even wound edges. |
| Laceration | A tearing of the skin by blunt trauma to the skin over a bony prominence, resulting in jagged, uneven wound edges. |
| Puncture | A small disruption in the skin, caused by a sharp, penetrating object. Puncture wounds should be carefully evaluated for possible injury to underlying structures. |
| Avulsion | A tearing off or complete disassociation of a portion of skin. |
| Compound fracture/dislocation | Disruption in the skin surface, secondary to penetration, by a displaced fracture fragment or joint dislocation. |

the heel or toe region is a common cause of blisters in physically active people. Gymnasts and baseball and softball players commonly get blisters on the hand as a consequence of repetitive friction and rubbing between the hands and the bar or bat. Signs and symptoms include pain, redness, and accumulation of fluid (may be clear, serous, or blood-filled) between the superficial skin layers. Although the injury the blister creates is usually quite minor, the pain can be extremely limiting. It is important to avoid puncturing or removing the superficial skin layer, as pain is often significantly increased with exposure of the deeper tissue layers. Early evaluation and recognition of "hot spots" on the skin showing areas of friction, as well as the use of proper padding, can help prevent a blister from forming.

• An **incision** is usually caused by a knife or sharp object that makes a "clean cut" through the full thickness of the skin. Signs and symptoms include an observable disruption in the skin, possible separation or gapping of the wound edges if the skin is under tension, and immediate bleeding. Even small incisions in areas that are highly vascularized, such as the face, can cause considerable bleeding initially, although such bleeding can be quickly controlled with direct pressure.

• A **laceration** differs from an incision in that the cause is a blunt, rather than a sharp, trauma. With a laceration, the skin basically "ruptures" when a blunt force is exerted against a bony prominence. An elbow hitting an opponent's cheek during a rebound, a ball striking the eyebrow region, and a blocker making contact with an opponent's chin are common mechanisms for lacerations. Signs and symptoms are consistent with those of an incision, except that because the tissue is torn rather than cut, the wound edges are more jagged.

• A **puncture wound** can result when a pointed, sharp object penetrates the skin. These injuries can be deceiving in that there seems to be little observable tissue damage, and bleeding is often minimal. Evaluating and caring for puncture-type wounds should involve two primary concerns. If the depth of penetration is beyond the thickness of the skin layers, deeper structures that are not visible may be injured or damaged. In addition, puncture wounds are particularly susceptible to infection because they are difficult to clean given the limited exposure of the involved tissue.

• An **avulsion** is characterized by the complete tearing away of a portion of skin. The range of severity and signs and symptoms can be quite large, depending on the structures involved and the amount of tissue damage. A simple skin avulsion, the most common type, typically results when the skin is either caught on an unyielding object or pinched between two objects. Depending on the mechanism and the offending trauma, underlying tissues such as muscle, tendon, bone, and even an entire limb (amputation) can be torn away along with the skin; but these severe injuries rarely result from trauma incurred during physical activity.

It is important to note that open wounds may be associated with an underlying (unexposed) injury. Paying careful attention to the way in which the injury occurred, as well as to signs and symptoms that may be in addition to or out of proportion with what you would expect of the open wound, is important when evaluating these injuries. An obvious example is a **compound fracture**, or **dislocation**. This injury occurs when a displaced fracture or joint penetrates the skin surface so that the bone or joint is exposed. Compound dislocations and fractures are most common in the fingers, but can occur with any joint dislocation or displaced long bone fracture. Crushing injuries that compress the soft tissue against the underlying bone and deeper tissue are another example of an open wound with an associated unexposed tissue injury.

!  Always wear gloves and follow Occupational Safety and Health Administration guidelines when caring for an open wound.

Also of importance in evaluating and caring for open wounds is the use of proper precautions in the presence of blood or seeping wounds. Open, or exposed, wounds are also susceptible to infection and should be monitored for signs and symptoms of increased pain, redness, swelling, heat, and red streaks running from the wound toward the trunk. If signs or symptoms of infection are present, the athlete should be referred for medical treatment and possible antibiotic therapy.

For further discussion of precautions in caring for open wounds, refer to *Introduction to Athletic Training* (Hillman 2000), chapter 8.

## SUMMARY

1. *Classify injuries as either acute or chronic based on the onset and duration of symptoms.*

   Injuries are generally classified as either acute or chronic. Acute injuries have a known mechanism and are of sudden onset; signs and symptoms usually surface immediately or shortly after the injury. Chronic injuries have a gradual onset and long duration. Often the person does not recall a specific mechanism of injury, and injury results from an accumulation or repetitive stress over time.

2. *Define the common chronic inflammatory conditions, including signs and symptoms.*

   Chronic inflammation conditions can result from repetitive overuse, mechanical loading, and/or friction. A variety of tissues are susceptible to chronic inflammation, including bone, bursa, capsule, muscle, and tendon. Terms used to describe inflammatory conditions of various structures contain the suffix "itis"—for example, "bursitis" (inflammation of the bursa) and "tendinitis" (inflammation of the tendon).

3. *Define the various classifications of closed soft tissue wounds, including degrees of severity.*

   Closed soft tissue wounds are generally classified as contusions (soft tissue compression), strains (stretching or tearing of muscle or tendon), and sprains (stretching or tearing of ligament). They are further classified by severity as first, second, or third degree. First-degree injuries, the least severe, are characterized by minimal pain and tissue disruption, and no loss of function. Second-degree injuries are injuries with moderate or partial tissue disruption. The signs, symptoms, and functional impairment associated with second-degree injuries can vary considerably, depending on the extent of tissue disruption. Third-degree injuries are the most severe; these are characterized by complete tissue disruption and severe functional impairment.

4. *Define and classify closed and open wounds of the bone and joint articulations.*

   Injuries involving the bone or joint articulation include fractures and dislocations. A fracture occurs when the continuity of a bone is disrupted. Fractures are typically classified by the type, location, and/or extent of bony disruption, which is often dictated by the impact mechanism. When disassociation of two articular surfaces of a joint occurs, the injury is classified as either a dislocation (complete disassociation) or subluxation (partial disassociation) and is often accompanied by varying degrees of disruption in the supporting ligaments. Fractures or dislocations can be classified as open (compound) or closed wounds, depending on whether the displaced bone or joint segment penetrates the surface of the skin.

5. *Classify nerve injuries according to mechanism, severity, and signs and symptoms.*

   Nerve injury can result from either compressive or tensioning forces placed on nerve tissues. Classifications for the extent of nerve disruption include neuropraxia, axonotmesis, and neurotmesis. Other terms used to describe more chronic nerve pathologies include neuralgia and neuroma. When an injury involves the nerve, there will be transient or permanent alterations in sensation and motor function, with signs and symptoms varying quite a bit depending on the extent of injury.

6. *Identify the classifications of open (exposed) wounds.*

   Open wounds, or injuries that involve a disruption in the continuity of the skin, are classified by the type of tissue disruption. Because the wound is exposed, the athletic trainer must use proper precautions when evaluating and treating these injuries and must closely monitor the wound for signs of infection.

# REVIEW QUESTIONS

1. Compare and contrast the following injury terms, giving three to four examples of each:
   - Sign versus symptom
   - Closed versus open wound
   - Acute versus chronic

2. What is the difference between a strain and a sprain? Include in your discussion the common mechanisms and the ways in which the severity of these injuries is defined.

3. In the young athlete, what type of fractures might you expect that you wouldn't see in an adult?

4. How are joint dislocations and subluxations related to joint sprains?

5. Describe the grades of nerve injuries and the signs and symptoms associated with each.

6. List and describe the classifications for open wounds. What are some of the precautions and/or complications that you should be concerned about when dealing with open wounds?

## CRITICAL THINKING QUESTIONS

1. An athlete comes to you complaining of chronic pain in the anterior aspect of the knee. Given the anatomical structures in this area, what types of chronic inflammatory conditions might you suspect? Do you think you might be able to differentiate which structure is involved based on the signs and symptoms? Why or why not?

2. A worker comes into the industrial clinic complaining of pain, paresthesia, and muscle weakness in the lower leg. What types of nerve injuries might be associated with these signs and symptoms? Can you give examples of acute and chronic injury mechanisms that may cause these symptoms?

3. Over the phone, you are asked by a physician to describe an ankle injury. What are some of the important terms you would use to classify the type and severity of the injury to provide the physician with as much information as possible?

4. You are called onto the track where a sprinter is lying on the ground complaining of pain in the posterior thigh. She tells you that she was doing 60 m time trials and felt a pop and immediate pain in the muscle. In your evaluation, you note immediate swelling and a palpable defect on the medial side of the midposterior thigh. The athlete is able to flex the knee with minimal discomfort, but she says it feels very weak. How would you classify this muscle injury? On the basis of these symptoms, how would you rate the severity of injury? Give reasons.

## CITED REFERENCE

Harris, R.B. 1983. *Textbook of disorders and injuries of the musculoskeletal system.* 2d ed. Baltimore: Williams & Wilkins.

## ADDITIONAL RESOURCES

Hillman, S.K. 2000. *Introduction to athletic training.* Champaign, IL: Human Kinetics.

*Taber's cyclopedic medical dictionary.* 1997. 18th ed. Philadelphia: Davis.

# CHAPTER TWO

# Principles
# of Assessment

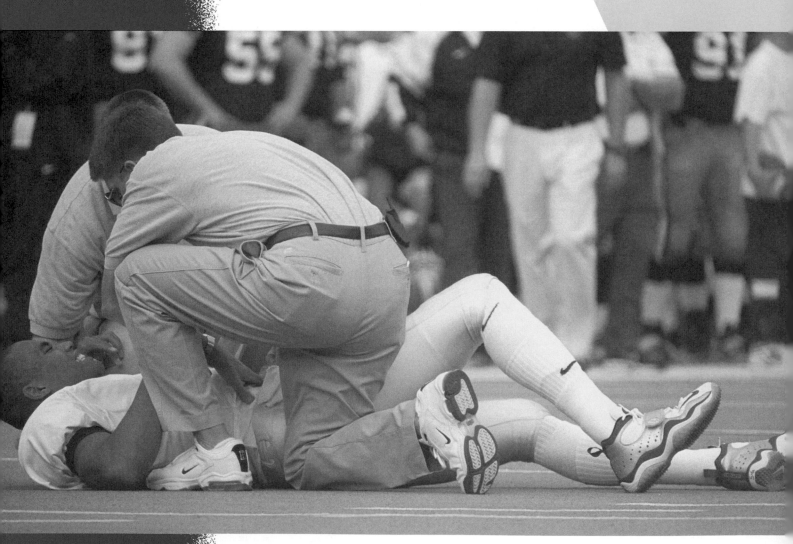

# OBJECTIVES

At the completion of this chapter, the reader will be able to do the following:

1. Identify the main goals and features of the on-field assessment

2. Explain the purpose and the components of the subjective assessment

3. Identify the general evaluation procedures of the objective assessment and the purpose for each

4. Identify the SINS factors of injury assessment

5. Discuss the goals, primary components, and evaluation sequence of the sideline assessment

6. Discuss the goals, primary components, and evaluation sequence of the off-field assessment

7. Explain the SOAP notes procedure for injury documentation

Bill had just sat down after a busy hour in the athletic training room getting the teams ready for practice.

Suddenly Ryan, the manager, came running in. "Bill! Come quick—Sara and Tina just went down on the soccer field!"

Bill leaped up and ran out with Ryan. As he was approaching the field he quizzed Ryan. "What's wrong? What happened?"

"I don't know, really. . . . I saw them both running full speed after the ball but wasn't watching when they made contact—I just came running when I saw they were down. . . . It looked kind of bad, though," Ryan explained.

As Bill approached, he surveyed the scene. All the athletes were gathered around the two young women on the ground. Tina appeared to be moving but was bleeding from the head. Sara was facedown and appeared to be unconscious. At that point, Bill was thinking, "Man, this does look bad—what do I do now, and who do I take care of first?"

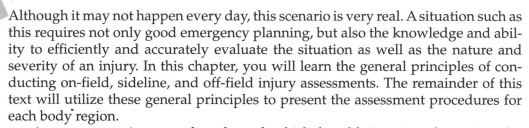

Although it may not happen every day, this scenario is very real. A situation such as this requires not only good emergency planning, but also the knowledge and ability to efficiently and accurately evaluate the situation as well as the nature and severity of an injury. In this chapter, you will learn the general principles of conducting on-field, sideline, and off-field injury assessments. The remainder of this text will utilize these general principles to present the assessment procedures for each body region.

An **assessment** is a procedure through which the athletic trainer determines the severity, irritability, nature, and stage of an injury. An **evaluation** is the systematic process that allows the athletic trainer to make the assessment. The assessment procedure and the evaluation techniques that are used to make the assessment are so closely aligned that the terms "assessment" and "evaluation" can be used interchangeably without confusion.

There are several purposes for an assessment of an athlete's injury:

- An assessment determines immediate care and transportation needs in situations involving life-threatening factors.
- It can identify the injury's **S**tage, **I**rritability, **N**ature, and **S**everity ("SINS").
- It can be used to evaluate changes before and after a treatment application.
- It can determine the athlete's course of treatment from the initial stage through the return to sport participation.

As an athletic trainer you will conduct assessments at various times in relation to the occurrence of an injury and for various purposes: (1) at the time of injury to determine first aid, emergency care measures, disposition (i.e., return to play, removal from play, medical referral, emergency medical services [EMS] referral), and transportation needs; (2) prior to initial treatment to determine the general and specific course for treatment; (3) during the treatment phase to determine the effectiveness of the treatment and the need for changes in treatment; and (4) before returning the athlete to full sport participation to assess the athlete's readiness to return. Other texts cover specific techniques for treatment and rehabilitation of an injured athlete.

For the assessment techniques you will use during the course of an injured athlete's treatment and rehabilitation, refer to *Therapeutic Exercise for Athletic Injuries* (Houglum 2000), chapter 4.

At the time of injury, the on-field assessment allows you to determine the presence of life-threatening conditions, as well as first aid and transportation needs. If you ascertain that the athlete does not need emergency care and that it is safe to get him to the sidelines, you will conduct a second and more detailed sideline assessment. If you did not see the injury happen and are consulted sometime later, you will perform an off-field assessment of the injury, which may or may not be recent. This chapter will focus on the general procedures and evaluation principles for each of these assessments. Later chapters will cover these assessment procedures in more detail as they relate to each body region.

# ON-FIELD ASSESSMENT

Before performing an on-field assessment, the athletic training staff should have an emergency plan in place for management and transportation of the injured athlete. Those plans are beyond the scope of this book. Whatever the emergency care plan, all athletes and coaching staff should be instructed not to move the injured athlete before the athletic trainer has attended to the person. Furthermore, those responsible should instruct any athlete who suffers a significant injury to remain down until adequate assessment of the injury has taken place.

For details of emergency plans and procedures, refer to *Introduction to Athletic Training* (Hillman 2000), chapter 8.

For game situations, it is also important that you know the rules regarding on-field assessment for each sport for which you provide medical coverage. Many sports have specific rules that apply in this situation. The rules for some sports won't allow you onto the field or court until the official has beckoned you, but other sports have very specific time frames within which a decision for care must be made before the team or athlete is penalized (i.e., charged with a time-out, removed from play, or disqualified). While such rules should never put you in the position of compromising your care and attention to the athlete, having a good knowledge of these rules will help you avoid unnecessary conflicts.

## GOALS AND PURPOSES

The purpose of the on-field assessment is to rule out life-threatening and serious injuries, determine the severity of the injury, and ascertain the most appropriate method of transporting the athlete off the field. Your goals are to make a quick and accurate assessment and to initially treat the injury in order to minimize its impact. These assessment decisions are among the most critical the athletic trainer must make, since an incorrect decision can have dire—even deadly—consequences. For example, allowing an athlete with a spinal cord injury to move may cause permanent paralysis; ignoring the signs of shock can result in death.

Even though on-field assessment often demands rapid decision making, it is imperative that you stay calm, take time to make the right determination, and yet be focused and efficient. Good evaluation skills and sound judgment along with knowledge and experience are essential, and you must make all decisions with the athlete's safety and health in mind. If you are ever unsure of the severity or nature of the athlete's condition, it is better to err on the side of caution and refer the athlete than to assume that this is not necessary. Always remember to stay within your scope of practice and training. Hippocrates said that those in medicine should "do no harm." Athletic trainers should adhere to that advice and never hesitate to call for assistance if the best course of action is unclear or the demands of the situation exceed their training or knowledge base.

## PRIMARY SURVEY

As you approach the injured athlete, you should make several observations. Quickly survey the surrounding environment to check for any objects that may have contributed to the injury or that pose a danger to the athlete or yourself. Observe the athlete where she is lying. Once at the athlete's side, conduct a **primary assessment** for life-threatening conditions. First check to see whether the athlete is responsive and assess the **ABCs** of emergency medical care: **A**irway, **B**reathing, and **C**irculation. If the athlete is unconscious, try to arouse her by speaking loudly, calling her name, or eliciting a pain response by pinching the soft tissue under her arm or rubbing your knuckle on her sternum. If you are unable to arouse the athlete, ask these questions first: Is the athlete's airway open? Is she breathing? Does she have a pulse? If the answer to any of these questions is no, cardiopulmonary resuscitation should be initiated immediately. If you did not observe the injury, you should assume a spinal cord injury until you have proven otherwise and should use the modified jaw thrust rather than the head-tilt/chin-lift method for rescue breathing. During the primary survey, you should also check and control for severe bleeding before proceeding.

For a further discussion of methods of rescue breathing, refer to *Introduction to Athletic Training* (Hillman 2000), chapter 8.

### Secondary Survey

If the athlete is breathing and any bleeding is under control, move on to a secondary assessment to evaluate for other serious or life-threatening injuries.

### History

When taking an on-field history, your primary goal is to quickly determine the mechanism, location, and severity of the injury. To establish the mechanism, ask how the injury occurred and what happened. If you were an eyewitness to the injury event, you may already have vital information regarding the mechanism and the forces involved. Seeing firsthand the athlete's initial response to the trauma can provide valuable information as well. If you did not witness the injury and the athlete is unconscious, ask bystanders what happened and how long the person has been unconscious.

If the athlete is conscious, you will attempt to obtain a history. In some cases this is a challenge; but the questioning may also help calm the athlete and help her focus on something besides her pain or fear, thus allowing you to proceed more easily with your assessment. You may find that the athlete has a very different perspective from your own or from that of other bystanders. For example, although observers on the sideline may not have heard a sound, the athlete may have experienced a pop or snap. Torque or rotational forces may also be experienced by an athlete, but not readily observed.

Questions regarding the location and intensity of the athlete's symptoms add to your picture of the injury, helping you determine its severity and decide on the method of transport off the field. Does the athlete have pain? If she complains of any neck or back pain and you suspect a spinal injury, ask if she is experiencing any numbness or tingling. If these symptoms are present, your evaluation should proceed accordingly (see chapters 3 and 7). Does the athlete complain of being dizzy, light-headed, or nauseated? This type of questioning will help you to quickly focus on the area of injury and allow you to make correct and appropriate decisions on the direction of your assessment.

You need not take a complete history during the on-field assessment. Instead, your goal is to gather the critical information necessary for determining the general nature and extent of the injury and the best course of immediate action. You can defer the rest of the history to the sideline evaluation once you know that it is safe to remove the athlete from the playing field.

### Observation

Your observation approach will differ depending on whether the athlete is conscious or unconscious.

*Decerebrate rigidity is a posturing of the body with all four extremities extended, indicating severe brain injury.*

*Decorticate rigidity is a posturing of the body in which the legs are extended and the arms are pulled in and flexed toward the trunk, indicating a severe brain injury.*

#### Unconscious Athlete

If the athlete is unconscious, check the position of the head, neck, and extremities. Again, until there is proof to the contrary, a spine injury should be suspected; the athlete should not be moved until spinal injury has been ruled out or the individual is properly stabilized. Determine presence, rate, depth, and rhythm of respirations and note any irregularities. Check the pupils for size, equality, and reaction to light, and note any abnormalities. Inspect the head, scalp, and neck for signs of swelling, deformity, discoloration, or fluid drainage from the ears (**otorrhea**) or nose (**rhinorrhea**). Note any unusual body posturing such as decerebrate or decorticate rigidity that would indicate a severe brain injury. (See chapter 13 for more details on evaluation of an unconscious athlete; for complete head injury evaluation, see chapter 11.) Finally, inspect the extremities for gross deformity, swelling, or discoloration. Assess for shock.

#### Conscious Athlete

If the athlete is conscious, is he moving? Check for abnormal positioning of the head, neck, or extremities. How is the athlete reacting to the injury? Is he able to move the injured part, protecting it, or not moving it at all? What are his facial expressions: do they show pain, fear, panic? Does he show no expression? Is his color pale, flushed, or normal? Does the athlete have bleeding from the head or other signs of head trauma? (See chapter 11 for more on head trauma.) If he suffered a severe blow to the trunk, especially the abdomen and chest, internal injuries should be immediately considered and evaluated as outlined in chapter 12. Evaluate the extremities for obvious signs of deformity, indicative of a fracture or dislocation. Also assess for signs of shock.

*Shock is the body's response to trauma, resulting in a collapse of the cardiovascular system.*

#### Assessment of Shock

Athletes with severe injuries, severe pain, or first-time injuries of any severity, as well as persons with poor tolerance for injury, are most susceptible to shock. The athletic trainer must understand the signs and symptoms of shock and must be prepared to take immediate action if necessary. Look for signs such as pale, cool, and clammy skin; rapid and shallow breathing; a weak and rapid pulse (thinking of a "wet, white, and weak" appearance may help you remember this); nausea; and falling blood pressure. An athlete exhibiting any of these signs should be treated for shock immediately and transported to an emergency medical facility. For a complete discussion of shock, see pages 428-429 in chapter 13.

In summary, in the presence of any life-threatening situations as noted in your initial on-field observation, the EMS system should be notified and emergency medical care initiated immediately, before further evaluation.

For more information on emergency medical care and transportation procedures, refer to *Introduction to Athletic Training* (Hillman 2000), chapter 8.

## SCREENING

Before moving the athlete, the athletic trainer must make an initial assessment of the severity of the injury through a few rapid evaluation techniques in order to select the appropriate transportation method. If you suspect a spinal injury, have the athlete's head stabilized while you perform a bilateral peripheral nerve assessment for sensory and motor innervations. Chapters 3 and 7 of this book and other texts in this series cover the specific techniques in more detail. If you suspect a peripheral nerve injury, perform sensory and motor testing for the specific nerve involved. For a suspected head injury, proceed with a head injury evaluation and ask questions to find out about the athlete's orientation to time, place, and person; this will help you determine how serious the condition is (see chapter 11). If the injury involves a bony region, palpate for possible fractures or dislocation; with confirmation of either, proceed with proper immobilization and splinting. If the athlete exhibits deformity, test for neurovascular compromise. Muscle injuries require a quick palpation for muscular defects and gross assessment of range of motion (ROM) and strength. For suspected injury of the ligamentous structures, perform immediate stress tests before transporting the athlete: muscle spasm will quickly set in and preclude accurate stress test findings, especially once the athlete is moved and pain becomes more severe. Other special tests may be necessary to determine the disposition, or whether it is safe to move the individual off the field. These tests will depend on the body region and will be discussed in the chapters on individual regions.

For a full discussion of management of suspected spinal injuries, refer to *Introduction to Athletic Training* (Hillman 2000), chapter 8.

In summary, your initial screen should give you sufficient information to determine the extent and severity of the injury and thus allow you to proceed with an immediate action plan. If at any time the athlete appears fearful or panicky, appears to be in significant pain, or presents other signs of apprehension, you can help calm him with a reassuring hand and by speaking quietly yet confidently to him throughout the assessment.

## IMMEDIATE ACTION PLAN

If the previous steps reveal any serious or life-threatening signs or symptoms, refer the athlete for further evaluation and treatment as needed. If you find that the athlete's injury does not require immediate medical care, have him transported off the field appropriately and proceed with a more detailed assessment on the sideline or in a more quiet environment such as a treatment facility.

The method of transporting the athlete off the field is selected on the basis of the injury, its severity, and the athlete's response to the injury. It is essential to make the decision that will result in the least additional insult to the injury and the most optimal outcome. The athletic training staff must be well rehearsed in the various methods of transport in advance so that when needed, transportation proceeds efficiently and effectively. Procedures for immediate treatment to minimize and control the injury, steps for immediate medical referral when indicated, and appropriate communication systems must all be in place in advance so that the athlete's care is optimal, efficient, appropriate, and correct.

## Checklist for On-Field Assessment

### Goals

- Rule out emergency conditions.
- Assess severity of injury.
- Determine transport method.

Begin every on-field assessment with a primary survey. Sometimes it will be immediately obvious that there is or is not a problem in one or all of these areas, but whether assessment is simply going through a checklist in your head or involves a more thorough process, never shortchange assessing

1. consciousness,
2. ABCs (airway, breathing, circulation), and
3. bleeding—pressure and severity.

Once you have assessed for and dealt with any immediately life-threatening problems, you may proceed with a secondary survey.

### Essential History

✓ From athlete, if conscious

✓ From bystanders, if athlete unconscious

### Observation

✓ Positioning or posturing

✓ Respirations (rate, depth, rhythm)

✓ Trauma
  - ✓ Observable signs of head injury
  - ✓ Gross deformity, swelling, or discoloration of the extremities
  - ✓ Signs of shock (wet, white, weak)

✓ Athlete's response to injury

### General Screening

✓ Sensory and motor testing for suspected spinal/nerve injury

✓ Neurovascular tests for suspected fracture/dislocation

✓ Assessment for head injury if suspected

✓ Orthopedic assessment
  - ✓ Palpation
  - ✓ ROM and strength screen
  - ✓ Special tests

✓ Continued monitoring for shock

# GENERAL PRINCIPLES OF NONEMERGENCY ASSESSMENT

In evaluating an injury, you are like a detective trying to solve a crime or a researcher attempting to discover whether or not a hypothesis is true. It is the investigator's responsibility to keep an open mind, to collect all the clues and data and place them in an order of significance, and to draw a reasonable conclusion from this information to either confirm or disprove a suspicion or hypothesis.

You must maintain an open mind throughout the evaluation process, not discounting possibilities until you have objectively eliminated them. Remember, do not assume. If you focus too narrowly, you may overlook or incorrectly identify an injury. The evaluation is important in that it sets the course for initial treatment and disposition. Correct, efficient, and effective initial and ongoing treatment depends upon an accurate evaluation.

## SUBJECTIVE AND OBJECTIVE SEGMENTS

Both sideline and off-field evaluations are divided into two parts, the subjective and the objective segments.

- The **subjective** segment involves the history portion of the evaluation or any information the athlete provides. This is the opportunity for the athlete to give you information that will help you formulate an initial impression of the injury. Components in the subjective assessment include items such as the athlete's impression of the onset of injury, the way the athlete felt at the time of the injury and feels at the time of the evaluation, and any relevant medical history including prior injuries to the involved segment. The subjective portion also includes your general observations regarding the athlete's response to the injury and the way she is moving or holding the injured body part, as well as observations of swelling, deformity, and skin coloration. You will use this subjective information to form a hypothesis about the nature and extent of the injuries. Your questioning should therefore be as complete as possible so that the information can serve as a guide for your objective assessment.

• During the **objective** segment, the athletic trainer performs the tests necessary to establish the severity and nature of the injury. If the objective tests do not confirm the hypotheses formed during the subjective segment, you must reassess for other possible injuries, and then retest to identify the injury or refer the athlete to another medical professional for further evaluation and diagnosis. But it is crucial that you also use common sense in deciding how aggressive the objective evaluation should be. If the athlete is in severe pain, do not perform a complete evaluation—only one or two tests may be needed in order to establish the most appropriate immediate treatment or referral. Further assessment can be deferred until the athlete is in less pain and the injury is less irritable. If the athlete is able to tolerate a more extensive evaluation, proceed—but only as necessity and her pain level dictate. Otherwise you will only aggravate her injury and will make her less confident of your ability to help her.

## TESTING DURING THE OBJECTIVE SEGMENT

The tests should elicit a negative response if the tissue or structure tested is not involved in the injury and a positive response if it is involved. A positive response indicates either a reproduction of the athlete's symptoms or an alteration of the symptoms. This reproduction of the athlete's complaint of pain with testing is sometimes called a **comparable sign** (Maitland 1991). During the objective phase, you will also use tests to appraise deficiencies in motion, strength, coordination, and agility resulting from the injury. Combine all these test results to establish a base for appropriate and justifiable treatment or referral.

In order to obtain reliable information from the tests, you need to understand the purpose of each test, compare the injured side with the uninjured side (**bilateral comparison**), and know what the "normal" response for each test is. You must also realize how changes in the athlete's positioning can affect test results. For example, consider how the results of strength testing of shoulder flexion may vary depending on whether the athlete is tested in sitting or supine. It is important to be efficient in completing the evaluation. If you do not understand the purposes of each test, you will tend to use more tests than necessary, prolonging the evaluation and perhaps further aggravating the athlete's condition.

## SINS

Combining the subjective and objective segments of an evaluation produces a total picture of an athlete's injury. The athlete's history along with your objective findings will allow you to define the injury's severity, irritability, nature, and stage (or **SINS**, from the first letter of each word) so you can select an appropriate course of treatment. While a sideline assessment includes investigation of only the severity and nature of the injury, an off-field assessment must address all the elements of SINS.

### *Severity*

The severity of the injury will determine whether or not the athletic trainer refers the athlete to a physician or other medical specialist. The most common injuries in athletics involve soft tissue: ligament, capsule, fascia, tendon, and muscle. These soft tissue injuries are more often overuse injuries or acute first- or second-degree injuries, less often third-degree injuries. While obviously you will refer the more severe injuries to the physician, you should never hesitate to refer if you are unsure of the severity or the proper disposition.

### Irritability

The irritability of an injury relates to its stage, its extent, the structures injured, and the athlete's pain tolerance level. When you have not witnessed the injury and see the athlete in the athletic treatment facility (off-field assessment), the athlete's history will give you an initial impression of the irritability. If the athlete reports frequent episodes of severe pain (7-10 on a 10-point scale) with little relief, is unable to sleep through the night because of pain, and is often uncomfortable even without activity, the injury is very irritable. On the other hand, if the athlete reports mild to moderate pain (0-3 or 4-6 on a 10-point scale) and is able to perform in his or her sport although perhaps not optimally, the injury is minimally irritable.

Irritability is an important factor to appreciate before you perform the objective segment of the evaluation. If the injury is very irritable, you will be unable to perform a complete evaluation because the athlete will be unable to tolerate it. In this case, use an abbreviated assessment that provides only the key information needed to begin treatment, deferring other tests until the irritability lessens. As a general rule, the less irritable the injury is, the more complete the evaluation process can be.

### Nature

The nature of the injury includes the type of injury and the type of structure involved. Is the injury caused by overuse? Is it a muscle strain or a ligamentous sprain? Is it a subluxation or a dislocation? Injury to inert tissue such as ligament, capsule, and bone causes pain with active and passive movement, whereas injury to muscle and tendon generally causes pain with active but not passive movement. Although the history is important in determining the nature of an injury, you must confirm any suspicions in this regard through the objective assessment.

### Stage

With an on-field or sideline assessment, the stage of the injury is obvious—since the injury has just happened, it is acute. In contrast, when the athlete presents to the athletic trainer at some time after the injury occurrence, the stage can range from acute to subacute to chronic.

Each stage of injury will present with different types of symptoms and signs. It is important to determine the injury's stage because the treatment approach will differ for each stage. Injuries fall into three stages or classifications: acute, subacute, and chronic. Although these classifications are based on the healing process, there is no clear-cut delineation between the end of one stage and the beginning of another.

- An **acute** injury results from a sudden onset of macrotrauma and has a wide range of recovery depending on severity. Although recovery from an acute injury may take some time, the primary initial symptoms that allow its classification as acute occur over the first 7 to 10 days following the onset.

- A **subacute** injury is at the interim stage between the acute and chronic stages and occurs around four to six weeks following the onset of trauma (American Academy of Orthopaedic Surgeons 1991).

• A **chronic**, or **overuse**, **injury** typically has a gradual but progressive onset of repetitive microtrauma that, without intervention, eventually results in symptoms sufficient to alter the athlete's performance. Chronic conditions are at least six to eight weeks in duration.

These terms—acute, subacute, and chronic—are not always applied in a hard-and-fast manner. The purpose of the classification is to help the athletic trainer understand the healing process and determine the appropriate treatment course. An acute injury is undergoing the inflammatory and proliferation healing stages, while the chronic injury is in the remodeling stage. The subacute injury is in transition and may be in either the proliferation or the remodeling stage, depending on the symptoms.

Now that we understand the importance of the subjective and objective segments that make up a total assessment process and know what information the assessment can yield, let's look at the specifics of each of these elements in both sideline and off-field assessments.

# SIDELINE ASSESSMENT

The sideline assessment will either follow the on-field assessment or will serve as the initial evaluation of an injured player who has walked off the field on his or her own power. The purpose is to determine more precisely the nature and severity of the injury so that an appropriate initial treatment can be administered. As with an on-field assessment, often you will have seen the injury occur and so will already know what segment was injured and whether or not the athlete's symptoms are referred from the site of injury or are localized. For this reason, you should usually perform palpation early in the sideline assessment. Because you already have a good idea of the segment injured, you should also do special tests early in order to confirm or disconfirm your suspicions and to determine the severity.

In a sideline assessment, the order of evaluation is as follows:

1. History
2. Observation
3. Palpation
4. Special tests
5. ROM
6. Strength
7. Neurological and circulatory tests (if necessary)
8. Functional tests (if appropriate)

## SIDELINE ASSESSMENT—SUBJECTIVE SEGMENT

The subjective segment gives the athletic trainer vital information regarding the injury and the athlete's response to it as well as any history that may be impacting the current situation. Again, your questioning should be complete enough to allow you to formulate a plan for the objective segment. The questions should not lead the athlete but instead allow her to answer as accurately as possible. For example, it would be leading to ask, "Did you feel a pop when you landed on your hand?" A better question would be, "Did you hear or feel anything when you landed on your hand?" As another example, avoid questions like "Is your pain more of a deep ache?" It would be better to ask, "How would you describe your pain?" Remember, the history is only as good as the questions asked.

### Current History

Once the athlete is removed to a location conducive to an accurate assessment, ask him about the impact and his reaction to the injury to add to the information regarding mechanism of injury that you obtained on the field. Your goal is to develop a good picture of the injury so that you can pay appropriate attention to the correct body segment during the objective assessment to come. Ask, for example, how the athlete landed or what position he was in when he received the blow. What position was the extremity in at the time of impact? Did the athlete hear any noise or feel any unusual sensations? Was the pain immediate? Did the pain shoot, or did it stay localized? Has the pain changed since it first began? Where is the pain? Can the athlete pinpoint the pain? How does the athlete describe the pain? What is its intensity on a 0- to 10-point scale (with 0 indicating no pain and 10 indicating "unbearable" pain)? Does the injury hurt only when the athlete moves it or while he's at rest as well?

Obtaining a good pain profile helps you determine the athlete's pain tolerance level and the severity and location of the injury. As noted earlier, it will also help establish how aggressive the objective assessment can be.

### Previous Injury History

Obtaining a history of prior injury or illness is important because it gives the athletic trainer a good idea of any previous medical problems or conditions that may impact the current injury. For example, if the athlete has a history of rotator cuff surgery and now suffers an elbow strain, could soft tissue tightness of the shoulder be related to the excess stress that may have precipitated this elbow injury? Or, if the athlete broke a leg two years ago and was casted for six weeks, could the secondary tightness in the calf (which was never completely resolved) have an effect on today's ankle sprain? Is the second baseman's diabetes well controlled?—the answer will influence one's level of concern about the laceration he received today when an opponent's cleat impacted his forearm. That an athlete has previously sprained the same knee may influence your findings during ligament stress testing (i.e., is the increased laxity due to this injury or could it be due in part to a previous injury?). It is also important to ask about the opposite, or "uninvolved," side. While the uninjured side is typically used as your benchmark for what is "normal" for a person, this may not provide an accurate comparison, depending on previous injuries.

---

### General Questions to Ask When Taking an Acute Injury History

What happened and how did it happen?

What position were you in when the injury occurred (i.e., how did you land, was the foot rotated in or out, etc.)?

Did you hear or feel any unusual sounds or sensations at the time of injury? (i.e., hear or feel a snap or pop)?

Do you have any unusual sensations now (i.e., numbness, tingling, burning)?

Where is the pain?

Can you describe the pain?

- Quality of pain (sharp, dull, achy)

- Intensity (scale of 1-10)
- Localized or diffuse
- Any referral
- Any changes in pain from when it started (intensified or lessened)

When does it hurt (i.e., all the time, only when moved, only when touched or stressed, etc.)?

Previous history of body region (information on nature, severity, duration of symptoms, treatment received)?

Previous history for opposite side?

Any other medical conditions to be aware of?

Ask, for example, "Have you had prior injuries to the same area or the surrounding area?" "Have you ever injured the other side?" "How long ago was the prior injury?" "How severe was the injury?" "What were the diagnosis and treatment?" "What was the outcome of the treatment?" "How long was the recovery?" "Have you had any problems with the injury since then?" "Are you taking any medications?" "Do you take, or have you taken, steroids or recreational drugs?" "Do you have any other medical conditions that may impact this injury?"

### Observation

**Observation** is a valuable skill of the athletic trainer, used throughout all phases and types of evaluations and treatments. Observing how the athlete responds provides useful information about the athlete's perception of the injury as well as additional clues to its nature and severity. Observation begins during the subjective segment of an assessment and continues throughout the objective portion. Facial expressions and the eyes are a window into the athlete's true response and should be carefully watched not only at the time of injury but also during the objective tests. The athletic trainer makes other observations including the athlete's general posture, the way in which the athlete holds or protects the injured part, and her willingness to move the injured segment. If she removes clothing to permit additional examination, how well does she perform the task? Does she have difficulty? Is she hesitant? Does she require assistance? Does she need help in moving, or does she substitute one segment function for another?

*Edema is swelling resulting from fluid accumulation in the interstitial tissues.*

Inspect the injured part visually before you perform additional examinations. Observe for contour and discoloration, and compare the right and left sides—they should be symmetrical. Are soft tissue and bony contours equal, or are there abnormalities because of edema, muscle spasm, subluxation, dislocation, or fracture? Is skin color normal and comparable with that of the surrounding skin or of the opposite extremity? Do alignments appear normal? Some malalignments are not abnormal or pathological, and you need to be aware of such normal anatomical discrepancies. For example, it is common for the dominant shoulder to sit lower than the nondominant one.

Observation of overall posture is important because poor posture can aggravate an injury. For example, a forward head posture can make a cervical sprain injury worse, and a round shoulder posture can negatively impact shoulder ROM. It is important to know what normal posture is in order to determine whether the athlete has dysfunctional posture that may have either aggravated, or resulted from, the new injury.

For a discussion on thorough posture evaluation, refer to *Therapeutic Exercise for Athletic Injuries* (Houglum 2000), chapter 11.

## SIDELINE ASSESSMENT–OBJECTIVE SEGMENT

If you are evaluating an injury with an open wound, you must wear gloves and observe Universal Precautions during your "hands-on" evaluation.

The objective assessment comprises all measurable evaluative techniques. The components of the sideline objective assessment include continued observation, as well as evaluation of the region by palpation, by special tests, and by ROM, strength, neurovascular status, and functional tests.

### Palpation

**Palpation** is a skilled application of the sense of touch to provide critical information regarding an injury. Since you will have a good sense of the segment that is injured, palpation is performed early in the sideline assessment.

### What to Palpate

Appropriately applied palpation can reveal information regarding the tension, thickness, and texture of soft tissue; the presence or absence of swelling; temperature, moisture, pulses, and muscle fasciculations; and general contours of soft tissue and bony prominences.

Soft tissue tension refers to the tone of an area. A segment that has a muscle spasm will have more tension than one that is relaxed. Soft tissue thickness can be an indication of swelling or edema, caused by fluid accumulation in the tissue or space. Different types of fluid formation in different areas will produce different types of soft tissue responses that can be distinguished with palpation.

- Synovial swelling produces a soft tissue, boggy response that feels spongy to palpation.
- Fluid formation within soft tissue feels softer and moves when palpated.
- Edema caused by blood formation is usually warmer than fluid-formation swelling and feels thicker or harder to palpation.
- Chronic swelling, or long-term swelling, can feel more leathery; in this condition, even cordlike fibrous band formations can be palpated. Recent soft tissue swelling that feels soft and will give or deform with pressure is called **pitting edema**, whereas long-term leathery swelling is called **brawny edema**

> **!** When a pulse cannot be palpated, the injury should be treated as a medical emergency.

Palpation for temperature, pulses, and muscle fasciculations provides valuable information regarding the area's general condition. Temperature will be elevated locally in comparison to that on the opposite side in the presence of infection and extravasation of blood in the area. Temperature is palpated by the fingertips or the dorsum of the hand. Pulses should be checked periodically with any severe injury, especially in areas such as joints where main blood vessels traverse; these vessels can either become injured from the direct trauma or be restricted due to secondary swelling that develops immediately following an injury. Any loss of pulse should be treated as an emergency situation.

Moisture on the skin is not normally a factor in athletes unless there is the possibility of a heat stress injury; and in these situations, assessment of skin moisture is key. Since sideline assessments usually involve an active athlete, skin moisture is usually present and is not a relevant factor in orthopedic injuries. During assessment of any injury, however, you must be cognizant of the risk of shock and should look to skin moisture as a key factor, especially when it is accompanied by other signs of shock.

**Muscle fasciculations**, or **tremors**, are involuntary muscle contractions that occur secondary to injury or pain. They can involve only a few muscle fibers that are innervated by one motor unit (fasciculations) or several motor units (tremors) and even the entire muscle (spasm); and they can involve either agonist or antagonist muscles. If present, they can usually be easily palpated in the segment that has been injured; more superficial muscles can be observed visually.

When you are palpating bony and soft tissue contours, you can easily recognize deformations through comparison with the uninvolved, contralateral side. Palpation of bony structures produces a hard, ungiving sensation. Depending on the contour and the area palpated, an abnormal bony palpation may be indicative of (a) displacement from a fracture, subluxation, or dislocation or (b) abnormal bone growth from an **osteophyte** (bone spur) or a calcification within a muscle (**myositis ossificans**). Palpable defects in soft tissue may also be identified with second- and third-degree strains.

### How to Palpate

Palpation should be performed in a systematic fashion so that all structures are included. If you establish your own routine, following the same pattern or progression for each evaluation, you are assured of doing a complete examination and will avoid inadvertently missing a structure. For an accurate palpation assessment, the athlete should be in a relaxed position with the injured segment supported. Before you begin, tell the athlete what you are going to do and ask her to report any pain during the palpation. Observe her facial expressions for visual signs of pain during palpation. The intensity and quality of the pain response observed are as important to identify as is the pain response reported. Remember to obtain a relative indication of the pain by asking the athlete to indicate on a 0- to 10-point scale the degree of pain.

You can sometimes perform palpation simultaneously on both right and left sides; but when this is not possible or convenient, you should palpate the uninvolved side first to find out what is "normal" for the athlete. Palpation of the uninvolved side first also allows the athlete to relax more with palpation of the injured area, since he will know what to expect after you have palpated the uninvolved side. When performing the palpation assessment, move from superficial to deeper structures and start with more outlying structures, palpating toward the specific site of injury. For example, if the glenohumeral joint is the site of the pain, begin at the sternoclavicular joint and anterior structures and move laterally; then palpate the superior-medial and posterior-medial areas and move laterally before going on to the glenohumeral joint.

Begin with light palpation of the skin temperature and general superficial soft tissue mobility; then move to deeper structures. How well does the skin move against the underlying subcutaneous and muscle tissue? Does it move freely in all directions, or is it restricted? Is the temperature normal compared to that on the other side? Palpation of the first layer of muscle is followed by palpation of underlying muscle layers. Each layer is assessed for tissue mobility, swelling, texture, congruity, pain with pressure, and spasm. Finally, the tendons, ligaments, and bony structures are palpated for tenderness, swelling, crepitus, and deformity.

Following these guidelines, the athletic trainer uses palpation to fill in the evaluation picture to further solve the mystery—the nature and severity of the athlete's injury.

## Special Tests

By the time you are prepared to use special tests, the history and palpation have suggested a narrow range of injury possibilities. Special tests are used to either eliminate or confirm a suspected condition, as well as to define the integrity of a structure or the extent of an injury. These tests stress the structure enough to either (a) demonstrate and allow you to grade an abnormal response or (b) reproduce the athlete's symptoms. The stress must be great enough to elicit an accurate response but not so great that it further aggravates the injury. For an inexperienced athletic trainer, finding this balance can be difficult at times.

Special tests by themselves do not provide a complete profile of the athlete's injury. Through the evaluation process, with every question, observation, and test, you are progressively focusing the picture and narrowing the possibilities of what the injury is. You must be careful not to make unfounded assumptions and rush the investigative process by focusing too quickly on one or two special tests.

Since the special tests are numerous and are unique to each body segment, they will not be described here but will be discussed in the chapters dealing with the various segments. There are, however, general principles related to the use of special tests that readers should understand at this point.

### Choosing the Tests

As noted earlier, deciding on the degree of stress or on which special test to use requires good judgment. It is sometimes neither necessary nor appropriate to use a special test to stress an injury—this is true, for example, in the case of an elbow dislocation. An athlete may simply be in too much pain to undergo a stress test; in this case it is better to defer the special test than to further aggravate the injury. If, on the other hand, the athlete has moderate pain with palpation over the lateral ligament structures of the elbow, ligament stress tests should be used to determine whether or not the injury involves the collateral ligaments of the elbow and to assess the degree of injury. Likewise, for an athlete who has moderate pain in the shoulder with weakness on active and resistive motion, special tests will help you ascertain whether the injury involves the rotator cuff, biceps, or other muscular support around the shoulder joint.

The special tests presented throughout this text are those most commonly used by certified athletic trainers because of their accuracy and demonstrated reliability. Readers must remember, however, that some of these tests may not be appropriate for some athletic trainers because of individual circumstances. For example, if you have a small hand and are evaluating a large athlete, a McMurray test for the knee may not be accurate or appropriate for assessing meniscus integrity, and you may find the Apley compression test more useful. You will need to determine the most appropriate tests for you, depending on the specific situation and your knowledge and skills.

### Good Testing Technique

Special tests take place only after you have explained to the athlete what will occur. The special tests are done on the uninvolved extremity first for two reasons, as already noted: (1) to familiarize the athlete with the procedure to reduce his apprehension and help him relax so that the result may be more accurate; (2) to provide knowledge of what is "normal" for that athlete. Since many special tests will produce different results from one individual to another, you must establish a baseline for each athlete in order to determine whether the test is positive or negative. Depending on the test, the result is considered positive if it produces different results on the involved side and on the uninvolved side in terms of laxity or stiffness, stability or instability, the presence or absence of sounds, restriction or ease of movement, strength or weakness, normal or abnormal function, and the presence or absence of pain.

### Factors in Accuracy of Test Results

Always remember that negative or positive results of a single special test do not necessarily indicate the absence or presence of a specific injury. A false-positive result may also occur, and other tests may be needed for confirmation. Your skills and your ability to perform the tests reliably can make a big difference in the test results; thus experience plays an important role in the accuracy of the results obtained from special tests. Another factor to consider is the accuracy of the specific tests themselves, as some are more sensitive than others. And, although for some injuries there are several tests, it is not necessary to use all available special tests. Remember, a special test is intended to reproduce the athlete's symptoms; so unless further confirmation is required, the use of only one or two tests for one structure is usually adequate and better tolerated by the athlete.

## Range of Motion

Range of motion of the injured segment is divided into active motion and passive motion. Active motion testing, performed first, assesses the integrity of the active or contractile tissue, the musculotendinous unit. Passive movement testing assesses inert structures around the joint. As with other tests, unless you are testing ROM on both sides simultaneously, test the uninvolved side first to obtain the athlete's normal motion and let her know what to anticipate. Wait until last to perform the motions that are most likely to cause pain. If performed first, these motions may exacerbate

When comparing bilaterally, make sure you have also taken a thorough injury history of the uninvolved side, as this may affect your interpretation of what is "normal" for that athlete.

the symptoms to the point where the athlete experiences a "pain overflow" into other tests that would otherwise not be painful, in addition to making the athlete more apprehensive during the remainder of testing.

Active and passive movements can be done in blocks or can be interspersed. That is, the athlete can perform all active motions within one sequence and then all passive movements, or can alternate between active and passive motions. The choice of method will depend on preference, on the amount of active motion available during the examination, and the athlete's level of comfort. As a rule of thumb, if the athlete has full active ROM without pain, you can perform the passive test immediately. However, if she has pain with limited ROM in one or several planes of motion, you may want to obtain an overall assessment of quality and quantity of active movement before performing specific passive movement tests, and to pay special attention to passive motions in those planes in which active movement was limited.

*Physiological motion is the active motion of the joint in planes of motion. Flexion, extension, abduction, adduction, and rotation are physiological motions.*

### Active Range of Motion Assessment

During **active ROM**, the athlete voluntarily moves the injured part without assistance through its full range while you observe for the quantity and quality of physiological motion. Is the athlete able to move through a full ROM, or is there restriction? And if so, when does it occur? Is the motion controlled and smooth? Does the athlete hesitate at any time during the ROM, and if so, why? What are his facial expressions during hesitation? These will often provide clues. If the athlete reports pain during movement, when does the pain start? Does it change as he moves through the range? Does the motion follow a normal pattern, or does the athlete move out of the plane of motion in order to complete the movement? Does he involve other joints to assist in the movement?

### Passive Range of Motion Assessment

**Passive ROM** is performed to assess inert tissue integrity without the participation of the athlete. These tissues include ligament, capsule, cartilage, bursa, and nerve structures. Information obtained from passive motion assessment includes quality and quantity of end-range physiological motion, end feel of the joint, and capsular status.

Rarely does active physiological motion equal full passive motion. You will typically be able to move the joint further passively than the athlete can actively. Therefore, passive movement tells you how much physiological motion remains once active motion has stopped, as well as whether the quality of that motion is smooth and free or is difficult, or whether the joint is hypermobile or restricted.

Once you determine that the active ROM is full, you can apply an **overpressure** at the end of a joint's physiological motion to assess end feel and ligamentous integrity. The normal response to overpressure is painless, but pathological joints will have pain with overpressure. The normal **end feel** of a joint will vary according to the reason for the end of joint motion. For example, a firm, springy sensation with an elastic give to it is most often the result of normal tissue stretch (i.e., muscle, ligament, and/or fascia) such as ankle dorsiflexion, and most extension movements such as knee extension. An end feel with a soft tissue **approximation** is experienced with normal elbow or knee flexion as the two muscle bellies come in contact with one another at the end of the motion. Occasionally you will observe a bony block, or bone-to-bone **approximation**, such as in elbow extension when the olecranon comes in full contact with the olecranon fossa.

Abnormal end feels can be caused by muscle spasm, loose bodies within a joint, joint instability, or joint stiffness due to ligamentous or capsular adhesions or muscle shortening. A springy sensation that occurs prematurely during end-feel testing usually occurs in joints that contain menisci, and may be the result of a tear in the meniscus that interferes with normal joint motion. Acute **muscle spasm** causes an end feel to occur suddenly and early in the motion and produces a definite hard end-feel sensation. An open or empty end feel lacks the normal approximation sensation at the end of the joint's motion, and occurs when capsular and ligamentous joint stability has been disrupted. An empty end feel can also occur when the athlete experiences the pain before the end of the motion. A **capsular restriction** can be either a soft or a hard soft tissue restriction, depending on the duration of the adhesions. You will not usually see this end feel in acute injuries unless preexisting joint adhesions are present, but you may see it in athletes who do not immediately report their injuries and are seen for the first time in the athletic injury treatment facility. The assessment of capsular status will be thoroughly discussed within the context of the off-field assessment. It is mentioned here simply to make you aware of this potential finding in the event that the acute injury you are evaluating was preceded by a previous injury or chronic condition.

In your passive assessment, you must answer questions similar to those you considered during active ROM testing: How much motion is available? Is the motion excessive or restricted? Do the motion and end feel match those of the uninvolved side? Does the athlete have pain-free active movement while reporting pain with passive end-motion movement, and if so, when does the pain occur? A strong knowledge of anatomy will aid you in your passive assessment, helping you visualize what specific structures are being stressed at the end ROM. In general, if pain occurs with both active and passive motion, or with passive motion only, a ligamentous or supportive structure is likely involved. Pain with only active motion is more indicative of contractile muscle tissue (i.e., muscle and tendon) involvement.

### Strength

Overall, the purpose of strength testing on the sideline is to assess the level of pain, the resistive capabilities, and the neuromuscular integrity in the active, contractile tissues surrounding the injured site. In the sideline assessment, isometric tests are typically performed first, followed by more specific manual muscle tests as warranted.

Isometric, or "**break tests**," are efficient and are usually performed with the joint in a neutral midrange position. This position limits the amount of stress applied to a joint and assures that a test for strength is obtained without interfering input from inert joint structures. After positioning the joint in midrange, instruct the athlete to hold that position, telling him "Don't let me move you" as you attempt to move the

*Additional confirmation of active tissue injury can be obtained through stretch of the muscle in the direction opposite to its motion. For example, if a positive strength test of pain and some weakness were obtained from the wrist extensors, pain may also be noted during stretch of the wrist extensors with passive wrist flexion and elbow extension.*

## Types of End Feel Encountered With Passive Overpressure

| End feel | Description |
| --- | --- |
| Tissue stretch | A springy or elastic sensation with normal stretch of soft tissue structures such as muscle, fascia, ligament, and capsule. |
| Soft tissue approximation | A soft end feel found often during flexion movements when two muscle bellies come in contact with one another. |
| Bony block | A hard, abrupt end feel caused by bone-to-bone approximation, can be normal or abnormal. |
| Muscle spasm | An abrupt, firm, springy resistance to motion caused by protective muscle spasm. |
| Capsular restriction | Can be a firm (leathery) or soft tissue restriction, depending on the maturity of the adhesions. |
| Open/empty | Lack of normal tissue approximation found with third-degree joint instabilities or where pain causes cessation of motion before the end of motion is reached. |

joint. Instead of a sudden application of a maximal force that overpowers him, the resistance you provide should build to a maximum as the athlete matches your resistance over 3-5 s.

Initial test results will yield one of four possibilities:

1. Strong and pain free, indicating a normal response (so the source of the athlete's injury is not neuromuscular)

2. Strong and painful, indicating a lesion in the muscle or tendon

3. Weak and pain free, indicating either a nerve injury or musculotendinous rupture

4. Weak and painful, indicating a serious injury that could range from a fracture to an unstable joint

The second category, strong and painful, is most commonly seen in acute injury evaluations and has a broad continuum of variation, ranging from slight weakness as compared to normal with some pain for a mild muscle strain, to moderate weakness with moderate pain for a second-degree strain, to little loss of strength with more pain for a tendinitis.

It is also important to note that pain strongly influences strength test outcomes. If the strength testing produces pain, the actual strength output may not be accurate. When the athlete reports pain with strength testing, you must realize that pain will cause an autonomic withdrawal so that she demonstrate less strength than she would without pain. In these cases, you should indicate on the evaluation that the test produced pain, and should be prepared to retest at a later date when the athlete does not have pain with the test.

In the event that isometric testing shows muscle weakness, more specific manual muscle tests can further delineate the location and reason for the weakness. For example, weak resisted elbow flexion can be caused by either the biceps, the brachialis, or the brachioradialis. Manual muscle tests can be used to define which specific muscle is causing the weakness. **Manual muscle tests** are graded on a 0- to 5-point scale with 5 being normal strength and 0 being no strength (table 2.1). Grades 0, 1, and 2 are not normally seen in acute athletic injuries except with musculotendinous ruptures or nerve disruptions. Grades 3, 4, and 5 are tested with the muscle working against gravity, with grades 4 and 5 tested against manually applied resistance. It is important to remember to apply a sufficient amount of resistance to make the manual muscle test accurate and reliable—this is the only way to obtain an accurate strength assessment.

For more detailed descriptions of manual muscle tests for the upper and lower extremities, refer to *Therapeutic Exercise for Athletic Injuries* (Houglum 2000), chapter 7.

### Neurological and Circulatory Tests

Neurovascular tests assess the integrity of the neurovascular structures. Because neurovascular compromise can have serious and even life-threatening consequences, it is essential to determine if the nerve and vascular structures are intact and functioning normally following an injury.

### Neurological Tests

*Referred symptoms are symptoms that are experienced away from the site of injury.*

A neurological exam is performed if a nerve injury is suspected and the athlete's symptoms include radiation of any numbness, tingling, shooting pain, deep pain, burning pain, or weakness. Radiating symptoms or referred symptoms can result from pathology in the spinal cord, nerve roots, or peripheral nerves secondary to disc herniations, fracture or dislocations, impingement or compression syndromes, nerve tensioning or stretch, or other nerve trauma.

| Table 2.1 | Comparison of Gravity-Resisted Muscle—Grading Criteria |
|---|---|
| **Medical research council** | **Daniels and Worthingham** |
| 5 (Normal) | Subject completes range of motion against gravity, against maximal resistance. |
| 4+ | Subject completes range of motion against gravity, against nearly maximal resistance. |
| 4 (Good) | Subject completes range of motion against gravity, against moderate resistance. |
| 4– | Subject completes range of motion against gravity, against minimal resistance, >50% range. |
| 3+ | Subject completes range of motion against gravity, against minimal resistance, <50% range. |
| 3 (Fair) | Subject completes range of motion against gravity with no manual resistance. |
| 3– | Subject does not complete range of motion against gravity but does complete more than half the range. |
| 2+ | Subject initiates range of motion against gravity or completes range with gravity minimized against slight resistance. |
| 2 (Poor) | Subject completes range of motion with gravity minimized. |
| 2– | Subject unable to complete range of motion with gravity minimized. |
| 1 | Subject's muscle contraction can be palpated but there is no joint motion. |
| 0 (Zero) | Subject exhibits no palpable contraction or joint motion. |

Data from Medical Research Council, 1943, *Aids to the investigation of peripheral nerve injuries*. 2nd ed. rev. (London: H.M.S.O.) and L. Daniels and C.A. Worthingham, 1980, *Muscle testing*, 4th ed. (London: W.B. Saunders).

*Dermatome is the area of skin that provides sensory input for a single spinal nerve root.*

*Myotome refers to the muscle(s) innervated by a single spinal nerve root.*

Neurological symptoms will vary with the level of nerve injury. Whereas unilateral symptoms are more indicative of a nerve root or peripheral nerve lesion, bilateral symptoms are more indicative of a central cord pathology. The symptoms will also be different for a nerve root versus a peripheral nerve injury. Nerve roots from the cervical and lumbar spine send branches to more than one peripheral nerve, so the profile of symptoms will be more diffuse with a nerve root lesion than with a peripheral nerve. For example, the C7 nerve root has branches that innervate the ulnar, median, and radial nerves, so an injury to the C7 nerve root will have various symptoms that could affect all three peripheral nerves, in contrast to an injury to the radial nerve that will affect primarily the posterolateral hand. It is important to understand these differential systems, as well as the innervation zones for each nerve root and peripheral nerve, for an accurate neurological assessment.

Although there are specific neurological tests for specific body areas, the three primary generic neurological tests involve assessment of sensory, motor, and reflex responses. These tests are designed for spinal cord and nerve root assessment, but sensory and motor results can also lead to peripheral nerve conclusions. Table 2.2 demonstrates dermatome, myotome, and reflex distributions for spinal and peripheral nerves for both the upper and lower extremities. You will need to know these levels of innervation in order to select appropriate testing for the sensory, motor, and reflex innervations.

### Sensory Tests

Sensory tests assess the integrity of afferent nerves and will show whether the sensory signal from the periphery is being received and processed centrally. Sensory perception includes a variety of sensory afferent receptors in the skin throughout the body, including those for light touch, pressure, vibration, temperature, and pain. Among those sensory receptors that can be tested, those that are most easily and

## Table 2.2 Nerve Root Dermatomes, Myotomes, and Reflexes

| Nerve root | Dermatome | Myotome | Reflex |
|---|---|---|---|
| C1 | Top of head | (Cervical flexion) | None |
| C2 | Temporal, occipital regions of head | Cervical flexion (longus colli, sternocleidomastoid, rectus capitis) | None |
| C3 | Neck, posterior cheek | Lateral neck flexion (trapezius, splenius capitis) | None |
| C4 | Superior shoulder, clavicular area | Shoulder shrug (trapezius, levator scapulae) | None |
| C5 | Deltoid patch, lateral upper arm | Shoulder abduction (deltoid), elbow flexion (biceps) | Biceps (brachioradialis) |
| C6 | Lateral forearm, radial side of hand, thumb and index finger | Elbow flexion (biceps, supinator), wrist extension | Brachioradialis (biceps) |
| C7 | Posterior lateral arm and forearm, middle finger | Elbow extension (triceps), wrist flexion | Triceps |
| C8 | Medial forearm, ulnar border of hand, ring, and little fingers | Ulnar deviation, thumb extension, finger flexion and abduction | None |
| T1 | Medial side of forearm | Finger abduction/adduction (hand intrinsics) | None |
| L1 | Back, over greater trochanter and groin | Hip flexion (psoas), iliacus, pectineus, sartorius | None |
| L2 | Back, wrapping around to anterior superior thigh, medial thigh above knee | Hip flexion (psoas), hip adductors | (Patellar tendon) |
| L3 | Back, upper gluteal, anterior thigh, medial knee and lower leg | Knee extension (quadriceps) | Patellar tendon |
| L4 | Medial gluteals, lateral thigh/knee, anterior medial lower leg, dorsomedial aspect of foot, big toe | Ankle dorsiflexion (tibialis anterior) | Patellar tendon |
| L5 | Lateral knee and upper lateral lower leg, dorsum of foot | Great toe extension (extensor hallucis) | Medial hamstring tendon |
| S1 | Buttock, posterolateral thigh, plantar surface of lateral foot | Ankle plantar flexion (gastrocnemius, soleus), ankle eversion (peroneals), hip extension (gluteals), knee flexion (hamstrings) | Achilles tendon (lateral hamstring tendon) |
| S2 | Buttock, posterior medial thigh, plantar surface of medial foot | Knee flexion (hamstrings), great toe flexion (flexor hallucis longus) | (Lateral hamstring tendon) |

most frequently examined are the light touch receptors. To perform the test, run your fingertips in light contact over the athlete's skin. Abnormal responses include an inability to feel anything (anesthesia), an altered response compared to that on the uninjured side (paresthesia), any sensation other than that of light touch, and sensation in an area other than the one touched. Comparisons are made right to left. The athlete closes her eyes or is positioned so that she cannot see when or where the light touch test is performed.

The sensory test serves as a scanning technique to quickly assess sensation. If the athlete reports any abnormal response, the next step is to perform a more detailed examination over a specific nerve root distribution and ask the athlete if he felt anything—and if so, what it was and how it compared to the sensation on the opposite side. Sometimes you will ask the athlete if he felt anything when in fact you did not perform any touch; the point is to assess whether or not the athlete is correctly perceiving the light touch. If the athlete's response is unclear, you should repeat the test over the questionable area before ending the sensory tests. If the sensory test is positive, other sensory tests assessing deep pressure or pain can be performed over the appropriate nerve distributions. For example, superficial pain is tested with a pinprick or pinwheel; deep pressure pain is tested with a pinch; temperature perception is tested with hot and cold objects placed against the skin; vibration is tested with a tuning fork on a bony prominence; proprioception is tested by passively moving a part and having the athlete indicate the direction of movement or position. If tools are not available for additional tests, these assessments can be deferred until the athlete is removed to the athletic training facility. A positive sign on any sensory test is an indication that the athlete may have a neurological injury, and referral to a physician for further evaluation is usually indicated.

*Proprioception is the awareness of position or movment of the body or body segment.*

Chapters 3 and 7 provide a map of the typical sensory distribution areas for the upper extremity and lower extremity, respectively. You will note in these figures that the sensory distribution (dermatome) for a nerve root is different from that for a peripheral nerve. It is also important to note that these sensory distribution zones may vary somewhat from one individual to another.

## Motor Tests

Motor tests are the manual muscle tests that follow the course of the cervical brachial or lumbosacral plexus. These muscle tests, which identify any neurological deficit that has affected the athlete's muscular function, are performed in the same way as the manual muscle tests previously described. The only difference between manual muscle tests for orthopedic assessment and those for neurological assessment is in the muscles tested. An orthopedic assessment deals with the muscles related to the joint and its function. In a neurological assessment, the manual muscle tests are used to identify the peripheral nerve or nerve root that is injured. For example, if an athlete has a suspected rotator cuff strain, you will use a manual muscle test to assess the strength of the rotator cuff muscles; but if she has suffered a cervical injury that has damaged the C6 and C7 nerve roots, you will use the manual muscle tests to identify which muscles have been affected. The specific motor tests for the upper and lower extremity will be discussed more thoroughly in chapters 3 and 7, respectively.

For more details on neurological testing, refer to *Therapeutic Exercise for Athletic Injuries* (Houglum 2000), chapter 4.

## Reflex Tests

**Deep tendon reflexes** are also tested as part of the neurological assessment. Technically, a test of any tendon could elicit a deep tendon reflex, but only a few are commonly used. Deep tendon reflexes identify the existence of an upper or lower motor neuron deficiency. They can serve as an adjunct to confirm suspected nerve injuries; but they should not be the sole tools for neurological assessment, since there are many variables that interfere with the results. For example, older and younger individuals can demonstrate less reflex activity than people in other age groups, and reflexes can become hyperactive when an individual exercises. Some individuals have normally diminished and others have normally excessive reflexes.

*Lower motor neurons are peripheral motor nerves that originate in the spinal column and innervate skeletal muscle.*

*Upper motor neurons are motor neurons that originate in the cerebral cortex and conduct stimuli from the brain to motor nuclei in the spinal cord.*

**Reflexes** are graded on a 0- to 4-point scale. They are listed as +1, +2, +3, and +4: +1 is a diminished reflex, +2 is a normal reflex, +3 is an excessive or exaggerated reflex, and +4 is a **clonus** or very brisk reflex response. A peripheral nerve or nerve root (lower motor neuron lesion) that is injured will demonstrate a diminished or absent reflex whereas a central nerve injury (upper motor neuron lesion) will produce an exaggerated reflex. Since most neural injuries seen in athletics are lower motor neuron lesions, diminished reflex responses are the most common observation.

The normal method of testing reflexes is with a reflex hammer, used against a tendon that is on slight stretch. Lightly tap the tendon to elicit a response, tapping five or six times to assess the reflex for nerve root involvement. If you have difficulty eliciting a reflex response, have the athlete isometrically pull crossed ankles apart (for an upper-extremity response) or pull clasped hands apart (for a lower-extremity response) (figure 2.1). This technique, called Jendrassik's maneuver, is used to increase the nervous system's sensitivity to allow an improved deep tendon reflex response.

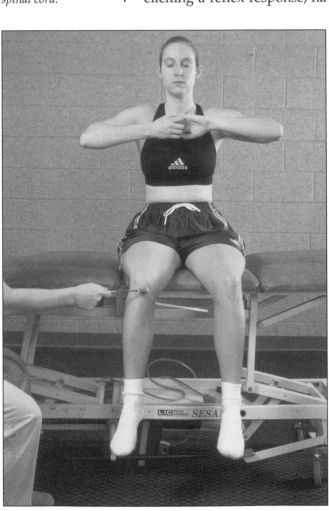

■ **Figure 2.1**   Jendrassik's maneuver.

### Circulatory Tests

Circulatory tests are performed to assess the integrity of the vascular system. Pulses are palpated to determine the presence of blood flow. When a pulse is palpated, it is assessed for presence, strength, and regularity. Dislocations and fractures can impair blood flow by occlusion or laceration, so in the case of these injuries a pulse should be routinely and periodically checked. If the pulse weakens or disappears, the situation is a medical emergency, and the athletic trainer must provide for immediate and emergency medical referral to prevent limb loss, or worse.

Remember that an athlete who has been engaging in a cardiovascular activity will have a normally elevated pulse rate and that an injury can increase pulse rate, especially if the athlete is in shock. You must be cognizant of these conditions and be aware of changes in the athlete's symptoms throughout the injury assessment process. For example, if the pulse rate remains significantly elevated after several minutes of rest, shock may be the cause.

Another sign of circulatory impairment is skin color. You will note pallor over areas of decreased blood flow or ischemia, such as would appear in the forearm if the brachial artery were occluded.

*Pallor refers to a loss of skin coloration due to decreased blow flow.*

You may also note generalized skin pallor with shock as blood is being shunted to the organs from the skin. Clearly, pulse and skin pallor are key signs that you need to monitor routinely in any ongoing evaluation when circulatory impairment is suspected.

### *Functional Tests*

Functional tests are used only when the athlete is ready to return to sport participation. This is the final testing, used to assess not so much the nature or severity of an injury, but rather the athlete's ability to safely return to full participation. Most commonly it is performed after a course of treatment following an injury rather than at the time of injury. Only in cases of mild injuries—if symptoms have subsided and all previous tests have demonstrated that the athlete is able to return to participation—is functional testing a part of the immediate evaluation process. In these cases, functional tests must be part of the assessment before the athlete is permitted to return to the field, track, or gym.

Functional testing will help you determine the athlete's confidence and physical readiness to return to participation beyond what you can learn from standard strength and ROM testing. Functional testing utilizes specific tasks and controlled skill movements that mimic the physical demands and joint stresses inherent in the sport. Simple examples are sprinting, cutting, and jumping maneuvers to stress the ankle or knee joint before return to basketball, and progressive throwing activities before a pitcher returns to full speed. By having the athlete perform these functional movements, you can assess the quality of performance in a more controlled environment and identify whether the athlete shows signs of apprehension or is compensating with other movements to protect the area and avoid pain. Functional assessment should begin with slow, controlled uniplanar movements that progress in speed and intensity, and then proceed to multiplanar movements that involve rotational stresses. In other words, start simple and slow; build to full speed and more complex movements, as long as the athlete tolerates them.

Specific functional tests are wide and varied. Obviously they will be unique to the athlete's sport and even the position played. For example, functional tests for a gymnast with a shoulder injury will be different from those for a tennis player with a similar injury because of the different demands these activities place on the shoulder. Likewise, functional activities for a football lineman who is blocking with the upper extremity will be different from those for a quarterback, who must perform an overhead throwing motion. Therefore, it is important to have a working understanding of the physical demands and stresses that a particular athlete will experience so that you can make the appropriate functional assessment.

For more discussion on functional assessment and readiness to return to activity, refer to *Therapeutic Exercise for Athletic Injuries* (Houglum 2000), chapter 4.

## OFF-FIELD ASSESSMENT

Many times you will not evaluate an injury immediately after it happens. More often, an athlete will report to the athletic treatment facility complaining of an injury that has occurred within the past few hours or days, or with an injury that has had no acute onset and has been getting progressively worse over time. Without the advantage of having witnessed an injury, your detective work must be broader but at the same time more detailed, as the picture of severity, irritability, nature, and stage can be much more complicated and thus less clear. The profile of an injury changes with time, and findings at the onset will not necessarily be the same as they are later. This makes accurate assessment and evaluation more complicated and difficult.

### GENERAL PRINCIPLES OF THE OFF-FIELD ASSESSMENT

Although the procedure in an off-field assessment follows a specific routine and includes many of the same components as the sideline assessment, some components

## General Evaluation Checklist for Sideline Assessment

**Goals**
- Determine nature of injury.
- Determine severity of injury.

**Subjective Segment**
✓ History
  ✓ Current
  ✓ Past
✓ Observation
  ✓ Skin coloration
  ✓ Swelling, deformity, ecchymosis

**Objective Segment**
✓ Palpation
✓ Special tests

✓ ROM
  ✓ Active
  ✓ Passive
✓ Strength
  ✓ General isometric tests
  ✓ Manual muscle testing
✓ Neurological tests (as appropriate)
  ✓ Sensory
  ✓ Motor
  ✓ Reflex
✓ Circulatory tests
  ✓ Pallor
  ✓ Distal pulse
✓ Functional tests (as appropriate)

are slightly altered and others are added. The signs to look for in the two assessments are comparable. As with the sideline assessment, the off-field assessment comprises subjective and objective segments. The following discussion covers the entire sequence of the off-field assessment, but refers only briefly to those components that are the same as for assessment on the sideline. Readers should refer back to the sideline assessment for a complete discussion of these. You will note that the sequence of the off-field assessment differs from that for the sideline assessment. The main difference is that palpation is performed much later in the off-field than in the on-field or sideline assessment.

In the off-field assessment, the evaluation order will be as follows:

1. Subjective (history)
2. Observation
3. ROM
4. Strength
5. Neurovascular tests
6. Special tests
7. Joint mobility
8. Palpation
9. Functional tests

## OFF-FIELD ASSESSMENT—SUBJECTIVE SEGMENT

You will ask many of the same questions during the off-field assessment that you ask at the sideline regarding the mechanism of the current injury and any history of prior injury and its treatment. You must first decide whether the injury is acute or chronic, so questioning about onset is important. When did the injury occur? Was the onset sudden, or did the symptoms come on gradually? If onset was sudden, when did it happen and how did it happen? If the symptoms came on gradually, when did they first appear and what was the athlete doing at the time? What activities aggravate the injury now? What makes it feel better? When in the athlete's workout do the symptoms come on, and how long do they persist? Do the symptoms interfere with daily activities, and if so, what activities? Where is the pain? Does it radiate to any other segment? How would the athlete describe the pain and other symptoms? The athlete should rate the intensity of the pain on a 0- to 10-point scale. Does the pain wake her up at night? Is there any time during the day that the pain is worse or less, or is the pain activity related? What treatment, if any, has the athlete self-administered? Later chapters will include other specific questions for particular regions.

If the athlete is unable to recall a particular injury or illness that has caused the current symptoms, special medically related questions may be appropriate to rule out general medical problems, some of which could be serious. Such special questions should include, for example, whether the athlete has experienced any unexplained weight loss recently or recurring incidents of night sweats. These signs could indicate any one of several life-threatening conditions, such as cancer or acquired autoimmune deficiency syndrome, that should not be ignored. Fever could suggest an illness needing medical attention. If the athlete is female and in her childbearing years, she should be asked if she is pregnant, as this may affect your treatment protocol. Other specific questions will depend on the athlete's symptoms. Generally, complaints of symptoms in and around the upper extremities and cervical regions include problems with dizziness, hearing or vision changes, coordination problems, unexplained weakness, or bowel or bladder dysfunction. These are symptoms of neurological pathology. Chapter 13 describes the signs and symptoms associated with a variety of common general medical conditions that you should also be familiar with.

## General Questions to Ask When Taking a History of a Nonacute Injury

What is the chief complaint?

When did the injury occur?

Was it a sudden onset, or did the symptoms appear gradually over time?

If sudden onset, does the individual know how it happened or what caused it?

If gradual, when did the symptoms first appear and what was the individual doing at the time?

Can you describe the pain?

- Quality of pain (sharp, dull, achy)
- Intensity (scale of 1-10)
- Localized or diffuse
- Any referral
- Any changes in pain from when it started (intensified or lessened over time)

When does it hurt?

Is the pain constant or intermittent?

Once the injury is irritated, how long does the pain last?

What activities make the pain worse?

How much do the pain or symptoms interfere with activity?

What activities make the pain better?

Any abrupt or significant changes in training?

- Change in intensity, duration, training surface, type of activity
- Any change in training implements (e.g., tennis racket grip, bat weight, shoes, etc.)

Previous history for body region (information on nature, severity, duration of symptoms, treatment received)?

Previous history for opposite side?

Any other medical conditions to be aware of?

- Change in diet or weight?
- Recent illness?
- Other signs and symptoms?
- Existing medical conditions?
- Taking any medications or receiving any treatment?

The information obtained in the subjective assessment should provide a clearer picture of the severity, irritability, nature, and stage (SINS) of the injury, and should determine how aggressive you can be in your objective assessment.

Begin your observation the moment the athlete enters the athletic injury treatment facility. The observations are the same as those made during the sideline assessment.

Remember, the goal with the subjective assessment is to obtain a profile of the SINS of the injury. As you complete the subjective assessment, you should have a good idea of stage and irritability. You should also have a more focused view of the particular nature and severity of the problem.

## OFF-FIELD ASSESSMENT—OBJECTIVE SEGMENT

Before you conduct the objective assessment on a postacute injury, it is always a good idea to caution the athlete that the evaluation may aggravate the symptoms. It is not unusual for an athlete to experience an increase in symptoms following the evaluation; assure the person that these should quickly subside. You should also instruct the athlete to inform you at the time of the next visit whether or not symptoms did increase after this examination.

### Differential Diagnosis

Since you did not see the injury occur, you may find it difficult to pinpoint the mechanism and nature of the injury, even with the athlete's history. The source of symptoms of some injuries can be difficult to discern, since more than one injury can be causing the profile the athlete presents. You must be able to delineate the possible causes and eliminate as many factors as possible. This process is called making a differential diagnosis.

**Differential diagnosis** should be a part of any off-field assessment in cases in which the injury is not obvious; and involvement of adjacent joints should be eliminated early in the evaluation before attention is focused on the area of complaint. The cervical region can refer symptoms to the shoulder, elbow, and wrist; the lumbar region can refer to the hip, knee, and ankle; any upper-extremity joint can refer to another upper-extremity joint; and any lower-extremity joint can refer to another lower-extremity joint. Therefore it is necessary to eliminate these referral segments as sources of the athlete's complaints.

Quick tests can often eliminate other areas or segments as the source of the symptoms. For example, if the athlete reports hip and back pain, you can have her perform a squat. If she reports no difficulty with the activity and performs the move smoothly through a full ROM, the problem may be related to the lumbar spine and not the hip. If she reports anterior thigh pain but is unable to recall a specific quadriceps injury, you can assess for a differential diagnosis with a quick test. In standing, the athlete performs lumbar flexion, extension, side-bending, and rotation movements. If she reports pain during any of these movements, you will more thoroughly investigate the lumbar spine to eliminate the possibility of a lumbar injury with nerve root dysfunction. If she reports symptoms in the shoulder but you are unsure whether they are related to a shoulder or cervical problem, you can perform a quick cervical screen of passive and active ROM before focusing on the shoulder. If the symptoms are related to the cervical region, they may be reproduced by these test motions.

### Range of Motion

Active and passive ROM is examined as in the sideline assessment to evaluate the quality and extent of physiological joint motion as well as end feel. Refer to the discussion of sideline assessment of ROM for details of the techniques and procedures.

Passive motion testing will also identify capsular-related problems that result in loss of motion and present with a capsular pattern of movement. A capsular pattern occurs when the joint's capsule becomes adherent. Secondary loss of motion creates a typical pattern of movement that is unique for each joint. A capsular pattern does not occur unless there is a limitation of normal capsular mobility. If a capsular pattern was noted during active motion, passive motion can confirm suspicions of capsule-related restriction through limitations of passive movement in a capsular pattern.

Capsular restriction is progressive. The more restricted the joint is, the less motion will be available. Although early capsular restriction may exhibit only slight loss of motion in one or two directions, more progressive restriction will include loss of motion in all directions and to greater degrees. For example, in early capsular restriction of the shoulder, it may be that only external rotation is limited; but in later stages, external rotation, abduction, and flexion will all be limited, with external rotation having the greatest limitation and flexion the least.

If the athlete demonstrates reduced ROM during active ROM testing but does not have a capsular pattern of movement, other structures besides the joint capsule may be responsible for the restricted motion. A variety of influences may cause a noncapsular restriction of motion, including ligamentous restriction, internal derangement, or extra-articular structure restriction such as muscle tightness, spasm, scarring, or myofascial restriction. If it is possible to assess passive overpressures, the quality of the end feel may help determine the cause of the restriction (see "Types of End Feel" on page 31).

### Strength

Remember, if the strength test causes pain, the athlete's strength will be inhibited and its assessment may not be accurate. Pain and apprehension with strength testing should be noted in your evaluation, and retesting should take place at a later date when the injury is less irritable.

As at the sideline, strength tests in the off-field assessment begin with isometric screening for any gross discrepancies and proceed to evaluation of specific muscles or muscle groups when bilateral differences have been noted. As with the sideline evaluation, manual muscle tests are the most convenient method of assessing strength. However, the off-field assessment may also incorporate instrumented strength-testing equipment to provide for more objective outcomes. Selection of equipment depends upon availability, preference of the athletic trainer, the muscle or muscle group being tested, and the athlete's condition. Equipment can range from isometric tensiometers to free and machine weights to isokinetic equipment. While manual muscle tests are the most efficient and readily available means of evaluating muscle strength, assessment using instrumented strength testing, when feasible and appropriate, provides a more objective and reproducible measure.

### Neurovascular Tests

Off-field neurovascular tests are the same as for the sideline assessment. Neurological assessment includes investigation of sensory, motor, and reflex responses to determine the integrity of afferent and efferent receptors within the neuromuscular system. Circulatory assessment includes palpation of the distal pulse for presence, rate, and rhythm and observance of skin coloration. All tests discussed in connection with the sideline assessment are used in the off-field assessment. If you note positive sensory responses with the light touch tests, you can perform other sensory tests if you wish, but they are not necessary. An athlete who demonstrates any positive neurovascular signs or symptoms should be referred to a physician for additional testing.

### Special Tests

Special tests as discussed for the sideline assessment are used off-field as well. Other tests may also be appropriate, depending on the athlete's history and the athletic trainer's preliminary findings from other objective tests. Because the off-field assessment is more likely than the sideline assessment to reveal chronic injuries, additional tests may be necessary to confirm the preliminary impression of the chronic nature of the injury. These additional special tests are joint specific and will be discussed in relation to off-field assessment in the chapters on the various body segments.

### *Joint Mobility*

Two factors determine a joint's ROM: physiological motion and accessory motion. **Physiological motion** is the active motion of the joint that occurs in the planes of motion. **Accessory motion** is the subtle, passive motion that occurs within and between the joint's inert structures and must be present in order for full physiological motion to occur. For example, the metacarpophalangeal joints flex, extend, abduct, and adduct actively; but for these motions to occur through their full ranges, the joint surfaces must also be able to passively glide and rotate on one another. Rotation and glide are not active motion at the metacarpophalangeal joints, but you can easily demonstrate them if you grasp the finger and passively rotate it. Accessory or passive joint movements are referred to as **joint play**.

Accessory movements must be assessed if the physiological joint motion noted during the ROM testing is not normal. They are evaluated through joint mobility assessment, also referred to as **joint mobilization** techniques. Joint mobility assessment is a passive movement evaluation, used primarily to assess the joint's capsular structures. Sideline assessments do not normally involve joint mobility except for special tests to determine instability or ligamentous injuries. Capsule-related problems usually stem from restriction of the capsule that develops because of chronic injury or disease, immobility, or limited use of the joint through its full motion.

### Capsular Patterns of Movement

When you observe a capsular pattern during active and passive movement testing, you should suspect a capsular restriction and use joint mobility assessment techniques for confirmation. These will more specifically determine the location and quality of restriction within the joint capsule.

### Joint Mobilization Techniques

Joint mobilization is a manual technique that is used both to assess and to treat a joint when restrictions are present. Although these techniques may be applied through use of either an oscillation or a sustained method, the techniques for assessment and treatment are similar. It is important to compare right to left sides to determine what is "normal" for each athlete. Each person has different "normal" joint play, which you must take into account along with what is considered normal for the age population of the athlete. The best way to learn what is normal for any given age group is to perform techniques on large numbers of athletes—experience is the best teacher of this base of knowledge.

> Capsular-related problems that result in loss of motion will present with a capsular pattern of movement. Each joint has its own characteristic capsular pattern of movement. When you observe a capsular pattern during active movement testing, suspect a capsular restriction and use joint mobility assessment techniques to confirm the suspicion.

> For information regarding the application of joint mobilization for treatment, refer to *Therapeutic Exercise for Athletic Injuries* (Houglum 2000), chapter 6.

*Loose-packed position is the position of the joint at the time the ligaments are at their resting length and under the least amount of tension.*

Perform joint mobility assessment with the athlete in a relaxed position, since muscle tension will prevent accurate assessment of joint play. The extremity being tested should be supported, and the joint is initially placed in a loose-packed position so that the ligaments are at a resting length and the joint's surface contact is reduced. One joint and one motion are assessed at a time. Apply the forces to the joint in the plane of the joint surface; use enough force to produce accurate findings but not enough to cause excessive pain. As with the other tests, assess the uninvolved side first. In the mobilization technique, one aspect of the joint is stabilized as the mobilization force is applied close to the joint at the other aspect.

Although joint mobilization techniques differ depending on the joint, some apply to most joints. With a **distraction**, or **traction**, technique, a longitudinal force is applied to the joint to separate the proximal from the distal portion. This assesses joint play and general capsular mobility and is usually used to obtain a general idea of overall mobility. If distraction produces a restricted feel, additional tests will be necessary for further identification of precise locations of restriction.

Most joints can also be assessed with anterior-posterior and posterior-anterior capsular mobilization techniques. These are both glide maneuvers in which one aspect of the joint is moved in a straight anterior-to-posterior (AP) or posterior-to-anterior (PA) direction on the opposing joint surface. This will assess the mobility of the anterior and posterior capsule in joints such as the shoulder, knee, and wrist. Lateral glides are applied in a manner similar to the AP and PA movements, but laterally instead of anteriorly or posteriorly. They are used to assess lateral stability or restriction of a joint such as the shoulder, ankle, wrist, and interphalangeal joints. Particular applications of these and other more specialized applications for each joint will be discussed in later chapters.

### *Palpation*

Appropriately applied palpation can reveal information regarding the tension, thickness, and texture of soft tissue; the presence or absence of swelling; temperature, moisture, pulses, fasciculations; and general contours of soft tissue and bony prominences.

The athletic trainer will perform palpation later in the off-field evaluation, after other portions of the evaluation have identified the source of the athlete's pain. Waiting to perform palpation until after you have completed the movement and special tests will provide you a more narrowed focus on the possible nature of the injury and allow you to concentrate attention on a specific area. If you perform palpation early in the evaluation, you may be palpating uninvolved tissue because the pain may in fact be referred from another source—something you will not know until you have performed other portions of the evaluation.

As at the sideline, palpation in the off-field assessment proceeds systematically, moving from superficial to deep structures and traversing the body segment in a routine such as from anterior to posterior, or superior to inferior. Palpation skills must be finely tuned to discriminate between normal and abnormal tissue. You must have knowledge of the tissue structures and an awareness of what is normal with respect to temperature, swelling, tenderness, restriction, and topography in order to distinguish normal from abnormal. Your hands should be warm, and your palpation should be confident and direct—with a pressure that is not so light as to tickle, but not so firm as to cause undue discomfort. Both you and the athlete should be relaxed.

Palpation of the structures is the same as in the sideline assessment. Carefully note areas of differences between the involved and uninvolved sides for soft tissue tension, spasm, restriction, temperature, moisture, swelling, thickness, texture, bony and soft tissue contours, and tenderness.

### *Functional Tests*

Functional tests mimic the physical demands and joint stresses inherent in the athlete's sport and position; the purpose is to define the athlete's physical and emotional ability to return to the sport with confidence and without undue risk of additional injury resulting from protective or compensatory movements.

As with the sideline assessment, functional tests are used in the off-field assessment to identify the athlete's readiness to participate in his or her sport, and the assessment itself is also the same.

### *Diagnostic Tests*

Additional diagnostic tests, usually ordered by a physician, may be indicated to either confirm or eliminate any suspected diagnosis. A variety of diagnostic tests are available. The specific tests one will use are determined in part by availability, physician preference, and the tissue involved. Laboratory tests such as blood and urine tests identify illness or organ injury; ultrasound scans can serve to rule out some organ and soft tissue injuries; and radiographic tests can identify bone, ligament, or other soft tissue injury. Common radiographic tests for evaluating orthopedic injuries include x-ray for fracture identification; magnetic resonance imaging and computed tomography scans for soft tissue, meniscal, and ligamentous injuries; and bone scans for hard-to-identify bone injuries such as stress fractures.

## General Evaluation Checklist for Off-Field Assessment

**Goals**
- Determine severity of injury.
- Determine irritability of injury.
- Determine nature of injury.
- Determine stage of injury.

**Subjective Segment**
- ✓ History
  - ✓ Current: Acute
  - ✓ Current: Chronic
  - ✓ Past
- ✓ Observation
  - ✓ Skin coloration
  - ✓ Swelling, deformity, ecchymosis

**Objective Segment**
- ✓ Differential diagnosis tests
- ✓ ROM: Active
- ✓ ROM: Passive

- ✓ Strength
  - ✓ General isometric tests
  - ✓ Manual muscle tests
  - ✓ Instrumented assessment
- ✓ Neurological tests (as appropriate)
  - ✓ Sensory
  - ✓ Motor
  - ✓ Reflex
- ✓ Circulatory tests (as appropriate)
  - ✓ Pallor
  - ✓ Distal pulse
- ✓ Special tests
- ✓ Joint mobility tests
- ✓ Palpation
- ✓ Functional tests

# DOCUMENTATION OF YOUR ASSESSMENT

A final ingredient of utmost importance in your assessment procedures is an accurate and thorough documentation of your findings. Injury documentation is essential for a number of reasons. From a medicolegal standpoint, you may need to reproduce records in the event of a legal dispute or for insurance claim verification. From a more practical standpoint, other colleagues may be in a position to care for your athlete when you are not available, and accurate assessment and injury records will ensure continuity of care. Injury documentation will also prove useful for re-evaluation of injuries, allowing you to compare your findings from one evaluation to the next. It is never wise to rely on your recall, as you may forget critical findings.

Your documentation should be thorough but concise. It is likely in most settings that you will perform multiple evaluations in a single day, so efficient documentation will be essential if you wish to avoid getting bogged down in paperwork. Many computerized injury-tracking systems are now available. But whether in written or computerized form, the information that you should provide is the same.

## SOAP NOTES

The simplest and most common documentation procedure is the use of "SOAP" notes. **SOAP notes** include documentation of your **S**ubjective findings, **O**bjective findings, overall **A**ssessment, and subsequent **P**lan for the athlete based on your assessment. The record does not need to include every aspect of your evaluation, but it should contain all information that might need to be recalled at a later date. The sample evaluation form in this chapter provides an idea of the kinds of information that may be included. Athletic trainers devise evaluation forms to suit their own preferences: some use an open-ended form like the one on page 46; others use a detailed "fill-in-the-blank" type of form that lists specific objective tests for each body region.

The **subjective** portion of the form will include the essential information from the history portion of the subjective assessment, such as chief complaint, mechanism of injury, and reported signs and symptoms. Your subjective documentation should provide a clear picture of the athlete's perception of the injury's SINS. The following is an example of documentation of the subjective evaluation:

> *The athlete reported to the athletic training room complaining of pain in her anterior knee. She stated that the pain had appeared gradually over the last 3-4 days and denied any mechanism of injury. The athlete is a freshman basketball player who in the last 2 weeks has begun intensive conditioning activities 2 hours a day in preparation for the season. Prior to this increase in activity, the athlete had been on vacation and physically inactive for the previous month. She described the pain as an "ache" just below the kneecap while pointing to the infrapatellar tendon. She stated that the pain is worse at the beginning of activity but improves somewhat with warm-up. Pain is worse during activities of jumping and squatting, and during rest after long sitting. She denies any previous injury to the involved or uninvolved knee.*

From this written history, you can determine the location and nature of the injury and also get a sense of what may have caused the injury, the degree of irritability, the stage or duration of the injury, and the level of severity.

The **objective** portion of your documentation should present all the findings of your objective assessment. This will include your observations as well as the results of pertinent objective tests such as ROM, strength, neurovascular, and special tests. The following is a continuation of the example just presented:

> *A slight limp was observed as the athlete walked into the athletic training facility. Upon inspection, mild swelling was noted just below the kneecap in the infrapatellar tendon region. No obvious deformity or discoloration was noted. Athlete was able to complete a full range of motion into flexion and extension, with some discomfort noted with active extension. There was no pain with passive motion, except in full passive flexion. Strength was 5/5 on manual muscle testing for both knee flexion and extension, with pain noted on extension. Neurological and special test evaluations were negative. Palpable tenderness and inflammation were noted over the infrapatellar tendon.*

Notice that not every test within the objective assessment is included in this account. Primarily, you want to report the important findings that clearly describe the injury. Although it is not necessary to document every negative finding, you may include the negative findings indicating that you ruled out other injuries or structures that would produce similar signs or symptoms. With practice, you will become more efficient in your written assessment and better able to discern what should be included.

The **assessment** portion of your documentation should include your impression of the injury. On the basis of the findings of your subjective and objective assessment, you should now have a good sense of what the injury is. Unless it is clearly definitive, often you may qualify your impression using wording such as "possible," "probable," or "rule out." To continue with our example:

> *Probable infrapatellar tendinitis.*

It is important to write down your impression, as it may change upon reevaluation or as symptoms progress or subside.

Finally, documentation of the plan provides a written account of your immediate treatment and referral plans for the athlete. If you referred the athlete for further medical evaluation or if EMS was called, this should be documented. If the athlete

# SOAP NOTES FORM

**ATHLETE'S NAME:** _____ **RECORD/ID#:** _____

**INJURY DATE:** _____ **RECORD DATE:** _____

**SPORT:** _____

Subjective (history, observation):

_____
_____
_____
_____
_____

Objective (palpation, ROM, strength,
neurological tests, special tests):

_____
_____
_____
_____
_____
_____
_____
_____
_____
_____
_____
_____
_____
_____
_____
_____
_____

Assessment (impression):

_____
_____

Plan (treatment and disposition):

_____
_____

From *Assessment of Athletic Injuries* by S.J. Shultz, P.A. Houglum, and D.H. Perrin, 2000, Champaign, IL: Human Kinetics.

was removed from activity, allowed to return to activity, or advised to rest, this should be noted as well. Additionally, any immediate treatment provided such as icing, immobilization, or wound cleansing should be reported. To finish our example:

> *The athlete was removed from activity, and ice was applied for 20 minutes. The athlete will rest over the weekend and will be reevaluated on Monday.*

Other essential information to include on your form is the athlete's name and identification number, date of initial injury, date of documentation, and sport. Physical characteristics such as age, height, and weight may be important in some instances. It is also helpful if the form includes a full-body diagram to mark the location of the athlete's pain and any referral pain patterns noted. Often it is easier to draw these pain patterns than to describe them verbally.

Write your documentation as soon after the injury evaluation as possible while the information is fresh in your mind. You can often document your findings as you proceed through an off-field assessment. With on-field and sideline assessments this is more difficult, as you will probably be unable to write the report during assessment. For this reason it is a good idea to have a notepad among your athletic training field supplies where you can jot down important findings that may be difficult to recall later.

# SUMMARY

1. *Identify the main goals and features of the on-field assessment.*

   The purpose of the on-field assessment is to identify or rule out life-threatening and serious injuries, determine the nature and severity of the injury, and determine the disposition and mode of transport from the field. Good judgment and sound decision-making skills are needed to provide an accurate and efficient assessment and an effective and correct response. The on-field assessment includes a primary survey to assess life-threatening injuries or conditions and a secondary survey to screen for other possible serious injuries.

2. *Explain the purpose and the components of the subjective assessment.*

   The subjective evaluation includes the history and observation portions of the injury assessment. Questioning of the athlete should yield an accurate picture of the injury including **what** the chief complaint is, **how** the injury happened, **where** and **when** it hurts, what the pain and other signs and symptoms are like, and what the previous history of injury and illness has been. Questions should be open-ended, not leading, allowing the athlete to provide full and accurate information about symptoms. The observation also provides valuable information on how the athlete is responding to the pain and how he moves or guards the injured area, as well as revealing signs of swelling, discoloration, and deformity of the injured area. The goal in the subjective assessment is to obtain sufficient information on which to base the objective assessment.

3. *Identify the general evaluation procedures of the objective assessment and the purpose for each.*

   In the objective assessment, you will continue to observe the athlete and use a variety of tests and measures to determine the nature and degree of severity of the injury. Although the subjective assessment guides the objective assessment, the objective tests may or may not confirm your original impressions. It is important to think broadly at the beginning in order to avoid missing any other conditions that may be producing the signs and symptoms, and only later to focus on the specific area of injury. Evaluation procedures in the objective assessment include palpation, active and passive ROM testing, joint mobility testing, strength evaluation, neurovascular assessment, special tests for identifying particular conditions, and functional tests.

4. *Identify the SINS factors of injury assessment.*

The combined subjective and objective portions of the injury assessment provide critical information on the SINS of the injury: severity, irritability, nature, and stage. Assessment of severity reveals the extent of the injury, establishes whether referral is needed, and indicates what medical care is appropriate. The assessment of irritability provides information on the stage of the injury and the degree of exacerbation of the symptoms, also indicating how aggressive you can be in the objective assessment. The nature of the injury includes the type of injury and the tissues or structures involved. Stage of the injury is determined according to whether the complaint is acute or chronic. Together, the SINS allow you to form an accurate impression of the injury and of the correct plan of action. Whereas the sideline assessment primarily evaluates the nature and severity factors, the off-field assessment thoroughly addresses all SINS factors. After completing an evaluation and on the basis of the SINS, the athletic trainer should be able to make appropriate decisions regarding referral to another medical authority, the appropriateness of return to full or partial participation, and the proper course of treatment. The treatment plan should not only include immediate treatment but also outline short-term and long-term treatment goals.

5. *Discuss the goals, primary components, and evaluation sequence of the sideline assessment.*

The sideline assessment will either follow an on-field evaluation or take place when an injured player has walked off the playing field under his or her own power. As compared to the on-field assessment, the sideline assessment more precisely defines the nature and severity of the condition. The sequence of evaluation techniques will be, as appropriate, history, observation, palpation, special tests, ROM, strength, neurovascular assessment, and functional tests.

6. *Discuss the goals, primary components, and evaluation sequence of the off-field assessment.*

The off-field assessment takes place when the athlete reports to the athletic training room, often at some delay after the injury has occurred. Therefore off-field assessments are for injuries ranging from acute to subacute to long-term chronic or overuse conditions. The order of the off-field assessment is slightly different from that for the on-field assessment: palpation is performed later, after the nature and location of the injury have been determined. The order of evaluative techniques for the off-field assessment will be, as appropriate, history, observation, active and passive ROM, strength evaluation, neurovascular tests, special tests, joint mobility, palpation, and functional tests.

7. *Explain the SOAP notes procedure for injury documentation.*

The purpose of injury documentation is to provide a record of the injury assessment—essential because such documentation may be needed for medicolegal verification and protection, for communicating findings with other health professionals, and for comparison of findings upon reevaluation. A SOAP notes form is commonly used to document the subjective findings, the objective findings, your impression or assessment of the injury, and the immediate plan of action. When documentation is not possible at the time of injury, it is important to have a pad of paper handy on the field so you can jot down the essential findings you will need to complete proper documentation.

# REVIEW QUESTIONS

1. How would your questioning in the history portion of the assessment differ for on-field, sideline, and off-field assessments?

2. Describe the sequence of steps in an on-field assessment. At which points will you make determinations regarding referral and/or mode of transport from the field?

3. What is the difference between physiological and accessory joint motion? How is each of these assessed?

4. What are the different types of end feels and what may they indicate? Is each of these end feels considered normal or abnormal?

5. What is a "comparable sign" and how is it determined? Why might a bilateral comparison be important in determining a comparable sign?

6. What is the purpose of palpation, and what information can be gained from this evaluation?

7. What is the difference between active and passive ROM? How is each assessed?

8. Describe the grading system for manual muscle tests. How do manual muscle tests differ from isometric, or "break," tests?

9. When (under what conditions and/or for what presenting symptoms) would a neurological assessment be performed? What are the three components of the neurological assessment?

10. What is the purpose of functional tests, and when would they be performed?

# CRITICAL THINKING QUESTIONS

1. An industrial worker comes into the clinic complaining of shoulder pain for the past five to seven days. What are some of the questions you might ask to determine the severity, irritability, nature, and stage of the injury?

2. You are called out to the track because an athlete has gone down. You know nothing else about the injury at this point. What is going through your mind as you run out to the field, and what steps will you take to quickly determine the nature and severity of the injury or illness? Be specific.

3. Let's revisit the scenario at the beginning of the chapter. You are the only athletic trainer available, and you need to quickly determine whom you should care for first. Given this scenario and the information gained in this chapter, how would you proceed in your assessment of these athletes?

4. You have an athlete who comes in complaining of a knee injury. In your history you find that the athlete had a second-degree sprain on the opposite knee just six months ago. How might this affect your evaluation and why?

# CITED REFERENCES

American Academy of Orthopaedic Surgeons. 1991. *Athletic training and sports medicine.* Rosemont, IL: American Academy of Orthopaedic Surgeons.

Maitland, D.G. 1991. *Peripheral manipulation.* Boston: Butterworth-Heinemann.

# ADDITIONAL RESOURCES

Caroline, N. 1995. *Emergency care in the streets.* Boston: Little, Brown.

Hillman, S.K. 2000. *Introduction to athletic training.* Champaign, IL: Human Kinetics.

Houglum, P.A. 2000. *Therapeutic exercise for athletic injuries.* Champaign, IL: Human Kinetics.

# CHAPTER THREE

# Cervical and Upper Thoracic Spine

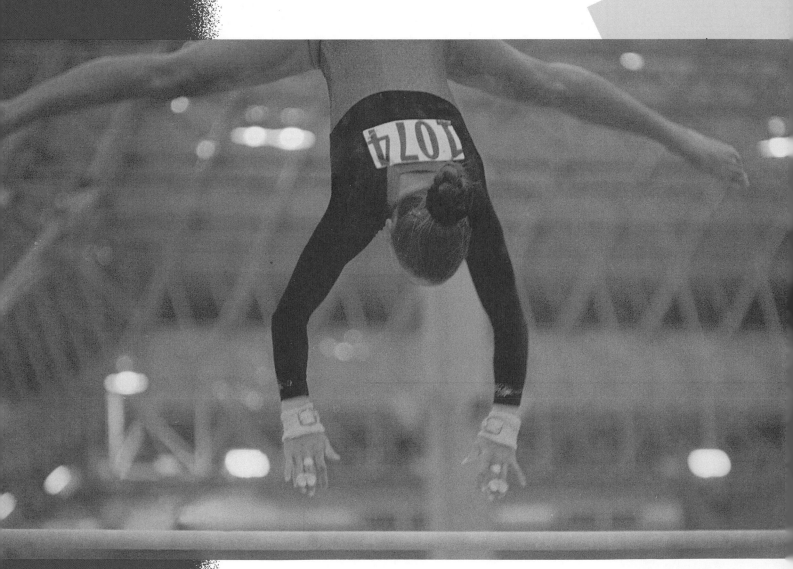

# OBJECTIVES

After completing this chapter, the reader will be able to do the following:

1. Identify the causes of cervical strain

2. Identify the various types of fractures in the cervical spine and the potential for spinal cord injury associated with each

3. Discuss the various causes of neuropathy in the upper extremity relative to cervical spine pathology

4. Conduct a neurological exam for the upper extremity, including sensory, motor, and reflex testing

5. Perform an on-field assessment for a suspected spinal cord injury and determine when a serious injury should be assumed

6. Perform a sideline assessment for the cervical spine region

7. Perform an off-field evaluation for the cervical spine region

Doug was the starting linebacker for his high school football team. He never missed a game, and the team relied heavily on him for his talent. During the game that evening, he went to make a tackle, using the top of his shoulder to make contact. Upon contact, he felt a shooting pain going down his arm. He was able to get up and walk off the field under his own power but immediately sought out Jeff, the athletic trainer who was covering the game.

"Jeff, I need your help, man," Doug said, holding his arm.

Jeff was already on his way toward Doug—he had seen the tackle. He had also observed that Jeff was a little slow to get up and noted that as Jeff walked off the field he was leaning to his right side with his arm hanging, appearing to be in some pain. "What happened?" Jeff asked, already having a good idea from what he had seen.

"I went to make this tackle and hit him with my shoulder. All of a sudden I got this shooting and burning pain going down my arm. It's kinda hard to lift my arm," Doug said.

"Do you have pain in your neck?" Jeff asked.

"No, just my arm—but you know what, the pain is letting up now. . . . Yeah, I think I'm all right . . . I'm ready to go back in," Doug said, as he had stopped feeling concerned and was anxious to get back in the game. As he was talking, he started to head for the coach to say he was good to go.

"Hold up a minute," Jeff said. "We need to take a look first and make sure you have your full strength back. You can wait a couple more plays." Doug was impatient, but cooperative. Upon completing his full evaluation, Jeff found that Doug's pain had not resolved, also noting some sensory changes in his lateral arm and weakness with shoulder abduction and biceps strength. Until these signs and symptoms subsided, Doug would remain a spectator.

Jeff thought to himself, "Boy, I'm glad I didn't just believe him and let him go back in. . . ."

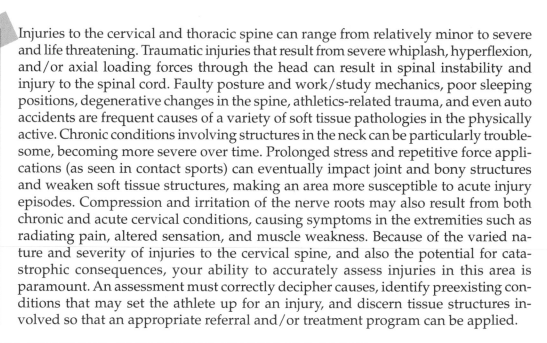

Injuries to the cervical and thoracic spine can range from relatively minor to severe and life threatening. Traumatic injuries that result from severe whiplash, hyperflexion, and/or axial loading forces through the head can result in spinal instability and injury to the spinal cord. Faulty posture and work/study mechanics, poor sleeping positions, degenerative changes in the spine, athletics-related trauma, and even auto accidents are frequent causes of a variety of soft tissue pathologies in the physically active. Chronic conditions involving structures in the neck can be particularly troublesome, becoming more severe over time. Prolonged stress and repetitive force applications (as seen in contact sports) can eventually impact joint and bony structures and weaken soft tissue structures, making an area more susceptible to acute injury episodes. Compression and irritation of the nerve roots may also result from both chronic and acute cervical conditions, causing symptoms in the extremities such as radiating pain, altered sensation, and muscle weakness. Because of the varied nature and severity of injuries to the cervical spine, and also the potential for catastrophic consequences, your ability to accurately assess injuries in this area is paramount. An assessment must correctly decipher causes, identify preexisting conditions that may set the athlete up for an injury, and discern tissue structures involved so that an appropriate referral and/or treatment program can be applied.

# INJURIES TO THE CERVICAL AND UPPER THORACIC SPINE

Although cervical and upper thoracic spine injuries represent only a small fraction of athletics-related injuries, they can be among the most devastating. Because stability is sacrificed for greater mobility in the cervical spine, this segment is more prone to injury than the more stable thoracic spine. This section will focus on the etiology and signs and symptoms of the more common traumatic injuries and chronic dysfunctions of the cervical and upper thoracic spine.

## ACUTE SOFT TISSUE INJURIES

Acute soft tissue injuries can result from direct contact, acute overstretch, or mechanical overload mechanisms. Sprains and strains make up the majority of athletics-related injuries seen in the cervical and thoracic spine. Because the mechanisms of injury and resulting symptoms are often quite similar, it can be difficult to differentiate a sprain from a strain. It is not uncommon for both to occur with traumatic injury mechanisms.

### Contusion

Contusions can result from a direct blow to either the soft tissue or bony prominences of the neck. Although cervical contusions are somewhat uncommon, they can cause considerable pain and a number of symptoms. Signs and symptoms include pain, muscle spasm, and decreased range of motion. A blow to the base of the neck can also traumatize the brachial plexus, resulting in additional signs and symptoms of numbness and weakness into the upper extremity.

### Sprains

Cervical and upper thoracic sprains involve the ligamentous and capsular structures that stabilize and connect the vertebrae and their facet joints. Sprains to the cervical and upper thoracic region most often result from compression, or "jamming," of the spine into extension. However, cervical sprains may also occur during forceful hyperflexion, hyperextension, or rotational movements. Typical signs and symptoms include neck or interscapular pain, or both, depending on the location of injury. Pain may also be noted in the muscles attaching near the site of the injured joint, particularly when the muscle is contracted. Range of motion will be restricted and painful, particularly into extension. Neurological symptoms are rarely associated with acute cervical sprains. If muscular weakness is present, it is usually secondary to an unwillingness to exert a full effort because of pain.

### Strains

Acute strains of the cervical and upper thoracic musculature are frequently seen in athletes. Commonly involved muscles include the levator scapula, trapezius, rhomboids, sternocleidomastoid, scalenes, and the extensor muscle group. Isolated muscular strains often result from a single episode of mechanical overload or from violent stretching into flexion, extension, or rotation. Chronic overuse or poor posture can be a precipitating factor in what appear to be acute strains, as chronic stress can fatigue postural muscles and thus make them more susceptible to mechanical overload. Signs and symptoms of cervical and thoracic strain include muscular pain, point tenderness, spasm, and decreased range of motion. It is not uncommon for these symptoms to be delayed or to gradually worsen up to 24 h following injury as soft tissue swelling increases. Pain will be reproduced with either stretching or contraction of the involved musculature. Depending on the severity of symptoms, the athlete is often seen "splinting," or stiffening the neck, rotating or flexing at the trunk rather than the neck to avoid painful motion. Although cervical and thoracic strains are rarely serious, when left untreated or poorly managed they can lead to muscular weakness or dysfunction, making the muscle more susceptible to recurrent injury.

# CHRONIC OR OVERUSE SOFT TISSUE INJURIES

Many chronic or overuse soft tissue injuries in the cervical and thoracic spine are caused by joint and muscular dysfunction resulting from poor posture and recurrent sprains or strains. The mobile cervical region is particularly susceptible to these chronic injuries, which can lead to permanent **degenerative** changes if left untreated. Therefore, any athlete complaining of chronic neck pain, decreased range of motion, or any hint of neurological symptoms with or without a recent or past history of trauma should be referred for a thorough cervical spine evaluation.

### Degenerative Disc Disease

*Annulus fibrosis is the outer fibrous covering of the intervertebral disc that acts to withstand tension and prevent distortion of disc material.*

Degenerative disc changes can occur with recurrent sprains and chronic joint dysfunction. The annulus fibrosis can be weakened or damaged with repetitive injury or stress, resulting in a loss of disc height and shock-absorbing capability. While the degenerative disc may be asymptomatic and unrecognized for some time, secondary problems resulting from the diminished disc space include impingement of the facet joints, degenerative changes of the bony surfaces, and increased susceptibility to nerve impingement within the intervertebral foramen (Wroble and Albright 1986).

### Facet Syndrome

Chronic inflammatory and degenerative changes can also affect the facet joints. Chronic inflammation, scarring, and fibrosis of the capsular structures can result from extension overload mechanisms, repetitive sprains, and impingement secondary to disc degeneration. Signs and symptoms include pain and decreased motion at the facet joints. Pain is usually exacerbated with extension and rotation to the involved side. Chronic inflammation of the facet joint can also cause irritation of the nearby nerve root.

### Chronic Cervical Joint Instabilities

As with any joint, a potential complication to be aware of with cervical sprains is chronic joint instability. Instability of the cervical spine has serious implications in that hypermobility can put the neurological structures at increased risk for injury. These instabilities are not easily identifiable during injury assessment and typically require radiographic examination in flexion and extension views. Therefore, athletes who sustain a cervical sprain should be referred routinely to a physician in order to rule out resulting instabilities.

# BONE AND JOINT PATHOLOGIES

Bone and joint pathologies are among the most potentially serious and life-threatening injuries of the cervical spine in the athlete. These structures are intimately associated with, and serve to protect, the spinal cord and nerve roots. Therefore, when forces exerted on the cervical spine are sufficient to displace bone and joint structures, catastrophic injury may result.

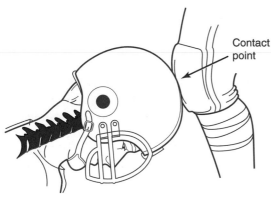

**I Figure 3.1**  Spearing with the head may result in buckling of the cervical spine.

### Cervical Spine Fractures, Dislocations, and Subluxations

The primary cause of cervical fractures, dislocation, and/or subluxations is headfirst contact, resulting in compression and buckling of the cervical spine as it is forced to decelerate the still-moving torso (figure 3.1). The mechanisms that contribute to various cervical spine pathologies are not necessarily based on head movement, but rather on the direction of the impact and resulting buckling/bending forces acting on the spinal segments (Winkelstein and Myers 1997).

Regardless of mechanism, immediate recognition of the signs and symptoms associated with cervical fracture and/or dislocation is paramount in order to avoid further injury. Signs and symptoms may include central spine pain, tenderness with palpation of the involved spinous process(es), muscle spasm, position deformity, and an unwillingness to move the neck. Neurologic symptoms of associated cord injury include bilateral sensory deficits (e.g., burning hands, paresthesia, numbness or loss of sensation), motor weakness, and paralysis in the upper and lower extremities. The level of spinal injury may be determined on examination by the patterns of sensory and/or motor weakness. Respiratory difficulty may be noted with fractures involving C3 and above.

## Compression Mechanisms

Impact to the top of the head, with or without the neck slightly flexed, poses the greatest risk for catastrophic spine injury. These injuries are seen most often in football but can also occur in any sport that involves head contact, such as ice hockey, wrestling, rugby, and gymnastics. Diving into shallow water and striking the head during recreational water activities represents the most frequent cause of activity-related, but not necessarily sport-related, injury. The cervical spine in its normal posture has a lordotic curve that allows greater energy-absorbing capacity. However, when the cervical spine is flexed to about 30°, the spine becomes a straight, segmented column. When an athlete makes contact with an opponent or immovable object with the top of his head and the spine in this position (i.e., "spearing"), stress is absorbed primarily by the vertebral bodies rather than the by neck musculature. Because the compressive force is acting perpendicular to the cervical spine, the head is unable to move to one side or the other and get out of the way of this compressive force (Winkelstein and Myers 1997). Once the maximum energy-absorbing capacity of the spinal column is reached, the spine will fail or buckle. Depending on the resulting bending or rotational forces acting on the spinal segment, a variety of fractures and/or dislocations may occur. Figure 3.2 provides a graphic example of the relationship between resulting forces and type of cervical spine injury that is typically produced.

Burst, wedge, and compression fractures of the vertebral bodies may occur at any level in the cervical spine. A **burst fracture** at C1, also known as a Jefferson fracture, rarely results in spinal cord damage, unless displacement is severe, because the spinal canal is rather large at this level. Similarly, a fracture of the pedicle or pars of C2 (hangman's fracture) can also occur without spinal cord injury. Signs and symptoms associated with C1 and C2 fractures in the absence of neurologic involvement include cervical pain and limited range of motion. Because the spinal canal narrows as it descends, burst fractures of vertebral bodies C3 and below commonly involve some level of cord pathology, and quadriplegia often results. When spinal cord injury occurs above C3, the injury is usually fatal, since respiratory muscle function is often lost.

| Posterior element fracture | ALL and anterior disc disruption | Compression injury | Burst fracture | Wedge compression fracture | Bilateral facet dislocation |

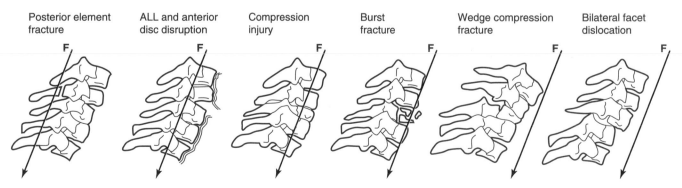

**❚ Figure 3.2** Cervical spine injuries resulting from various forces.

Reprinted, by permission, from B.A. Winkelstein and B.S. Myers, 1997, "The biomechanics of cervical spine injury and implications for injury prevention," *Medicine and Science in Sports and Exercise* 29 (7 suppl): S246-255.

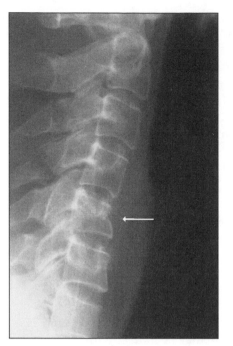
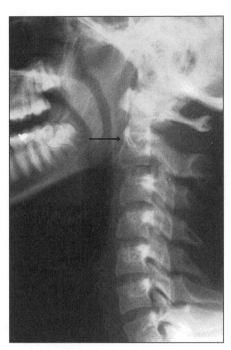

*a*                                                    *b*

**▌ Figure 3.3**    (a) Compression fracture of C5 and dislocation of C3-C4, and (b) subluxation of C2 on C3.

Dislocation of the cervical vertebrae can occur with or without fracture because of the **transverse** orientation of the facet joints (figure 3.3, a-b). Typically, the superior vertebrae will translate anteriorly, causing the superior facets to ride forward and lock anterior to the inferior facets. Isolated unilateral facet dislocations occur most often when axial loading is combined with rotational and forward flexion moments. Neurological involvement is likely with this injury and may involve both the nerve root and spinal cord. Bilateral facet dislocation typically results from flexion buckling of the spine with axial loading, and almost certainly causes some level of spinal cord injury, particularly in the absence of an associated fracture.

### Hyperflexion and Hyperextension Mechanisms
Although impact to the face or the back of the head poses a substantially lower risk to the cervical spine than impact directed through the top of the head, this type of impact can nevertheless cause significant injury. With pure hyperflexion injuries, the anterior body can be compressed and the posterior ligaments torn. Since the contact of the chin with the chest will limit further flexion, dislocation and neurological involvement are less common with isolated flexion mechanisms (Marks, Bell, and Boumphrey 1990). With hyperextension mechanism, resulting from face-first contact, athletes who have normal cervical spines are at a low risk for fractures or neurologic injury. However, athletes with spinal stenosis or osteophytes may have an increased injury risk for neurologic compression with pure extension mechanisms.

### *Spinous Process Fractures*
Although uncommon, spinous process fractures of the cervical and thoracic spine can result from either hyperflexion or extension mechanisms. Contact or impingement of adjacent spinous processes can result in a push-off fracture with hyperextension mecha-

nisms. **Avulsion** fractures secondary to traction of attaching ligaments may occur with hyperflexion injuries (figure 3.4). Signs and symptoms associated with spinous process fractures include localized pain, tenderness to palpation, and pain with extreme flexion and extension movements. Neurological injury is not typically associated with these fractures.

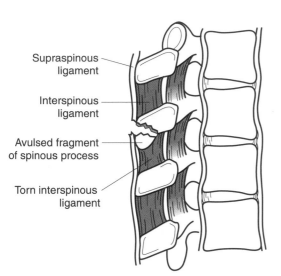

Supraspinous ligament

Interspinous ligament

Avulsed fragment of spinous process

Torn interspinous ligament

■ **Figure 3.4** Spinous process avulsion fracture.

*Neuropraxia refers to transient loss of nerve function caused by trauma.*

### Defects and Abnormalities Secondary to Trauma or Repetitive Stress

Although degenerative joint conditions are more commonly seen in older adults, athletes can also exhibit degenerative bony changes resulting from traumatic injury or repetitive insult. These changes are most commonly seen in contact sports such as football and rugby. Complications associated with the degenerative bony changes to be described include structural malalignment, narrowing of the spinal canal or intervertebral foramen resulting in nerve compression, and increased risk of nerve injury.

### Osteophytes

**Osteophytes**, or **bone spurs**, can arise from the uncinate processes of the vertebral bodies secondary to degenerative disc changes that increase wear and compression of the joint surfaces. Osteophytes are most commonly found posterior-laterally but can also be found anteriorly. Posterior-lateral osteophytes can cause narrowing of the intervertebral foramen, resulting in nerve root compression and increased susceptibility to brachial plexus neuropraxia (figure 3.5). Osteophytes can also cause straightening of the spinal column, which reduces its capacity for axial loading. Signs and symptoms associated with osteophytic changes may include decreased range of motion, postural changes, neck discomfort that increases with lateral rotation and extension, and increasing complaints of neurological symptoms as intervertebral narrowing progresses.

### Spinal Stenosis

**Spinal stenosis** is characterized by a developmental or congenital narrowing of the cervical spinal canal. Spinal stenosis is of particular concern in contact sports and may disqualify an athlete from participation because of the increased risk of spinal cord injury. Because of the narrowed spinal canal, the athlete is at a greater risk for cord compression and injuries resulting from hyperextension or hyperflexion mechanisms. When these are coupled with secondary complications such as cervical spine instability or disc herniation, the risk for spinal cord injury is increased further.

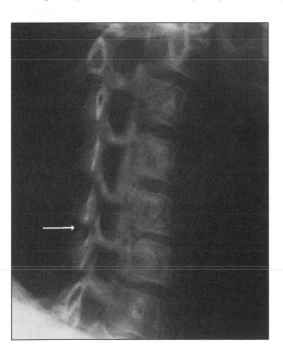

■ **Figure 3.5** Posterior-lateral osteophytes and narrowing of the intervertebral foramen.

# NERVE AND VASCULAR INJURIES

Nerve and vascular injuries associated with the cervical spine are typically caused by encroachment of bony or soft tissue into spinal canal or intervertebral foramen spaces, causing compression of the neurovascular structures that run through that space (figure 3.6).

## Spinal Cord Injury and Transient Neuropraxia

Although the spinal cord is well protected within the spinal column, neurological complications can result from either acute trauma or chronic degenerative changes. As previously discussed, spinal cord injury can be a consequence of acute fractures and dislocation of the cervical and upper thoracic spine, ranging from contusions to complete severance of the cord. Central cord compression and **transient neuropraxia** can also result secondary to posterior disc herniation, spinal stenosis, congenital fusion, or instability in the cervical spine. Signs and symptoms of transient neuropraxia include sensory changes, such as burning, tingling, or numbness, and/or motor changes ranging from weakness to temporary paralysis in both the upper and lower extremities (Torg et al. 1996). These symptoms usually subside within a few minutes but may persist for one to two days. Regardless of the cause, bilateral neurological symptoms in both the upper and lower extremities or bowel/bladder dysfunctions are indicative of central cord involvement; and any athlete presenting with any of these symptoms should be immediately referred for further evaluation.

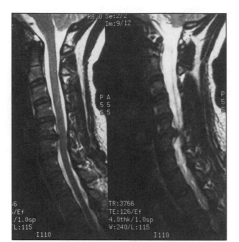

■ **Figure 3.6** Encroachment and compression of the spinal cord and nerve root by a herniated disc.

## Nerve Root Injury and Compression Syndromes

Nerve root injury can be caused by either stretch or compressive mechanisms resulting from acute trauma or chronic mechanical stress. Injury may involve a single nerve root due to encroachment of a herniated disc or osteophyte formation, or may involve multiple nerve roots with brachial plexus traction injuries.

### Intervertebral Disc Herniation

Cervical disc **herniation** is relatively uncommon in athletics but can result from acute trauma causing compression or flexion/extension of the cervical spine. More often, it is caused by a gradual weakening or failure of the annulus fibrosis over time, secondary to chronic or repetitive mechanical stress. Examples of mechanical stress conditions include poor posture, excessive or limited segmental mobility, and degenerative changes. The levels most often affected are C4-C5 and C5-C6, involving the C5 or C6 nerve root, respectively, because of their exceptional mobility and susceptibility to everyday stress. Because the disc is stronger anteriorly and the posterior longitudinal ligament is firmly attached to the central-posterior body of the vertebrae and disc, most herniations occur posterior-laterally (figure 3.7). As a result, the herniated disc material typically protrudes into the intervertebral foramen, causing compression and irritation of the exiting nerve root. Occasionally, if the posterior longitudinal ligament is disrupted, the disc material may protrude centrally into the spinal canal, causing cord compression. Symptoms associated with the neurological compression typically cause the athlete to seek help.

Signs and symptoms of cervical disc herniation and associated nerve compression include pain and discomfort that

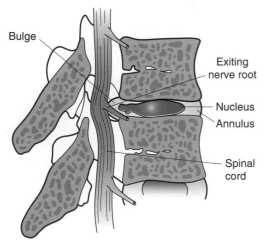

Bulge

Exiting nerve root

Nucleus

Annulus

Spinal cord

■ **Figure 3.7** Posterior lateral disc herniation resulting in compression of the exiting nerve root.

improves with cervical distraction and worsens with extension and rotation to the involved side. The athlete will exhibit decreased range of motion and muscular "splinting," with the head tilted away from the involved side to avoid compressive and painful positions. With nerve root compression, pain will be referred along the distribution of the nerve involved. Neurological deficits such as sensory deficits, motor weakness, and/or diminished reflex may also be present. Muscle atrophy may be observed in chronic cases. If the disc protrusion causes narrowing in the spinal canal, additional signs and symptoms associated with spinal cord compression include bowel and bladder dysfunction, sensory or motor changes in the lower limbs, and episodes of decreased coordination or tripping with no apparent cause. Identification of disc herniation and neurological encroachment is typically confirmed with radiographic evaluation such as computed tomography, magnetic resonance imaging, or myelogram studies.

### Brachial Plexus Injury

Brachial plexus injury involves mechanical deformation of the C5 through T1 nerve roots as they exit the cervical spine (figure 3.8). Injury to the brachial plexus occurs most frequently in football but can also occur with wrestling, rugby, and water skiing at high speeds. Brachial plexus injury can result from either traction or compression mechanisms. A "pinch"-type injury occurs when the head is rotated, laterally flexed, and compressed or extended to the same side of the shoulder, closing down the intervertebral foramen and impinging the nerve roots. Compression injuries can also occur secondary to a direct blow to the base of the neck, particularly when the head is flexed away and the brachial plexus is on stretch. Conversely, a "stretch" injury occurs when the head is forced laterally away from the shoulder while at the same time the shoulder is forced downward. Although these forces can be sufficient to severely or seriously disrupt the integrity of the nerve (**neurotmesis**), typically the injury results in a transient functional block due to mechanical deformation with little or no structural disruption (neuropraxia).

Brachial plexus injuries are often termed "**stingers**" or "**burners**" because of the classic symptoms of immediate sharp, burning pain radiating down into the arm at the time of injury. The athlete will also complain of temporary weakness or inability to move the arm. Symptoms may be reproduced with lateral flexion away from the stabilized shoulder, or with flexion and extension toward the involved side. Symptoms associated with brachial plexus injury are usually short-lived, and full function of the extremity is typically restored within minutes. However, neurological symptoms may persist

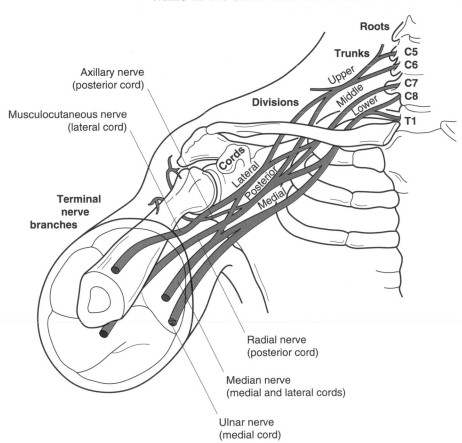

Axillary nerve
(posterior cord)

Musculocutaneous nerve
(lateral cord)

**Terminal
nerve
branches**

**Roots**

**Trunks**    C5
C6

Upper
Middle    C7
**Divisions**    Lower    C8

T1

Cords
Lateral
Posterior
Medial

Radial nerve
(posterior cord)

Median nerve
(medial and lateral cords)

Ulnar nerve
(medial cord)

∎ **Figure 3.8**  Brachial plexus nerve roots as they exit the cervical spine into the upper extremity.

for a few days or even months, depending on the severity of nerve disruption. In rare cases involving sufficient trauma to cause a neurotmesis, permanent neurological deficits and muscle wasting will result. The distribution of motor and sensory weakness will localize the level of the nerve root lesion. Since injury most often involves the upper trunk, or nerve roots C5 and C6, residual numbness and motor weakness will most often be noted in the deltoid, biceps, and internal and external shoulder rotators. Wrist and thumb extensor weakness is also common.

Note an important distinction between brachial plexus injury and cervical spine injury: brachial plexus injuries typically do not result in central cervical spine pain or loss of cervical motion. Therefore, when these symptoms are associated with a suspected brachial plexus injury, further evaluation for possible cervical spine involvement is warranted before return to activity. In athletes who experience repeated or recurrent brachial plexus injuries, the cervical spine should also be carefully evaluated for spinal stenosis or other degenerative conditions that may increase the potential for nerve tractioning or impingement.

> **!** The cervical spine should also be carefully evaluated in athletes who suffer repeated or recurrent brachial plexus injuries to rule out spinal stenosis or other degenerative conditions that may increase the potential for nerve tractioning or impingement.

### Vascular Compression—Thoracic Outlet Syndrome

**Thoracic outlet syndrome** (TOS) is a clinical term that describes compression of the neurovascular structures as they exit through the thoracic outlet. The thoracic outlet is marked by the anterior scalene muscle anteriorly, the middle scalene posteriorly, and the first rib inferiorly. Structures that exit through the thoracic outlet into the upper extremity include the brachial plexus and the subclavian artery (figure 3.9). As these neurovascular structures proceed into the axillary region, there are three primary locations where compression may occur due to encroachment of either bony or soft tissue structures. The most proximal and common site of compression is the interscalene triangle. In this location, compression can be caused by hypertrophy, tightness, or fibrotic bands within the anterior or middle scalene muscles or, in rare cases, by the presence of a cervical rib. Moving further distally, compression may occur within the costoclavicular space between the first rib and the posterior clavicle. Narrowing within this space can result from hypertrophy of the subclavian muscle, or from encroachment of a posterior angulation and/or callous formation following a clavicular fracture. The third common location of compression is the insertion of the pectoralis minor at the coracoid process. As the neurovascular structures pass under the tendon, compression can occur between the tendon and the coracoid process, particularly when the arm is abducted.

Incidence of TOS is more common in women than in men. Thoracic outlet syndrome is also more prevalent in individuals with postural imbalances, such as rounded or depressed (i.e., drooping) shoulders, which can strain the scapular stabilizing muscles and further traction the neurovascular bundle. In many cases, TOS occurs secondary to a previous trauma or injury that results in residual swelling, muscular imbalance, or altered shoulder or scapular mechanics. Neurological structures are involved more often than vascular structures, with compression of the lower trunk of the brachial plexus being the most common pathology. Because of the multiple anatomical sites where compression can occur and the neurovascular structures that can be involved, symptoms can vary considerably. Therefore, signs and symptoms may include pain anywhere between the neck, face, and occipital region or into the chest, shoulder, and/or upper extremity. The athlete may also complain of altered or absent sensation, weakness, fatigue, or a feeling of heaviness in the arm and hand. There may also be swelling and discolora-

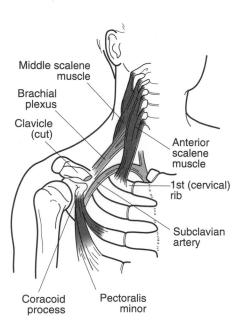

Middle scalene muscle

Brachial plexus

Clavicle (cut)

Anterior scalene muscle

1st (cervical) rib

Subclavian artery

Coracoid process    Pectoralis minor

**Figure 3.9** Location and structures involved in thoracic outlet syndrome.

tion. Signs and symptoms are typically worse when the arm is abducted overhead and externally rotated with the head rotated to either the same or the opposite side. As a result, activities such as overhead throwing or serving a tennis ball may exacerbate symptoms. Because of the complexity of symptoms and their similarity to other cervical-related conditions, determination of TOS is often difficult.

## STRUCTURAL AND FUNCTIONAL ABNORMALITIES

Postural deviations are commonly seen in the cervical and thoracic spines. Postural deviations may be functional, resulting from pain, muscular imbalance, and/or poor postural habits; or they may involve permanent structural changes that can be quite debilitating and disfiguring.

### Forward Head Posture

The most common acquired postural deviation is a forward head posture. This posture is characterized by a forward alignment of the head relative to the shoulders, rounded shoulders, and increased extension of the lower cervical spine in order to maintain an upright head position (figure 3.10). This posture can be caused by pain avoidance secondary to cervical injury but more commonly results from training imbalances or poor postural mechanics. Training imbalances can occur when athletes strengthen the anterior pectoral muscles and ignore the upper back muscles. This results in tight pectoral muscles and weakened rhomboid and trapezius muscles, which make maintaining an upright posture more difficult. Other contributing factors include poor sitting posture (i.e., slouching) and studying habits. Regardless of the contributing factor, the posterior postural muscles have to work much harder against gravity in order to keep the head upright as compared to the situation with a neutral posture. Therefore it is not uncommon for these individuals to report muscular discomfort secondary to chronic overuse and muscular fatigue. If the underlying postural mechanics and muscular imbalances are not recognized and corrected, degenerative disc and joint changes can result from increased mechanical stress over time.

### Torticollis

**Torticollis** is a deformity characterized by a lateral curvature of the cervical spine. In the thoracic spine, this lateral curvature is commonly known as scoliosis. These deformities may be either structural or functional. Structural deformities are characterized by permanent structural changes in the bone and are usually congenital. Structural changes may also be caused by degenerative osteophytes that disrupt the normal contours and motions of the spine. Functional deformities do not involve permanent bony changes; they result from mechanical dysfunctions consequent to poor posture, leg length discrepancy, joint inflammation, nerve root irritation, or muscular imbalance. These conditions are marked with observable postural deformity and loss of spinal range of motion. A distinguishing factor of functional as opposed to structural curvatures is the disappearance of the functional curvature with forward flexion of the spine. Because of the muscular imbalance and compensatory changes created by these spinal curvatures, individuals with torticollis often complain of pain, muscular fatigue, and spasm in the postural muscles.

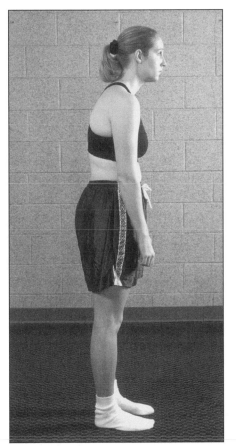

■ **Figure 3.10**    Forward head posture.

## INJURY ASSESSMENT

As an athletic trainer, you will likely experience sometime in your career an on-field assessment of a serious neck injury. Although these injuries don't occur often, your ability to accurately and efficiently determine the nature and extent of the injury could mean the difference between life and death or between full recovery and permanent paralysis for the athlete. Therefore, periodic practice of your on-field assessment skills will keep you sharp and ready for when the time comes. Most of the time, however, you will be asked to evaluate a postacute or chronic cervical injury. Assessment of these injuries is sometimes difficult, as they may result from chronic postural or repetitive stresses that are unrelated to physical activity. In all cases, whether acute or chronic, knowledge of which symptoms and findings dictate immediate medical referral versus conservative care is essential for each of the on-field, sideline, and off-field assessment procedures.

## ON-FIELD ASSESSMENT

As explained previously, it is important to observe the downed athlete as you approach. Noting the position of the head and neck and observing whether the athlete is moving or lying motionless are among the most important things you do before reaching the athlete.

### Primary Survey

Upon arriving at the athlete's side, do a **primary survey** to check for consciousness as well as airway, breathing, and circulation. If the athlete is facing down and not breathing, you will need to carefully logroll him to a supine position, while supporting and protecting the cervical spine, in order to initiate cardiopulmonary resuscitation. If the athlete is unconscious, treat him as if he had a spinal cord injury.

### Secondary Survey

If the primary survey is cleared and the athlete conscious, place a reassuring hand on his shoulder to keep him calm, quiet, and still and to help him to focus on your immediate questions. When a cervical injury is suspected, the athlete should be evaluated in the position that he is lying in, and an assistant should immediately stabilize his head while you assess his condition. Until you have made your assessment and proven otherwise, you must assume that the athlete has suffered a spinal cord injury.

Before the athlete is moved, it is crucial to know whether he has any neck pain or is experiencing any numbness, burning, or tingling in any extremity. Is he having any difficulty moving his extremities? Is he having any difficulty breathing or swallowing? A quick sensory test for light touch over the hands and lower legs, with comparisons of right and left sides, can confirm any suspicions. Areas to test on the hand are over the lateral thumb for C6, over the middle finger for C7, and over the little finger for C8. In the lower extremity, light touch tests can be performed over the distal anterior thigh for L3, over the anteromedial lower leg for L4, over the lateral lower leg for L5, and over the posterolateral lower leg for S1. If any of these signs are positive, you must assume a serious neck injury. Figure 3.11 shows the full sensory distribution pattern for the cervical spine and the brachial plexus.

If all tests to this point are negative and the athlete has only neck pain, check for tenderness and deformity in the cervical region and perform a quick muscle test for strength and function. Ask the athlete to squeeze your hands, and look for good and equal strength left to right. Can she dorsiflex the ankle against manual resistance equally left to right? Again, if these tests are positive, serious neck injury is assumed.

If all findings so far are negative, have the athlete demonstrate slow, active cervical range of motion. It sometimes happens that the athlete has no pain as long as she lies quietly but that once she moves, pain will appear. If the athlete is unwilling to

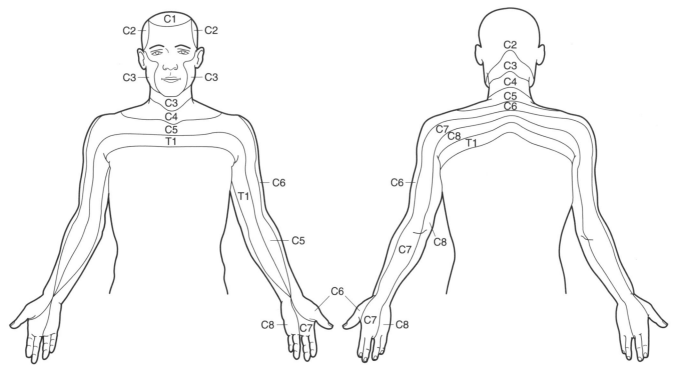

■ **Figure 3.11**   Sensory distribution for the cervical spine and the brachial plexus (C1-T1).

## Checklist for On-Field Assessment of Cervical and Upper Thoracic Spine

### Primary Survey

As you approach,

✓ check surroundings and environment,

✓ gain history of event from bystanders if you did not witness, and

✓ note position of head and neck.

Do necessary checks:

✓ Consciousness

✓ Airway, breathing, and circulation

✓ Severe bleeding

### Secondary Survey (Evaluate in the Position Found)

If athlete is unconscious, manage as a serious spinal injury. If conscious, assess the following:

✓ Presence of neck pain

✓ Sensations of numbness, tingling, or burning

✓ Difficulty with breathing

✓ Difficulty in moving extremities

If any of the above are positive, assume serious spine injury. If neck pain only

✓ palpate for tenderness and deformity and check for grip and dorsiflexion strength.

If signs are positive, assume serious neck injury. If signs listed are negative

✓ assess slow active range of motion of cervical spine and assess for sensory changes with motion

If positive, assume serious neck injury. If negative, move to sideline for further assessment. Throughout primary survey and secondary surveys

✓ continue to monitor vitals and continue to check sensory and motor function in extremities.

move, if neck pain is increased, or if there are sensory changes, your evaluation ceases and serious neck injury is assumed.

If at any time in your evaluation a serious neck injury is assumed, no further evaluation is necessary; emergency medical services (EMS) should be notified, and the athlete should be properly stabilized and secured to a spine

!  If at any time in your evaluation a serious neck injury is suspected, do not proceed with evaluation; notify EMS at once, and see that the athlete is properly stabilized and secured to a spine board for transportation.

board for transportation. Even if the symptoms appear minor (i.e., the athlete has only minimal sensation or strength deficits), you must follow procedures for a serious spine injury. In other words, any positive test should be regarded as indicative of a possible spinal cord injury, and the athlete should be transported accordingly. Before EMS arrives, it is important to monitor vital signs and use a reassuring voice to help keep the athlete calm during the waiting period and during transport.

For further discussion of transportation procedures for a serious spine injury, refer to *Introduction to Athletic Training* (Hillman 2000), chapter 8.

## SIDELINE ASSESSMENT

Only if the on-field assessment is negative (i.e., sensory, motor, palpation, cervical motion, strength) can the athlete leave the field under his own power for further assessment on the sideline.

### History

Once the athlete comes off the field, it is important to obtain a thorough history. Appropriate questions can determine the mechanism, symptoms, location of the involved tissue, and severity of the injury. You can sometimes judge from the history—even before performing an objective assessment—whether or not a referral to a physician is necessary. Can the athlete describe the mechanism of injury? Did he hear any noises at the time of injury? Where was the pain at the time of injury, and has it changed? Have the athlete describe the pain in terms of type and intensity using the 10-point scale. Does the athlete have any unusual sensations now? Does he have any dizziness or light-headedness? Has he had any prior injury to the area? Does he have a headache?

Headaches can originate from the cervical spine or may result from an associated head injury if the mechanism involved contact with the head. The athletic trainer should suspect a neck-related headache if the area of pain is in the suboccipital region at the base of the neck, if neck motion changes the headache pain, or if the athlete reports sensory changes in the suboccipital area. Cervical muscle-related headaches can also create symptoms in the occipital area, temporal area, and frontal area of the head. Occasionally eye pain, ear pain, or jaw pain is related to cervical muscle dysfunction. It is important to differentiate these symptoms from those caused by a head injury (see chapter 11).

### Observation

In your observation, note how the athlete holds her head and whether it is in good posture and alignment. Is there a normal concave curve of the cervical spine, or is it flattened from muscle spasm? Note how the athlete moves her head. Are movements slow or guarded, or are they normal and without apparent hesitation? Does the athlete move her head freely, and is she able to look side to side by turning her head rather than her body (rotating the trunk rather than the neck is an indication of pain and muscle guarding)? Does she move her arms and legs normally, or is any guarding or weakness noticeable? Is the gait normal? Is the athlete able to sit, stand, and move normally?

## Palpation

Sideline palpation is a cursory palpation to determine the presence and intensity of muscle spasm. Pain referred to the head, base of the skull, and posterior scapular areas can be secondary to muscle spasm. Muscle spasm is palpated as a rigidity of the muscle, and the muscle in spasm exhibits tenderness to pressure. Muscle spasm can also be confirmed with a reduced active cervical range of motion. Palpated muscle spasm should receive immediate treatment of at least ice and rest with the athlete in supine. An in-depth palpation sequence for both soft tissue and bony structures is described for the off-field assessment.

*Intrathecal pressure is pressure within the spinal canal.*

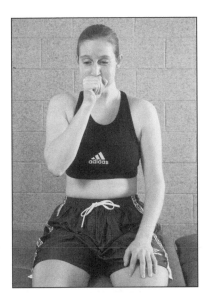

**Figure 3.12** Valsalva maneuver.

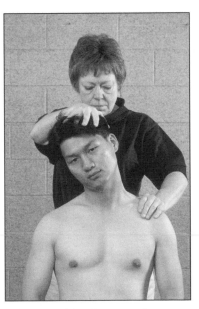

**Figure 3.13** Compression test with downward compression on the side of the head.

## Special Tests

If a positive result occurs with any of these tests, referral to a physician is indicated. If any test produces a positive sign, there is no need to continue testing.

### Valsalva Test

In a **Valsalva test**, the athlete holds her breath and bears down, or similarly blows into a closed fist (figure 3.12). These activities increase intrathecal pressure, so if the space has been reduced by swelling or a disc bulge, the increase in pressure will cause a radiation of symptoms down the distribution of the compromised nerve root.

### Compression Test

A compression test can be performed in various positions. In the first position, the athlete is sitting and the athletic trainer applies a downward compression force on the top of the head with the neck in a neutral position. If this test is negative, the athlete side-bends his head, and a downward compression force—not a lateral force—is applied as in the first test (figure 3.13). If this test is negative, the athlete can position his neck in extension and rotation to the side of complaints; a directly downward compression force as in the other tests is applied. This last test position is also known as **Spurling's test**. If the athlete reports symptoms down the arm of the cervical concavity with either position, a nerve root compression is indicated. In the neck, pain referred down the arm from nerve root compression is known as **cervical radiculitis**. If he reports pain or sensory changes on the convex side, the problem is probably muscle or soft tissue related. If he reports pain in the neck without radiation, the injury is probably related to soft tissue in the neck and is a negative test result.

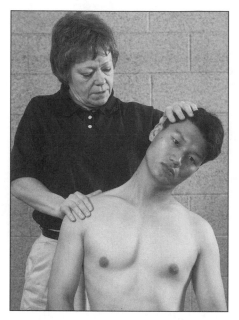

■ **Figure 3.14** Shoulder depression test.

## Shoulder Depression Test

If a brachial plexus stretch is suspected, perform the test to assess this injury with the athlete in sitting. The athlete's neck is laterally flexed to the shoulder opposite the side with symptoms, and a downward pressure is applied to the involved shoulder while a lateral pressure is applied to the head (figure 3.14). A positive sign (reproduction of the athlete's symptoms) will confirm a brachial plexus injury.

## Nerve Root Compression Relief Test

If a nerve root compression or disc injury is suspected, a relief test can be used to assess for these injuries. The athlete, seated, places the hand that is on the side of symptoms on top of her head (figure 3.15). In this position, the nerve root pressure is decreased as the traction caused by the weight of the hanging limb is reduced. A reduction in the athlete's symptoms is a positive sign for nerve root compression or disc injury. If the symptoms increase, they may be secondary to TOS.

## Cervical Distraction Relief Test

If the athlete complains of burning, tingling, numbness, or weakness into the upper extremity, a cervical distraction relief test will confirm suspicion of a nerve root compression injury. Place one hand at the base of the athlete's skull and the other under the chin with the athlete in sitting. Gradually apply an upward distraction force to the neck by slowly lifting the head (figure 3.16). A positive sign occurs if the symptoms subside. Nerve root pressure can be further reduced with a decrease in symptoms if the athlete is instructed to abduct the shoulder during the test.

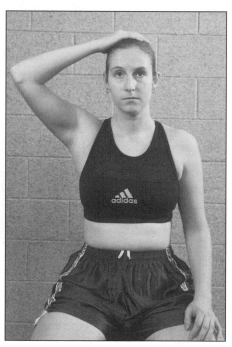

■ **Figure 3.15** Nerve root compression relief test.

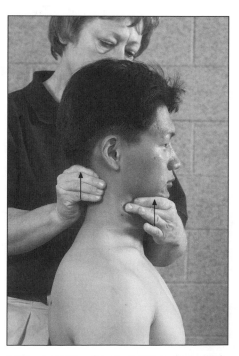

■ **Figure 3.16** Cervical distraction relief test.

### Range of Motion

Full active motion should be available in all cervical motions. As the athlete performs the motions, there should be no hesitation of movement. Watch for changes in the athlete's facial expressions for indications of pain or difficulty with the motion. Full cervical flexion allows the athlete's chin to touch the chest (figure 3.17a); extension will produce a head position such that the eyes point straight to the ceiling, or will produce a straight vertical line from the chin down the throat (figure 3.17b); lateral flexion should create a 45° angle between a vertical line and a line through the nose and chin in both left and right end motions (figure 3.17c); and the athlete should be able to place the chin almost in line with the tip of the shoulder in rotation (figure 3.17d). Observe neck flexion and lateral flexion from the posterior view to observe the spine motion during these movements. These motions should create a roundness of the spine. If the spine appears flat in any portion, there may be either facet blockage or muscle spasm restrictions.

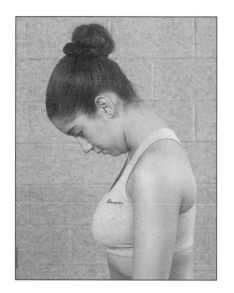

a

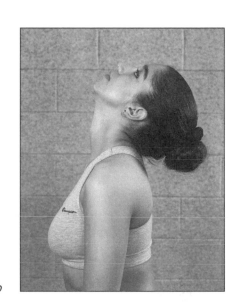

b

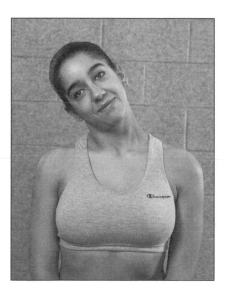

c

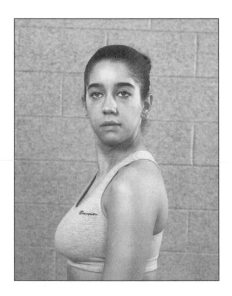

d

∎ **Figure 3.17** Cervical range of motion: (a) flexion, (b) extension, (c) lateral flexion, and (d) rotation.

If the athlete complains of pain or sensation changes in the neck or extremities with active motion, passive overpressure motions should not be performed.

Passive motion tests can be performed either after the athlete has completed all active motions or after each active motion test. The aim in passive overpressure motion tests is to attempt to reproduce the athlete's pain. Passive **overpressure** motion is applied gently on the head to move the neck in the desired direction. The motion is not quick or severe but controlled, slow, and gentle until an end point is felt. However, if the athlete complains either of pain in the neck or of pain or sensation changes in the extremities with active motion, passive overpressure motions should not be performed. Likewise, if you suspect that the cervical spine itself may have an injury such as a fracture or subluxation or may be unstable, do not perform passive overpressure motion tests.

### Strength

Isometric strength tests are performed against cervical flexion, extension, lateral flexion, and rotation with resistance provided at the head. To test flexion, the resistive hand is placed on the forehead. To test extension, the resistive hand is placed on the posterior head. For lateral flexion it is placed on the side of the head with the stabilizing hand on the same-side shoulder. (The hands are placed on the sides of the forehead, not the jaw, since resistance at the jaw can aggravate any temporomandibular joint dysfunction the athlete may have.) To test rotation strength, use both hands to provide the resistance. With each test position, stabilize the athlete's upper trunk by placing a hand on the shoulder. You can perform these motions in a midrange position. Use a slow buildup of force until a maximum resistance is created; also release the force slowly. Be sure to tell the athlete what to expect before executing each movement.

### Neurological Examination

Once you have conducted a gross examination of range of motion and strength, you will perform specific neurological tests for dermatome, myotome, and reflex parameters if the athlete reports any sensory disturbances or weakness distal to the acromion. If the athlete reports no numbness, tingling, burning, or weakness distal to the acromion, a neurological assessment is not necessary.

#### Sensory Assessment

**Dermatome** distributions of the cervical spine are shown in figure 3.11 and described in chapter 2, table 2.2. Test for light touch in one of two ways: either lightly graze the skin over the innervated surface and compare right to left for quality of sensation, or use a pin to perform a pinprick test for sharp discrimination. These tests assess abnormalities in sensory perception.

#### Motor Assessment

Myotome assessment is performed using specific muscle strength tests of muscles that are innervated by the cervical nerves. The muscle is placed in a midposition, and the athlete is instructed to work against the athletic trainer's resistance to movement. C1-2 nerve root innervates the neck flexor muscles (figure 3.18a); C3 innervates lateral cervical flexor muscles (figure 3.18b); C4 innervates the muscles that shrug the shoulders (figure 3.18c); C5 innervates shoulder abductors (figure 3.18d); C6 innervates elbow flexors (figure 3.18e) and wrist extensors; C7 innervates elbow extensors (figure 3.18f) and wrist flexors; C8 innervates thumb extensors and wrist ulnar deviators (figure 3.18g); and T1 innervates hand intrinsic muscles (i.e., finger abduction) (figure 3.18h).

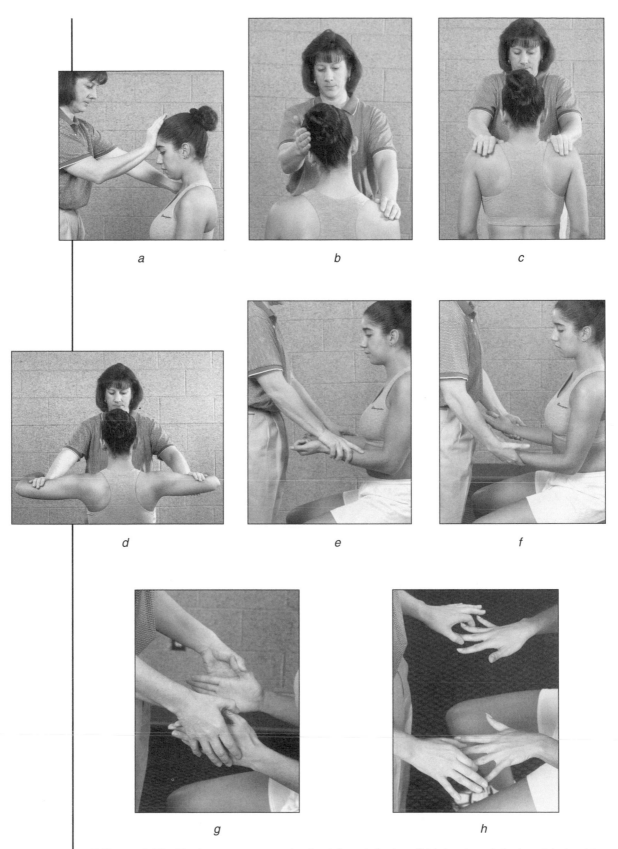

**Figure 3.18** Myotome assessment using (a) neck flexion, (b) lateral neck flexion, (c) shoulder shrug, (d) shoulder abduction, (e) elbow flexion, (f) elbow extension, (g) thumb extension, and (h) finger abduction.

## Reflex Assessment

Perform reflex assessment using a reflex hammer to test biceps (figure 3.19a), brachioradialis (figure 3.19b), and triceps (figure 3.19c) reflexes. Conduct a **clonus test** for the lower extremities by applying a sudden dorsiflexion force to the ankle. A positive result occurs if the motion results in several rapid contractions of the ankle plantarflexors so the foot twitches from plantar flexion to dorsiflexion. A positive result indicates an upper motor neuron injury.

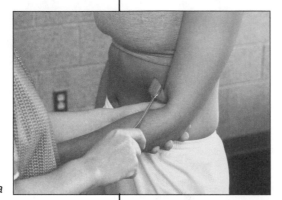
a

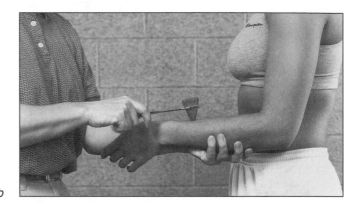
b

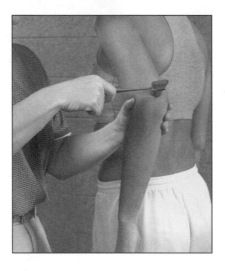
c

∎ **Figure 3.19**   Reflex assessment of the (a) biceps, (b) brachioradialis, and (c) triceps.

### *Functional Tests*

Only if all previous tests are negative should the athlete undergo functional tests to determine physical and psychological readiness to return to participation.

These functional tests should include some basic tests and some sport-specific assessments. A basic test might include a functional sensory assessment such as having the athlete tie her shoe with her eyes closed. This requires adequate sensory feedback from the fingers and also tests balance if the athlete is in a standing position with the foot up on a bench or chair.

Sport-specific functional activities are skill execution drills that mimic the athlete's sport. A drill may involve agility, coordination, power, and flexibility from the extremity (upper, lower, or both), depending on the athlete's sport and position within the sport. Observe for flow of movement without hesitation, coordination and agility during the execution, and demonstration of adequate flexibility, movement, and strength throughout the drill. It is important in functional assessment of cervical injuries to observe carefully whether the athlete moves the head easily and naturally in all directions without guarding.

## Checklist for Sideline Assessment of Cervical and Upper Thoracic Spine

### History
✓ Mechanism of injury
✓ Unusual sensations at time of injury and currently
✓ Location, quality, and intensity of pain
✓ Symptoms of headache, dizziness, or light-headedness
✓ Previous injury

### Observation
✓ Presence of cervical lordosis
✓ Observable spasm, swelling, discoloration
✓ Bilateral assymetry
✓ Evidence of pain or restricted movement
✓ Position of head

### Palpation
✓ Evidence of body tenderness
✓ Evidence of muscle tenderness, spasm, trigger point
✓ Bilateral comparison

### Special Tests
✓ Valsalva test
✓ Compression test
✓ Shoulder depression test
✓ Nerve root compression relief test
✓ Cervical distraction test

### Range of Motion
✓ Active range of motion
  ✓ Flexion, extension, rotation, and lateral flexion
✓ Passive range of motion
  ✓ Flexion, extension, rotation, and lateral flexion

### Strength Tests
✓ Flexion, extension, rotation, and lateral flexion

### Neurological Tests
✓ Dermatome
✓ Myotome
✓ Reflex

### Functional Tests

## OFF-FIELD ASSESSMENT

It is common for an athlete to have a cervical injury but to have no complaints at the time it occurs, especially if it involves cervical muscles or ligaments. In these cases, however, muscle spasm and other symptoms will often surface later. In a typical example, a football receiver is tackled from the side as he makes a sudden cut into the unseen opponent. As he falls to the ground the opponent's impact forces him in one direction, but his momentum continues to move his neck in the opposite direction and causes a cervical whiplash. The athlete feels a brief pain in the side of his posterior neck, but it is not enough to interrupt his participation. His neck may feel slightly stiff after the game, but he thinks little of it and continues in his normal daily activities. The next morning, his neck is stiff, painful, and difficult to move because muscle spasm has become predominant.

When this athlete enters the athletic injury treatment facility, a complete evaluation is warranted. The athlete may be able to recall the injury in yesterday's game, but he may or may not be able to identify any additional factors since the occurrence of the injury that may have also contributed to the condition. There also may be other preexisting factors that can add to the problem (e.g., previous unresolved injury) or additional problems that may have developed secondary to the injury and to the subsequent lack of treatment.

The off-field assessment is more complex than the sideline assessment for several reasons: there are more potential conditions to consider; there are complications that occur with untreated symptoms; and masking of original symptoms and over-riding of new symptoms occur after the injury incident. The athlete may present with an acute injury or an injury caused from repetitive stress. Causes and effective treatment of repetitive stress injuries can be more difficult to identify and more frustrating to resolve. Acute injuries that are not immediately treated usually develop additional symptoms, and the severity of the symptoms increases. This can change the injury's profile and can complicate assessment. As an athletic trainer you must be aware of additional possible injuries and changes in the symptoms of acute injuries, and you must make an accurate and total assessment so these potential problems are not overlooked. To ensure adequate treatment, you must both take a careful history and attempt to reproduce the athlete's symptoms using objective tests to clearly identify the injury's SINS (**S**everity, **I**rritability, **N**ature, and **S**tage).

## History

If the athlete is able to recall the injury specifically, ask for the details related to the occurrence. The mechanism of injury, sensations experienced in the neck and surrounding area at the time of injury, postinjury activity, and previous injuries are all important factors to be gleaned from the athlete. The history should identify the location of the athlete's pain and/or symptoms. Is there any radiation of the pain, or is it localized? What kind of sensation is it? A sensation of burning, stinging, tingling, or heaviness may indicate a nerve-related problem. An ache or sharp pain may indicate a muscle, joint, or ligament injury. Does the pain increase with coughing, laughing, or sneezing? These activities increase intrathecal pressure and can be signs for disc dysfunctions. Does the pain change with activity or time of day? What activities aggravate the symptoms, and what activities ease them? Does the athlete have headaches, tinnitus, or blurry vision? These signs can indicate either a cranial nerve injury that affects the sympathetic system or myofascial referred pain. Does the pain awaken the athlete, and does he have difficulty returning to sleep? Sleep disturbances with difficulty returning to sleep are an indication of an irritable injury. What position does the athlete sleep in? Prone sleeping is very stressful on a neck, especially an injured neck. How many pillows does the athlete use? More than one pillow under the head can increase cervical curvature and maintain a poor cervical alignment to add to the cervical stress. As with other injuries, the athlete's pain profile will provide insight into the intensity, irritability, and possible tissue involved. If the athlete is unable to identify when, how, or why his symptoms started, a good history can also point to the stage of the injury: is it acute, subacute, or chronic?

*Tinnitus refers to a sensation of ringing or similar noise in the ear.*

If the athlete complains of pain or sensory changes distal to the acromion process, a neurological examination is warranted, since the changes may result from nerve root compression or injury. If the pain is severe, ranked 7 or higher on a 10-point scale, the injury may be easily irritated, so an abbreviated evaluation may be warranted. If the athlete indicates the pain to be less than 7, it is permissible to use a more aggressive assessment. If you detect neurological changes (sensory, motor, or reflex), you should refer the athlete to a physician.

## Observation

Throughout the history-taking process, note the athlete's movements and watch for hesitation in cervical or extremity movement, incomplete motions, restricted motions in one or more directions, and grimacing or facial expression changes with movements; also note whether or not the athlete must change positions frequently and seems unable to find a comfortable position. Watching the athlete remove his sweatshirt or shirt will also indicate how guarded and painful his movements are.

*Lordosis is a curvature of the spine characterized by an excessive anterior convexity.*

Observe the athlete's posture. Some cervical lordosis is normal, but excessive lordosis or a flat cervical spine can indicate either generally poor cervical posture or muscle spasm. In normal cervical posture, the earlobe is in alignment with the acromion process from a lateral view, and the nose is in line with the manubrium and xiphoid process of the sternum from a frontal view. A forward head position with the earlobe anterior to the acromion process is frequently combined with rounded shoulders and can indicate either poor posture, muscle spasm, or pain that restricts the athlete's normal posture. Head tilt to one side can indicate pain or spasm. Reduced mobility or guarded movements are also possible signs of muscle spasm, pain restricting movement, or both. If the athlete supports an upper extremity, there may be a nerve root irritation that is aggravated if the arm is allowed to hang at the side normally.

### Differential Diagnosis

There are many common referral patterns that both emanate from and centralize into the cervical area. Whenever an athlete presents in the treatment facility with cervical complaints, other possible sources of pain must be eliminated. This is especially true if the athlete reports symptoms distal to the acromion process. Other causes that you must eliminate include nerve root lesions, disc injuries, brachial plexus lesions, peripheral nerve injuries, upper extremity joint or muscle injuries, and myofascial irritations. Special tests for these injuries are discussed in the special test and palpation subsections later in the chapter.

### Range of Motion

As discussed in relation to the sideline assessment, range of motion of the cervical spine is tested in all planes with the athlete in sitting. The quantity and quality of cervical movement should be assessed, as well as the presence or absence of a capsular pattern or movement. The **capsular pattern** for the cervical spine is equal limitation of lateral flexion and rotation, with less restriction into extension. Active motion should be performed slowly and smoothly through a full range of motion; note changes in the athlete's facial expressions to indicate pain or difficulty with the cervical movement.

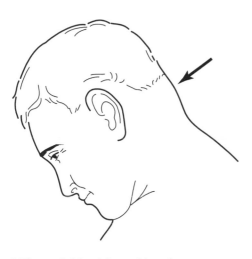

If the athlete experiences no pain with the active movement, each active motion is followed by a gentle, yet full-motion passive movement that the athletic trainer produces. For example, after the athlete moves his neck into full flexion, ask whether the motion causes pain. If the answer is no, apply an additional force to the top of the head to move the neck into additional flexion. Ask whether pain occurs with this movement while you assess the end feel of the motion. Before applying passive motion, observe whether a bulge occurs in the upper posterior spine during cervical flexion. If it does, you should not apply passive overpressure, since this is a sign for a possible atlas subluxation (figure 3.20). In this case you should refer the athlete to the physician without additional examination.

**Figure 3.20**    Atlas subluxation.

Figure 3.17, a-d, demonstrates normal full range of cervical motion. After each active cervical motion, apply a passive overpressure and ask whether the motion reproduced the athlete's pain. If all positions with overpressure are negative, then place the head into a **quadrant position** with the neck in end-range extension, rotation, and side-bending to the same side as the symptoms; then apply an overpressure force to the head in this position. If the athlete reports pain either in the neck or into the upper extremity, these are positive signs and an indication of either a facet syndrome or a nerve root pathology.

### Strength

Test cervical muscle strength with the athlete reclined and the muscle working against gravity for each cervical movement. The trunk is stabilized with the athlete lying on the examination table. With the athlete supine, neck flexion is resisted; lateral flexion is tested in side-lying; and cervical extension is tested with the athlete prone and her head over the end of the table. It is important that the neck begin in good alignment. For example, to test cervical extension, the athlete first places her head in proper posture alignment (i.e., without a forward head or excessive lordosis) and then moves the neck into extension against manual resistance. The resistance is gradually built up to a maximum with the neck in proper alignment and in a midrange position for each motion tested.

Scapular elevation and retraction movements are manually resisted to assess the upper and middle trapezius.

Because of the possibility of injury with machine resistance, isokinetics and other instrumented strength evaluations are not usually used for cervical strength testing, and manual muscle tests are the assessment of choice.

### Neurological Tests

If the athlete reports symptoms distal to the acromion, neurological tests are indicated. Sensory, motor, and reflex tests are performed to eliminate neural injury as the cause of peripheral symptoms. If these tests are negative, the tissue involved is probably not neural; but if any of these tests is positive, neural structures are probably involved. Remember, not all neurological tests need to be positive to indicate pathology. Except in severe or prolonged cases, it is not usual for all three types of neurological tests to be positive at the same time, and sensory deficits are often noted before motor deficits.

Sensory tests include light touch and pinprick. Other sensory tests are for temperature, deep pressure, and pain, but most often light touch or pinprick is used.

### Sensory Test Points

Figure 3.11 demonstrates the dermatome distribution for the brachial plexus (see also chapter 2, table 2.2). Although it is important to remember that sensory distribution patterns can vary from one person to another, each area outlined in the figure can be used as a guideline for sensory testing. Compare sensation from left to right. If the athlete reports a difference between the two sides, more detailed neurological investigation and referral to a physician is indicated.

### Myotome Sensory Test Points

Myotome tests can be quickly and efficiently performed with the athlete in sitting. Moving from proximal to distal innervation, myotome tests for the cervical nerves include the resisted muscle tests that were described for the sideline assessment. These tests are illustrated in figure 3.18.

### Special Tests

Since an injury evaluated in the athletic injury treatment facility may have originated from other factors in addition to the acute injury mechanism, special tests besides those used in the sideline assessment will be necessary for differential diagnosis to rule out other types of injuries. The athletic trainer will have narrowed the possibilities through the history and objective criteria used thus far, so not all tests will be necessary.

Tests mentioned in connection with the sideline assessment may also be indicated in the off-field assessment (refer to the special test section of the sideline assessment). These include the Valsalva test, compression tests, shoulder depression test, nerve root compression relief test, and cervical distraction relief test. In addition to these tests, tests for neuropathy may be included in the off-field examination.

#### Special Tests for Neuropathy

If the athlete reports "nerve pain," brachial plexus neuropathy tests are indicated. Nerve pain is any pain symptom that is likely to be caused by nerve irritation, and presents as complaints of numbness, tingling, burning, or shooting. Nerve pain is usually constant or persistent, with few episodes of relief.

Indications of a positive nerve tension test are a difference in symptoms between the right and the left, reproduction of the symptoms with a test, or a change in the symptoms with a test. Since other soft tissue structures are stretched along with the

Remember, the objective of the special tests is to reproduce the athlete's symptoms during the evaluation. Tests that reproduce the athlete's symptoms are positive. Positive tests will provide answers regarding type of injury and tissue involved and will indicate whether or not referral to a physician is necessary.

nerve, it is not uncommon for the athlete to complain of a stretch sensation or ache in the anterior shoulder, cubital fossa, wrist, or forearm with the stretch application. Since the nerve is placed on stretch, sometimes a normal response will be a tingling sensation in the fingers; but this is different from the symptomatic results of a positive test and is usually noted bilaterally.

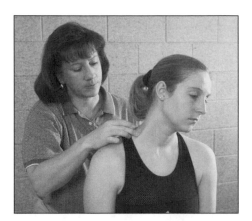

**■ Figure 3.21** Tinel's sign test.

## Tinel's Sign

Pain or radiation of symptoms reproduced with nerve percussion (**Tinel's sign**) indicates the presence of pathology in the brachial plexus. To perform the test, have the athlete in a seated position with the neck slightly flexed. Then use a finger to tap each nerve root at the transverse processes (figure 3.21).

## Passive Upper Limb Tension Tests

Neuropathy tests also include upper limb tension tests. Various limb positions are used to place each nerve of the brachial plexus on stretch. Although the position also stretches other soft tissue, symptoms elicited will indicate the tissue affected. If the athlete reports an increase in symptoms since their onset or if the injury is very acute, these tests are contraindicated because they can aggravate the condition.

The athlete is in supine for these tests, with the shoulder at the edge of the examination table. Passively depress the athlete's shoulder girdle for each test by placing your hand on the top of the shoulder and pulling caudally. Test the median, ulnar, and radial nerves by passively placing the elbow, wrist, and hand in different positions to place the nerve on its bias, or stretch:

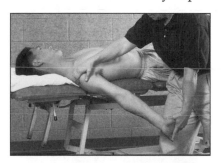

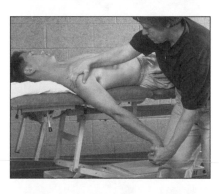

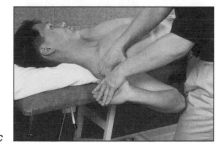

**■ Figure 3.22** Nerve bias tests of the (a) median nerve, (b) radial nerve, and (c) ulnar nerve.

- **To place the median nerve on bias**, the shoulder is in slight abduction, external rotation, and full extension; the elbow is in full extension; the wrist is in extension; and the fingers are placed in extension (figure 3.22a).

- **To place the radial nerve on bias**, the shoulder is placed in slight abduction, internal rotation, and extension; the elbow is in full extension; the wrist is in flexion and ulnar deviation; and the fingers are in flexion (figure 3.22b).

- **To place the ulnar nerve on bias**, the shoulder is placed in abduction and external rotation; the elbow is in flexion; the wrist is in extension and radial deviation; and the fingers are in extension (figure 3.22c).

Once each nerve bias test is completed and the athlete reports minimal or no symptoms, ask him to laterally flex his head to the opposite side. Apply each joint position one at a time for each nerve bias, each time asking the athlete if any symptoms are reproduced. There is no need to continue the nerve bias test if positive results occur at any time during the test.

### Active Upper Limb Tension Tests

These nerve tension tests can also be performed actively as a quick assessment prior to the passive bias tension tests:

- **For the ulnar nerve.** With the athlete in sitting, the athlete abducts the shoulder and places his hand behind his head with the shoulder in full external rotation. The elbow is kept behind the body's midline (figure 3.23a).

- **For the median nerve.** The athlete places the arm in 90° abduction with the elbow in full extension. The shoulder is then fully externally rotated and moved posteriorly into horizontal extension (figure 3.23b).

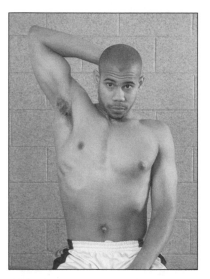
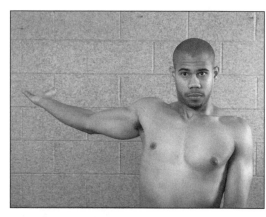

*a*          *b*

**∎ Figure 3.23**   Correct position for the (a) active ulnar nerve tension test and the (b) active median nerve tension test.

### Special Tests for Vascular Compromise

### Vertebral Artery Test

The aim of the vertebral artery test is to evaluate compression of the vertebral artery. Perform it with the athlete in sitting or supine. Passively move the athlete's head into extension and lateral flexion, and then rotate it to the same side (figure 3.24). This position is held for 30 s. The test is positive if the athlete reports dizziness or if nystagmus occurs. **Nystagmus** is an involuntary lateral oscillatory movement of the eyes.

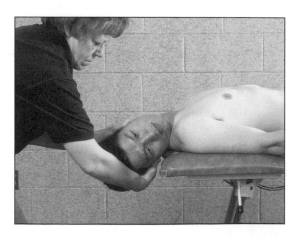

**∎ Figure 3.24**   Vertebral artery test.

### Thoracic Outlet Tests

Tests for TOS are explained in chapter 4. Thoracic outlet syndrome can result from neck or shoulder pathology. Thoracic outlet tests should be performed during both shoulder and cervical examinations.

### Palpation

Palpation is best performed with the athlete supine for enhanced relaxation of supporting muscles. If the athlete is uncomfortable in this position, you can perform palpation either prone, with the athlete on a table that has a face hole, or with the athlete sitting and leaning forward with her head and arms supported on a structure of appropriate height. Palpation begins superficially with notation of any restricted movement of skin and fascia and proceeds from superficial muscles to deep muscles. A systematic approach is the best method to avoid omitting any muscle. Palpation can begin in the superior posterior neck at the occiput and move distally to the upper thoracic region. The lateral neck and then the anterior neck are systematically assessed from a superior to an inferior approach.

The spinous processes can be palpated posteriorly. C2, C6, C7, and the upper thoracic spinous process are usually easily palpated; but C3, C4, and C5 usually lie more anterior and can be difficult to differentiate. The spinous processes are palpated for point tenderness. The base of the occiput and ligamentum nuchae are also palpated for tenderness and restriction. The upper trapezius, levator scapulae, spleni group, and paraspinal muscles are all palpated for areas of tenderness, soft tissue restriction, trigger points, and muscle spasm.

Palpation of lateral structures includes lateral fibers of the upper trapezius and sternocleidomastoid muscles. The C1 transverse processes can be palpated slightly inferiorly and laterally from the mastoid process behind the ear. These are slight nubs and are commonly tender; but when palpated, the right and left transverse processes should feel balanced, with the same degree of protrusion and tenderness on each side.

Anterior structures to palpate are the distal insertion of the sternocleidomastoid, scalenes, first rib, and carotid artery. The scalenes are often tender to palpation in persons with a forward head posture. These muscles lie lateral to the sternocleidomastoid and superior to the clavicle.

For more information on locating the sternocleidomastoid and scalene muscles and assessing trigger points through therapeutic exercises, refer to *Therapeutic Exercise for Athletic Injuries* (Houglum 2000), chapter 16.

*Trigger points are a focal hyperirritable area in the muscle or fascia that develops due to compensatory overload and overuse. They will result in referred symptoms of pain, particularly when pressure is applied.*

Cervical muscles in spasm or with active trigger points can refer pain into other areas such as the head, base of the skull, and posterior scapular areas, thus mimicking nerve pain. Figure 3.25 illustrates some of the more common referral patterns of cervical muscles. In the presence of referred pain symptoms, the athletic trainer must investigate to determine whether the pain is secondary to neural or muscular dysfunctions. A precise evaluation can help determine the injury source. If palpation of muscle structures reproduces the athlete's pain, it is likely that the pain is soft tissue related. If, however, the pain is reproduced by some of the special tests discussed previously, the pain is neurological in origin.

### Functional Tests

Functional tests were discussed in connection with the sideline assessment. If the athlete complains that any daily or sport-related activities are difficult because of the injury, assessment of the athlete's performance is in order. If previous assessment tests were positive, functional tests are deferred. Functional tests should be a part of the final assessment, however, before the athlete is allowed to resume full sport participation.

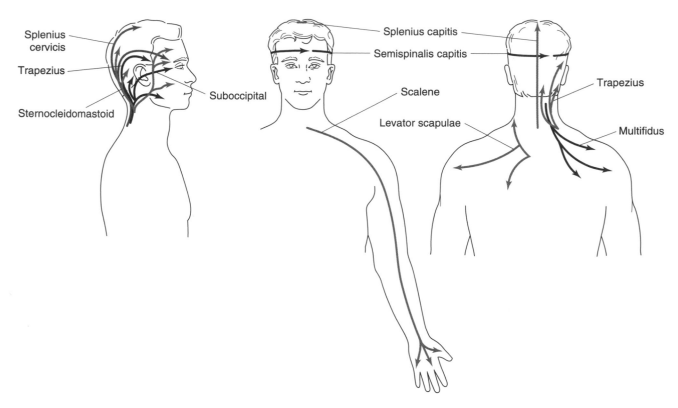

**Figure 3.25** Common referral patterns of cervical muscles.

Specific functional tests are dependent upon the athlete's specific sport and position within the sport. Since the cervical and upper thoracic spine can impact both upper and lower extremities, the athlete should perform functional tests for all extremities. These might be specific running, jumping, and agility drills for the lower extremities or throwing, dribbling, and other coordination activities for the upper extremities.

## Checklist for Off-Field Assessment of Cervical and Upper Thoracic Spine

### History

✓ Mechanism of injury
✓ Unusual sounds or sensations?
✓ Previous injury
✓ Type and location of pain
✓ Numbness and tingling
✓ Chief complaint

If chronic, ascertain:

✓ Aggravating and easing factors
✓ Onset and duration of symptoms
✓ Effects of time of day on symptoms

### Observation

✓ Posture
✓ Restriction, guarding, or hesitation in movement

✓ Facial expressions
✓ Visible swelling, discoloration, spasm, assymetry

### Differential Diagnosis

Refer to palpation procedures and special tests listed below.

### Range of Motion

✓ Active ROM: cervical flexion, extension, lateral flexion, and rotation and shoulder motions
✓ Passive ROM: end-range cervical flexion, extension, lateral flexion, and rotation
✓ Shoulder motion as appropriate

### Strength

✓ Manual resistance to cervical flexion, extension, lateral flexion, and rotation

**Neurological Tests**

✓ Dermatome (C5-T1)
✓ Myotome (C5-T1)
✓ Reflex (biceps, brachioradialis, triceps)

**Special Tests**

✓ Valsalva test
✓ Compression test
✓ Shoulder depression test
✓ Nerve root compression relief test
✓ Tinel's sign
✓ Upper limb tension tests
✓ Vertebral artery test
✓ TOS test

**Palpation**

✓ Soft tissue mobility
✓ Cervical and upper thoracic spinous process
✓ Transverse processes
✓ Posterior, lateral, and anterior cervical and upper back muscles

**Functional Tests**

Check for normal unrestricted movement with

✓ Sport-specific activity
✓ Overhead and upper-extremity movements
✓ Balance and coordination lower-extremity drills

# SUMMARY

1. *Identify the causes of cervical strain.*

   Cervical strains, which are common in physically active persons, can result from both acute trauma and chronic stresses. Acute causes are sudden mechanical overload and/or violent overstretching into rotation, flexion, or extension (i.e., whiplash). Chronic overuse, postural faults, and poor mechanics can be precipitating factors that can make the cervical spine susceptible to acute strains. Signs and symptoms will include muscular pain and spasm, tenderness, and decreased range of motion.

2. *Identify the different types of fractures in the cervical spine and the potential for spinal cord injury associated with each.*

   Fractures in the cervical spine can result from hyperflexion, hyperextension, and axial loading mechanisms. The primary cause of cervical fractures resulting in catastrophic spinal cord trauma is headfirst contact with or without the spine flexed, resulting in axial loading and buckling of the cervical spine. Compression fractures, burst fractures, fracture dislocations, and facet dislocations are the most serious spinal fractures and have a high probability for spinal cord involvement. Contact to the back of the head and face can also result in avulsion fractures of the spinous processes, but these rarely have associated neurological pathology.

3. *Discuss the various causes of neuropathy in the upper extremity relative to cervical spine pathology.*

   Neurological symptoms into the upper extremity can have as their cause a variety of mechanisms resulting in either tractioning or compression of the spinal cord and nerve roots. Spinal cord compression, caused by acute fractures and dislocations as well as by severe degenerative conditions (stenosis), can result in bilateral neurological symptoms. Nerve root compression—causing radiating symptoms, sensory impairment, and motor weakness into one extremity—can result from brachial plexus stretch and compression mechanisms, thoracic outlet syndromes, degenerative disc disease, acute disc herniations, and osteophytes, leading to stenosis in the intervertebral foramen. These conditions can be differentiated by means of special tests to assess sensory, motor, and reflex responses, as well as tests for various compression syndromes.

4. *Conduct a neurological exam for the upper extremity, including sensory, motor, and reflex testing.*

   A neurological exam consists of sensory testing, motor testing, and reflex testing. Each nerve root exiting the cervical spine has a specific sensory, motor, and reflex distribution (table 2.2). Sensory testing typically involves the assessment of sensory acuity with light touch applied over the dermatome for each nerve root. Motor tests are performed with manual muscle testing of specific muscles that have a single nerve root as their primary innervation. Reflex testing of the biceps, brachioradialis, and triceps muscle will also provide information on the type and location of nerve pathology. Depending on the nerve pathology, one or all of these tests may be positive. An athlete with any positive neurological sign should be referred to a physician for further evaluation.

5. *Perform an on-field assessment for a suspected spinal cord injury and determine when a serious injury should be assumed.*

   Acute cervical injuries can be life threatening or can cause paralysis, so immediate on-field assessment must establish the severity of the injury, including whether or not possible spinal cord injury is present. A primary survey for level of consciousness, ABC (**A**irway, **B**reathing, **C**irculation) assessment, and body position is followed by tests for cervical spine pain, sensation impairment, motor weakness, and palpable defects to determine the nature of the injury and to ascertain whether a serious spine injury should be suspected. If any positive signs are present with these tests, EMS is called and the athlete is transported off the field with a spine board. See page 63 for an evaluation checklist.

6. *Perform a sideline assessment for the cervical spine region.*

   If emergency transportation is not warranted, a more complete assessment can take place on the sideline or in the athletic training room. This includes continued observation of the athlete's movements; a more detailed history of the injury; evaluation of range of motion, strength, and neurological parameters; and special tests. These special tests include the Valsalva test and compression test for disc or nerve root injury, shoulder depression test for brachial plexus stretch, and nerve root compression test and relief tests for nerve root injuries. Palpation of the cervical and upper thoracic areas should also be performed to determine specific areas of tenderness, muscle spasm, active trigger points, and soft tissue restriction. If the athlete has no positive results on any of these tests, a functional assessment is performed to determine the ability to return to sport activities. See page 71 for an evaluation checklist.

7. *Perform an off-field evaluation for the cervical spine region.*

   When the athlete enters the sport injury treatment facility with complaints about a neck injury or neck pain, assessment must be more complete since there are additional possibilities for causes and types of injuries. There can also be other injuries that must be eliminated through differential diagnosis. Additional objective assessment tools include evaluation of active and passive range of motion, strength, neurological parameters if symptoms are present distal to the acromion process, and special tests that include those performed in the sideline assessment as well as others. The additional special tests include those for cervical neuropathy (Tinel's sign, upper limb tension tests), vertebral artery test, and tests for TOS. Palpation then determines the precise location of pain and assesses bony and soft tissue structures. Functional tests are not commonly performed when the athlete is initially assessed, but they are necessary prior to the athlete's return to normal sport participation. See pages 78-79 for an evaluation checklist.

# REVIEW QUESTIONS

1. What are the dangers associated with "spearing" in football?

2. Describe some of the degenerative changes that can occur in the cervical spine and the symptoms and potential complications they may cause over time.

3. What is TOS? Describe the etiology and signs and symptoms associated with this injury. What other cervical spine conditions may result in similar symptoms?

4. In an on-field evaluation of a cervical spine injury, when can you determine that it is safe for the athlete to move and leave the field under his or her own power?

5. What is considered the normal posture and active range of motion of the cervical spine?

6. What are the contraindications to performing passive overpressures in the cervical spine?

7. Describe the special tests used in the off-field assessment to evaluate for nerve root compression.

8. Describe the special tests used in determining brachial plexus injury. What would a positive result for each of these tests indicate?

# CRITICAL THINKING QUESTIONS

1. Think back to the scenario at the beginning of the chapter. What injury did Doug likely have? Based on the location of his symptoms, what specific structures were likely involved? Finding that he was not being completely honest in reporting his pain, what specific tests did Jeff use to determine that Doug had weakness and sensory changes? If you were Jeff, how would you have gone about your evaluation, and what other tests would you have performed to rule out other related conditions?

2. A 35-year-old computer analyst comes into the clinic complaining of an increasing amount of pain and discomfort in her neck and some achiness into her left arm. She does not remember any specific injury but states that over the past six months she has often awakened in the morning with a "stiff neck" and has an increasing amount of discomfort at work when sitting at the computer for long periods of time. She also is an avid swimmer and weight lifter who spends 5 h a week in the gym. Given her chief complaint, how would you go about taking a history on this physically active individual? Given the type of work and training that she does, what are some questions you could ask and observations you could make to obtain some clues to possible overload stresses that may be causing her pain?

3. How might you differentiate between referred pain into the arm caused by a chronic muscle condition versus a nerve compression syndrome? In your evaluation, discuss some of the special tests you would use to make this determination.

# CITED REFERENCES

Marks, M.R., Bell, G.R., and Boumphrey, F.R. 1990. Cervical spine injuries and their neurologic implications. *Clin Sports Med* 9:263-278.

Torg, J.S., Naranja, R.J., Palov, H., Galinat, B.J., Warren, R., and Stine, R.A. 1996. The relationship of developmental narrowing of the cervical spinal canal to reversible and irreversible injury of the cervical spinal cord in football players. *J Bone Jt Surg* 78A:1308-1314.

Winkelstein, B.A., and Myers, B.S. 1997. The biomechanics of cervical spine injury and implications for injury prevention. *Med Sci Sports Exerc* 29:S246-255.

Wroble, R.R., and Albright, J.P. 1986. Neck and low back injuries in wrestling. *Clin Sports Med* 5:295-325.

# ADDITIONAL RESOURCES

Cantu, R.C. 1998. Neurologic athletic head and neck injuries. In *Clinics in sports medicine.* Philadelphia: Saunders, 210.

Durham, J.R., Yao, J.S., Pearce, W.H., Nuber, G.M., and McCarthy, W.J. 1995. Arterial injuries in the thoracic outlet syndrome. *J Vasc Surg* 21:57-69.

Hershman, E.B. 1990. Brachial plexus injuries. *Clin Sports Med* 9:311-329.

Hillman, S.K. 2000. *Introduction to athletic training.* Champaign, IL: Human Kinetics.

Houglum, P.A. 2000. *Therapeutic exercise for athletic injuries.* Champaign, IL: Human Kinetics.

Nichols, A.W. 1996. The thoracic outlet syndrome in athletes. *J Am Board Fam Prac* 9:246-55.

Spencer, C.W. 1986. Injuries to the spine. In *Clinics in sports medicine.* Philadelphia: Saunders, 410.

Torg, J.S. 1987. Head and neck injuries. In *Clinics in sports medicine.* Philadelphia: Saunders, 222.

# CHAPTER FOUR

# Shoulder and Arm

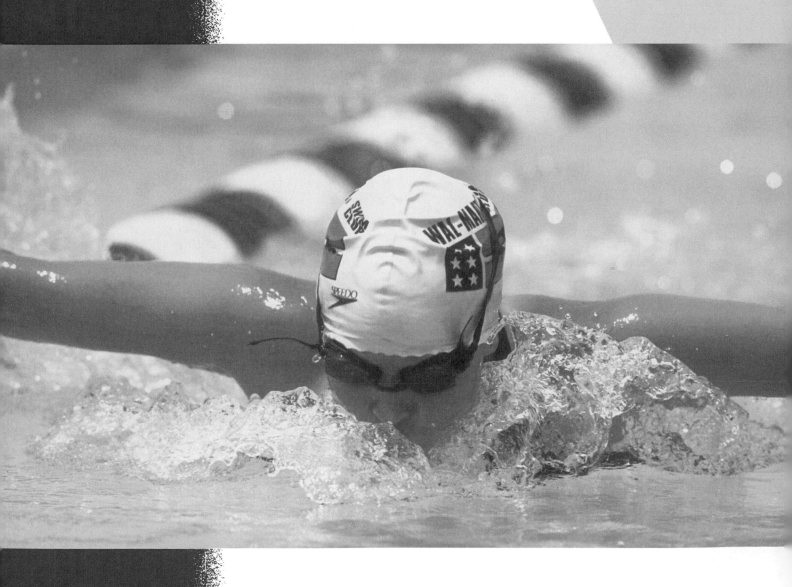

# OBJECTIVES

After completing this chapter, the reader will be able to do the following:

1. Discuss the types of overuse injuries that commonly result from repetitive overhead throwing activities

2. Identify the signs and symptoms associated with various stages of rotator cuff impingement

3. Demonstrate an on-field assessment for the shoulder and upper arm, and discuss criteria for immediate referral and mode of transportation from the field

4. Perform a thorough and sequential sideline assessment for the shoulder and upper arm, and discuss criteria for determining return to activity

5. Perform a thorough and sequential off-field assessment, including considerations for differential diagnosis from cervical pathologies

6. Describe and perform the various special tests for evaluation of glenohumeral instabilities

7. Describe and perform the various special tests for assessment of rotator cuff pathology

Janet was a senior student athletic trainer who was looking forward to taking her certification exam in six months and getting her first real job. One day, Darin, her supervising athletic trainer, asked Janet to perform a shoulder evaluation on Kevin, one of the swimmers. After Janet had done the assessment, she and Darin sat down to discuss her impressions of the injury.

"Well, Janet, what did you think?" Darin asked.

"It seems pretty clear to me that Kevin is having some shoulder impingement. All the impingement tests I performed reproduced his pain." Janet felt pretty confident in her assessment.

"What do you think is causing it?" Darin asked as he reflected on her evaluation and his own observations.

"Causing it? Well, uh . . . I guess his swimming? But he didn't report any unusual changes in his swim workouts." Janet was not so confident now.

"Did you notice his posture?"

"Uh, no, not really—what would that have to do with it?"

"Well," Darin explained, "I noticed his posture is not the greatest. His head is forward and his shoulders are pretty rounded; a posture like this can be a result of muscle imbalance and can also be a contributing factor to impingement. How about his weight training? Any problems there?"

"His weight training? I didn't really ask him about that, but I see him in the weight room all the time. Oh, he did say it hurts a bit on bench press, but I don't think strength is an issue." Janet wasn't sure what Darin was looking for.

"It may not be a strength issue as much as a muscle balance issue. It is not unusual for athletes to work hard on bench press and other chest exercises, but when it comes to exercises for the back, they are not always quite so faithful. I saw his weight program last week. He has about one back/posterior shoulder exercise for every three chest/anterior shoulder exercises. Between that and being a breaststroker, I would bet he is pretty tight anteriorly and weak posteriorly, and that's probably contributing to his problem," Darin suggested.

"Okay, I see what you mean now," Janet said thoughtfully. "I guess I got so focused on his pain and symptoms, I really didn't look at the big picture to see what might be causing it. I'll keep that in mind next time . . . thanks, Darin, for the pointers!"

The shoulder is a highly mobile joint that allows a large range of motion in all planes to perform a variety of overhead activities. Statically, the glenohumeral joint is supported by the capsule, capsular ligaments, and glenoid labrum. However, to allow freedom of movement, these ligaments have to be relatively lax. As a result, the glenohumeral joint relies on the deltoid and rotator cuff muscles for dynamic stabilization.

The shoulder complex as a whole is unique in that it relies very little on bony and ligament structures for stability—with the majority of support coming from the 18 muscles acting on the shoulder complex. The only direct attachment of the upper extremity to the axial skeleton is through the sternoclavicular (SC) joint. The scapula, completely suspended by muscles, serves as a mobile yet stabilizing platform to facilitate glenohumeral motion. When scapular muscles are weak or atrophied, normal scapular motion is affected, and this can have a significant impact on shoulder mechanics and function. This dysfunction—combined with the high stress demands placed on the shoulder's static and dynamic stabilizing structures with repetitive overhead throwing activities—is a common cause of soft tissue injuries and instability in the shoulder region. Therefore, it is important that you consider the shoulder complex as a whole when performing a shoulder assessment.

# INJURIES OF THE SHOULDER COMPLEX AND UPPER ARM

The shoulder joint is particularly susceptible to injuries because of its great mobility and inherent instability. The heavy reliance on soft tissue structures and balanced muscular control for stabilization through a large range of motion places considerable demands on these structures, resulting in both acute and chronic injuries. Because of the interplay of the muscles acting on the shoulder, injury recognition is sometimes difficult.

## ACUTE SOFT TISSUE INJURIES

Acute soft tissue injuries can result from direct trauma, movements forcing the joint beyond its normal range, and forceful muscle contraction during activity.

### Contusions

During sports such as football, wrestling, and soccer, direct contact with other players and the ground can result in contusions to both bony anatomy and the superficial musculature. The clavicle and acromion are two bony structures with little soft tissue protection. Contusion of the acromion is often referred to as a "shoulder pointer." Contusions to these isolated bony structures are rarely disabling, with signs and symptoms typically limited to localized swelling, pain, and point tenderness. Contusions to the musculature can be more disabling, since hematoma formation and pain can limit muscular function. A complication of biceps muscle contusion is **myositis ossificans**, or calcification within and around the biceps. Myositis ossificans can result from an unresolved hematoma in cases with large hematoma formation, repetitive insult, or continued use following the initial contusion. In most cases, this can be prevented with proper rest and treatment.

### Sprains and Dislocation

Sprains involving the ligaments and capsule of the shoulder complex are relatively common. Ligamentous and capsular disruption can result from both compressive and tractional forces that force the joint beyond its normal range of motion. Sprains of the glenohumeral and acromioclavicular joint occur more frequently than SC joint sprains do.

#### Glenohumeral Joint Sprains

In order to provide the mobility inherent in the glenohumeral joint, the capsule and ligament structures are comparatively lax throughout most of glenohumeral motion. Therefore, the capsule and ligaments are minimally involved in maintaining joint stability throughout most of the range, with tensioning and potential injury to these structures occurring at the extreme ranges of motion. As a result, mild to moderate (first- and second-degree) glenohumeral sprains are fairly uncommon. However, forces exerted at the end ranges of motion that are sufficient to tear the glenohumeral ligaments will often cause subluxation or dislocation of the humeral head because of its shallow articulation with the glenoid.

#### Acromioclavicular Joint Sprains

Within the shoulder complex, the acromioclavicular (AC) joint is the most commonly sprained or "separated" joint. Ligament injuries to this joint typically result from a fall or from direct contact to the "point" of the shoulder, driving the acromion down underneath the clavicle. Forces may also be transmitted through the arm with a fall on an outstretched hand. **First-degree** sprains are characterized by localized pain, point tenderness, and swelling over the joint. The injured individual may complain of mild to moderate pain with shoulder motion, particularly with abduction above 120° and horizontal adduction. **Second-degree** injuries involve partial tearing of one or both of the acromioclavicular and coracoclavicular ligaments. The athlete will have increased complaints of pain, swelling, and disability with arm motion above horizontal. The distal end of the clavicle may or may not be elevated, depending on the extent of disruption of one or both of the associated ligaments (acromioclavicular and coracoclavicular portions). **Third-degree** injuries are characterized by complete disruption of both the acromioclavicular and coracoclavicular ligaments. The athlete will complain of severe pain at the time of injury and demonstrate an unwillingness to raise the arm, typically protecting it at his or her side. Obvious swelling and elevation of the distal clavicle relative to the acromion will be noted (figure 4.1).

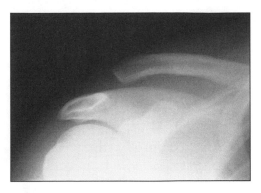

**I Figure 4.1**    Third-degree acromioclavicular separation.

### Sternoclavicular Joint Sprains

The SC joint is quite stable, and sprains are infrequent. Injury to the SC joint involves disruption of both the sternoclavicular and costoclavicular ligaments. Injury can occur as a result of an anteriorly directed force, or direct blow, but more commonly results from forces transmitted along the long axis of the clavicle. Signs and symptoms of SC sprains include localized pain, swelling, and point tenderness directly over the joint. Pain will increase with forward rotation of the shoulders and horizontal adduction, which will act to compress the joint. With a first-degree sprain there is minimal tearing of the ligaments, with no laxity or joint displacement. Second-degree sprains involve partial tearing of both the sternoclavicular and costoclavicular ligaments, resulting in some displacement of the proximal clavicle from the sternum. Third-degree sprains are readily observed and are characterized by complete separation of the SC joint with complete rupture of both ligaments. In most cases, the proximal clavicle will be displaced anteriorly and superiorly in relation to the sternum secondary to its joint contour. However, on occasion, an anteriorly directed force will cause the clavicle to be displaced posteriorly. With posterior displacement, secondary injury to the trachea and vascular structures underlying the proximal end of the clavicle may occur and cause breathing and vascular complications.

### *Strains*

The muscles of the shoulder complex provide much of the stability for the shoulder through most of its normal range. Consequently, acute muscle and tendon strains frequently occur with ballistic arm activities secondary to overstretching, forceful concentric contractions with limb acceleration, and excessive eccentric loading during limb deceleration. Improper warm-up, poor conditioning, and muscular fatigue can also make the muscles more susceptible to acute strain. Any of the 18 muscles acting within the shoulder complex are susceptible to injury. Signs and symptoms will be typical of any first-, second-, or third-degree muscle injury, and the specific muscle involved may be identified through isolated manual muscle testing.

### Rotator Cuff

The rotator cuff muscles are among the most commonly injured, and rotator cuff injury can result in significant disability. In addition to the mechanisms previously mentioned, acute rotator cuff injuries can also result from a fall on the shoulder or an outstretched hand, forcing the humeral head into the acromion. These compressive-type injuries result in contusion and inflammation of the underlying surface of the rotator cuff tendons. Conversely, falling on the point of the shoulder and driving the humeral head downward can traction and tear the supraspinatus near the myotendon junction. Signs and symptoms of acute rotator cuff injury resulting from these mechanisms include anterior-lateral shoulder pain, point tenderness, decreased range of motion, and loss of strength consistent with the severity of injury. Pain may radiate down the lateral arm but usually stops at midhumerus. Pain is often increased at night while the individual is lying on the affected side.

Only rarely is acute trauma responsible for full-thickness tears of the rotator cuff. More often, complete tears are secondary to an underlying accumulative microtrauma. In young athletes, complete tears rarely occur without bony avulsion, since the myotendinous structures are often stronger than the bone.

### Biceps Tendon Injuries

Rupture of the long head of the biceps is easily observed as a "bulging" of the muscle in the anterior arm, particularly when contracted. Acute rupture may be caused by a one-time traumatic event but more typically results from repetitive microtrauma and degeneration that weakens its tensile strength over time. Consequently it is more commonly seen in older athletes. When the biceps tendon is ruptured, the athlete will usually complain of experiencing a sudden sharp pain in the anterior shoulder and may experience a "pop" or snapping sensation. Muscular weakness will also result.

The biceps tendon can subluxate or dislocate within the bicipital groove if there is tearing of the transverse humeral ligament or attachment of the subscapularis tendon that stabilizes the tendon within the groove. The mechanism most often associated with dislocation of the biceps tendon is a rapid and abrupt external rotation of the humerus while the biceps is under tension. The athlete will complain of anterior shoulder pain and a painful popping or snapping sensation as the tendon slips in and out of the groove during internal and external rotation. Tenderness will be noted directly over the biceps tendon.

## CHRONIC OR OVERUSE SOFT TISSUE INJURIES

Given the repetitive nature of overhead motions that physically active individuals typically perform, the rotator cuff, biceps tendon, and associated bursa are particularly susceptible to chronic inflammatory and degenerative conditions.

### *Biceps Tendinitis*

The long head of the biceps can be involved in a number of pathologies. Tendinitis can result from repetitive overloading and friction as the long head of the biceps passes through the bicipital groove and under the transverse humeral ligament on its way to its attachment on the superior glenoid labrum (figure 4.2). Tractioning of the tendon's attachment on the glenoid labrum can also occur with forceful contraction during deceleration phases of throwing. In cases of glenohumeral instability, the biceps and the subscapularis may be overloaded as they are called on to provide more of the anterior restraint to glenohumeral motion. This can cause inflammation and pain within the substance of the tendon and at its attachment to the superior glenoid labrum. Biceps tendinitis occurs infrequently as an isolated injury and is typically associated with a shoulder impingement syndrome. Signs and symptoms may include diffuse anterior shoulder pain with point tenderness specifically over the bicipital groove and proximal tendon. Pain can be elicited with passive stretching of the biceps tendon and with contraction of the biceps while resisting supination. The throwing motion may also be painful, particularly during late cocking and acceleration phases.

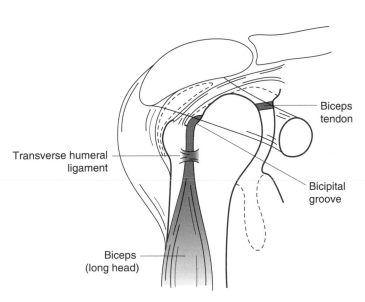

Transverse humeral ligament

Biceps tendon

Bicipital groove

Biceps (long head)

**■ Figure 4.2** The biceps tendon passing through the bicipital groove to its attachment on the glenoid rim.

### Rotator Cuff

As previously mentioned, the rotator cuff acts both as a prime mover for shoulder rotation and as a primary stabilizer for normal glenohumeral function. Therefore it is prone to overuse. In cases of glenohumeral instability, the increased demands on the rotator cuff as a glenohumeral stabilizer make it susceptible to chronic strains and inflammatory conditions. With overhead throwing activities, repetitive forceful muscle contraction during deceleration phases of throwing can result in eccentric injuries to the midsubstance and undersurface of the supraspinatus and infraspinatus portions of the cuff (Meister and Andrews 1993). Signs and symptoms include pain during throwing motion, tenderness over the supraspinatus and/or infraspinatus, and mild weakness of the external rotators. Atrophy of the infraspinatus may also be noted in long-standing chronic cases. Other chronic rotator cuff tendon pathologies and strains typically result secondarily to an impingement syndrome.

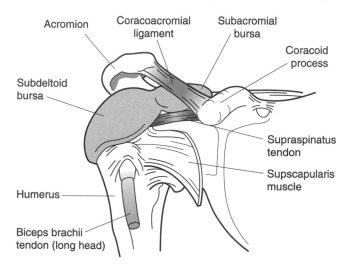

Acromion — Coracoacromial ligament — Subacromial bursa

Coracoid process

Subdeltoid bursa

Supraspinatus tendon

Supscapularis muscle

Humerus

Biceps brachii tendon (long head)

■ **Figure 4.3** Anatomy of the subacromial arch.

### Impingment Syndrome

Impingement syndrome is caused by encroachment in the subacromial space that decreases the space through which the supraspinatus and subacromial bursa pass underneath the subacromial arch (figure 4.3). Impingement is most commonly seen in occupations and sporting activities involving repetitive overhead shoulder motions. The rotator cuff in older adults is also more prone to injury as it becomes less vascular with age. Impingement, which has been categorized as either primary or secondary, can result from a variety of mechanisms including acute injury, glenohumeral instability, muscle weakness, inflammation secondary to chronic overuse, and bony abnormalities.

Primary impingement is caused by direct encroachment within the subacromial space and is most often seen in adults. Anatomical or bony encroachment can occur with variations in the contour of the acromion. A more curved or "hooked" acromion is more often found in association with rotator cuff pathologies. Weakness in the rotator cuff, particularly the infraspinatus and subscapularis, can disrupt the deltoid/rotator cuff force couple, causing the head of the humerus to ride too far superiorly and compress the supraspinatus tendon against the coracoacromial arch. Weakness of the supraspinatus lessens its ability to "hug" and depress the humeral head against the glenoid fossa, which also may cause the humeral head to ride too far superiorly. In older adults, the more likely cause of primary impingement is degenerative changes to the bony surface and soft tissue structures caused by chronic inflammation that decrease the subacromial space. These degenerative changes include scarring and weakness in the avascular zone of the supraspinatus tendon, spur formation on the undersurface of the acromion, and thickening of the subacromial bursa. Acute injuries with unresolved inflammation and resultant scarring and weakness can also result in muscular dysfunction and decreased subacromial space.

Secondary impingement results from encroachment due to other shoulder pathologies such as glenohumeral instability, and is the most frequent mechanism associated with impingement in the young athlete. Jobe and Pink (1993) describe an "instability continuum" in which anterior instability leads to subluxation, which in turn leads to impingement and eventual rotator cuff tears. Many times, the instability is not noted until symptoms of impingement and rotator cuff pathology are present. Glenohumeral instability increases the demands on the rotator cuff, increasing its role in shoulder stabilization. This can lead to overuse, fatigue, and repetitive microtrauma, which may cause inflammation and disrupt normal functioning of the rotator cuff. With anterior glenohumeral instability, range of motion is often lost with internal rotation, secondary to tightness of the posterior capsule.

In 1973, Neer described three stages of impingement:

- **Stage I** is found most often in younger athletes and is characterized by edema and hemorrhage within the rotator cuff. Symptoms include pain only with activity and little or no weakness; range of motion is unrestricted. If impingement is recognized and treated during this early stage, permanent tissue injury can be avoided.

- **Stage II** is characterized by thickening and fibrosis of the subacromial bursa and supraspinatus tendon. There will be pain both during and after activity, including activities of daily living, and perhaps also at night. Because degenerative changes have occurred, stage II impingement is not thought to be reversible with conservative treatment.

- **Stage III** degeneration has progressed to partial- or full-thickness tears of the rotator cuff tendons; there will also be bony changes to the surface of the humerus and anterior acromion located within the subacromial space. The athlete will complain of continuous pain and restricted range of motion.

Biceps tendinitis often occurs secondarily to impingement because of the close proximity of the proximal biceps tendon to the joint capsule and rotator cuff insertion. The subacromial bursa, which separates the coracoacromial arch from the underlying rotator cuff, also becomes inflamed (subacromial bursitis) and further compromises the subacromial space. As impingement progresses, the bursa will thicken and become fibrotic.

Pain and weakness associated with impingement will be most pronounced in midrange, from 60° to 120° of abduction and flexion. The athlete will typically complain of a dull or deep pain underneath or near the acromion. Point tenderness may be noted just anterior lateral to the acromion and at the insertion of the supraspinatus tendon. The athlete may also complain of pain radiating down the anterior (biceps) and lateral (supraspinatus) aspects of the upper arm.

## TRAUMATIC FRACTURES

**!** Because of the close proximity of the neurovascular structures to the shoulder joint and humerus, always check neurovascular status in the upper extremity with any suspected fracture.

Fractures within the shoulder and upper arm are usually caused by traumatic forces; stress fractures are rare. Traumatic fractures can result from both direct contact and indirect forces. Because of the relatively weak ligamentous and capsular support of the glenohumeral joint, dislocation typically will occur before a fracture. However, in the young athlete, fractures are more of a concern because of the weakness and immaturity of the growth plate.

### *Clavicle*

Within the shoulder complex, the clavicle is the most commonly fractured bone. The clavicle can fracture as a result of a direct anterior blow—or more often as a result of a force transmitted through the shoulder. Forces transmitted through the shoulder include those resulting from a fall on an outstretched hand and from landing on the shoulder with the arm adducted. Usually the fracture occurs at the distal one third where the contour of the bone changes. Signs and symptoms include pain, localized swelling, and point tenderness. The bone may or may not be displaced. However, since the clavicle is so superficial, any deformity is easily noted. Any time a force is transmitted through the shoulder and there is localized point tenderness over the clavicle, a fracture should be suspected.

### Humerus

Fractures of the proximal humerus and humeral shaft are usually caused by a direct blow but may also result from a fall on an outstretched hand. Fractures caused by this type of fall are more commonly seen in older adults. In young adults, the ligament and capsular structures will usually fail first, resulting in dislocation rather than fracture. In some cases, both glenohumeral dislocation and fracture of the anatomical neck may result. Signs and symptoms include severe pain, swelling, and disability. There may also be deformity and crepitus near the fracture site. In cases of fracture to the anatomical neck, the deformity may resemble a glenohumeral dislocation.

Epiphyseal fractures of the proximal humeral growth plate, or "Little Leaguer's shoulder," are usually associated with skeletally immature throwing athletes. These injuries occur most often during the deceleration phase of throwing. The primary sign of impending epiphyseal injury is severe shoulder pain with hard throwing.

Spiral fractures of the humeral shaft can result from torsional forces associated with the throwing mechanism, particularly during the acceleration phase (Ogawa and Yoshida 1998). Throwing fractures are most prevalent in young adult pitchers. At the time of injury, the fracture is often audible enough to be heard by others. Pain may be experienced anywhere in the midshaft and may extend to the elbow or shoulder. Deformity may be noted if displacement occurs.

A potential complication of humeral shaft fractures is involvement of and injury to the radial nerve, or "radial nerve palsy" (figure 4.4). Anatomically, the radial nerve exits the axilla and passes posteriorly from medial to lateral along the radial groove of the humeral shaft. If the fracture is displaced, the radial nerve can be contused or injured. In cases of radial nerve involvement, there will be numbness or tingling down the distribution of the nerve into the dorsal forearm and hand. Weakness or paralysis may be noted in the wrist and thumb extensors.

### Scapula

The scapula is one of the least commonly fractured bones of the upper extremity, primarily because of the presence of numerous muscles protecting the bony surfaces, as well as the scapula's mobility on the posterior chest wall. Because the scapula is so well protected, fracture usually does not occur unless there is a significant and direct trauma. Thus scapular fractures are often associated with other more serious injuries to thoracic structures. On very rare occasions, less traumatic mechanisms such as intensive and prolonged muscular action can result in stress fractures (Deltoff and Bressler 1989). Initial signs and symptoms include diffuse aching over the posterior shoulder region and musculature and an unwillingness to move the arm. The pain may become more localized, with tenderness and swelling noted over the scapula. People with this injury will typically hold their arm to the side and demonstrate significant weakness when abduction is attempted. Because of the overlying musculature, stress-related scapular fractures may mimic signs and symptoms of rotator cuff and other muscular injuries, depending on the location of the fracture.

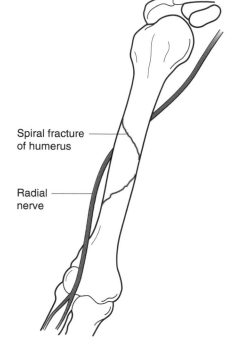

Spiral fracture of humerus

Radial nerve

■ **Figure 4.4**   Spiral fracture with potential radial nerve compression.

## BONY OR CARTILAGINOUS LESIONS SECONDARY TO REPETITIVE STRESS

Athletes complaining of pain and a sensation of "clicking" or "catching" with overhead throwing motions may have sustained an injury to the glenoid labrum. The glenoid labrum deepens the glenoid fossa to increase glenohumeral stability (figure 4.5). Glenoid labral tears are usually associated with glenohumeral instability and can result from either acute trauma/dislocation or chronic instability. Stresses related to throwing can also disrupt the labrum, particularly near the attachment of the biceps tendon. Swimmers, softball and baseball players, javelin throwers, and volleyball players are all susceptible to labral tears.

## DISLOCATION AND SUBLUXATION

The glenohumeral joint is considered the most commonly dislocated joint in the body. Glenohumeral dislocations are named according to the direction in which the humeral head is displaced in relation to the glenoid (figure 4.6, a-c). Dislocations and subluxations can result from both acute traumatic events and chronic shoulder instability. Many times, acute dislocations will result in permanent joint laxity, and recurrent episodes of subluxation or dislocation are common.

### *Acute Anterior Dislocation*

Anterior glenohumeral dislocations represent the large majority of all glenohumeral dislocations. Anterior subluxations and dislocations typically occur with the arm in an abducted and externally rotated position. Hyperextension of the joint in this position, or a force applied to the posterior or lateral aspect of the humerus, can stress the anterior and inferior glenohumeral ligaments and capsule and cause them to fail. At lower applied forces the capsular ligaments may be partially stretched, and the person feels a slipping or

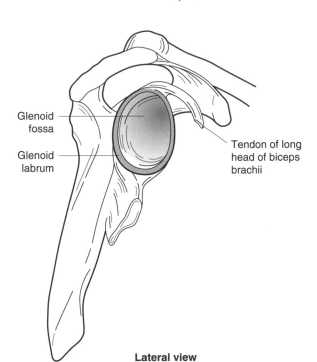

**Lateral view**

■ **Figure 4.5**  Glenoid labrum.

Glenoid fossa

Glenoid labrum

Tendon of long head of biceps brachii

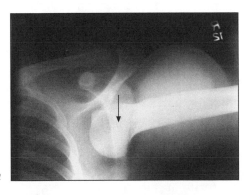

*a*

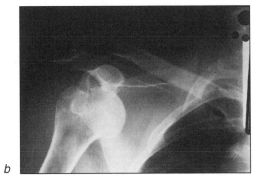

*b*

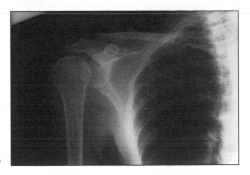

*c*

■ **Figure 4.6**  Three directions of glenohumeral dislocations: (a) anterior-inferior, (b) anterior, (c) posterior.

giving sensation that indicates a subluxation or spontaneous relocation. As these static restraints are further stretched and torn, the humeral head is displaced anteriorly and usually lodges between the anterior inferior glenoid rim and the coracoid process (see figure 4.6b).

An athlete with an anterior dislocation will typically present with the arm slightly abducted and supporting the injured extremity. The acromion will be prominent, and the deltoid will appear flattened. The humeral head will appear as a prominence in the anterior-inferior aspect of the shoulder or may be palpable in the axilla. The athlete will complain of pain and will be unwilling to move the extremity. In cases of subluxation or spontaneous reduction, he will be apprehensive and complain of pain when the arm is abducted and externally rotated. Because of its close proximity to the humeral head in the axilla, the axillary nerve may also be injured. In this case, there will be impaired sensation and motor function in the deltoid.

### Posterior Dislocation

Posterior dislocations are less frequent but can occur when the arm is forward flexed and a posteriorly directed force is applied along the length of the humerus. Straight arm blocking and falling on the elbow with the shoulder in a forward and flexed position are examples of this type of mechanism. This mechanism drives the humeral head through the posterior capsule, allowing it to dislodge between the posterior glenoid and the posterior cuff muscles (see figure 4.6c). Posterior dislocations are not as obvious as anterior dislocations, as they often spontaneously reduce and the deformity associated with humeral head displacement is not as pronounced. Athletes with a posterior dislocation will typically present with the arm adducted and internally rotated. The anterior-lateral portion of the deltoid may or may not appear flattened, and the coracoid process may be prominent. The humeral head may be palpable posteriorly. There will also be signs and symptoms of pain and swelling and an unwillingness to move the extremity.

### Inferior Dislocation

Displacement of the humeral head directly inferior to the glenoid is fairly uncommon. More often, the displacement will be anterior-inferior (see figure 4.6a). Mechanisms associated with inferior dislocation include forced abduction with stress applied to the inferior joint capsule.

### Chronic Instability

Chronic glenohumeral instability is commonly seen in physically active persons because of the inherent mobility and weak static stabilizing structures of the shoulder. **Chronic instability** is also classified by the direction of excessive humeral head translation (anterior, inferior, posterior, and multidirectional). Chronic instability can result from an initial traumatic event but also may be unrelated to any previous history of trauma or dislocation. Repetitive overload caused by overhead throwing can also stress and slacken the anterior and inferior ligaments and capsule.

Young athletes involved in overhead activities such as baseball, swimming, javelin, tennis, volleyball, and even golf can place tremendous stress on the anterior structures of the glenohumeral joint. If the musculature (i.e., pectoralis major, subscapularis, latissimus dorsi, and teres major) that supports the anterior capsule becomes fatigued or weak or is injured, the anterior capsule can become stretched and lax, allowing the humeral head to translate anteriorly. Over time, this anterior laxity can result in tightening or shortening of the posterior capsule and subsequent impingement syndrome (Jobe and Pink 1993). This posterior tightening will further encourage anterior translation.

Athletes with chronic instability are most susceptible to episodes of subluxation or dislocation when the arm is positioned in abduction and external rotation. Signs and symptoms include pain and a sensation of joint slippage while the glenohumeral joint is subluxating during overhead activity. The athlete may also complain of weakness, numbness, and tingling following the subluxating event.

Resultant from the glenohumeral instability, secondary injuries involving degeneration of the glenoid labrum, overuse syndromes of the dynamic stabilizers (rotator cuff muscles and biceps tendon), and shoulder impingement syndromes are common. Signs and symptoms of these secondary injuries may be more pronounced than those associated with the instability and may represent the first indication of a possible instability.

## NEUROVASCULAR INJURIES

Because of the close proximity to the shoulder of the brachial plexus and axillary vessels, neurovascular injury is a concern with significant shoulder trauma (figure 4.7). Associated nerve injuries are more common than vascular injuries at the shoulder. However, any time there are changes in skin coloration, diminished distal pulses, numbness, tingling, weakness, or loss of motor function, neurovascular trauma or compression should be suspected and traced to its origin.

Axillary and radial nerve palsy associated with fractures and dislocations of the humerus (page 92) have been previously discussed. Brachial plexus injuries and thoracic outlet syndrome were discussed in chapter 3 (pages 59-61) but are equally pertinent in the assessment of shoulder injuries.

Other peripheral nerves that may be involved with trauma at the shoulder include the suprascapular, long thoracic, and spinal accessory nerves. The suprascapular nerve is vulnerable to injury through both direct blow and traction mechanisms. Signs and symptoms include diffuse posterior shoulder pain and weakness of the supraspinatus and external rotators. Pain and a burning sensation may also be produced with horizontal arm adduction across the front of the body (Silliman and Dean 1993). For these reasons, the signs and symptoms of suprascapular nerve injuries may be confused with those of rotator cuff injuries. Entrapment of the *suprascapular nerve* occurs most often as it passes through the suprascapular notch. Direct pressure or percussion over the notch will often elicit suprascapular nerve pain and symptoms. Atrophy of the supraspinatus and/or infraspinatus may be noted, depending on the duration of symptoms and the location of nerve compression or injury.

The *long thoracic nerve* is also prone to both traction- and compressive-type injuries. It is particularly vulnerable to direct blows as it runs superficially along the lateral chest wall to innervate the serratus anterior muscle. Injury to the long thoracic nerve may or may not be associated with pain in the posterior shoulder and scapular regions. Injury may remain unrecognized until serratus anterior weakness and subsequent "**winging of the scapula**" are noted.

The *spinal accessory nerve* innervates the trapezius muscle and runs near the posterior triangle of the neck. Injury to this nerve can result from a direct blow to the

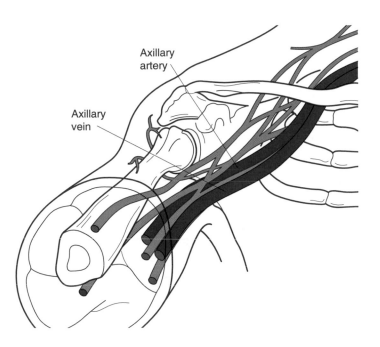

Axillary artery

Axillary vein

**▮ Figure 4.7** Note the close proximity of the brachial plexus (light blue) and axillary vessels (darker blue) to the shoulder joint.

base of the lateral neck or with traction and depression of the shoulder. Signs and symptoms include pain, weakness with shoulder elevation, and rotatory winging of the superior angle of the scapula (Silliman and Dean 1993). The trapezius muscle may also show atrophy with time.

## STRUCTURAL AND FUNCTIONAL ABNORMALITIES

Structural deformities are usually congenital, whereas functional deformities result from prior injury or musculoskeletal dysfunction. Although these conditions may be rarely seen in people who are physically active, it is important that you are able to recognize them, as they can have significant impact on normal mechanics of the shoulder.

### Adhesive Capsulitis

A concern with immobility following any shoulder injury is **adhesive capsulitis**, or a "frozen shoulder" syndrome. If the arm is either volitionally held or purposely immobilized for an extended period of time, the inflamed shoulder capsule may develop adhesions and subsequent contractures, causing severe limitations in range of motion. Adhesive capsulitis can usually be avoided through proper treatment and rehabilitation following shoulder injury.

For more information on adhesive capsulitis, refer to *Therapeutic Exercise for Athletic Injuries* (Houglum 2000), chapter 17.

### Sprengel's Deformity

**Sprengel's deformity** is the most common congenital deformity of the shoulder. It is characterized by an underdeveloped scapula that sits high on the posterior chest wall (figure 4.8). Often the scapula will be medially rotated and the scapular muscles will be poorly developed. This deformity is caused by a failure of the scapula to descend properly and may be associated with other congenital abnormalities. Sprengel's deformity may be found both unilaterally and bilaterally. Depending on severity, shoulder abduction range of motion may be affected. Muscle imbalance or dysfunction created by underdevelopment of the scapular muscles may be a precipitating factor for other shoulder joint pathologies.

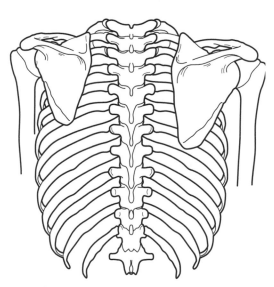

**❚ Figure 4.8**　Sprengel's deformity.

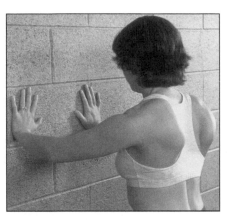

**I Figure 4.9**    Scapular winging.

### *Scapular Winging*

**Scapular winging** is characterized by a protrusion of the vertebral border away from the posterior chest wall (figure 4.9).

The scapula is stabilized against the posterior chest wall primarily by the joint function of the serratus anterior and trapezius muscles. If the serratus anterior or trapezius muscles are weak because of deconditioning or muscle imbalance, slight to moderate scapular winging may be present. Severe winging can occur with injury to the spinal accessory (trapezius) or long thoracic (serratus anterior) nerve. Given that scapular stabilization is imperative for proper glenohumeral function, scapular winging may be an important finding in the evaluation of glenohumeral joint pathology.

## INJURY ASSESSMENT

By now you should have a good appreciation for the variety of acute and chronic conditions commonly seen in people who are physically active. This knowledge, along with a good background in anatomy, will help you interpret the findings of your assessment.

## ON-FIELD ASSESSMENT

On-field assessment can be the most efficient when the athletic trainer has observed the injury occur. You can glean much from seeing the mechanism of injury, including an immediate impression of the severity and the athlete's immediate physical and emotional response. As you approach the athlete, observe the surroundings as well as the position and response of the athlete. Is the athlete moving, holding the arm to protect his shoulder, or keeping his arm in the position of injury? Is the shoulder in abduction, close to the side, or does it appear deformed? Is the athlete in excessive pain or able to control his response to the pain?

Once you are at the athlete's side, check ABCs and for obvious signs of deformity or severe bleeding. Place a reassuring hand on the athlete to calm him while he provides you with necessary history regarding the location and severity of the pain.

Palpation for a distal pulse and sensory perception (C5-T1 nerve roots) should be routine with more severe injuries, particularly with suspected fractures or dislocations that may compromise the neurovascular structures. If signs of neurovascular compromise are present, activate EMS and immediately refer the athlete for emergency care. Next, palpate the shoulder's bony and soft tissue structures, comparing them to the ones on the uninvolved side, to reveal any gross deformities and areas of tenderness around the shoulder (see sideline assessment for the complete palpation sequence). Check for any flattening of the deltoid that would indicate a dislocation or subluxation. If there is no deformity, ask the athlete to slowly move the arm. You can place a hand on his shoulder during active motion to palpate for any crepitus or abnormal movement. If the athlete is able to move his arm, shows no sign of serious injury, and is not in extreme pain, assist him to a seated position and then to a standing position, making sure not to pull on the injured arm. Be sure to support the arm—or have the athlete support it with his uninvolved hand—before he stands and ambulates off the field. The athlete then moves to the sideline for a more detailed evaluation.

For most upper-extremity injuries, athletes will be able to move to the sidelines under their own power, without the need for passive transport. However, passive

Remember, an athlete does not have to have a severe injury to suffer shock. You should always be aware of the athlete's reaction to the injury and observe for signs of shock. If the athlete appears to be going into shock, the injury should be stabilized and immediate emergency care is indicated.

transport may be necessary in the case of fracture or dislocation or if the athlete is in severe pain, is light-headed, or is nauseous because of the injury. If a fracture or dislocation is suspected, the arm should be immobilized before the athlete is moved. Safety of the athlete is always the primary concern in the decision about the mode of transportation from the field. Although efficiency is also a concern, it should never compromise the athlete's health and welfare.

# SIDELINE ASSESSMENT

Once the athlete is off the field and you have determined that the injury is not severe enough to warrant immediate physician referral, a sideline assessment will enable you to determine the severity of the injury, the specific tissue or structure involved, and the ability of the athlete to return to participation.

## History

Ask the athlete to provide a history of the injury even if you saw the injury happen. Many times the athlete can provide information about the direction of forces applied that people on the sideline cannot observe. The injured person also has information about the sounds and sensations heard or felt at the time of injury and immediate sensations after the injury. Specific questions may include the following: How did the athlete land? Did she hear or feel anything (i.e., a snap or pop) at the time of the injury? Was there immediate pain? Has the pain changed? Ask the athlete to describe the location, quality, and intensity of the pain. Do the pain or symptoms radiate up to the neck or down the arm? If so, what are the sensations? This is also the time to ask about any prior injuries to the shoulder. If the athlete was previously injured, what was the nature of the injury and what treatment, if any, did she receive? Had she had any problems with the shoulder before that, or has she had any since?

## Observation

Throughout the history-taking portion of the evaluation, observe the athlete's actions and response to the injury. Observe for signs of swelling, discoloration, deformity or abnormal contours, pain, and guarding. Does the athlete gesture freely with the arm or hold and support it? Is he able to remove his shirt without difficulty, or does he require assistance or hesitate to move the arm overhead?

---

### Checklist for On-Field Assessment of the Shoulder and Arm

**Primary Survey**
- ✓ Consciousness
- ✓ Airway, breathing, and circulation
- ✓ Severe bleeding

**Secondary Survey**

History
- ✓ Mechanism, location, and severity of pain
- ✓ Information from bystanders

Observation
- ✓ Deformity, swelling, discoloration
- ✓ Athlete's response to injury
- ✓ Unusual positioning of limb

Palpation
- ✓ Deltoid contour
- ✓ Bony tenderness
- ✓ Bone and joint deformity or crepitus

Neurovascular assessment
- ✓ Sensory (C5-T1)
- ✓ Motor (C5-T1)
- ✓ Distal pulse (radial)

Active ROM
- ✓ If all tests negative, remove athlete from field.

If a severe injury is suspected, it is advisable to cut the athlete's clothing and equipment away rather than move the shoulder into positions that might cause further injury or pain. Once the shirt is removed, observe the shoulder for contour and balance in comparison to the uninvolved side. Check for any flattening of the deltoid that may indicate a subluxation or dislocation. Also assess the posture of the shoulder, neck, and upper back, since poor posture can either aggravate or be caused by an injury. The head should be in the midline position in an anterior and posterior view. The acromions, SC joints, inferior border of the scapulae, and scapular spines should be level bilaterally. However, it is common for the dominant shoulder to be slightly lower than the nondominant, so this difference, if not exaggerated, would not be considered abnormal. The shoulders should be rounded and have equal contour left to right. In normal shoulder alignment, the inferior tip of the scapula is in line with T7, and the superior medial ridge is in line with T2. The medial border of the scapula is 2 to 3 in. (5.1 to 7.6 cm) from the thoracic spinous processes.

Since it is usually difficult for people to keep from revealing pain through facial expressions, continue to observe the athlete's facial expressions throughout the examination to help determine the athlete's level of discomfort.

### *Palpation*

Palpation is best performed with the athlete in sitting. This allows you to move from the anterior to the lateral to the posterior aspect of the shoulder without requiring the athlete to change positions. If the athlete has a difficult time relaxing during palpation, it may be advantageous for her to recline and to move from supine to prone as you perform the palpation portion of the evaluation.

Look for areas of tenderness or differences between the right and left sides in contour, muscle spasm, and soft tissue mobility. Superficial muscles to palpate are the pectoralis major anteriorly; the trapezius and supraspinatus superiorly; the trapezius, rhomboids, levator scapula, teres major, latissimus dorsi, and posterior cuff muscles posteriorly; and the deltoid laterally. The muscles are palpated for tenderness, spasm, and defects.

The anterior shoulder palpation begins at the SC joint and moves laterally along the clavicle to the AC joint. The coracoid process is located about 1 in. (2.5 cm) inferior to the junction of the lateral one-third and medial two-thirds of the clavicle where it is most concave. The sternum, costicartilage, and ribs should be palpated if the athlete complains of anterior chest tenderness or symptoms or has received an anterior impact injury.

The lateral shoulder is palpated beginning with the acromion process. Directly inferior to the acromion process is the greater tubercle, and immediately medial to the greater tubercle is the bicipital groove. The lesser tubercle is immediately medial to the bicipital groove. The bicipital groove and lesser tubercle are sometimes easier to palpate if the arm is externally rotated. In full external rotation, the bicipital groove lies directly under the acromion. The rim of the lesser tubercle is the attachment site of the subscapularis tendon. If the athlete places her hand in the small of her back, you can palpate the supraspinatus tendon about .8 in. (2 cm) inferior to the anterior acromion. If the shoulder is passively positioned in end hyperextension, you can palpate the subacromial bursa immediately anterior to the anterior acromion (figure 4.10).

Palpation of the posterior shoulder begins with bony structures: the spine of the scapula, lower cervical and upper and middle thoracic spinous processes, and inferior and superior angles of the scapula. The triceps tendon can also be palpated. If the athlete is positioned prone with the elbows slightly medial to the shoulder and rotated inward, the

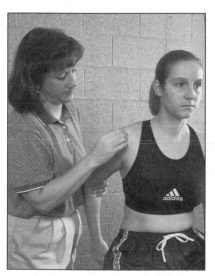

**■ Figure 4.10** Palpation of the subacromial bursa.

infraspinatus tendon can be palpated immediately inferior to the most lateral aspect of the scapula.

When you passively abduct the athlete's shoulder to about 30° to 40°, you can palpate the axillary structures. The muscles must remain relaxed for this palpation. The anterior wall is formed by the pectoralis major; the posterior wall is the latissimus dorsi; and the medial wall is the ribs and anterior serratus. Each of these structures should be palpated for tenderness and abnormalities. The brachial artery can also be palpated in the axilla.

## Special Tests

Since several joints and soft tissue structures comprise the shoulder complex, you must examine many elements in order to evaluate the shoulder thoroughly. The special tests you select will be based on the cumulative results of your assessment thus far. It may be useful to briefly pause in your assessment to consider your impressions before proceeding. For example, if you have eliminated the possibility of acromioclavicular injury, then there is no need to perform the special tests for it.

### Glenohumeral Stability Tests

Several tests are used to determine instability of the glenohumeral joint. The glenohumeral joint can be unstable anteriorly, posteriorly, inferiorly, and in multiplanar directions. There is a different test for each of these instabilities. The more commonly used ones will be presented here.

A positive sign of a special test has been obtained when the test elicits or reproduces the athlete's complaints. If the athlete's pain is not reproduced to some degree with the test, the test is negative.

Remember to perform the tests on the uninvolved side first to make the athlete less apprehensive and more relaxed when you are testing the involved side. Testing the uninvolved side first will also help you to determine what is normal for the athlete.

### Load and Shift Test

Anterior shoulder pain is an indication for the load and shift test to assess anterior and posterior instability. Unless you are an experienced examiner, perform each test separately to get a clear result—that is, perform a separate anterior movement and a separate posterior movement rather than gliding from one to the other. Although anterior instability is a common problem of throwing athletes, it can also occur in other athletes.

The load and shift test can be performed with the athlete sitting or supine. In sitting, the athlete's arm rests on his thigh, and the athletic trainer stands at the athlete's side and slightly behind him. To perform the test, use one hand to stabilize the scapula and clavicle and the other as the test hand. Place your test hand on the athlete's shoulder with your thumb over the posterior humeral head and your fingers over the anterior humeral head. Load the humerus by pushing the humeral head into the glenoid fossa to seat it in its proper neutral position. While maintaining the humeral head in a seated position, you shift the humerus forward by applying an anterior force to assess anterior instability. Apply a posterior force to assess posterior instability (figure 4.11). Some movement in each direction is normal, but it should not be more than 25% of the humeral head size. Grade I instability is present if the humeral head moves 25-50% in either direction; grade II is present with more than 50% movement with spontaneous reduction when the force is stopped; and grade III is present when the humeral head shows more than 50% movement, but without spontaneous reduction, and remains dislocated (Hawkins and Mohtadi 1991). A combination of laxity and reproduction of the athlete's symptoms determines whether or not the test is positive.

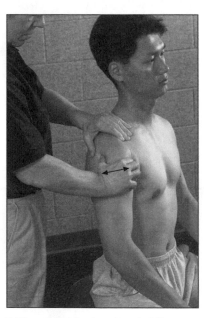

∎ **Figure 4.11**    Load and shift test.

## Relocation Test and Apprehension Test

The relocation test is also known as the **Fowler test** or the **Jobe relocation test**. It is used to further assess anterior instability. The apprehension test, also called the crank test, assesses anterior shoulder dislocation (figure 4.12a). With the athlete in supine, the shoulder is positioned in 90° abduction and maximum degrees external rotation; it is when the athlete is in this position that the test is referred to as the crank test, or apprehension test. A positive apprehension is present if the athlete either has an apprehensive look on her face or resists further movement. To continue with the relocation test, create the position slowly to minimize the athlete's apprehension and the risk of dislocation (figure 4.12b). If the position is painful, apply an anterior-to-posterior force to the shoulder to relocate the humerus in the glenoid; the pain will diminish if the test is positive.

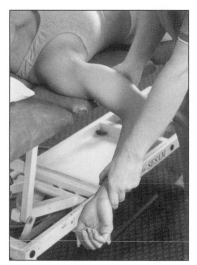
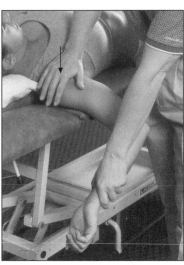

*a*  *b*

**▌Figure 4.12** (a) Crank, or apprehension, test and (b) relocation test.

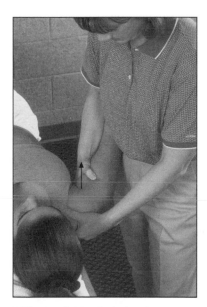

**▌Figure 4.13** Anterior drawer test.

## Anterior Drawer Test

There are many variations of the anterior drawer test. The primary feature is the application of a posterior-to-anterior **glide force** to the shoulder to provide stress to the joint's anterior structures. With the athlete supine and her shoulder over the edge of the table, place her hand between your upper arm and your side to support the arm. The athlete's arm should be relaxed. The athlete's arm is positioned in midrange abduction and some forward flexion and external rotation, about 20-30° each. Your stabilizing hand is placed on the scapula so that your fingers and thumb secure the scapula at the spine of the scapula and the coracoid process. With the test hand supporting the posterior upper arm, pull the athlete's arm anteriorly to apply a posterior-to-anterior glide force to the glenohumeral joint (figure 4.13). If a click is heard during the maneuver, the glenoid labrum may be torn, or the joint is sufficiently lax to allow the humeral head to glide over the glenoid labrum rim.

## Posterior Drawer Test

The posterior drawer test assesses posterior glenohumeral laxity. As with the anterior drawer test, there are several variations. The intent with each is to apply a force sufficient to stress the soft tissue structures that stabilize the posterior joint; this will enable you to determine the presence and degree of laxity.

The athlete lies supine with her arm relaxed. Use one hand to support the athlete's arm and position her shoulder in midrange abduction and about 30° flex-

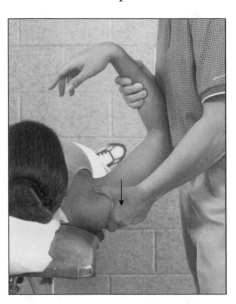

ion. Place your other hand on the humerus just off the acromion. As you move the athlete's shoulder into more flexion, apply an anterior-to-posterior force to the humeral head (figure 4.14). A positive test may not produce pain, but laxity is obvious. The athlete may demonstrate signs of apprehension.

■ **Figure 4.14**  Posterior drawer test.

## Sulcus Sign

The **sulcus sign** is used to assess inferior instability. With the athlete in sitting or standing, the arm is hanging relaxed at the side. Palpate the shoulder by placing your thumb and fingers on anterior and posterior aspects of the humeral head. Your testing hand grasps the elbow and applies a distal distraction force (figure 4.15). As you apply the force, observe the skin over the surface inferior to the

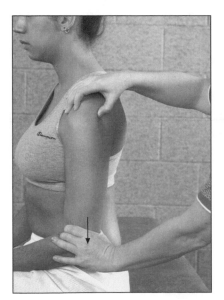

acromion. If the sulcus sign is positive, a dimpling may occur between the acromion and humeral head as the humeral head moves inferiorly with distraction force. The distance between the humeral head and acromion—and thus the amount of dimpling—will be dependent on the degree of laxity. Movement of the humeral head less than .4 in. (1 cm) distally is a grade +1 sulcus sign; movement of .4 in. is grade +2; movement of .6 in. (1.5 cm) or more is grade +3. If the shoulder demonstrates laxity inferiorly, it may also be multidirectionally unstable, so you should also perform anterior and posterior stability tests.

■ **Figure 4.15**  Sulcus sign test.

## Clunk Test

The clunk test assesses glenoid labrum integrity. With the athlete supine, position his arm in full flexion over his head. Place one hand under his shoulder and the other on the distal upper arm. As you apply an anterior force with the hand under the athlete's humeral head, use your distal hand (hand on the upper arm) to move his shoulder into external rotation (figure 4.16). A positive test produces a grinding or clunk in the shoulder.

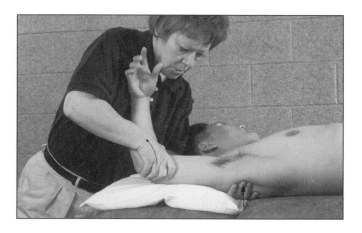

∎ **Figure 4.16** Clunk test.

### Acromioclavicular Stability Tests

There are two tests to assess stability of the AC joint, the shear test and the compression test. These tests can be used if an AC joint injury is suspected but is not severe enough to produce disruption or displacement of the joint such that abnormal joint position is readily apparent.

## Shear Test

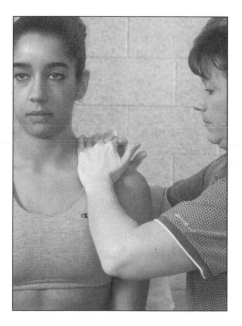

Perform the shear test with the athlete in sitting and her arm relaxed with the forearm supported in her lap. Stand at the athlete's side and place your hands over the top of her shoulder. The heel of one of your hands is on the distal clavicle, and heel of the other is on the lateral scapular spine. Squeeze the bases of the hands together to move the distal clavicle and spine of the scapula toward each other (figure 4.17). A positive test produces pain or laxity in comparison to the other side.

∎ **Figure 4.17** Shear test.

For the acromioclavicular compression test, the athlete is sitting. The athlete places the hand from the involved side on the opposite shoulder, with the elbow positioned at shoulder level (figure 4.18). To perform the test, horizontally adduct the shoulder by passively moving the elevated elbow toward the opposite shoulder to further compress the AC joint. A positive sign is elicited if pain occurs either with or without the passive movement.

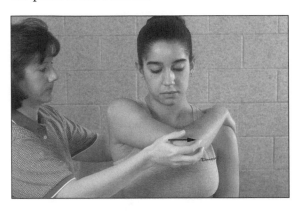

**▮ Figure 4.18** Acromioclavicular/ compression test.

## Rotator Cuff

Rotator cuff injuries can result from inflammation, instability, and acute stress. Since this discussion centers on acute injuries that are commonly evaluated on the sideline, only the drop arm test, a special test for an acute rotator cuff injury, will be presented here. Inflammation- and instability-based problems are more commonly seen in nontraumatic situations in which the athlete reports to the athletic injury treatment facility because of repeated or prolonged pain, discomfort, or interference with performance.

**Drop Arm Test**

The **drop arm test** assesses the integrity of the rotator cuff. A positive sign is an indication of a rotator cuff tear. Place the athlete's arm passively in 90° of abduction. Then instruct the athlete to slowly lower her arm to her side (figure 4.19). Normal movement is precise and controlled. A rotator cuff tear will produce pain during movement, or the athlete will be unable to control movement throughout a slow motion.

Acute tears of the rotator cuff are not usual in a young athlete; they are more common in athletes who are older. A young throwing athlete may experience a rotator cuff tear, but it is usually secondary to instability and impingement.

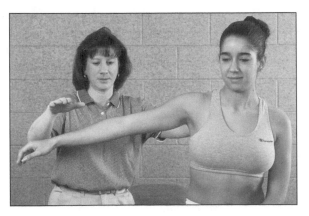

**▮ Figure 4.19** Drop arm test.

### Biceps Tests

As with some rotator cuff tests, some biceps tests are assessments for chronic bicipital tendinitis. The tendinitis tests will be presented in the section on off-field assessment. Speed's and Ludington's tests, however, will be discussed here, since their results can indicate a tear as well as a tendinitis. If you do not readily observe a biceps tear, the preferred test to assess biceps tendon tears is Ludington's test.

### Speed's Test

**Speed's test** is used to examine the integrity of the biceps tendon. Since the biceps is an integral part of the shoulder joint, it can often be the site of injury in the athletic shoulder. A positive result can indicate either a tendinitis or a rupture of the biceps tendon, depending on the severity of the response. If significant weakness is present, the tendon may be ruptured. If the primary result of the test is pain, the injury is probably bicipital tendinitis.

Have the athlete sitting with her elbow in full extension, and palpate the bicipital groove; use your other hand to resist the athlete's attempt to forward flex the shoulder (figure 4.20). The test should be performed with the forearm in supination and repeated with the forearm in pronation. This test is also referred to as a straight arm test or biceps test.

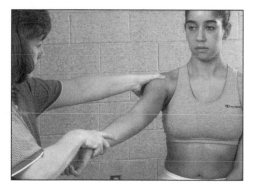

**Figure 4.20** Speed's test.

### Ludington's Test

A positive result from Ludington's test indicates a tear of the tendon of the long head of the biceps. With the athlete sitting, instruct her to place both hands behind her head and to relax the arms by letting her interlocked hands support her arms in this position. Stand behind the athlete and palpate the bicipital groove (figure 4.21). Then instruct her to alternate contraction of right and left biceps as you palpate the tendons. In a positive test, the uninjured tendon can be palpated, but the involved one cannot.

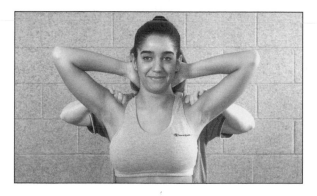

**Figure 4.21** Ludington's test.

### Range of Motion

Range of motion of the shoulder is first performed actively and then passively. Active motion is performed in all planes: flexion and extension (figure 4.22, a-b), abduction and adduction (figure 4.22, c-d), horizontal adduction and abduction (figure 4.22, e-f), and internal and external rotation (figure 4.22, g-h). These motions can be performed in sitting unless the athlete displays less than grade 3 (against gravity) strength. Observe for full motion that is controlled, painless, and smooth. Glitches in the movement because of either pain or difficulty with the motion indicate an abnormal movement and call for further evaluation. Incomplete motion or substituted motions are also abnormal and require further investigation as to cause.

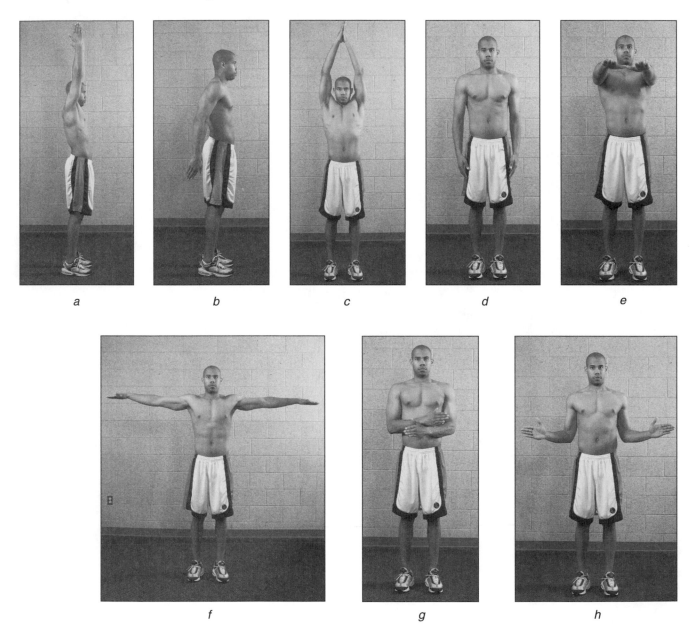

a    b    c    d    e

f    g    h

▌**Figure 4.22**   Active range of motion for (a) flexion, (b) extension, (c) abduction, (d) adduction, (e) horizontal adduction, (f) horizontal abduction, (g) internal rotation, and (h) external rotation.

It is often best if the athlete performs the motions simultaneously with right and left arms. The athletic trainer can compare flow of movement and ranges of motion at the same time. Substitutions can be more easily noted, too. Observe motions from anterior, lateral, and posterior views for complete comparisons. From the posterior view, you should also observe scapular motion during these movements. Although the scapula does not act alone, you should observe scapular movement bilaterally during the shoulder motions just described, checking for smooth and equal movement bilaterally. Movement that is not symmetrical may indicate muscle substitution (compensatory movement) or chronic dysfunction. Scapular motions to assess during active range of motion testing of the shoulder include depression and elevation, retraction and protraction, and upward and downward rotation. See table 4.1 for muscles involved in these scapular movements.

You may note in your evaluation that the dominant arm has slightly less motion than the nondominant arm. This is normal. Some athletes may also exhibit excessive motions in specific planes (i.e., **hypermobility**), which may also be considered normal. For example, pitchers will have more than the "normal" 90° of external rotation—and if they have less than 90°, this would be considered abnormal for them.

Pain through the arc of motion into shoulder flexion can indicate either pathology in the subacromial soft tissue structures (biceps tendon, bursa, or rotator cuff), if the pain occurs during the mid-arc portion of the motion, or acromioclavicular pathology if pain occurs at the end of the motion. If pain occurs with horizontal adduction, the pathology may be in the AC joint.

Perform passive movements when the active motion is less than normal in order to assess full range of motion and end feel. Normal end feel for shoulder motions is most often a sensation of a soft tissue stretch. However, it is not abnormal to feel a bony restriction at the end of shoulder abduction. Any abnormal restriction either in end feel or limitation in motion should be noted.

End feel can identify abnormal tissue restriction that may be limiting range of motion. At the end of each active motion, move the athlete's arm into the end degrees of the motion. This is usually a few more degrees than the athlete is able to move actively (see chapter 2, "Types of End Feel Encountered With Passive Overpressure").

| Table 4.1 | Muscles Involved in Scapular Movement | | |
|---|---|---|---|
| **Elevation** | **Depression** | **Protraction** | **Retraction** |
| Trapezius | Pectoralis minor | Pectoralis minor | Rhomboids |
| Levator scapula | Lower trapezius | Serratus anterior | Medial and lower trapezius |
| Sternocleidomastoid | Subclavius | | |
| Rhomboids | | | |
| **Upward rotation** | **Downward rotation** | | |
| Upper and lower trapezius | Levator scapula | | |
| Serratus anterior | Rhomboids | | |
| | Pectoralis major and minor | | |
| | Latissimus dorsi | | |

## Apley's Scratch Test

A combination of movements can also be tested by means of Apley's scratch test. For example, placing the hand behind the back and up on the spine requires shoulder extension, adduction, and internal rotation (figure 4.23a), while placing the hand behind the head involves shoulder flexion, abduction, and external rotation (figure 4.23b).

### Strength

The athlete can perform strength tests in sitting unless he has less than grade 3 strength. The resistance should be applied with the shoulder stabilized. The resistance should gradually build to a maximum level and then gradually decrease: note that it should not be suddenly released. Resistance to internal and external rotation is commonly provided with the athlete's elbow stabilized at his side.

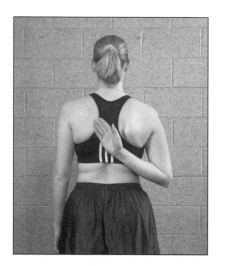
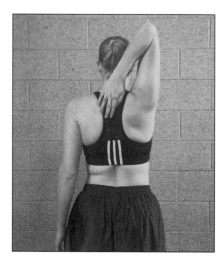

*a*     *b*

▌**Figure 4.23**   Apley's scratch test (a) shoulder extension, adduction, and internal rotation, and (b) shoulder flexion, abduction, and external rotation.

For a review of all positions of muscle testing for shoulders with the various muscle grades, refer to *Therapeutic Exercise for Athletic Injuries* (Houglum 2000), chapter 7.

Glenohumeral motions of flexion and extension, abduction and adduction, internal and external rotation, and horizontal adduction and abduction are routinely tested. Scapular motions should also be tested. These motions are elevation and depression and upward rotation (figure 4.24, a-b), scapular retraction (figure 4.24c), protraction (figure 4.24d), and downward rotation (figure 4.24e). Scapular elevation is tested with a shoulder shrug. Depression and upward rotation are tested with the athlete prone and the arm overhead; the resistance is given to the scapula as the athlete elevates the shoulder. Scapular retraction is tested with the athlete prone. Resistance is given at the scapula against scapular adduction. Scapular protraction is resisted with the athlete in sitting with the shoulder flexed to 90-120°. As the athlete attempts to push his arm forward and upward, the athletic trainer offers resistance to the movement. Scapular downward rotation is tested with the athlete prone, his hand behind his back. He elevates his hand to the ceiling as the athletic trainer offers resistance at the scapula.

Since the biceps and triceps also influence the shoulder and can be involved in shoulder injuries, they should also be tested for strength deficiencies. The athlete can be sitting. With the elbow at 90° flexion, test the biceps as well as the triceps with isometric resistance.

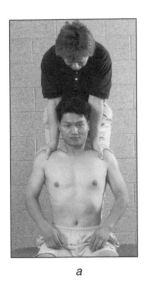

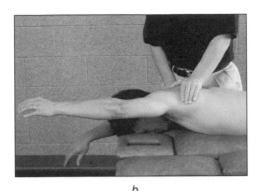

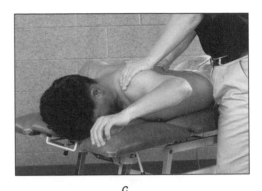

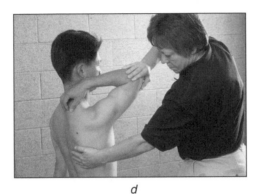

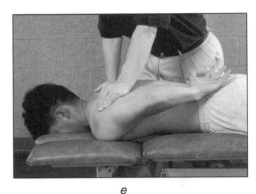

*a*

*b*

*c*

*d*

*e*

▌**Figure 4.24** Scapular motion strength tests for (a) elevation, (b) depression and upward rotation, (c) retraction, (d) protraction, and (e) downward rotation.

### Neurovascular Tests

Distal pulse should be periodically checked with all dislocations and fractures. If the athlete reports numbness, tingling, burning, or shooting pains distal to the acromion, a neurological assessment should also be part of the evaluation. The neurological tests include assessment of sensory, motor, and reflex components. These tests were discussed in chapter 3 on pages 68-70.

### Functional Tests

If the athlete's symptoms have subsided during the course of your evaluation and you determine that the injury was minor, you should perform functional tests before allowing the athlete back into the game or practice.

Functional tests for the injured shoulder, as for other body segment injuries, should accurately demonstrate the athlete's readiness to return to activity. These tests, then, should include specific activities particular to the athlete's sport. For example, if the athlete is a wrestler, functional tests can include handstands, resisted push-ups, and full-motion activities against resistance. If the athlete is a volleyball player, then overhead hitting, quick lateral overhead movements, and blocking shots will be part of the functional tests.

## OFF-FIELD ASSESSMENT

Often the athlete with shoulder pain will not seek treatment or evaluation immediately following injury. Soreness may not set in until hours later or even the next day. Signs and symptoms related to repetitive stress will also appear gradually over time. Therefore it is likely that the majority of your shoulder assessments will be for postacute and chronic injuries.

## Checklist for Sideline Assessment of the Shoulder and Arm

### History

Ask questions pertaining to the following:

✓ Chief complaint
✓ Mechanism of injury
✓ Unusual sounds or sensations
✓ Type and location of pain or symptoms
✓ Previous injury
✓ Previous injury to opposite extremity for bilateral comparison

### Observation

✓ Check for visible facial expressions of pain.
✓ Check for swelling, deformity, abnormal contours, or discoloration.
✓ Does athlete let arm hang and swing, or does he or she hold or splint it?
✓ Observe overall position, posture, and alignment (anterior, lateral, and posterior).
✓ Check muscle development—areas of muscular atrophy.
✓ Make bilateral comparison of acromions, SC joints, inferior border of scapula and scapular spine.
✓ See whether inferior tip of scapula is level with T7, superior medial ridge is at T2.

### Palpation

Palpate for pain, tenderness, and deformity over the following:

✓ SC joint, clavicle, AC joint, acromion, coracoid process, subacromial bursa, greater tuberosity, lesser tuberosity, bicipital groove
✓ Spine, superior and inferior angles of scapula, lower cervical and upper thoracic spinous processes

✓ Rotator cuff insertion
✓ Sternocleidomastoid muscle, pectoralis muscle
✓ Biceps tendon and muscle
✓ Trapezius muscle, rhomboid muscle, latissimus dorsi, serratus anterior
✓ Axillary structures

### Special Tests

✓ Glenohumeral stability tests
✓ Acromioclavicular stability tests
✓ Rotator cuff
✓ Biceps tests

### Range of Motion

✓ Active ROM for shoulder flexion/extension, abduction/adduction, horizontal adduction/abduction, and internal/external rotation
✓ Scapular elevation/depression, retraction/protraction, upward/downward rotation with motions just listed
✓ Passive ROM for shoulder motions listed
✓ Passive ROM for scapular motions listed
✓ Bilateral comparison

### Strength Tests

✓ Perform manual resistance against same motions as in AROM.
✓ Check bilaterally and note any pain or weakness.

### Neurovascular Tests

✓ Sensory
✓ Motor
✓ Distal pulse

### Functional Tests

### *History*

Gaining a good history from the athlete is essential in the off-field shoulder assessment, particularly when the athlete presents with chronic conditions.

In addition to the typical questions you will ask about the mechanism, nature, and severity of the injury, activity history is important if there was no specific injury and the pain has progressed over time. Does the athlete recall what activity he was performing when he first noticed the pain? Did the pain last through the rest of the activity? When does the pain occur now? Does it last all the way through the activity, persist after the activity, or interfere with other areas of daily life? Have there been any abrupt changes in training or weight-lifting practices? Do other activities aggravate or ease the symptoms? If there is a previous history of injury, when was the first and last occurrence; how often does the injury recur; what treatment was provided; and what was the outcome of treatment? Even if prior injuries were different from the current complaint, they can provide insight into potential causes of this new injury. For example, if the athlete's only prior injury was a clavicular fracture and the present injury seems to be related to the rotator cuff, perhaps the shoulder following the clavicular injury was never strengthened after a period of immobilization, resulting in weakness in cuff muscles and making them more susceptible to injury. These and other questions for postacute, chronic, or overuse injuries can help you identify the stage of the injury, its severity, and its irritability.

By the time you have finished taking the athlete's history, you should have a good idea of whether the injury is acute, subacute, or chronic (**S**tage), how irritable the injury is (**I**rritability), what structure is probably involved (**N**ature), and how severe the injury is (**S**everity). Once you have determined these SINS factors, you will have a better sense of the special tests that you should perform and how aggressive you can be.

### Observation

Observe how the athlete moves the shoulder, holds the arm, and removes a jacket or shirt; also note the general posture. Observe facial expressions both during relaxed sitting and during active movement.

The best observations of the injured shoulder are made with both shoulders exposed. Comparisons of symmetry are made from anterior and posterior views. Clavicle, scapular levels, and the balance, contour, and position of other structures as discussed for the sideline assessment are evaluated in the off-field assessment. Muscle atrophy is an indication of a more chronic problem, whereas discoloration indicates more acute injuries. Atrophy can be an indication of either muscle disuse or neural damage resulting in weakness.

### Differential Diagnosis

The shoulder and cervical regions are closely related, and it is sometimes difficult to identify whether the source of the injury is in the shoulder or the cervical area. The brachial plexus can also be a site of shoulder-related symptoms, since the complex runs through the axilla and can be damaged either during a shoulder injury (i.e., fracture or dislocation) or secondary to cervical trauma. You should eliminate these sources of shoulder symptoms any time the athlete's pain is distal to the acromion and you did not witness the injury.

Quick tests can eliminate the cervical and brachial plexus as sources of shoulder symptoms. These quick tests include cervical range of motion with overpressure at each end range (see chapter 3). If the symptoms are not reproduced with overpressure of these motions, you can perform an additional quick test in the cervical quadrant position. Place the athlete's head in lateral flexion, rotation, and extension to the side of symptoms and apply overpressure in the end position. The athlete may experience some discomfort in the neck, but a positive sign occurs only if any of the symptoms are reproduced.

Thoracic outlet syndrome (TOS) is another condition that you should eliminate if the athlete's signs and symptoms lead you to suspect this injury (see chapter 3). Specific tests for TOS will be discussed later, in the special tests section of this chapter.

### Range of Motion

In the athletic treatment facility, use the same range of motion tests as for the sideline assessment, checking for both quality and quantity of movement. Note whether the limitation is due to stiffness or pain. Note any capsular patterns of movement if the athlete's motion is incomplete. The shoulder's capsular pattern includes more limitation in external rotation than in abduction, more limitation in abduction than in flexion, and more limitation in flexion than in internal rotation. If the athlete's reduced range of motion follows a capsular pattern, you must perform a joint mobility assessment (see page 117) to establish locations and quantity of capsular restriction. If, for example, the athlete has no restriction of external rotation motion but is limited in abduction and flexion, a capsular pattern is not present, and reduced range of motion is caused by another factor.

### Strength

Manual muscle tests discussed in connection with the sideline assessment can also be used in the off-field examination. In addition, instrumented tests can more objectively define strength deficiencies. Use of instrumented strength tests will depend on the injury's severity and irritability, as maximal strength tests can further aggravate an easily irritated injury.

In cases in which machine assessment of strength is appropriate, isokinetic testing is frequently used to obtain objective results. Isokinetic machines can evaluate muscle activity (concentric and eccentric) in a variety of motions and joint positions, all at different speeds (figure 4.25).

You can obtain other objective strength measures with one-repetition maximum assessment using dumbbells or weight machines. If you use these, you should indicate on the evaluation form the position in which the athlete was tested, since different positions may produce different results. For example, when the athlete performs shoulder flexion in standing with a dumbbell, the maximum resistance will occur at 90° flexion, whereas in the supine position the maximum resistance occurs at the start of the motion; therefore different results can occur with the same weight lifted.

If the injury is very irritable or is severe enough to prevent an accurate test, it may be more prudent to defer the strength tests until the injury has calmed down sufficiently to produce more accurate results.

For more information on therapeutic exercise and the relationship between levers and resistance, refer to *Therapeutic Exercise for Athletic Injuries* (Houglum 2000), chapter 3.

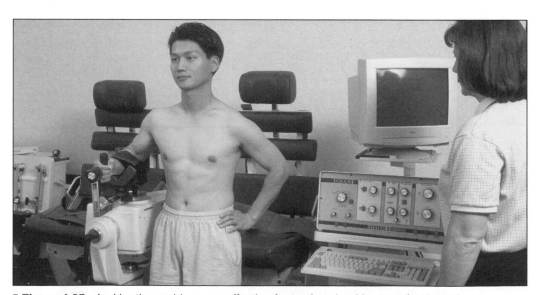

∎ **Figure 4.25**   Isokinetic machines are effective for testing shoulder muscle strength.

### Neurovascular Tests

The aim of neurological tests is to establish any differential diagnosis or evidence of neurological compromise. These tests include assessment of sensory, motor, and reflex components. As mentioned with reference to the sideline assessment, these tests should be performed on any athlete who reports symptoms of nerve pain including radiating pain down the arm, burning, tingling, or sharp pain or numbness. The specific tests are those described in the chapter on the cervical spine. Neurovascular tests associated with thoracic outlet syndrome are discussed later in this chapter beginning on page 116.

### Special Tests

By the time you reach this point in the evaluation, you should have a good idea which special tests are necessary to confirm or disprove your preliminary impressions. The special tests discussed in relation to the sideline assessment are also performed in the off-field assessment. In addition, you may need other special tests to assess chronic inflammatory and overuse conditions.

#### Rotator Cuff and Impingement Tests

Special tests for acute rotator cuff injuries were discussed in connection with the sideline assessment. Those tests described here are for suspected inflammation-based injuries. Since inflammatory conditions (tendinitis and bursitis) can be secondary to impingement of the rotator cuff, various impingement tests are discussed here.

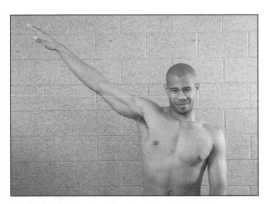

**I Figure 4.26**   Active impingement test.

### Active Impingement Test

This test identifies impingement of the active structures in the shoulder with the presence of a painful arc of motion. The athlete stands and actively abducts or flexes the shoulder through a full range of motion (figure 4.26). A positive test occurs when the athlete reports pain in the mid-arc of the motion.

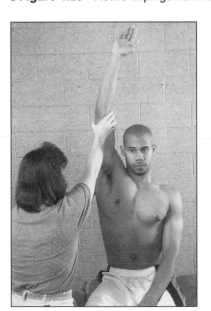

**I Figure 4.27**   Neer impingement test.

### Neer Impingement Test

The Neer impingement test is named after the orthopedic surgeon who first described it. It compresses the supraspinatus and biceps tendons and the subacromial bursa between the anterior acromion and greater tubercle. The athlete flexes the shoulder as far as possible, and the athletic trainer then passively flexes the shoulder to its end motion (figure 4.27). A positive sign occurs if the athlete has pain with the test, indicating impingement of either the biceps or supraspinatus tendon.

## Hawkins-Kennedy Test

This test is also referred to as the Hawkins test. This impingement test compresses the supraspinatus tendon against the coracoacromial ligament. With the athlete's arm flexed to 90°, forcefully move the shoulder into internal rotation (figure 4.28). A positive sign occurs when the athlete reports pain with the test and indicates impingement of the supraspinatus tendon.

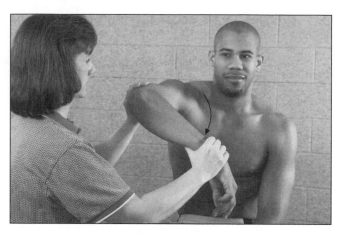

**Figure 4.28**   Hawkins-Kennedy Test.

## Empty Can Test

This test, also called the supraspinatus test, assesses the integrity of the supraspinatus. A positive result indicates a possible muscle tear or, more likely, tendon or suprascapular nerve pathology. The test is performed with the athlete sitting. The shoulder is placed in a position of scaption (abduction to 90° in a scapular plane, about 30° anterior to the frontal plane). Apply a downward force against the athlete, who attempts to prevent shoulder motion (figure 4.29). A positive result occurs when the athlete is unable to resist the force.

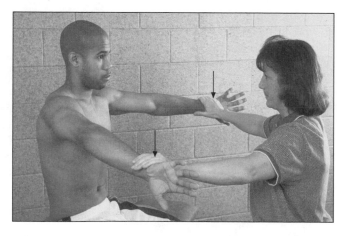

**Figure 4.29**   The Empty Can Test.

## Impingement Relief Test

If other active and passive impingement tests are positive, the impingement relief test (Corso 1995) can help you identify the involved structures. The athlete repeats the active impingement test three to five times and reports where the painful arc of motion begins with each movement, as well as how much pain is present on a 0- to 10-point scale. The active impingement test is then repeated: immediately to the onset of the painful arc, apply an inferior glide for an abduction movement (figure 4.30) or a posteroinferior glide with a flexion movement. If a complete resolution of the painful arc occurs with the test, the source of the injury is deficiency within the contractile tissues. Either the muscles that depress the humerus in the glenohumeral joint or the scapulothoracic muscles that rotate the scapula or create scapulohumeral rhythm are weak, imbalanced, or uncoordinated in their firing patterns.

If the athlete experiences some but not complete relief of the painful arc, both contractile tissue and inert tissue may be involved. In addition to the deficiencies already listed, you should suspect inert tissue tightness, especially in the inferior or posteroinferior capsule.

If the test produces no relief of pain, you should suspect inert tissues as the source of the athlete's painful arc of motion. Tightness of the capsule and glenohumeral ligaments may be the primary source of restriction.

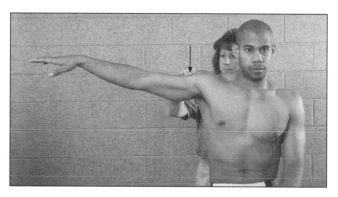

**∎ Figure 4.30** Impingement relief test with inferior glide for shoulder abduction.

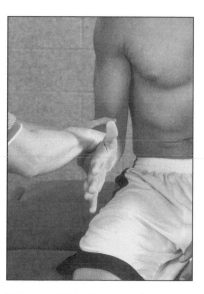

**∎ Figure 4.31** Yergason's test.

## Other Muscle and Tendon Pathology Tests

### Yergason's Test

**Yergason's test** is used to assess bicipital tendinitis and subluxation. It is not as effective as Speed's test for tendinitis, since the tendon does not move within the bicipital groove as much during this test. The elbow is positioned in 90° flexion, and the forearm is pronated. The athletic trainer resists the athlete's attempt to supinate the forearm and externally rotate the shoulder (figure 4.31). A positive test will produce bicipital pain during the resistive movement. If the transverse humeral ligament is torn, an audible or palpable "pop" may occur as the biceps tendon subluxes over the lesser tuberosity

## Pectoralis Major Contracture Test

This test is used to evaluate the tightness of the pectoralis major. Tightness in this muscle can impact shoulder impingement, so you should evaluate chronic shoulder injuries for pectoralis major tightness. The athlete lies supine with his hands behind his head. With your assistance, he should then attempt to lower his elbows to the table (figure 4.32). A positive test occurs if the elbows do not reach the table.

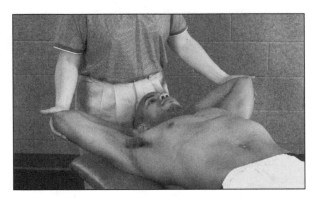

■ **Figure 4.32**  Pectoralis major contracture test.

## Acromioclavicular Compression Test

This test assesses the integrity of the AC joint. With the athlete sitting, passively flex her shoulder to 90° and horizontally adduct the shoulder (see figure 4.19). A positive sign is pain in the AC joint. Crepitus may also be present.

### Thoracic Outlet Syndrome Tests

There are a number of tests for TOS. As has been mentioned, TOS can result from brachial plexus or subclavian artery compression from a number of primary causes. In assessing TOS you should attempt to either reproduce the athlete's symptoms or reduce circulation, so you must observe for the presence of either of these signs. Since there are several causes for TOS, there are also several tests for identifying it. Some of the more common ones will be presented here.

## Adson's Test

Palpate the radial pulse of the involved side, and instruct the athlete to rotate his head to the same side. Then as he extends his neck, extend and externally rotate his arm (figure 4.33). In this position, the athlete takes a deep breath and holds it while you palpate for a pulse. If the pulse is diminished or gone, the test is positive.

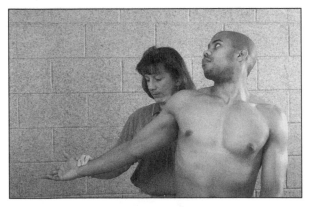

■ **Figure 4.33**  Adson's test.

## Allen Test

Locate the athlete's radial pulse and then position his arm with the elbow at 90° flexion and the shoulder in external rotation and horizontal abduction. The athlete then rotates his head away from the tested arm (figure 4.34). The test is positive if the pulse is diminished or absent.

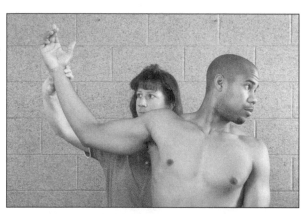

**▌ Figure 4.34**  Allen test.

## Military Brace Position

The military brace position test is also called the costoclavicular syndrome test. Palpate the athlete's radial pulse with his elbow and shoulder in full extension. Position the arm into hyperextension and external rotation; the athlete then rotates the head away from the side being tested (figure 4.35). A positive test occurs if the pulse is diminished or absent.

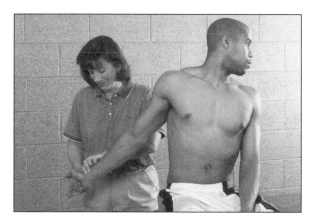

**▌ Figure 4.35**  Military brace position.

### Joint Mobility

As noted in chapter 2, joint mobility is divided into two types, physiological and accessory (see page 42). Whereas physiological movements are assessed earlier, during range of motion testing, accessory movements are assessed after completion of the special tests, using joint mobilization techniques.

Assessment of accessory joint mobility of the glenohumeral, scapulothoracic, and clavicular joints is performed with the athlete reclined in a comfortable position. Most of the techniques are performed with the athlete supine; but in a few the athlete is side-lying, and in some the athlete is prone. Supine positioning is preferred for most glenohumeral motions because it permits stabilization of the scapula and relaxation of the surrounding muscles; this increases the chances of an accurate assessment. Joint play in various directions is assessed by comparison of the involved side to the uninvolved side for each of the joints. A positive result occurs if the injured shoulder has different joint play than the uninvolved side or if movement reproduces the athlete's symptoms. These tests determine mobility of the joint capsule in the various planes of movement. Joint capsular restriction will limit shoulder range of motion. For example, if the inferior posterior capsule is limited, the athlete will have limited shoulder flexion and internal rotation. On the other hand, if the anterior capsule has excessive mobility, the joint will have anterior instability that can affect shoulder stability during follow-through in throwing. If the anterior capsule is lax, it is also likely that the athlete's symptoms may include shoulder impingement.

### Glenohumeral Joint Mobility

The loose-packed position of the glenohumeral joint is 55° flexion and 20-30° horizontal abduction, so many of the joint assessment techniques are initially performed in this position. This allows the greatest passive movement possible and provides a reference point for comparison with the uninvolved shoulder and with future assessments.

The loose-packed position is the position of the joint at which the ligaments are at their resting length and under the least amount of tension.

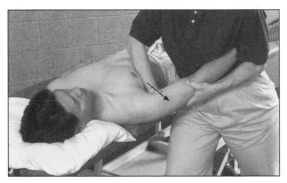

**■ Figure 4.36**   Glenohumeral distraction test.

### Distraction

The technique of distraction is typically used first to provide a general idea of mobility—an overall impression of tightness or looseness in the joint. With the athlete supine, stand between the athlete's side and his arm. Support his arm with one hand while placing your mobilizing hand high in the axilla with your fingers on the posterior arm and your thumb on the anterior arm just distal to the shoulder joint (figure 4.36). Apply a lateral force to move the humerus away from the glenoid fossa, and assess the quality and quantity of mobility compared to those for the opposite shoulder.

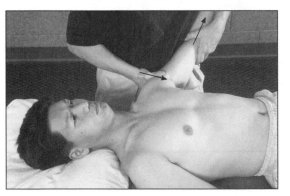

**■ Figure 4.37**   Glenohumeral caudal (inferior) glide.

### Caudal Glide

This maneuver, also called an inferior glide, assesses mobility of the inferior capsule. Limited abduction, caused by a restricted capsule, will demonstrate tightness in this test. A glenohumeral joint with a history of inferior dislocations may have an abnormally loose glide.

With the athlete lying supine, stand at his side on the lateral side of his arm. Passively place the arm in the shoulder's loose-packed position. Place the mobilizing hand on top of the athlete's shoulder immediately lateral to the acromion. The stabilizing hand applies a slight distraction of the glenohumeral joint, and the mobilizing hand applies a caudally directed force (figure 4.37).

## Posterior Glide

The posterior glide is used to evaluate the mobility of the posterior capsule. If the athlete's posterior capsule is restricted, physiological motions of horizontal abduction, internal rotation, and flexion will be limited.

The athlete lies supine with his shoulder over the edge of the table. Standing between the athlete's side and his arm, support the shoulder in a loose-packed position with the athlete's arm secured between your side and your stabilizing arm (figure 4.38). Place your mobilizing hand over the anterior shoulder just distal to the acromion. As you apply some joint distraction with your stabilizing hand, apply a downward force with the mobilizing hand to assess posterior capsule movement.

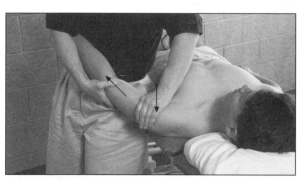

**Figure 4.38** Posterior glide test.

## Anterior Glide

This maneuver is used to assess anterior capsule mobility. An athlete with a restricted anterior capsule will present limited shoulder extension, horizontal abduction, and external rotation. If the anterior capsule is lax, a profile of impingement, anterior instability, or glenoid labrum tear may be present.

The athlete lies prone with his shoulder over the edge of the table. Stand alongside him, facing the top of the table with your supporting hand; position his arm in a loose-packed position. Place your mobilizing hand on the posterior shoulder just distal to the posterior acromion. As your stabilizing hand applies a slight distraction force, the mobilizing hand applies a posterior-to-anterior force to the glenohumeral joint (figure 4.39).

### Scapulothoracic Joint

The scapula rests against the rib cage, separated from the ribs by muscles. It is not a true joint in the sense of two bones supported by ligaments, but restricted glenohumeral movement can cause limitation of normal scapular motion on the thorax. If the athlete demonstrates reduced glenohumeral physiological motion, the mobility of the scapula on the ribs should be assessed.

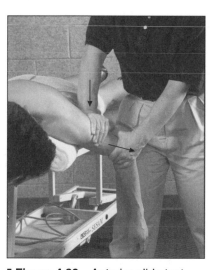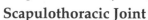

**Figure 4.39** Anterior glide test.

The scapula moves on the thorax in several planes. It glides superiorly and inferiorly, glides laterally and medially, and rotates. For assessment of these motions, the athlete is in side-lying with the shoulder that will be examined on top. The athletic trainer supports the arm by placing his or her own forearm under the athlete's upper arm, and grasps the athlete's scapula at its superior aspect and inferior angle. The hands alternate in applying the mobilizing force and assessing the scapular movement. For example, when you are assessing scapular inferior mobility, your

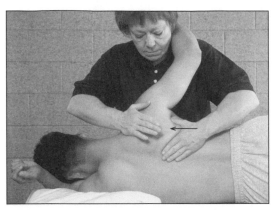

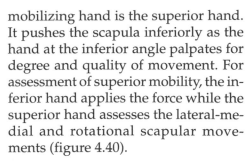

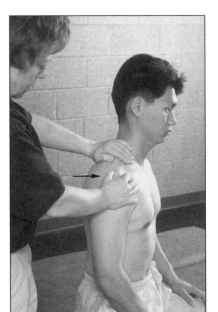

**Figure 4.40** Scapulothoracic joint mobility test.

mobilizing hand is the superior hand. It pushes the scapula inferiorly as the hand at the inferior angle palpates for degree and quality of movement. For assessment of superior mobility, the inferior hand applies the force while the superior hand assesses the lateral-medial and rotational scapular movements (figure 4.40).

### Clavicular Joints

Both the AC and the SC joints should be assessed if glenohumeral physiological motions are limited. These joints should also be assessed if an injury to either joint is suspected.

### Acromioclavicular Joint

With the athlete sitting, stand behind him and place a stabilizing hand over the glenohumeral joint and the thumb of your mobilizing thumb on the posterior aspect of the lateral clavicle (figure 4.41). Apply an anteriorly directed force to the posterior clavicle just medial to the AC joint.

### Sternoclavicular Joint

For assessment of the SC joint, the athlete is supine and the athletic trainer stands either at the head or at the side of the table facing the athlete. Although the joint can be assessed in various maneuvers, a commonly used technique is the posterior glide. To perform this, place the pads of one or both of your thumbs directly over the anterior surface of the clavicle, just lateral to the sternum (figure 4.42), applying an anterior-to-posterior force.

**Figure 4.41** Acromioclavicular joint mobility test.

### *Palpation*

Palpation is performed as outlined for the sideline assessment. Comparison of right and left structures for symmetry, atrophy, nodules, and areas of tenderness or crepitus is important. Even though the athlete's injury may not be recent, spasm may still be present. You may also find active trigger points with palpation. Follow a systematic routine to palpate all aspects of the shoulder region and its related structures. As with the sideline assessment, a logical

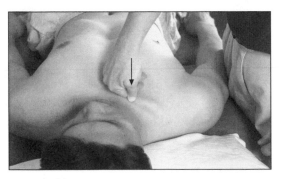

**Figure 4.42** Sternoclavicular joint mobility test.

progression would be to start at the anterior shoulder and progress laterally and to finish palpation in the posterior aspect. If the athlete's area of pain is the anterior shoulder, however, it may be better to begin at the posterior shoulder and progress to the anterior shoulder area to complete the palpation in the region of primary complaint.

### *Functional Tests*

Functional tests are critical for the shoulder region. Because of the high velocity and strong eccentric actions inherent in overhead throwing motions, pain and symptoms may occur during these dynamic activities that were not present, or were relatively mild, during your assessment. For this same reason, functional tests for the overhead athlete should be conducted in a gradual progression in skill complexity and velocity. For example, the gymnast may be asked initially to perform a regular push-up. If this activity does not reproduce her symptoms, an inverted push-up may be the next test. If she performs these exercises without symptoms, she then may be asked to perform an activity such as a front walkover or a more aggressive activity such as a running pass with multiple handsprings or other maneuvers.

Remember to tailor your functional tests to the specific demands of the athlete's sport and position. Consider the different forces and stresses that would be placed on the shoulder within a sport (i.e., breaststroke vs. butterfly specialist), as well as between sports (i.e., gymnast vs. thrower vs. tennis player vs. lineman).

For guidelines and examples of functional tests to use prior to the return of an athlete to full participation, refer to *Therapeutic Exercise for Athletic Injuries* (Houglum 2000), chapter 1.

---

### Checklist for Off-Field Assessment of the Shoulder and Arm

**History**

Ask questions pertaining to the following:

✓ Chief complaint
✓ Mechanism of injury
✓ Unusual sounds or sensations
✓ Type and location of pain or symptoms
✓ Previous injury
✓ Previous injury to opposite extremity for bilateral comparison

If chronic, ascertain:

✓ Duration of onset
✓ Aggravating and easing activities
✓ Training history

**Observation**

✓ Check for visible facial expressions of pain.
✓ Check for swelling, deformity, abnormal contours, or discoloration.
✓ Does athlete let arm hang and swing, or does he or she hold or splint it?
✓ Observe overall position, posture, and alignment (anterior, lateral, and posterior).
✓ Check muscle development bilaterally—areas of muscular atrophy.

✓ Make bilateral comparison of acromions, SC joints, inferior border of scapula and scapular spine.
✓ Check scapular position (inferior tip of scapula is level with T7, superior medial ridge is at T2).

**Differential Diagnosis**

✓ Clear cervical region with overpressure tests—quadrant position.
✓ Eliminate thoracic outlet and brachial plexus pathologies.

**Range of Motion**

✓ Active ROM for shoulder flexion/extension, abduction/adduction, horizontal adduction/abduction, and internal/external rotation
✓ Scapular elevation/depression, retraction/protraction, upward/downward rotation with motions just listed
✓ Passive ROM for shoulder motions listed
✓ Passive ROM for scapular motions listed
✓ Bilateral comparison

**Strength Tests**

✓ Perform manual resistance against same motions as in AROM.
✓ Check bilaterally and note any pain or weakness.

*(continued)*

## Checklist for Off-Field Assessment of the Shoulder and Arm *(continued)*

**Neurovascular Tests**

✓ Sensory

✓ Motor

✓ Reflex

✓ Distal pulse

**Special Tests**

✓ Glenohumeral stability tests

✓ Acromioclavicular stability tests

✓ Rotator cuff and impingement tests

✓ Biceps tests (Speed's and Yergason's)

✓ Pectoralis major contraction test

✓ Acromioclavicular stability tests

✓ TOS tests

**Joint Mobility**

✓ Glenohumeral joint

✓ Scapulothoracic joint

✓ Clavicular joint

**Palpation**

Palpate for pain, tenderness, and deformity over the following:

✓ SC joint, clavicle, AC joint, acromion, coracoid process, subacromial bursa, greater tuberosity, lesser tuberosity, bicipital groove

✓ Spine of scapula

✓ Rotator cuff

✓ Sternocleidomastoid muscle, pectoralis muscle

✓ Biceps tendon and muscle

✓ Trapezius muscle, rhomboid muscle, latissimus dorsi, serratus anterior

✓ Axillary structures

**Functional Tests**

# SUMMARY

1. *Discuss the types of overuse injuries that commonly result from repetitive overhead throwing activities.*

   The considerable velocity and eccentric forces that occur repetitively over a large range of motion during overhead throwing activities are a common cause of chronic conditions of the shoulder. Strains in the rotator cuff and biceps tendon that act to decelerate the arm during throwing are common. Traction forces of the biceps tendon attachment to the glenoid labrum during deceleration can cause bicipital tendinitis and tears of the glenoid labrum. Glenoid labral tears can also result from chronic instability. In addition, throwing athletes often experience chronic instability and shoulder impingement.

2. *Identify the signs and symptoms associated with various stages of rotator cuff impingement.*

   Rotator cuff impingement is caused by encroachment in the subacromial space that has decreased the space through which the supraspinatus and subacromial bursa pass underneath the subacromial arch. Impingement is most commonly seen in occupations and sporting activities involving repetitive overhead motions. Signs and symptoms for impingement range from mild pain with activity and no loss of strength or range of motion (stage I) to degenerative changes and full thickness tears of the rotator cuff, resulting in considerable pain and disability (stage III).

3. *Demonstrate an on-field assessment for the shoulder and upper arm, and discuss criteria for immediate referral and mode of transportation from the field.*

As with other injuries, an on-field assessment of a shoulder injury requires that the athletic trainer be observant in approaching the athlete. Following a primary survey, the injured part is palpated to determine obvious signs of fracture or dislocation. The athletic trainer must determine the injury's severity, assess the level of pain, evaluate for shock, and establish neurovascular integrity of the limb before a decision can be made on how to transport the athlete off the field.

4. *Perform a thorough and sequential sideline assessment for the shoulder and upper arm, and discuss criteria for determining return to activity.*

In the sideline assessment, the athletic trainer can perform a more specific and detailed evaluation of the severity of the injury in order to determine the athlete's ability to return to sport participation that day. The sideline assessment includes a thorough palpation, an investigation of the shoulder's active and passive range of motion, strength, neurovascular status, and assessment of specific structures. Palpation determines the presence of spasm, deformity, and tissue restriction. Special tests of these structures address tissue integrity, joint stability, and pathology that would warrant excluding the athlete from immediate return to participation. Only if findings are negative or the injury is deemed minor are functional tests performed.

5. *Perform a thorough and sequential off-field assessment, including considerations for differential diagnosis from cervical pathologies.*

Athletes commonly report to the athletic trainer with an injury that either occurred at some delay following acute trauma or with a gradual onset over a period of time. In either case, the athletic trainer must thoroughly assess the athlete's shoulder to define the SINS of the injury. These results will determine the treatment program. It is important to obtain a complete history from the athlete, including information on training and activities of daily living. The athletic trainer closely observes the athlete throughout the process to note any abnormal posture or any restricted use of the shoulder or arm. Differential diagnoses to eliminate other sources of the symptoms that may emanate from the cervical region should be part of the off-field assessment. In addition to the tests used in the sideline assessment, additional tests and joint accessory assessment are incorporated to assess chronic overuse and inflammatory conditions.

6. *Describe and perform the various special tests for evaluation of glenohumeral instabilities.*

Several tests are used to determine instability of the glenohumeral joint, which can occur in anterior, inferior, posterior, or multiplanar directions. The more frequently used tests include the load and shift test, relocation and apprehension test, anterior drawer test, posterior drawer test, sulcus sign, and clunk test.

7. *Describe and perform the various special tests for the assessment of rotator cuff pathology.*

Special tests for rotator cuff pathology include those for acute strains and those for chronic impingement syndromes. For acute injuries, the drop arm test assesses tears in the rotator cuff. Impingement tests include the active impingement, Neer impingement, Hawkins-Kennedy, empty can, and impingement relief tests.

# REVIEW QUESTIONS

1. What is the difference between primary and secondary impingement? Which is more commonly seen in the young athlete?

2. Why would glenohumeral instability be a contributing factor to an impingement syndrome?

3. What is the role of the scapula in glenohumeral motion, and what impact could scapular dysfunction have on shoulder injuries?

4. Name three peripheral nerve injuries that may occur with trauma to the shoulder. What are the signs and symptoms associated with each? How would you test for them?

5. What are the primary conditions that you would want to rule out in an on-field shoulder assessment before moving the athlete from the field?

6. What tests are used to determine glenohumeral joint mobility? How do you determine whether instability or restriction exists?

# CRITICAL THINKING QUESTIONS

1. In your off-field assessment, how would you differentiate between a primary and secondary impingement? Discuss what special tests you would use to distinguish between these conditions and what findings you would expect for each.

2. You are called out onto the football field and find an athlete down in considerable pain, holding his arm. He is the quarterback and states that he had his arm cocked back to throw and was hit on his arm. Upon palpation, you feel up underneath his shoulder pads and feel a flattening of the deltoid muscle. What injury might you suspect, and how would you proceed with your evaluation?

3. A 15-year-old pitcher comes to you complaining of pain in his shoulder, particularly with hard throwing. He states that sometimes when he throws a fastball he gets a "twang" in the shoulder, followed by a tingling sensation down his arm. What shoulder conditions might you suspect in this young athlete? What types of questions would you ask, and how would you proceed with your evaluation?

4. An 18-year-old soccer player comes into the athletic training room holding his arm at this side. He states he was out "goofing around" on the field and fell on his shoulder. He points to pain at the tip of his shoulder and is unable to raise his arm because of pain. You have already noted some swelling over his acromion. What type(s) of injuries might you suspect given this history? What tests might you perform, and how would you determine the severity of this injury?

# CITED REFERENCES

Corso, G. 1995. Impingement relief test: An adjunctive procedure to traditional assessment of shoulder impingement syndrome. *J Orthop Sports Phys Ther* 22(5):183-192.

Deltoff, M.N., and Bressler, H.B. 1989. Atypical scapular fracture. *Am J Sports Med* 17(2):292-295.

Hawkins, R.J., and Mohtadi, N. 1991. Clinical evaluation of shoulder instabilities. *Clin J Sports Med* 1:59-66.

Jobe, F.W., and Pink, M. 1993. Classification and treatment of shoulder dysfunction in the overhand athlete. *J Ortho Sports Phys Ther* 18(2):427-432.

Meister, K., and Andrews, J.R. 1993. Classification and treatment of rotator cuff injuries in the overhand athlete. *J Ortho Sports Phys Ther* 18(2):413-421.

Neer, C. 1973. Impingement lesions. *Clin Orthop* 173:70-77.

Ogawa, K., and Yoshida, A. 1998. Throwing fracture of the humeral shaft. *Am J Sports Med* 26(2):242-246.

Silliman, J.F., and Dean, M.T. 1993. Neurovascular injuries to the shoulder. *J Ortho Sports Phys Ther* 18(2):442-448.

## ADDITIONAL RESOURCES

Houglum, P.A. 2000. *Therapeutic exercise for athletic i5njuries.* Champaign, IL: Human Kinetics.

Jensen, K.L. 1999. The shoulder. In D.H. Perrin (ed.), *The injured athlete* (3d ed., pp. 241-280). Philadelphia: Lippincott-Raven.

Magee, D.J., and Reid, D.C. 1996. Shoulder injuries. In J.E. Zachazewski, D.J. Magee, and W.S. Quillen (eds.), *Athletic injuries and rehabilitation* (1st ed., pp. 509-542). Philadelphia: Saunders.

# CHAPTER FIVE

# Elbow
# and Forearm

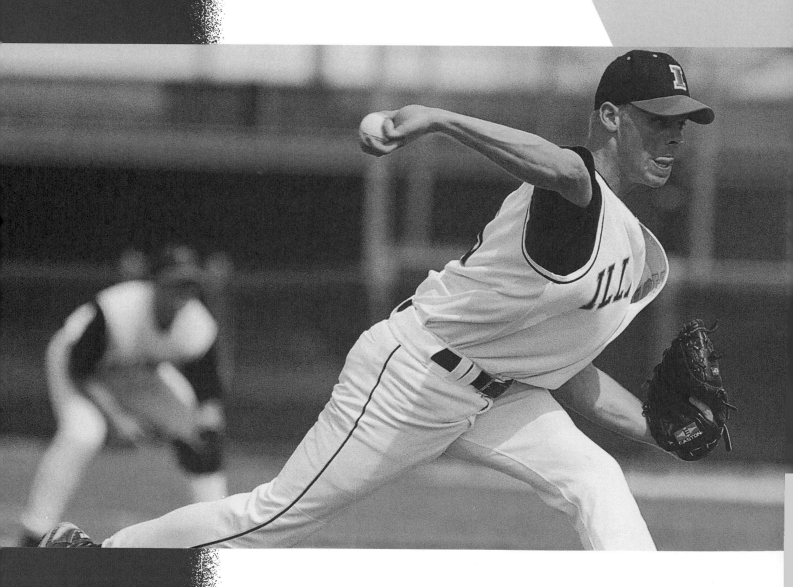

# OBJECTIVES

At the completion of this chapter, the reader will be able to do the following:

1. Describe the etiology, signs and symptoms, and potential complications associated with acute and chronic injuries of the elbow and forearm commonly encountered in physically active people

2. Identify the common pathologies associated with repetitive valgus overload stresses in the throwing athlete

3. Identify potential causes of forearm compartment syndrome and the 5 P's of neurovascular compromise

4. Identify the various anatomical sites and signs and symptoms associated with nerve compression syndromes

5. Describe the normal anatomical alignment, carrying angle, and range of motion of the elbow joint

6. Demonstrate an on-field assessment for the elbow and forearm, and determine criteria for immediate medical referral and mode of transportation from the field

7. Perform a sequential and thorough sideline assessment of the elbow and forearm, noting criteria for referral and return to activity

8. Perform a sequential and thorough off-field assessment of the elbow and forearm, noting considerations for differential diagnosis

Randy was a 14-year-old baseball player who lived for Saturdays when he pitched for his Little League team. As he was warming up for a big game, he felt that same pain on the inside of his elbow that he had been noticing for months. He wasn't overly worried about it—a friend of his dad's had looked at it and said it was just some tendinitis that would eventually go away. This was someone who should know, after all, because he was an avid golfer and had once had the same symptoms.

In the second inning, Randy noticed that his arm was more sore than usual. But he was facing the toughest batter on the other team, so he decided to throw a hard, fast ball for a strikeout that would end the inning. As Randy wound up and threw the ball, he felt a "snap" and tremendous pain in his elbow.

The news at the emergency room wasn't good. Randy had avulsed a piece of bone off of his medial elbow and would be out of action for a very long time.

On Monday, he went by and saw Jill, the athletic trainer at his high school, and told her what had happened.

"Why didn't you tell me you were having pain, Randy?" asked Jill.

"I just thought it was tendinitis. . . . A friend of my dad's had the same thing and I figured it would just go away on its own. . . . I didn't know something like this could happen," Randy said, dejected.

"Randy, you're young and your bones are still growing," Jill explained. "They will be weaker in certain areas than your muscles and tendons until you get a few years older. As a young athlete, you will have different injuries than an older adult. So even though your pain may be the same, your injury probably isn't. . . . Pain is never something you should ignore, particularly when it is near a bone. Next time something is painful, you should tell me right away—understood?"

"Yes," said Randy. "I promise to tell you right away next time . . . if there is a next time."

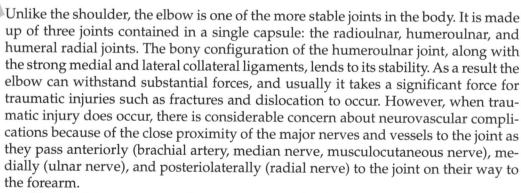

Unlike the shoulder, the elbow is one of the more stable joints in the body. It is made up of three joints contained in a single capsule: the radioulnar, humeroulnar, and humeral radial joints. The bony configuration of the humeroulnar joint, along with the strong medial and lateral collateral ligaments, lends to its stability. As a result the elbow can withstand substantial forces, and usually it takes a significant force for traumatic injuries such as fractures and dislocation to occur. However, when traumatic injury does occur, there is considerable concern about neurovascular complications because of the close proximity of the major nerves and vessels to the joint as they pass anteriorly (brachial artery, median nerve, musculocutaneous nerve), medially (ulnar nerve), and posteriolaterally (radial nerve) to the joint on their way to the forearm.

Chronic injuries commonly occur as a result of physical activity. A variety of medial stress injuries can occur in both young and older athletes due to valgus overload forces associated with overhead throwing activities. Individuals engaging in sports such as tennis and golf also frequently experience repetitive stress injuries. As you will find, and as the scenario suggests, the young, competitive athlete will present unique pathologies that should always be considered in the evaluative process. As you read this chapter, consider the common types of repetitive stress injuries and the variety of conditions that can be associated with each. Through the assessment techniques you will learn in this chapter, you will be able to identify and differentiate between the involved structures.

# INJURIES OF THE ELBOW AND FOREARM

The ability to perform athletic skills involving the upper extremities is dependent on the integrity of the bones, ligaments, and muscles of the elbow and forearm to help position the hand for functional activity. In order to allow full mobility at the elbow joint, the elbow and forearm are typically unprotected during athletic activity and thus exposed to a variety of contact injuries. Injuries associated with the repetitive forces inherent in overhead throwing and racket sports are also quite common.

## ACUTE SOFT TISSUE INJURIES

Acute soft tissue injuries at the elbow and forearm include contusions, ligament and capsular sprains, and muscle/tendon strains.

### Contusions

During sport activity, contusions frequently occur to the muscles of the forearm and to the superficial bony surfaces of the elbow because of direct contact with another player (e.g., blocking in football), a sport implement (e.g., lacrosse stick or pitched ball), or the ground. Signs and symptoms include point tenderness localized over the area of contact and ecchymosis. Direct blows to the olecranon process of the ulna will frequently cause inflammation or bleeding in the overlying olecranon bursa resulting in significant bursal swelling, mild to moderate pain, and limited elbow flexion. Because of the superficial course of the ulnar nerve between the medial epicondyle of the humerus and the olecranon process of the elbow, this nerve is vulnerable to contusions. With direct blows to the ulnar nerve, the athlete will complain of radiating pain down the medial aspect of the forearm, the hand, and into the fourth and fifth fingers. Contusions to the extensor or flexor muscle masses of the forearm may produce symptoms of decreased range of motion (ROM) and pain during muscular stretch or active motion. Although contusions to the forearm muscles are rarely serious or debilitating, it is important to realize that severe bleeding within a muscular compartment can cause a significant rise in intracompartmental pressure and compromise neurovascular structures. The resulting **compartment syndrome**, a very serious limb-threatening condition, will be discussed later in this chapter.

*Varus is a laterally directed force or angulation of a joint.*

*Valgus is a medially directed force or angulation of a joint.*

### Sprain

The elbow is a relatively stable joint because of its bony configuration and strong collateral ligaments. However, acute stretching or tearing of ligament and capsular structures can occur in sport due to excessive joint loading resulting from rotational, hyperextension, and varus and valgus forces imposed on the elbow. These high-level joint forces can be created both internally by muscular forces within the body and externally through contact with another player or object.

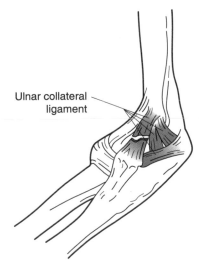

Ulnar collateral ligament

**Figure 5.1** Ulnar collateral ligament tear.

#### Ulnar (Medial) Collateral Ligament Sprains

Acute stretching or tearing of the ulnar collateral ligament (UCL) most often occurs as a result of a traumatic valgus force (figure 5.1). The anterior band of the UCL is the primary structure that limits or resists valgus forces and thus is more commonly injured than the posterior or transverse bands. Excessive valgus force can be created when an individual falls on an outstretched hand; these forces also occur in sports such as wrestling or football in which the athlete is bearing weight on the hands and contact is made to the lateral aspect of the elbow. Acute ruptures of the UCL can also result from overhead throwing motions such as baseball pitching and javelin throwing. However, these ruptures typically occur secondary to an underlying chronic condition of repetitive valgus loading during the late cocking/early acceleration phases of the throwing motion. This repetitive traction force on the medial structures can weaken the ligament over time until it eventually fails. In these cases, the athlete typically will have experienced medial elbow pain for months prior to the acute injury (Jobe, Stark, and Lombardo 1986). It is important to recognize UCL injuries, particularly in throwers, to ensure adequate healing and to avoid chronic instability problems.

Signs and symptoms of UCL sprains include sudden pain following a valgus-type force to the elbow. A sensation of a "pop" may or may not be reported. There will be point tenderness over the anterior band of the UCL. Depending on severity, there may be significant swelling and decreased ROM, with the athlete holding the elbow in a flexed position for comfort. Pain is reproduced with valgus stress, and instability may or may not be noted with second- and third-degree sprains. Because of the close communication of the ulnar nerve with the medial elbow, it is not uncommon to have associated symptoms of ulnar nerve irritation with these injuries.

### Radial (Lateral) Collateral Ligament Sprains

Injuries to the lateral collateral ligament occur much less frequently than medial collateral ligament injuries, since direct traction or varus forces to the lateral aspect of the elbow are rare during athletic activity. Isolated injuries to the lateral collateral ligament are thought to occur most often with the elbow hyperextended and forearm supinated (Tyrdal and Olsen 1998). This mechanism can occur with a fall on an extended elbow or in an athlete who stretches out his arm to stop a ball or an opponent. Although infrequent, lateral traction forces at the elbow during extension follow-through or deceleration phases of throwing can also injure the lateral collateral ligament (Andrews and Whiteside 1993).

Signs and symptoms associated with injuries to the lateral collateral ligament include pain, point tenderness, and swelling to the lateral aspect of the elbow. Pain may be reproduced with forced hyperextension and supination of the forearm and with varus stress. Instability is rarely noted with straight varus stress testing. If left unchecked, lateral collateral ligament tears can lead to posterolateral rotary instability of the elbow, and the athlete may complain of painful and recurrent locking or snapping with activity (Behr and Altchek 1997).

### Anterior Capsular Sprains

Anterior capsular sprains can occur with forced hyperextension of the elbow (Andrews and Whiteside 1993). Typical mechanisms for forced-hyperextension injuries include using an outstretched arm to stop a ball or an opponent, and falling with the arm outstretched and elbow extended. Young athletes with hyperlaxity of the joint and insufficient muscular strength may be more prone to hyperextension injuries than other athletes are (Andrews and Whiteside 1993). Signs and symptoms include pain and tenderness in the anterior compartment, with the athlete often apprehensive of fully extending the joint. The athlete may also complain of pain posteriorly where the olecranon process has been "jammed" or forced into the olecranon fossa. Severe hyperextension force mechanisms can also result in collateral ligament sprains, elbow dislocations, and fractures.

## Strains

Acute strains of the muscles and tendons around the elbow joint can result from a one-time episode of excessive overload or stretch.

### Flexor/Pronator and Extensor/Supinator Mass Strains

Strains to the wrist flexor/pronator muscle mass can occur with any activity that produces a forceful "snapping" of the wrist into flexion and pronation, such as a tennis serve, javelin throw, or racquetball forehand. Excessive eccentric loads that force the wrist into extension and supination during active wrist flexion and pronation movements, such as the impact of the ball forcing the racket back, can also result in strain to this muscle mass. Similarly, wrist extensor/supinator muscle mass strains typically result from forceful wrist extension movements and eccentric loads forcing the wrist into flexion and pronation while the wrist is concentrically extending or supinating. These extension injuries are often associated with backhand stroke mechanics in racket sports.

Signs and symptoms for acute strains to the forearm muscles include acute pain and tenderness over the involved muscle mass, typically near its proximal attachment and the myotendon junction. Consequently a strain near the origin may be difficult to distinguish from an acute tendinitis or epicondylitis (see section on tendinitis and epicondylitis further on). The athlete will complain of pain with active and resistive motion and with passive stretch. Severity of symptoms and disability will be consistent with those of a first-, second-, or third-degree muscle strain, although third-degree strains of the wrist flexor and extensor masses are quite rare.

### Distal Biceps Tendon

Injuries to the distal biceps tendon near or at its insertion at the radial tuberosity are rare in comparison to injuries at its proximal attachment. Distal biceps tendon strains are usually associated with a violent eccentric extension force or a ballistic flexion force against a heavy or immovable resistance. Distal biceps tendon injuries occur most often in heavy resistance training and competitive weight lifting. Injury may also occur during a football tackle or wrestling takedown when the elbow is forcibly hyperextended while the biceps is contracting. Signs and symptoms of tendon strain include immediate burning or pain in the anterior cubital area with point tenderness near the insertion on the radial tuberosity. There may be weakness and pain with active or resistive elbow flexion and supination. With tendon rupture (figure 5.2),

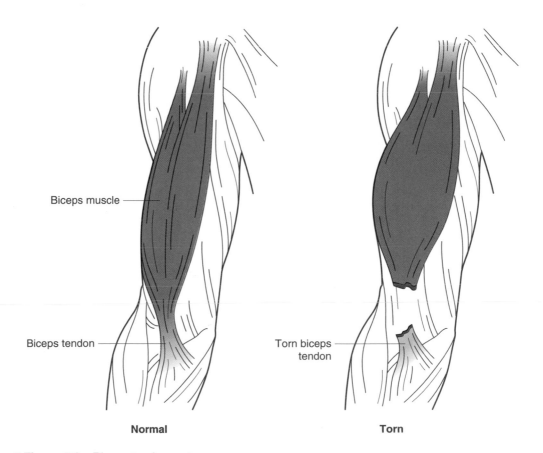

Biceps muscle

Biceps tendon

Torn biceps tendon

**Normal**

**Torn**

**∎ Figure 5.2** Biceps tendon rupture.

the athlete will often complain of feeling a pop or immediate sharp pain, or both, at the time of injury. A palpable defect and deformity will be observed anteriorly as the muscle retracts proximally into the upper arm. Antecubital swelling is often present. The athlete will demonstrate marked weakness with elbow flexion and supination.

### Distal Triceps Tendon

Strains and rupture of the distal triceps tendon are extremely rare but can occur with forced flexion during active extension, elbow dislocation, or a direct blow to the posterior elbow (Alley and Pappas 1995). Signs and symptoms include localized pain, swelling, and ecchymosis. The athlete will demonstrate a diminished capacity or an inability to extend the elbow against resistance. There may be a palpable defect in the distal tendon near its insertion to the olecranon.

## CHRONIC OR OVERUSE SOFT TISSUE INJURIES

Chronic or overuse soft tissue injuries, the most commonly occurring elbow injuries, are typically associated with overhead throwing motions or racket sports. During these activities, the soft tissue structures of the elbow are susceptible to repetitive overuse and microtrauma that can result in chronic inflammatory conditions, fibrotic changes within the tissue, or instabilities due to stretch or weakening of joint stabilizing structures.

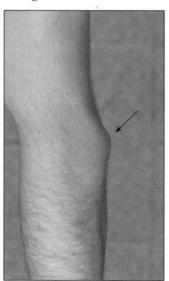

**▌Figure 5.3** Olecranon bursitis.

### Bursitis

Olecranon **bursitis** is an inflammatory condition of fluid accumulation in the subcutaneous **bursa** overlying the olecranon process (figure 5.3). Olecranon bursitis is common in sports such as football and wrestling in which the elbow is susceptible to repetitive friction and direct trauma. It is thought to occur more frequently on artificial turf than on natural turf (Larson and Osternig 1974). The athlete will present with a large, localized fluid-filled bursa; motion can be limited as the pressure within the bursa increases during flexion of the elbow. The bursa may be warm to the touch in the acute stages and is usually painless. If the athlete does not receive treatment and the condition persists, the fluid can thicken within the bursal walls and thus become difficult for the body to reabsorb.

### Tendinitis and Epicondylitis

Tendinitis and epicondylitis are overuse injuries to the tendinous attachments of the flexor/pronator group at the medial epicondyle or the extensor/supinator group at the lateral epicondyle (figure 5.4). Whereas **tendinitis** is associated with a simple inflammatory response, **epicondylitis** is usually associated with a degenerative condition in which increased fibroblastic activity and formation of granulation tissue are present within the tendon (Nirschl 1993). Nirschl used the term "tendinosis" to differentiate this pathological condition from simple tendinitis. Epicondylitis is often referred to as **"tennis elbow"** because of its high in-

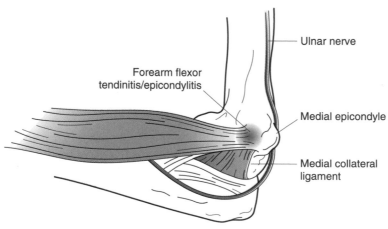

Ulnar nerve

Forearm flexor tendinitis/epicondylitis

Medial epicondyle

Medial collateral ligament

**▌Figure 5.4** Anatomical sites of medial epicondylitis/tendinitis at common flexor/pronator.

cidence in that sport. As many as 50% of athletes playing tennis will complain of tennis elbow symptoms at some point; the majority of cases are lateral and are seen in persons over 30 years of age. However, this chronic condition is also commonly seen in golf, baseball, throwing field events, swimming, and a number of occupational activities involving repetitive wrist motion and torque. Anyone engaged in activity that results in prolonged, high-intensity, and repetitive forearm muscle use is susceptible. Contractile overloads, occurring either concentrically or eccentrically, that chronically tension or stress the tendon near its attachment on the humerus are the primary cause of epicondylitis.

### Lateral Epicondylitis ("Tennis Elbow")

In most cases, lateral epicondylitis involves primarily the extensor carpi radialis brevis and usually results from activities that tension and stress the wrist extensor and supinator muscles. The backhand in tennis, for example, can place tremendous stress on the wrist extensor muscle group. Factors such as faulty mechanics, inadequate muscular strength and endurance, and poor racket fit (improper string tension, grip size, or racket weight or size) may further contribute to excessive contractile overload. Wheelchair athletes, especially marathon racers, may also suffer from lateral epicondylitis due to repetitive wrist flexion and pronation as the elbow extends during the push phase. Signs and symptoms include gradual onset of pain over the anterior aspect of the lateral epicondyle with the majority of tenderness localized to the origin of the extensor carpi radialis brevis tendon. Pain can be reproduced or aggravated with gripping and wrist extensor activities, as well as passive movement into flexion and pronation with the elbow extended. Observable swelling and discoloration are rare. Pain at rest, decreased ROM, and a weakened grip strength are symptoms characteristic of severe or prolonged cases.

### Medial Epicondylitis

Medial epicondylitis occurs much less frequently than the lateral condition. Repetitive wrist flexor and pronator muscle activity, as in baseball pitching, golf swings, overhead tennis serve and forehand racket motions, and pull-through swimming strokes, is the primary cause of medial epicondylitis (also referred to as "**golfer's elbow**"). Faulty mechanics or changes in technique with these activities can further increase stress at the flexor/pronator origin. Signs and symptoms may include pain and mild swelling over the medial epicondyle. Pain is reproduced with palpation just distal and lateral to the epicondyle over the flexor/pronator muscle group origin, and with resisted wrist flexion and forearm pronation. Passive extension of the wrist and supination of the forearm with the elbow extended may also reduce pain. Symptoms of ulnar nerve irritation are often associated with medial epicondylitis.

Due to skeletal immaturity, medial epicondylitis in young athletes usually involves stress or disruption at the bone rather than the tendon. Therefore, adolescents who present with symptoms of medial epicondylitis should be evaluated for traction avulsion apophysitis, discussed later in this chapter.

### *Periostitis*

*Shinsplints is a general term used to describe pain and inflammation of the musculotendinous unit and/or periosteum along the anteromedial border of the tibia.*

Although **periostitis** is more commonly associated with shinsplints in the lower extremity, it can also occur in the forearm. Forearm periostitis, or **forearm splints**, typically an early-season inflammatory reaction of the muscle insertion at the **periosteum**, have been seen in weight lifters, gymnasts, and pitchers prone to repetitive stress and overuse of the forearm muscles (Grossfield et al. 1998; Wadhwa et al. 1997; Weiker 1995). Signs and symptoms may include diffuse aching in the forearm with pain exacerbated with activity and relieved with rest. Pain may be reproduced with repetitive or resisted action of the involved musculature, and there will be tenderness with deep palpation between the ulna and radius (Grossfield et al. 1998; Weiker 1995). A bone scan can help to differentiate periostitis from other forearm stress injuries, demonstrating increased uptake along the bony margin that indicates a periosteal reaction (Grossfield et al. 1998; Wadhwa et al. 1997).

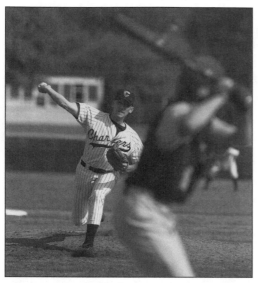

**■ Figure 5.5** The late cocking and early acceleration phase in pitching demonstrates valgus loading of the elbow.

### *Valgus Overload Instabilities*

During late cocking and early acceleration phases of overhand throwing mechanics, the medial elbow is subject to considerable valgus forces (figure 5.5). Repetitive and excessive valgus forces result in tractioning forces to the medial joint, causing progressive microtrauma and weakening of the UCL. Eventually, the UCL becomes stretched and valgus instability results. Chronic valgus overload, rather than acute trauma, is the major cause of medial collateral ligament ruptures in the throwing athlete. On exam, the athlete will complain of chronic pain with throwing that has persisted for months, and of point tenderness located approximately .8 in. (2 cm) distal to the medial epicondyle (Caldwell and Safran 1995). There will also be pain and instability with valgus stress testing. However, undersurface tears of the UCL have been observed with little or no evidence of laxity on clinical examination (Timmerman and Andrews 1994). As a consequence of ligament instability, stress normally absorbed by the ligament will be transferred to the bony articulations, resulting in injury pathology to these structures as well. Therefore, early recognition is essential.

## TRAUMATIC FRACTURES

*Intra-articular refers to a location within the joint capsule.*

Because of the potential for neurovascular injury, a neurovascular examination should always be performed with suspected fracture.

Traumatic fractures at the elbow, relatively uncommon in adults, occur much more frequently in children and skeletally immature adolescents. Traumatic fractures can occur anywhere within the elbow complex from either direct or indirect forces imposed on the bony structures. Since the majority are intra-articular, you must be concerned about the possible impact of these fractures and their healing mechanisms on elbow mechanics and function. The following paragraphs deal with some of the more common or significant fractures. Signs and symptoms common to all fractures include significant pain, swelling, crepitus, and tenderness over the fracture site. If bony fragments are displaced, there may also be deformity. Because of the potential for neurovascular injury, always perform a neurovascular examination with suspected fracture.

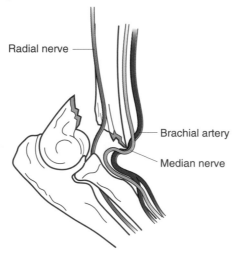

Radial nerve

Brachial artery

Median nerve

**■ Figure 5.6** Supracondylar fracture with potential injury of neurovascular structures.

### *Distal Humeral Fractures*

Condylar fractures can result from a direct blow, from a fall on a outstretched hand, or from a traumatic valgus or varus force applied to the elbow. Supracondylar fractures (transverse fractures just superior to the condyles), which occur more frequently in children than in others, typically result from a fall on an outstretched hand with the elbow extended. Displacement is a significant concern with these fractures. The proximal fragment of the humerus is often displaced anteriorly, and the potential for injury to the primary neurovascular structures (brachial artery; median, ulnar, and radial nerves) is high (figure 5.6). Suspected injury to these structures represents a medical emergency, as serious complications and permanent disability can result if the injury is not recognized and treated immediately.

### Radial Fractures

Radial head and neck fractures usually result from a fall on an outstretched arm with the forearm pronated, causing an axial compression of the radius against the capitellum (Alley and Pappas 1995; Morrey 1993). Radial head fractures may also result from traumatic elbow dislocations (figure 5.7). Signs and symptoms include swelling and pain over the lateral elbow. The athlete will complain particularly of pain with palpation of the radial head and pronation and supination movements of the forearm.

### Olecranon Fractures

A direct blow to the posterior elbow is the primary cause of traumatic olecranon fractures (figure 5.8). Fracture may also occur secondary to a violent pull of the triceps, although this is rare. Most fractures of the olecranon are intra-articular, and therefore joint instability may result (Cabanela and Morrey 1993). Signs and symptoms may include pain, point tenderness, and swelling, as well as crepitus and deformity over the posterior elbow.

### Forearm Fractures

Fractures of the forearm result from forces transmitted along or across the shaft of the radius and ulna. Axial forces, a consequence of falling on an outstretched hand, may cause a fracture of one or both bones. Transverse forces, caused by a direct blow to the forearm from an opponent or a stick, are common in contact sports such as football, hockey, and lacrosse (Griggs and Weiss 1996). In addition to the typical signs and symptoms of fracture, there may be pain and crepitus with active wrist motion.

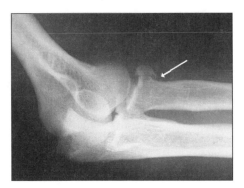

**■ Figure 5.7**  Radial fracture of the head.

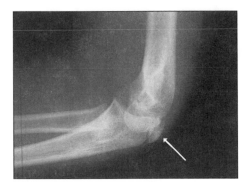

**■ Figure 5.8**  Traumatic fractures of the olecranon process.

## BONY LESIONS SECONDARY TO REPETITIVE STRESS

Chronic, repetitive valgus forces at the elbow joint can also result in progressive bony lesions, particularly in skeletally immature youth. As discussed previously, these forces are typically associated with throwing mechanics. With excessive valgus loading, traction forces are applied at the bony attachments of ligament and tendon on the medial side, while compression forces are exerted on the lateral joint structures.

### *Traction Apophyseal and Epiphyseal Injuries ("Little League Elbow")*

The medial apophysis is a nonarticular growth plate in adolescent athletes that serves as the attachment site for the flexor/pronator muscle group as well as the UCL. In skeletally immature athletes, valgus traction forces applied during the late cocking/early acceleration phases of throwing will stress the apophyseal plate rather than the tendon or ligament. The resulting injury, commonly known as "**Little League elbow**," may start out as an inflammatory response, or "**apophysitis**," and progress to an avulsion of the apophysis if the repetitive stress continues (figure 5.9). Athletes with this condition will report a prolonged history of pain with throwing. Signs and symptoms include point tenderness and swelling over the medial epicondyle, and pain with valgus stress localized directly over the medial apophysis (Andrews and Whiteside 1993). A flexion contracture may also be present.

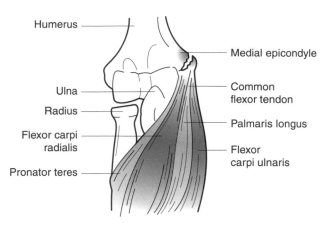

Humerus
Medial epicondyle
Ulna
Common flexor tendon
Radius
Palmaris longus
Flexor carpi radialis
Flexor carpi ulnaris
Pronator teres

**I Figure 5.9**   Traction apophyseal fracture of the medial epicondyle.

Other less common epiphyseal traction injuries involve the olecranon and the lateral apophysis. These traction apophyseal injuries can result from extension and pronation traction forces during the acceleration and follow-through phases of throwing. The athlete will present with signs and symptoms similar to those just described: prolonged pain with throwing, tenderness over the involved epiphyseal site, and decreased elbow extension (Lowery et al. 1995).

### *Osteochondral Defects*

**Osteochondritis dissecans** appears to result from compressive forces that damage the vascular supply to the osteochondral surface, causing vascular insufficiency and aseptic necrosis. Osteochondritis dissecans at the elbow, most often seen in young throwing adolescents (ages 10-15), primarily affects the capitellum and radial head (figure 5.10). The main cause for this pathology is repetitive throwing in which the radial capitellar joint is subject to compressive and shear forces secondary to chronic valgus overload during the late cocking and early acceleration phases. However, osteochondritis dissecans has also been observed in young gymnasts (Andrews and Whiteside 1993). Lateral joint compression is further intensified in the presence of medial instability. This degenerative process is characterized by changes in the articular surface, including flattening of the subchondral bone, fragmentation of the articular cartilage, and loose body formation (see next section). Signs and symptoms include chronic elbow pain, tenderness over the capitellum, flexion contracture, and articular changes seen on radiographic examination (Bennett 1993; Takahara et al. 1998). Intermittent locking or incomplete motion may occur if loose bodies are present (Alley and Pappas 1995). Early articular changes, thought to precede osteochondritis dissecans of the capitellum, include impaction of the subchondral bone and alterations in ossification of the epiphysis (Takahara et al. 1998). Many regard these early changes as a distinct condition known as **osteochondrosis**

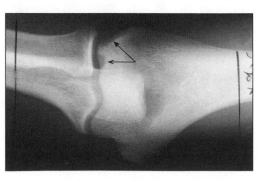

**I Figure 5.10**   Osteochondritis dissecans of the capitellum.

### *Osteophytes and Loose Bodies*

Osteophytes (bone spurs) or loose bodies may form at the posterior tip and posterior medial aspect of the olecranon as a result of medial instability and chronic valgus extension overload forces (figure 5.11). Valgus extension overload occurs during late acceleration and follow-through phases of the throwing motion, causing impingement of the posterior medial aspect of the olecranon on the posterior medial surface of the olecranon fossa. This impingement and resulting bony hypertrophy of the olecranon can further result in chondromalacia of the articular surface of the olecranon fossa (Wilson et al. 1983). The athlete's chief complaint will typically be pain experienced between acceleration and follow-through phases of the pitching motion, rendering them ineffective (Wilson et al. 1983). Other signs and symptoms may include pain over the posterior and/or posterior medial aspect of the olecranon process and pain with forced extension and valgus stressing. A flexion contracture may also be present.

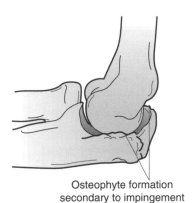

Osteophyte formation
secondary to impingement

**▌Figure 5.11** Osteophyte formation on the posterior tip and posteromedial aspects of the olecranon.

## DISLOCATION AND SUBLUXATION

Elbow joint dislocations are among the more common dislocations seen in sport. In common injury scenarios, a baseball player slides into base headfirst, or a wrestler or gymnast stretches out his or her arm to break a fall. Elbow dislocations can range from simple cases involving isolated ligament disruption to more complicated cases involving associated fractures, neurovascular complications, or both. In simple cases, conservative treatment of elbow dislocations produces excellent results, and recurrent dislocation or chronic instability is rarely a concern.

### *Humeroulnar Joint*

In athletics, posterior dislocations of the ulna and radius on the humerus are significantly more common than anterior dislocations. The prevailing mechanism associated with a posterior dislocation of the humeroulnar joint is a hyperextension force during axial loading, typically resulting from a fall on an outstretched or extended elbow. With this mechanism the olecranon process is jammed into the olecranon fossa, which acts as a fulcrum by which the trochlea is forced over the coronoid process. Because the annular ligament is usually left intact, the ulna and radius are displaced together. The displacement can be directly posterior (figure 5.12, a-b), posterolateral (most common), or posteromedial. Minimally, the medial collateral and lateral collateral ligaments are usually ruptured. However, if the hyperextension force is accompanied by valgus and rotatory forces, then associated

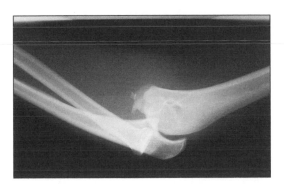
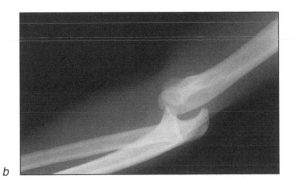

*a*      *b*

**▌Figure 5.12** Humeroulnar dislocation (a) with a fracture and (b) without a fracture.

> **!** The potential for occlusion of the brachial artery or entrapment of the median or ulnar nerves with humeroulnar dislocation (and/or with subsequent reduction) is a very real concern, indicating a medical emergency.

fractures of the radial head and neck, coronoid process, or medial epicondyle may also result (Alley and Pappas 1995). Additionally, the potential for occlusion of the brachial artery or entrapment of the median or ulnar nerves with humeroulnar dislocation (and/or with subsequent reduction) is a very real concern, indicating a medical emergency. Signs and symptoms of elbow dislocation include immediate pain, swelling, deformity, and an unwillingness to move the extremity. Signs and symptoms of associated arterial injury include excessive swelling of the forearm and hand, diminished or absent distal pulses, pale or cyanotic skin coloration, paresthesia, and pain with passive finger extension (Slowik, Fitzimmons, and Rayhack 1993).

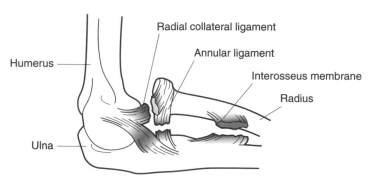

**■ Figure 5.13** Radioulnar joint dislocation and tearing of the ligamentous structure.

### Radioulnar Joint

Isolated dislocation of the radioulnar joint is rare in adults, and subluxations are more commonly seen in children. In adults, radioulnar dislocation does not appear to result from one single mechanism, but can occur from a direct blow to the lateral elbow (Takami, Takahashi, and Ando 1997). Dislocation is typically preceded by tearing of the annular ligament, distal radioulnar joint capsule, and interosseous membrane (figure 5.13). Signs and symptoms may include pain, limited ROM, elbow effusion, tenderness over the antecubital region, and inability to supinate the forearm.

In young children, a traction force or longitudinal pull with accompanying pronation of the forearm can result in subluxation or dislocation of the radioulnar joint, commonly know as **nursemaid's elbow**. With this injury mechanism, the radial head is pulled down into and becomes caught in the annular ligament. Usually the annular ligament is not torn in young children, but in older children it can be. Signs and symptoms include pain, holding the forearm in a pronated position, and unwillingness to move the elbow.

## NEUROVASCULAR INJURIES SECONDARY TO TRAUMA

As mentioned previously, a serious complication of supracondylar fractures and elbow dislocations is injury to the brachial artery and peripheral nerves, which can severely compromise blood flow and function of the forearm and hand.

### General Neurovascular Injury

> **!** Signs and symptoms of arterial injury and resulting ischemia include pain out of proportion to what is expected for the injury, diminished or absent distal pulses, poor skin coloration, and decreased skin temperature.

> **!** Signs and symptoms of nerve trauma include loss of sensation and motor function over the involved nerve's distribution.

Neurovascular injury should always be suspected and carefully evaluated with these injuries and with other severe trauma to the elbow and forearm. Signs and symptoms of arterial injury and resulting ischemia include pain out of proportion to what is expected for the injury, diminished or absent distal pulses, poor skin coloration, and decreased skin temperature. Signs and symptoms of nerve trauma include loss of sensation and motor function over the involved nerve's distribution. There may also be additional signs and symptoms associated with ischemic complications resulting from an acute compartment syndrome.

### Forearm Compartment Syndrome

Arterial injury as well as severe posttraumatic swelling can lead to a compartment syndrome in the forearm. In this condition a muscular compartment, enclosed by its relatively inelastic surrounding fascia, is subject to excessive swelling and increas-

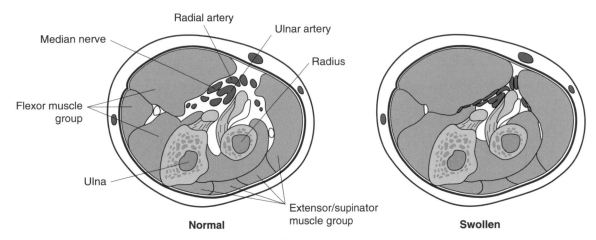

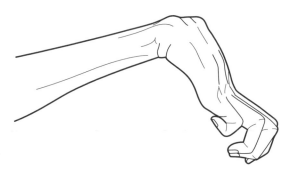

**Figure 5.14** Severe forearm compartment swelling.

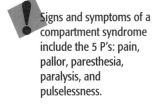

**Figure 5.15** Volkmann's ischemic contracture.

> Signs and symptoms of a compartment syndrome include the 5 P's: pain, pallor, paresthesia, paralysis, and pulselessness.

ing pressure (figure 5.14). As pressure exceeds that of the vessel walls within the compartment, vascular collapse occurs and circulation to the muscles and nerves is compromised. Since venous pressure is lower than capillary pressure, the veins will collapse first; this will further increase pressure within the compartment since blood can still flow in, but cannot flow out. Eventually, as pressure continues to rise, the capillary walls will collapse, causing ischemia to the surrounding muscles and nerves. If ischemia persists for more than 6-12 h, tissue necrosis and permanent loss of nerve and muscular function will ensue. The final complication is a **Volkmann's ischemic contracture** of the forearm, resulting from the replacement of the nonviable, necrotic muscle with an inelastic and contracted scar tissue (figure 5.15).

Signs and symptoms of a compartment syndrome include the 5 P's (Pain, Pallor, Paresthesia, Paralysis, and Pulselessness). The earliest and most reliable symptom of a compartment syndrome is unrelenting pain, often out of proportion to the injury. Severe pain will also be present with stretching of the ischemic muscles. The compartment will be tense and tender to palpation and may begin to take on a whitish skin color (pallor) or shiny appearance due to decreasing circulation. There will be paresthesia as the nerve becomes ischemic. As nerve ischemia progresses, the individual will experience diminished sensation (**hypoesthesia**) and motor weakness—and eventually, numbness and complete loss of motor function (paralysis). Pulselessness may also be present if the compartment syndrome is a result of arterial occlusion. Otherwise, there may still be distal pulses, since intracompartmental pressure rarely exceeds that of major arterial vessels. Any one of the foregoing signs or symptoms is indicative of a medical emergency. You must refer the athlete for surgical decompression and restoration of blood flow in order to avoid a Volkmann's ischemic contracture.

## NERVE COMPRESSION SYNDROMES

Nerve compression syndromes are common around the elbow, frequently resulting from repetitive compression or traction mechanisms seen in sports such as throwing and tennis. This section will deal with the more common compression syndromes of the major peripheral nerves of the forearm.

### Ulnar Nerve

The elbow is the most common site for ulnar nerve compression and injury. The ulnar nerve passes the elbow superficially between the medial epicondyle and the medial border of the olecranon. Because of its superficial course and anatomical constraints as it passes the medial elbow, it is prone to contusions, subluxation, traction and frictional forces, compression syndromes, and irritation caused by surrounding chronic or degenerative conditions. Ulnar nerve contusions can result from a direct blow to the medial surface of the elbow where the nerve passes superficially, particularly when the elbow is in a flexed position. Recurrent subluxations can result when the overlying retinaculum, which holds the nerve within the epitrochlear (ulnar) groove, becomes stretched or torn. **Cubital tunnel syndrome** (the term collectively describes ulnar neuropathy and compression) can result from a variety of conditions, such as inflammation or scarring of the nerve, muscle hypertrophy, occupying lesions, fractures, dislocations, or any pathology that narrows the nerve's passageway as it crosses the elbow. Common sites of anatomical compression include the arcade of Struthers, medial intermuscular septum, cubital tunnel, flexor carpi ulnaris aponeurosis, and the deep flexor/pronator aponeurosis (figure 5.16). Chronic traction and frictional forces resulting from valgus overload and medial instability associated with throwing can also cause nerve irritation. Other inflammatory conditions such as chronic medial epicondylitis, flexor/pronator tendinitis, and UCL injuries can also cause ulnar neuropathy.

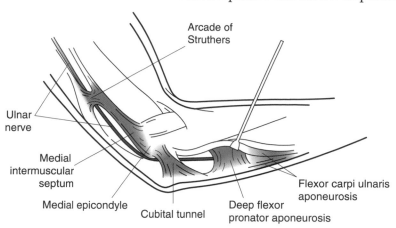

**Figure 5.16** Common anatomical sites for ulnar nerve compression syndrome.

Regardless of the underlying cause, the signs and symptoms of ulnar neuropathy will be similar. Symptoms may begin gradually with chronic and degenerative conditions, or acutely with traumatic injury. Signs and symptoms include pain or aching originating at the medial elbow and radiating down the lateral forearm into the fifth and the medial surface of the fourth digit. The nerve may be tender when palpated just posterior to the medial epicondyle. Subluxation or dislocation of the nerve can often be reproduced with flexion and extension of the elbow, and the athlete may complain of "clicking" over the posteromedial aspect of the elbow. With chronic compression syndromes, the athlete will present with paresthesia over the ulnar distribution of the forearm and hand, which may advance to numbness if symptoms progress. Symptoms usually worsen when the elbow is in a flexed position, since anatomical structures become stretched over the cubital tunnel and space within the tunnel significantly decreases in this position. Radiating pain or paresthesia may be reproduced with light tapping over the irritated or inflamed nerve (**Tinel's sign**). In severe compressive or traumatic cases, muscle atrophy, motor weakness, and loss of function may also be present in the intrinsic muscles of the hand. There may also be loss of pinch or grip strength.

### Median Nerve

Compression of the median nerve at the elbow, or pronator teres syndrome, can occur between the two heads of the pronator teres secondary to muscle hypertrophy or tight fibrous bands (figure 5.17). Pronator teres syndrome is most often seen in sports such as weight lifting, rowing, golf, and racket sports as a consequence of repetitive pronation and sustained gripping. Median nerve compression is characterized by aching and pain in the volar aspect of the forearm that is exacerbated with flexor/pronator muscle activity (Andrews and Whiteside 1993). Signs of paresthesia and motor weakness over the median nerve distribution of the thumb and the second and third digits may be present in later stages. A Tinel's sign over the volar aspect of the proximal forearm may also be positive.

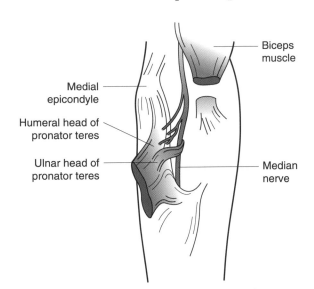

**Figure 5.17** Sites for pronator teres syndrome.

### Anterior Interosseous Nerve

The anterior interosseous nerve is a motor branch off the median nerve that runs along the interosseous membrane, passing between the flexor digitorum profundus and flexor pollicis longus on its way to the pronator quadratus. Occasionally this nerve is compressed by the forearm muscles or overlying fibrous bands, secondary to forceful muscle contractions. Compression of the anterior interosseous nerve will cause pain and motor weakness in the proximal forearm. The prevailing sign is loss of pinch strength between the tips of the thumb and index finger.

### Radial Nerve

The radial nerve runs from the medial to the lateral aspect of the posterior humerus and crosses the lateral epicondyle, where it passes through the radial tunnel and divides into deep and superficial branches. Radial nerve compression, or radial tunnel syndrome, can occur within the radial tunnel, which extends anteriorly from the radial head to the supinator muscle (Andrews and Whiteside 1993) (figure 5.18). Radial tunnel syndrome is typically caused by repetitive or vigorous wrist extension and forearm pronation and supination. It is often incorrectly identified as lateral epicondylitis but can be differentiated from this condition with careful evaluation. With radial tunnel syndrome, tenderness is present several centimeters distal to the lateral epicondyle, within the supinator/extensor muscle mass of the proximal forearm (Behr and Altchek 1997). Other symptoms include pain radiating into the forearm extensors and pain reproduction with resisted supination or resisted extension of the middle finger. Motor weakness is usually not found on clinical examination.

### Posterior Interosseous Nerve

The deep branch of the radial nerve continues as the posterior interosseous motor nerve supplying the wrist and finger extensors. Just distal to the radial tunnel, the posterior interosseous nerve can be compressed under the arcade of Frohse. The **arcade of Frohse** is a fibrous band located at the proximal edge of the supinator muscle, near the edge of the extensor carpi radialis brevis and radial capitellar joint

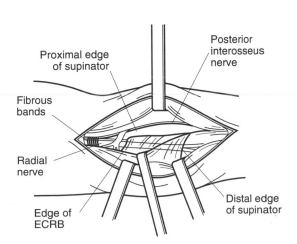

**Figure 5.18** Location of radial tunnel syndrome.

(Andrews and Whiteside 1993; Behr and Altchek 1997) (figure 5.19). Signs and symptoms include deep aching in the extensor muscle mass and proximal forearm after repetitive activities such as weight lifting, throwing, and grasping. Palpable tenderness is noted approximately 2 in. (5 cm) distal from the lateral epicondyle, near the site where the nerves passes through the arcade of Frohse. What differentiates compression of the posterior interosseous nerve from radial tunnel syndrome is a primary finding of motor weakness in the wrist and finger extensors.

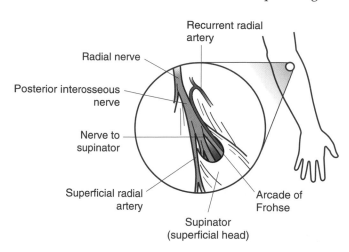

■ **Figure 5.19**   Arcade of Frohse.

## STRUCTURAL AND FUNCTIONAL ABNORMALITIES

Cubital varus and cubital valgus are two structural abnormalities of the elbow's carrying angle. The normal carrying angle of the extended elbow is slightly valgus—approximately 5° for males (see figure 5.22a, page 144) and 10-15° for females. **Cubital valgus** is a carrying angle that is greater than the normal 5° or 15° valgus angulation (figure 5.20). Cubital valgus can result from an epiphyseal plate injury secondary to fracture of the lateral epicondyle. Potential complications of an increased valgus angle include decreased ROM and delayed ulnar neuropathy. **Cubital varus**, or **gunstock deformity**, is a carrying angle less than the normal valgus angle, usually taking on a varus angulation (see figure 5.21). Cubital varus, which is more common than cubital valgus, is most often a result of a supracondylar fracture during childhood that either disrupts the growth plate or heals with a malalignment of the distal humerus. Little consequence or functional impairment is associated with this deformity. Note that structural abnormalities, particularly cubital valgus, are potential contributory mechanisms in chronic conditions of the elbow.

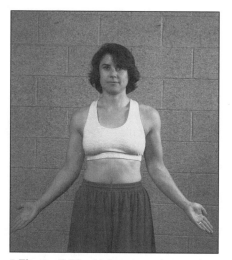

■ **Figure 5.20**   Valgus carrying angle of the elbow.

## INJURY ASSESSMENT

As you have likely noted, multiple conditions involving a variety of structures can result from similar mechanisms. Through the assessment techniques covered in the following sections, you will be able to identify and differentiate between the potential structures involved.

### ON-FIELD ASSESSMENT

The need for an on-field assessment for an elbow injury most often arises from either direct contact, a fall on an outstretched hand, hyperextension, or a severe valgus or varus mechanism. As always, your goal is to quickly determine the nature and severity of the injury and check for any conditions that would indicate a medical emergency. As you approach the athlete, observe his response to the injury, his willingness to move the injured limb, and the position of the limb.

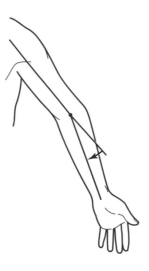

**Figure 5.21**
Gunstock deformity resulting from an epiphyseal fracture.

### History and Observation

As you reach the athlete, ask him or any bystanders what happened if you did not witness the injury. Observe closely for signs of immediate swelling, discoloration, and deformity. A gunstock deformity or varus angulation of the joint in a young athlete may indicate an epiphyseal fracture (figure 5.21). Check to see if the olecranon process is more pronounced posteriorly, indicating the possibility of a posterior humeroulnar dislocation.

### Palpation

If you note a deformity, immediately palpate for distal pulse. Also at this time, assess the sensory distribution of the peripheral nerves in the hand. If neurovascular findings are positive, immediately refer the athlete and stabilize the elbow—in the position in which it was found—for emergency transport.

If neurovascular structures are intact, proceed with a palpation of the bone and joint structures of the posterior, medial, and lateral elbow, the distal humerus, and the proximal radius and ulna to check for bony tenderness, crepitus, or subtle deformities that would indicate a fracture or subluxation. Fractures and dislocations are usually easy to detect because of the superficial nature of joint structures. However, tenderness over the superficial bony structures will also be present with severe contusions due to direct contact, which also may result in considerable acute pain.

### Range of Motion

If no obvious signs of fracture or dislocation and no severe bony tenderness are present, and all neurovascular signs are negative, have the athlete slowly flex and extend the elbow. If pain does not increase or becomes severe with movement, assist the athlete off the field for continued evaluation on the sideline. Since any muscle spasm will have little effect on stress testing at the elbow, you can defer ligament stress tests until the sideline evaluation. If for any reason the athlete has difficulty standing, is in enough pain to make ambulation difficult, or shows signs of shock, provide assisted transportation.

## SIDELINE ASSESSMENT

Once the athlete has been removed to the sideline (as also in the case of an injured athlete who has left the field on her own power to seek evaluation), you will perform a more detailed assessment.

### History

Determining the mechanism of injury will help you identify the nature of the injury. Was the athlete throwing at the time, and in what position did the pain occur? Did the injury occur because the athlete put her hand out to break a fall or because of direct contact by an opponent or sport implement? Was there a torque or twisting motion or a traction force, or was the elbow forced in an unnatural direction? Have the athlete identify the specific location of the injury and rate the intensity of the pain from 1 to 10 for later comparison. Determine whether she heard or felt anything at the time of injury. A pop or snap in the joint could indicate a tendon or ligament rupture or a fracture. As always, the more thorough your history taking, the more information you will have on which to base your objective assessment.

## Checklist for On-Field Assessment of the Elbow and Forearm

### Primary Survey

✓ Airway, breathing, and circulation

✓ Severe bleeding

✓ Check for unusual positioning of the limb

✓ Assess for shock

### Secondary Survey

History

✓ Chief complaint

✓ Mechanism of injury

✓ Location and severity of pain

✓ Information from bystanders

Observation

✓ Note deformity, swelling, discoloration, pallor.

✓ Note unusual positioning of the limb.

✓ Assess for shock.

Palpation

✓ Check for bony tenderness, crepitus, and deformity along the medial supracondylar ridge, medial epicondyle, olecranon process and proximal ulna, lateral supracondylar ridge, lateral epicondyle, radial head, and proximal radius

Neurovascular assessment

✓ Sensory

✓ Motor

✓ Distal pulse

Gentle, active ROM

✓ Elbow flexion, extension

✓ Pronation, supination

If all tests are negative, remove athlete from field for continued evaluation on the sideline.

### *Observation*

As the athlete comes to the sideline, observe how he is holding his elbow and look for any guarding or obvious expressions of pain. Note the location and degree of swelling and discoloration by comparing to the uninvolved side. If you conducted an on-field assessment, has there been any change in appearance since that time? Diffuse and rapid swelling of the elbow and/or forearm can occur with elbow injuries and lead to a compartment syndrome, so you need to monitor closely for signs of excessive swelling and impending neurovascular compromise. If the athlete fell hard or received a direct blow to the posterior elbow, check for localized swelling of the olecranon bursa.

Next, check for alignment and the relationship of structures to one another, noting any differences between the right and left sides. Alignment includes the carrying angle and the relationship between the olecranon process and the epicondyles. Normal carrying angle is about 5° in males and 10-15° in females, so the valgus angle of the elbow in extension is 175° in men and 165-170° in women (figure 5.22a). When the elbow is flexed, the carrying angle disappears (figure 5.22b). An abnormal carrying angle can be the result of a fracture or epiphyseal separation.

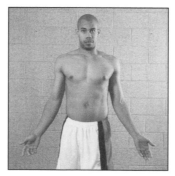
*a*

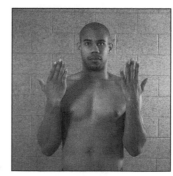
*b*

❚ **Figure 5.22**  Normal carrying angle in (a) full elbow extension and (b) full elbow flexion.

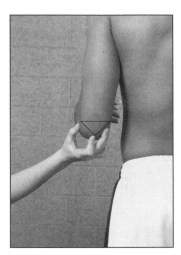 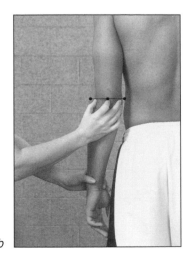

*a*                                    *b*

∎ **Figure 5.23**    (a) Normal elbow alignment at 90° and (b) full extension.

With the elbow flexed to 90°, the olecranon process and medial and lateral epicondyles should form an isosceles triangle (figure 5.23a). When the elbow is in full extension, these same structures should form a straight line (figure 5.23b). If this alignment is not present, there may be a fracture, subluxation, or dislocation.

### Palpation

After your observation, do the palpation before performing functional testing. Gently palpate around the injured area to detect temperature variations and soft tissue tightness or soft tissue texture differences that may be occurring with the advent and progression of edema. Temperature changes will occur naturally over different areas such as bony prominences compared to muscle bellies, but changes that are abnormal are most appropriately identified by comparison to the uninjured (contralateral) side. Check distal pulses again to ensure continued circulatory integrity.

Palpation of the elbow structures is best performed with the elbow in a flexed, relaxed position. Palpate for tenderness, swelling, and subtle deformities over the medial epicondyle, medial supracondylar ridge, olecranon process, olecranon fossa, proximal ulna, lateral epicondyle, supracondylar ridge, and radial head. Palpation of soft tissue is best performed regionally. Palpate for inflammation and tenderness of the flexor/pronator muscle mass and origin, the ulnar nerve within its groove, and the medial collateral ligament (medial aspect); the olecranon bursa and triceps insertion (posterior aspect); the extensor/supinator muscle mass and origin, brachioradialis, lateral collateral ligament, and annular ligament (lateral aspect); and from lateral to medial, the biceps tendon, brachial artery, and median nerve (anterior aspect).

Depending on the mechanism of injury, you may note tenderness on opposite sides of the joint. Diffuse tenderness anteriorly along with pain within the olecranon fossa posteriorly is common with hyperextension mechanisms. With valgus forces, you will note tenderness over the medial structures that have been stressed, as well as lateral tenderness due to compression. When pain is experienced on both sides of the joint with these mechanisms, the injury is typically more severe than if only one side of the joint is tender.

### Special Tests

Special tests for the elbow that you would typically use in the sideline assessment are those that assess joint stability.

## Medial and Lateral Stress Tests

Medial and lateral stress tests are applied to the collateral ligaments of the elbow joint. With the athlete's elbow in a partially flexed position (15° to 20° from full extension), place your stabilizing hand on the distal medial forearm and the stress-applying hand on the lateral elbow to apply a **valgus stress** to the medial collateral ligament (figure 5.24a). The lateral collateral ligament stress test is applied similarly, but the stress-applying hand is placed on the medial elbow and a **varus stress** is applied while the distal forearm is stabilized (figure 5.24b).

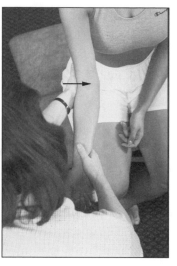
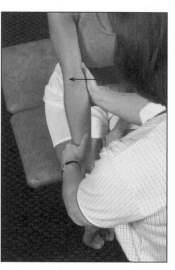

a
b

**▌Figure 5.24** (a) Medial (valgus) stress test and (b) lateral (varus) stress test.

## Radioulnar Joint Test

To assess the integrity of the proximal radioulnar joint, apply an anterior-to-posterior stress to the joint. Place your stabilizing hand on the proximal aspect of the ulna, holding the athlete's forearm between your side and your arm. With the other hand, position your thumb over the anterior radial head and your index finger over the posterior aspect. Then apply stress with the hand grasping the radial head in an anterior-to-posterior and posterior-to-anterior direction (figure 5.25).

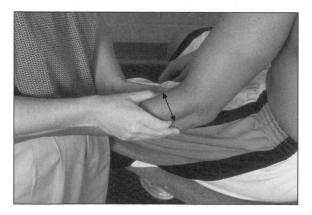

**▌Figure 5.25** Radioulnar stress test.

### Range of Motion

Active ROM is assessed through a full range for elbow extension and flexion, as well as for forearm supination and pronation. You may also wish to have the athlete perform active wrist flexion and extension, since the origin for the extrinsic muscles responsible for these motions crosses the elbow joint. Normal active ROM of the elbow is from 0° at full extension to 145° of flexion (figure 5.26, a-b). Full supination should be approximately 90° and pronation slightly less, at 85° (figure 5.26, c-d). Having the athlete grasp a pencil or pen in his hand when performing supination and pronation movements may help you better observe the degree of motion. Observe for both quality and quantity of movement, looking for any signs of apprehension or pain with movements. If pain is present during any active motions, note where in the motion and over what range it occurs. As a rule of thumb, the earlier in the motion the pain occurs and the greater the pain is, the more serious the injury. Incomplete motion can be due to pain, weakness, or a bony block.

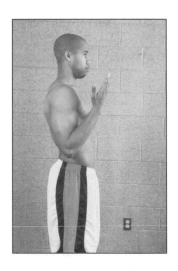
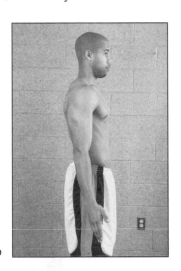
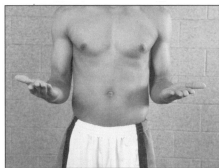
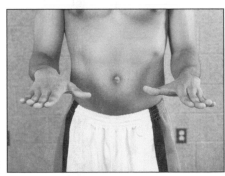

**∎ Figure 5.26**   Active ROM of the elbow into (a) flexion, (b) extension, (c) supination, and (d) pronation.

Passive motion can be assessed either after the athlete has completed the full series of active ROM tests or at the end of each completed active motion.

Next, perform passive ROM tests to assess the end feel of the joint and to determine the cause for any limitations in active ROM. Passive movement will normally be about 5° to 10° greater than active motion in elbow extension and forearm motions. It is not unusual for elbow flexion to increase as much as 15° up to a full range of 160° passively. Full passive motion without full active motion indicates weakness that can result from either muscle or nerve injury or pain. Incomplete passive motion is the result of a blockage that restricts motion. End feels will vary depending on the reason for the end movement. Elbow extension should have a firm end feel as the olecranon process moves against the olecranon fossa. Elbow flexion, however,

If pain occurs with active and passive motion, a ligamentous or supportive structure is usually involved, but if pain occurs only with active motion, a muscle or tendon is often its source.

should have a soft, springy end feel as the forearm makes contact with the belly of the biceps brachii muscle.

### Strength

Strength of the elbow musculature is commonly tested in midposition. Manual resistance tests should also be performed for wrist flexion/extension as well as shoulder flexion/extension, depending on the pathology. These tests are discussed in chapters 6 and 4, respectively. It is important to examine the shoulder to eliminate any possible referred pain from the shoulder into the elbow. Assessing wrist strength is important because an elbow injury may affect wrist function and strength, as many of the elbow muscles function at the wrist.

### Elbow Flexion

To test elbow flexion, flex the elbow to 90°, stabilize the elbow with one hand, and place your other hand on the distal forearm just proximal to the wrist. Then provide an isometric resistance to the elbow flexors, instructing the athlete to attempt to bend the elbow further against your resistance. This test is performed in three positions:

Always test strength of the uninvolved side first to familiarize the athlete with the test and to provide a baseline for comparison when testing the involved side.

- In forearm neutral to isolate the brachioradialis muscle

- In pronation to isolate the brachialis

- In supination to isolate the biceps as the primary elbow flexor

Then test triceps strength with the elbow in the same position (90° flexion): reverse the hand on the forearm to the posterior aspect, and instruct the athlete to try to straighten his elbow against your resistance.

### Supination and Pronation

Supination and pronation are evaluated with the elbow at 90° to eliminate shoulder motion. To test pronation strength, stabilize the elbow at the athlete's side, and grasp the distal forearm with the forearm in midrange supination. Instruct the athlete to pronate (medially rotate) the forearm while you attempt to supinate the forearm. Then place the forearm in a pronated position and test supination by asking the athlete to laterally rotate the forearm into supination against your resistance.

### Neurological Tests

If at any time the athlete complains of numbness, tingling, or referred pain into the elbow or forearm as a result of an elbow injury, a complete neurological examination should follow to assess integrity of both the primary nerve trunks and the peripheral nerves of the elbow and forearm (i.e., median, radial, musculocutaneous, and ulnar). To assess sensation around the elbow and forearm, provide light touch over the lateral aspect of the elbow (C5), lateral forearm (C6), medial forearm (C8), and medial aspect of the elbow (T1) (see chapter 3, page 63). For injuries occurring at the elbow joint or below, you should also assess sensation over the distributions of the peripheral nerves; the distal lateral fifth finger (ulnar), radial aspect of the second finger (median), dorsal web space (radial), and lateral forearm (musculocutaneous) (figure 5.27).

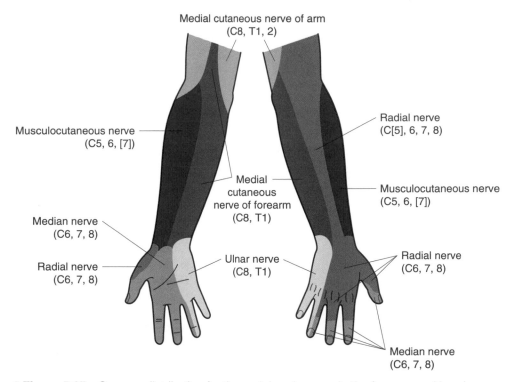

Medial cutaneous nerve of arm
(C8, T1, 2)

Musculocutaneous nerve
(C5, 6, [7])

Radial nerve
(C[5], 6, 7, 8)

Medial
cutaneous
nerve of forearm
(C8, T1)

Musculocutaneous nerve
(C5, 6, [7])

Median nerve
(C6, 7, 8)

Radial nerve
(C6, 7, 8)

Ulnar nerve
(C8, T1)

Radial nerve
(C6, 7, 8)

Median nerve
(C6, 7, 8)

■ **Figure 5.27**   Sensory distribution for the peripheral nerves in the forearm and hand.

To assess motor function, perform isometric tests for each peripheral nerve. Use thumb opposition and pinch strength to test the median nerve (figure 5.28a); abduction of the fifth finger to assess the ulnar nerve (figure 5.28b); and wrist extension/thumb extension to assess the radial nerve (figure 5.28c). Past the elbow the musculocutaneous nerve has no muscle innervation, so there is no motor testing for this nerve, only sensory testing. If any shoulder or cervical involvement is suspected, you should evaluate also for nerve root myotomes (see chapter 3).

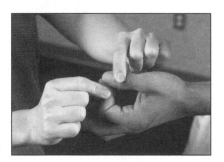

a

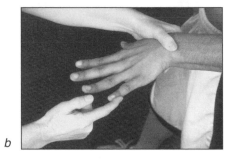

b

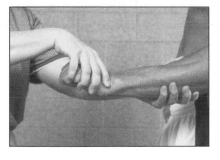

c

■ **Figure 5.28**   Motor testing of (a) thumb opposition (median), (b) 5th finger abduction (ulnar), and (c) wrist extension (radial).

The athletic trainer must have an understanding of the athlete's sport and position, and must determine on the basis of the athlete's performance of the functional tests whether or not he or she is able to safely return to participation.

Reflex testing is performed on the biceps tendon (C5-6), triceps tendon (C7-8), and brachioradialis (C5-6) (chapter 3, figure 3.19, a-c). Perform these tests with the muscles relaxed and near midrange. The best way to obtain the biceps and brachioradialis reflexes is to place your thumb over the tendon and hammer tap the thumbnail. You can obtain the triceps reflex directly over the tendon just proximal to the olecranon process.

### Functional Tests

If your evaluation demonstrates no positive findings that would indicate cessation of activity, and pain has sufficiently subsided, you will perform functional tests to assess readiness to return to activity. Examples of functional tests include swinging a bat, throwing, swimming with strokes specific to the athlete's competitive events, tennis serve, handstand or walkover, and discus throw. Execution of the activity

---

## Checklist for Sideline Assessment of the Elbow and Forearm

### History
Ask questions pertaining to the following:

✓ Chief complaint
✓ Mechanism of injury
✓ Unusual sounds or sensations
✓ Type and location of pain or symptoms
✓ Previous injury
✓ Previous injury to opposite extremity for bilateral comparison

### Observation
✓ Check for visible facial expressions of pain.
✓ Check for swelling, deformity, skin coloration, abnormal contours, or discoloration.
✓ Note whether athlete lets arm hang and swing, or whether he or she holds or splints it.
✓ Observe overall position, posture, and alignment.
　✓ Carrying angle
　✓ Alignment of the medial and lateral epicondyle and olecranon process (extended and flexed elbow)
　✓ Flexed elbow posture
✓ Check muscle development—areas of muscular atrophy.
✓ Make bilateral comparison.

### Palpation
Palpate for pain, tenderness, and deformity over the following:

✓ Medial epicondyle and supracondylar ridge
✓ Olecranon process, olecranon fossa, and proximal ulna
✓ Lateral epicondyle and supracondylar ridge, radial head

✓ Flexor/pronator group, ulnar nerve, medial collateral ligament
✓ Olecranon bursa, distal triceps
✓ Extensor/supinator muscle group, brachioradialis, lateral collateral ligament, annular ligament
✓ Biceps tendon, brachial artery, median nerve

### Special Tests
✓ Collateral stress tests
✓ Radioulnar joint stress test

### Range of Motion
✓ Active ROM for elbow flexion/extension, forearm pronation/supination
✓ Active ROM for shoulder flexion/extension and wrist flexion/extension as appropriate
✓ Passive ROM for same motions as for active ROM
✓ Bilateral comparison

### Strength Tests
✓ Perform manual resistance against same motions as in AROM.
✓ Check bilaterally and note any pain or weakness.
✓ Perform manual resistance for wrist flexion/extension and shoulder flexion/extension as appropriate.

### Neurovascular Tests
✓ Sensory, motor, and reflex of nerve roots C5, C6, C7, C8, and T1
✓ Sensory and motor for peripheral nerves: median, ulnar, musculocutaneous, and radial
✓ Distal pulse

### Functional Tests

should be pain free and normal in movement flow and joint excursion, without hesitation, deficiency, or any unusual outcome. If you are ever uncertain whether the athlete is ready to return to activity, it is better to err on the side of caution for the sake of the athlete's health.

## OFF-FIELD ASSESSMENT

The off-field evaluation is very similar to the sideline assessment, but it includes additional evaluation techniques for the assessment of chronic and postacute conditions.

### History

Questions regarding the onset of symptoms, duration, aggravating and easing factors, past history of both involved and uninvolved sides, and previous rehabilitative care are as important as the questions you asked in the sideline assessment. In particular, ask about the athlete's sport and other activities that may indicate excessive or repetitive wrist flexion/extension or pronation/supination movements. Does the pain worsen or improve with activity? Is it sufficient to interfere with activity, and has it stayed the same over time or has it gotten progressively worse? Be sure to ask whether there have been any recent changes in either training equipment or practice routines. For instance, if you are evaluating a tennis player, has she recently changed racket style or grip size? All these questions, in addition to those asked in the sideline assessment, will give you a good idea of the **SINS** (**S**tage, **I**rritability, **N**ature, **S**everity) and your evaluation objectives.

### Observation

Observe how the athlete holds his elbow. Does it hang freely when he walks, or is he guarding it and supporting it with the other hand? If he is maintaining the joint in a flexed position, this may be a sign of joint swelling or pain in either the anterior capsule or olecranon fossa with full extension. This elbow posture is common with hyperextension injuries. Also notice whether the athlete uses the arm to open doors or carry heavy objects such as books. Upon direct observation, look for signs of swelling, redness or ecchymosis, changes in skin coloration, or any structures that appear abnormal in size or contour.

### Differential Diagnosis

The quadrant position places the neck in end-range extension, rotation, and lateral flexion to the same side as the symptoms before the athletic trainer applies overpressure to the head.

Elbow pain can also be referred from the shoulder and cervical regions. You must differentially rule out these areas as possible sources of the athlete's complaints before focusing on the elbow. Active ROM with overpressure at the end ranges for cervical and shoulder motions will eliminate these areas as possible referral sites. If straight-plane motions with overpressures for the cervical spine are negative, include in your assessment the quadrant position discussed in chapter 4. If the athlete's complaints are reproduced with any of these cervical or shoulder motions, you should further investigate the site reproducing the complaints before moving on to the elbow.

### Range of Motion

Range of motion tests as discussed for the sideline assessment, both active and passive, are also performed in the off-field assessment. As with the sideline assessment, the athlete can either perform each passive motion immediately after each active motion or can perform all the active motions and then all the passive motions.

### Strength Tests

Manual strength tests are also the same as those for the sideline assessment. In addition, you should pay special attention to resisted wrist flexion and extension tests.

Elbow pain, especially subacute and chronic pain, can emanate from either the medial or the lateral epicondyle. Since these sites are the origin of the common wrist flexor and extensor tendons, the athlete with epicondylitis will experience pain at the elbow with resisted movements of the wrist.

The treatment facility may also provide tools that you do not have on the field for a more objective assessment of strength. These include a cable tensiometer for elbow flexion and extension and weight machines or dumbbells to determine a one-repetition maximum for strength. Dynamometers used to evaluate grip strength and pinch strength can also help you determine weakness emanating from an elbow injury, since the muscles providing these activities originate at the elbow (figure 5.29). Isokinetic testing for both elbow and wrist strength can also further define specific strength output for elbow flexors and extensors, forearm pronators and supinators, and wrist flexors and extensors.

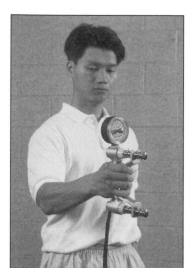

**▌Figure 5.29** Grip strength testing in the treatment facility.

### Neurological Tests

If the athlete complains of burning, tingling, numbness, radiating pain, or weakness into the elbow, wrist, or hand, you should include a neurological examination to assess sensory, motor, and reflex components as described for the sideline assessment (pages 148-150). With chronic conditions, sensory or motor deficits are likely due to a nerve compression syndrome.

### Special Tests

Stress tests for the elbow's collateral ligaments and the proximal radioulnar joint are consistent with those outlined in the sideline assessment. Check for presence of pain and instability with stress application and compare bilaterally.

**Lateral Epicondylitis Test**

You can perform both active and passive testing for lateral epicondylitis or tendinitis. The active test elicits pain with resisted wrist extension with the elbow flexed and forearm pronated (figure 5.30a). Adding radial deviation to the resisted motion will increase the pain. Pain will also occur with passive flexion of the wrist with the elbow extended (figure 5.30b). Pain will increase when combined with ulnar deviation.

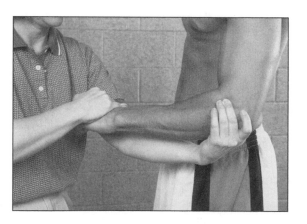
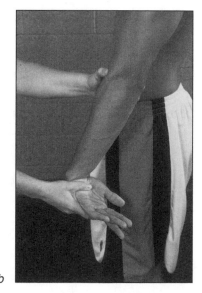

a                    b

**▌Figure 5.30** Lateral epicondylitis tests: (a) active and (b) passive.

## Medial Epicondylitis Test

Both passive and active tests can be used to evaluate medial epicondylitis. For the active test, apply resistance to wrist flexion with the elbow flexed and forearm supinated (figure 5.31a). For the passive test, extend the wrist, with the elbow extended and forearm pronated (figure 5.31b). In severe cases of epicondylitis, the athlete will complain of pain if he simply shakes hands or pulls open a door.

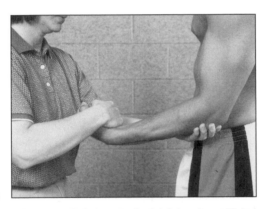
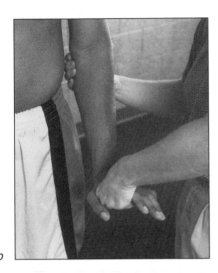

a

b

■ **Figure 5.31** Medial epicondylitis tests: (a) active and (b) passive.

## Tinel's Sign

Tinel's sign identifies ulnar nerve compression or transmission interference at the elbow. Tap the ulnar nerve where it passes through the ulnar groove between the olecranon process and the medial epicondyle. The test is positive if it elicits a tingling or shooting sensation into the lateral forearm, hand, and fifth finger (figure 5.32).

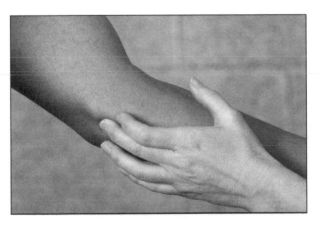

■ **Figure 5.32** Tinel's test over the ulnar groove.

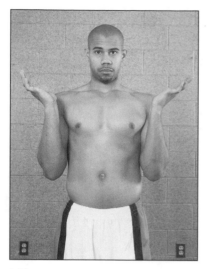

**Figure 5.33** Elbow flexion test for ulnar nerve entrapment.

### Elbow Flexion Test

You can assess ulnar nerve compression or entrapment in the cubital tunnel with the elbow flexion test. For this test, the elbow is maximally flexed with the forearm neutral and wrists fully extended. The test is positive if paresthesia is noted along the medial border of the forearm and hand (figure 5.33).

### Pronator Teres Test

To check for median nerve compression due to muscle hypertrophy of the pronator teres, apply sustained resistance against forearm pronation. In a positive test, symptoms of pain and paresthesia are reproduced along the median nerve distribution in the hand.

## Joint Mobility

You will have already tested physiological joint motion during ROM assessment. If the athlete lacks full joint motion, that limitation may be related to restriction within the joint capsule. This determination is made in two ways: observation of a capsular pattern of movement and assessment of joint accessory motion. A capsular pattern of the elbow is more limited with flexion than with extension and is equally limited in supination and pronation. In other words, a capsular restriction is present if the joint displays a loss of motion greater in flexion than extension. Supination and pronation may also be restricted, but will be restricted equally. Assessment of joint accessory motion is performed on the humeroulnar and radioulnar joints.

### Humeroulnar Joint Mobility Test

With the athlete sitting or lying comfortably, stabilize the humerus and distract the ulna in a longitudinal caudal motion to assess the humeroulnar joint (figure 5.34).

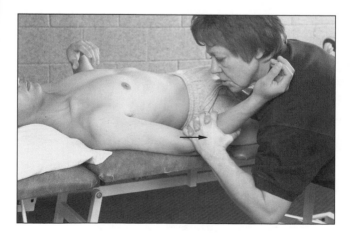

**Figure 5.34** Humeroulnar joint mobility test.

### Radioulnar Joint Mobility Test

To assess the proximal radioulnar joint, grasp the ulna with your stabilizing hand and the radial head with your mobilizing hand. Apply an anterior-to-posterior force to the radius, similar to the movement for testing joint stress (figure 5.35).

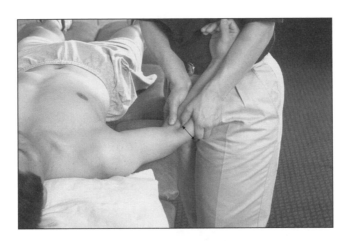

∎ **Figure 5.35**   Radioulnar joint mobility test.

### *Palpation*

Palpation in the off-field situation is similar to that for the sideline assessment. As you begin your palpation, have the athlete positioned comfortably. Often the most comfortable position is supine or sitting. If the athlete presents with tenderness over the medial or lateral epicondyle, pay special attention to assessing tenderness and any crepitus in the common flexor or extensor tendon, since the problem may be an epicondylitis. Soft tissue assessment into the muscle bellies of these muscles can also elicit pain, especially if the athlete's injury has become chronic. Tendon palpation should begin lightly and then move deeper. Tendinitis can be very isolated, so start in a small area and progress outward from the initial palpation site. Once you locate the source of pain, continue palpating distally along the tendon and into the muscle for evidence of pain and soft tissue restriction. Comparison to the other elbow is crucial for accurate assessment of soft tissue restriction.

---

## Checklist for Off-Field Assessment of the Elbow and Forearm

### History

Ask questions pertaining to the following:

✓ Chief complaint

✓ Mechanism of injury

✓ Unusual sounds or sensations

✓ Type, location, onset, and duration of pain or symptoms

✓ Previous injury

✓ Previous injury to opposite extremity for bilateral comparison

If chronic, ascertain:

✓ Aggravating and easing activities

✓ Training history (changes in training or equipment)

✓ Activity restrictions

✓ Treatment if any

### Observation

✓ Check for visible facial expressions of pain.

✓ Check for swelling, deformity, abnormal contours, or discoloration.

*(continued)*

## Checklist for Off-Field Assessment of the Elbow and Forearm (continued)

### Observation (continued)

✓ Does athlete let arm hang and swing, or does he or she hold or splint it?

✓ Observe overall position, posture, and alignment.

  ✓ Carrying angle

  ✓ Alignment of the medial and lateral epicondyle and olecranon process (elbow flexed and extended)

  ✓ Flexed elbow posture

✓ Check muscle development—areas of muscular atrophy.

✓ Make bilateral comparison.

### Differential Diagnosis

✓ Clear cervical region with overpressure tests in straight planes and quadrant position.

✓ Clear shoulder region wtih passive overpressures in all ranges.

### Range of Motion

✓ Active ROM for elbow flexion/extension, forearm pronation/supination

✓ Passive ROM for same motions

✓ Active ROM for shoulder flexion/extension, wrist flexion/extension as appropriate

✓ Passive ROM for same motions

✓ Bilateral comparison

### Strength Tests

✓ Perform manual resistance against same motions as in active ROM.

✓ Check bilaterally and note any pain or weakness.

✓ Perform instrumented strength tests.

### Neurovascular Tests

✓ Sensory, motor, reflex of nerve roots C5, C6, C7, C8, and T1

✓ Sensory and motor of peripheral nerves: median, ulnar, radial, and musculocutaneous

✓ Distal pulse

### Special Tests

✓ Collateral stress tests

✓ Radioulnar joint stress test

✓ Epicondylitis tests (active, passive)

✓ Nerve compression tests

### Joint Mobility Assessment

Note capsular restriction and end feel.

✓ Humeroulnar

✓ Radioulnar

✓ Bilateral comparison

### Palpation

Palpate for pain, tenderness, and deformity over the following, remembering to make bilateral comparisons:

✓ Medial epicondyle and supracondylar ridge

✓ Olecranon process, olecranon fossa, and proximal ulna

✓ Lateral eipcondyle and supracondylar ridge, radial head

✓ Flexor/pronator group, ulnar nerve, medial collateral ligament

✓ Olecranon bursa, distal triceps

✓ Extensor/supinator muscle group, brachioradialis, lateral collateral ligament, annular ligament

✓ Biceps tendon, brachial artery, median nerve

### Functional Tests

# SUMMARY

1. *Describe the etiology, signs and symptoms, and potential complications associated with acute and chronic injuries of the elbow and forearm commonly encountered in physically active people.*

Both acute and chronic injuries commonly occur at the elbow as a result of physical activity. Acute muscle strains and tendon ruptures of the biceps, triceps, and wrist flexor and extensor groups can result from violent muscle contractions. Traumatic injuries such as sprains, fractures, and dislocations most often occur as a result of extreme valgus, varus, and hyperextension forces; falls on an outstretched hand; and direct contact. Because of the close proximity of the major nerves and vessels to the elbow joint, neurovascular compromise can result as a complication of these traumatic injuries. Chronic overuse injuries are also prevalent, particularly in athletes engaged in overhead throwing sports and in sports such as tennis and golf that involve repetitive wrist motions. A variety of medial stress injuries can occur in both young and older athletes due to valgus overload forces associated with overhead throwing activities. A careful assessment is required in order to identify and differentiate which structure is involved.

2. *Identify the common pathologies associated with repetitive valgus overload stresses in the throwing athlete.*

During the late cocking phase of throwing, tremendous valgus forces are placed on the elbow, resulting in traction-type injuries on the medial aspect and compression-type injuries on the lateral aspect of the joint. In the adult athlete, injury is usually to the ligament or tendon, resulting in medial epicondylitis and valgus instability. In the young athlete, injury more often involves the medial humeral apophysis and can result in apophysitis—and eventually a traction apophyseal fracture if the stress is allowed to continue. Osteochondritis dissecans of the radial head as a result of medial compression with valgus overload can also occur in the young athlete who performs throwing activities.

3. *Identify potential causes of forearm compartment syndrome and the 5 P's of neurovascular compromise.*

Forearm compartment syndrome can result from any injury that compromises the vascular structures. Laceration or occlusion of the brachial artery secondary to fracture or dislocation, or any trauma that causes rapid, excessive swelling in the elbow and forearm, will compromise blood flow to the forearm, ultimately resulting in venous collapse and tissue necrosis. Signs and symptoms of compartment syndrome include pulselessness, pallor, pain out of proportion to the injury, paresthesia, and eventual paralysis. With traumatic injuries, it is essential to assess neurovascular status immediately and to monitor it often.

4. *Identify the various anatomical sites and signs and symptoms associated with nerve compression syndromes.*

The peripheral nerves of the forearm and hand travel across the elbow through anatomical spaces created by bone, fascia, and muscle. Nerve compression can occur if these spaces are compromised due to excessive muscle hypertrophy, scar formation, fascial restriction, and swelling. Signs and symptoms are common to all, with pain, paresthesia, and possible muscle weakness along the involved nerve's distribution. Special tests that reproduce these signs and symptoms are positive for nerve compression syndromes.

5. *Describe the normal anatomical alignment, carrying angle, and range of motion of the elbow joint.*

To perform an accurate assessment of joint position and motion, it is important to have a good understanding of the normal anatomical alignment of the elbow. In the anatomical extended position of 0°, the carrying angle of the elbow is slightly valgus (with females having a slightly greater angulation than males), and the medial and lateral epicondyle and olecranon process form a straight line. The elbow is capable of flexing about 145° actively and about 155-160° passively. In the flexed position, the valgus angulation disappears, and an isosceles triangle is formed by the olecranon process and medial and lateral epicondyles.

6. *Demonstrate an on-field assessment for the elbow and forearm, and determine criteria for immediate medical referral and mode of transportation from the field.*

The immediate aims in an on-field assessment of an elbow injury are to assess the joint for possible dislocation, fracture, and compromised vascular supply, as well as the athlete's overall condition. When obvious deformities are present, neurovascular status must be immediately assessed; and if the findings are positive, medical referral is made without delay because of the potential complications. If gross deformities are not present, the athletic trainer performs palpation to check for any bony tenderness, crepitus, or subtle deformities that may indicate less serious fractures. If the injury is not serious, the athlete is removed from the field for a more thorough evaluation on the sideline.

7. *Perform a sequential and thorough sideline assessment of the elbow and forearm, noting criteria for referral and return to activity.*

Once the athlete is on the sideline, the athletic trainer determines whether he or she is able to return to sport participation using a more thorough evaluation of the severity of the injury, the structure involved, and the athlete's functional ability. This includes a more detailed history, observation, and palpation assessment. Because of the superficial nature of many of the soft tissue and bony structures of the elbow, careful palpation is an important tool in identifying the specific structure(s) involved. In addition, the sideline assessment includes active, passive, and resistive ROM tests in elbow flexion, extension, pronation, and supination. Joint stability tests to determine medial and lateral collateral ligament integrity also take place at this time, as do neurovascular tests as appropriate. If the evaluation reveals no significant injuries, functional tests mimicking the forces and movements required of the upper extremity are performed to determine readiness to return to activity.

8. *Perform a sequential and thorough off-field assessment of the elbow and forearm, noting considerations for differential diagnosis.*

Many conditions at the elbow are chronic and are often first reported in the athletic treatment facility. The off-field assessment for the elbow is similar to the sideline assessment, with the addition of special tests to evaluate more chronic conditions such as epicondylitis, tendinitis, and nerve compression syndromes. Differential tests to rule out cervical and shoulder pathologies are also performed, as these pathologies may refer symptoms to the elbow. The off-field assessment may also incorporate joint mobility tests to identify any joint or capsular restriction and to assess joint end feel.

# REVIEW QUESTIONS

1. What is the normal carrying angle of the elbow? What is a "gunstock" deformity, and what are some of its potential causes?

2. What causes olecranon bursitis? What are the signs and symptoms associated with this condition?

3. Define the terms tendinitis, epicondylitis, and tendinosis. What are the differences among these conditions, and how would their signs and symptoms differ?

4. Identify the specific injuries that cause a compartment syndrome. Describe the continuum of this pathology and the characteristic deformity that results if care is not immediate.

5. Discuss the causative factors, signs and symptoms, and structures involved in cubital tunnel syndrome. What special tests might you use to confirm this condition?

6. What are some secondary conditions that can result from chronic valgus overload in an athlete with valgus instability? Think about the other structures that could be tractioned or compressed as a consequence of increased ligament laxity. What signs and symptoms would you expect if these structures were involved, and what special tests would you use to confirm their involvement?

7. What test is used to test the integrity of the medial (ulnar) collateral ligament? How would you grade and determine the severity of the ligament injury?

8. Identify the peripheral nerve pathology that would cause the following symptoms:

   • Weakness in pinch strength

   • Paresthesia over the dorsal web space

   • Deep ache in the extensor muscle mass with repetitive gripping

   • Paresthesia over the distal, radial aspect of the second digit

   • Intrinsic muscle weakness

# CRITICAL THINKING QUESTIONS

1. You are asked to evaluate an 18-year-old pitcher who has had medial elbow pain for six weeks. His history reveals that he has been a pitcher for six years and has no previous injury. He complains of pain with hard throwing. Upon palpation, it is difficult for you to tell whether his tenderness is over the medial collateral ligament, medial condyle, or the musculotendinous origin of the flexor/pronator group. You also note that he has mild lateral joint pain. Given his age and his sport, which condition(s) might you most likely suspect and why? What special tests would you use to differentiate the potential structures involved?

2. Identify the type of end feel you might find with the following pathologies and passive motions:

   • Posterior lateral osteophyte of the olecranon process with elbow extension

   • Valgus instability with valgus stress test

   • Biceps rupture with elbow extension

   • Acute anterior capsular strain with elbow extension

   • Lateral epicondylitis with pronation

3. You are covering soccer practice and you see an athlete fall onto his outstretched hand. You arrive at his side to find that he is in considerable pain, and you observe an obvious deformity. You immediately check distal pulse and find it absent. You know this is a medical emergency, and the coach's car is parked right next to the field. The coach offers to take the athlete immediately to the emergency room. Do you take him up on this offer to get the athlete medical attention sooner, or do you wait for emergency medical services? Discuss what decision you would make and give the reasons.

# CITED REFERENCES

Alley, R.M., and Pappas, A.M. 1995. Acute and chronic performance related injuries of the elbow. In A.M. Pappas (ed.), *Upper extremity injuries in the athlete* (pp. 339-364). New York: Churchill Livingstone.

Andrews, J.R., and Whiteside, J.A. 1993. Common elbow problems in the athlete. *J Orthop Sports Phys Ther* 17(6):289-295.

Behr, C.T., and Altchek, D.W. 1997. The elbow. *Clin Sports Med* 16(4):681-704.

Bennett, J.B. 1993. Articular injuries in the athlete. In B.F. Morrey (ed.), *The elbow and its disorders* (2d ed., pp. 581-595). Philadelphia: Saunders.

Cabanela, M.E., and Morrey, B.F. 1993. Fractures of the proximal ulna and olecranon. In B.F. Morrey (ed.), *The elbow and its disorders* (2d ed., pp. 405-428). Philadelphia: Saunders.

Caldwell, G.L., and Safran, M.R. 1995. Elbow problems in the athlete. *Orthop Clin N Am* 26(3):465-485.

Griggs, S.M., and Weiss, A.-P.C. 1996. Bony injuries of the wrist, forearm and elbow. *Clin Sports Med* 15(2), 373-400.

Grossfield, S.L., Heest, A.V., Arendt, E., and House, J. 1998. Pitcher's periostitis. *Am J Sports Med* 26(2):303-307.

Jobe, F.W., Stark, H., and Lombardo, S.J. 1986. Reconstruction of the ulnar collateral ligament in athletes. *J Bone Joint Surg* 68A:1158-63.

Larson, R.L., and Osternig, L.R. 1974. Traumatic bursitis and artificial turf. *J Sports Med* 2:183.

Lowery, W.D., Kurzweil, P.R., Forman, S.K., and Morrison, D.S. 1995. Persistence of the olecranon physis: A cause of "Little League Elbow." *J Elbow Shoulder Surg* 4(2):143-147.

Morrey, B.F. 1993. Radial head fracture. In B.F. Morrey (ed.), *The elbow and its disorders* (2d ed., pp. 383-404). Philadelphia: Saunders.

Nirschl, R.P. 1993. Muscle and tendon trauma: Tennis elbow. In B.F. Morrey (ed.), *The elbow and its disorders* (2d ed., pp. 537-552). Philadelphia: Saunders.

Slowik, G.M., Fitzimmons, M., and Rayhack, J.M. 1993. Closed elbow dislocation and brachial artery damage. *J Orthop Trauma* 7(6):558-561.

Takahara, M., Shundo, M., Kondo, M., Suzuki, K., Nambu, T., and Ogino, T. 1998. Early detection of osteochondritis dissecans of the capitellum in young baseball players. *J Bone Jt Surg* 80A(6):892-897.

Takami, H., Takahashi, S., and Ando, M. 1997. Irreducible isolated dislocation of the radial head. *Clin Orthop Rel Res* 345:168-170.

Timmerman, L.A., and Andrews, J.R. 1994. Undersurface tear of the ulnar collateral ligament in baseball players. A newly recognized lesion. *Am J Sports Med* 22(1):33-36.

Tyrdal, S., and Olsen, B.S. 1998. Combined hyperextension and supination of the elbow joint induces lateral ligament lesions. An experimental study of the pathoanatomy and kinematics in elbow ligament injuries. *Knee Surg, Sports Traum, Arthro* 6(1):36-43.

Wadhwa, S.S., Mansberg, R., Fernandes, V.B., and Qasim, S. 1997. Forearm splints seen on bone scan in a weightlifter. *Clin Nuclear Med* 22(10):711-712.

Weiker, G.G. 1995. Upper extremity gymnastic injuries. In J.A. Nicholas and E.B. Hershman (eds.), *The upper extremity in sports medicine* (2d ed., p. 840). St. Louis: Mosby.

Wilson, F.D., Andrews, J.R., Blackburn, T.A., and McCluskey, G. 1983. Valgus extension overload in the pitching elbow. *Am J Sports Med* 11(2):83-87.

# CHAPTER SIX

# Wrist and Hand

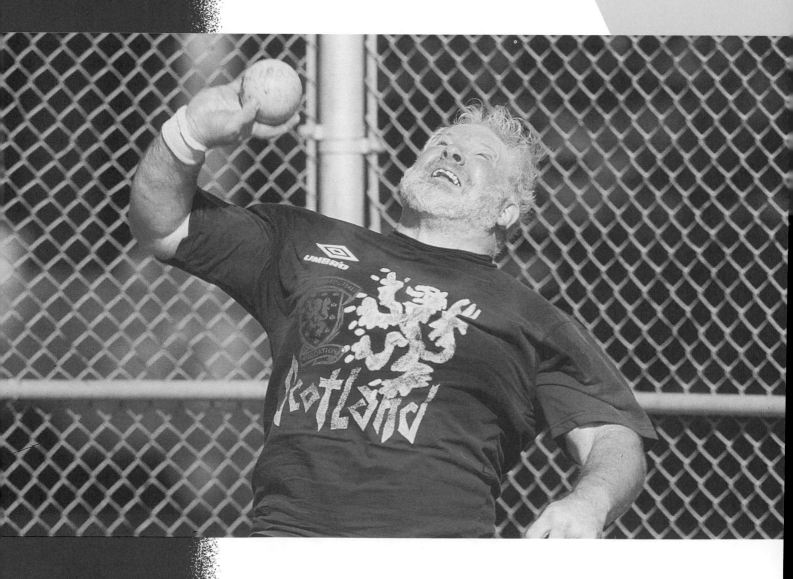

# OBJECTIVES

After completing this chapter, the reader will be able to do the following:

1. Describe the general types and mechanisms of acute and chronic injuries of the wrist and hand that physically active people commonly experience

2. Describe the potential complications and deformities that can result from seemingly simple sprains and strains

3. Identify the common sites of nerve compression injuries, as well as the common signs and symptoms associated with each

4. Discuss the common fractures that occur in the wrist and hand and their characteristic deformities, signs, and symptoms

5. Perform an on-field assessment of the wrist and hand, being able to identify which conditions warrant immediate referral

6. Perform a sideline assessment of the wrist and hand, including special tests used to evaluate acute conditions

7. Perform an off-field assessment of the wrist and hand, including evaluation techniques to assess injuries that are more chronic

John was in his first year as an assistant athletic trainer at California State University and was excited to be with his team in Oklahoma City for the NCAA National Championships in women's softball. Before the game, the coach from UCLA, the reigning national champions, approached John and informed him that their athletic trainer was back at the hotel with the flu.

She then asked, "Would you mind helping us out by coming onto the field if one of my players gets hurt during the game?"

John didn't see this as a problem, and injuries were so rare in softball anyway. "Sure, I'd be glad to help . . . just let me know if you need me."

It was the top of the seventh inning and CSU was behind by one run. UCLA was currently up to bat with one out, and their All-American pitcher (and fastest runner) was on first. On the next pitch, she made an attempt to steal second, sliding into the bag headfirst with hands outstretched. She was safe, but she was also obviously in a great deal of pain and was holding her hand. John realized he was needed and ran out to the injured player. It took only a moment to recognize that she had a dislocation of her fifth proximal interphalangeal joint.

"Put it back in," she cried. "I've already come out of the game once and I have to pitch this last inning." The coach also chimed in, "We need her—please take care of it for us."

John really wasn't sure quite what to do—it appeared to be a simple dislocation, and he knew how important this player was to the team. He certainly didn't want to be accused of not helping her because they were the opponent. He knew he had to make a decision quickly. . .

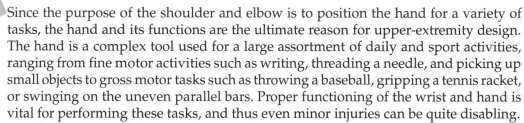

Since the purpose of the shoulder and elbow is to position the hand for a variety of tasks, the hand and its functions are the ultimate reason for upper-extremity design. The hand is a complex tool used for a large assortment of daily and sport activities, ranging from fine motor activities such as writing, threading a needle, and picking up small objects to gross motor tasks such as throwing a baseball, gripping a tennis racket, or swinging on the uneven parallel bars. Proper functioning of the wrist and hand is vital for performing these tasks, and thus even minor injuries can be quite disabling.

The structure of the wrist and hand represents a complex network of multiple bones, joints, ligaments, and both intrinsic and extrinsic muscle actions functioning together to provide the precision, coordination, mobility, and strength required to perform various tasks. Because of the anatomical complexity of the wrist and hand, you are encouraged to review the structures and functions of this body region before continuing with the assessment procedures in this chapter. As with any body region, a thorough knowledge of anatomy is essential for accurate assessment and interpretation of your findings.

# INJURIES TO THE WRIST AND HAND

The dexterity and precision that the wrist and hand must have for fine motor control often leaves them unprotected and vulnerable to injury during sport activity. Contact with the ground, an opponent, and balls and other sporting implements represents the primary mechanism for acute injury of the wrist and hand. The hand and wrist are also prone to repetitive stress injuries, as well as chronic conditions that may result from ignored or untreated acute injuries.

## ACUTE SOFT TISSUE INJURIES

Physically active people commonly experience contusions, sprains, and strains, primarily as a result of direct contact, falls, and other forces that either compress or tension the soft tissue structures.

## Contusions

Because of the many bony prominences and superficial tendons exposed in the wrist and hand, contusions resulting from direct contact may be quite bothersome. Pain and swelling from contusions to the tendons and ligaments can result in decreased range of motion and loss of function. Rarely are these injuries serious, and pain and dysfunction usually dissipate rather quickly. Pain and loss of motion that continue for more than a few days should raise a high suspicion of bony contusion, fracture, or both.

## Sprains

Because of the multiple bones and joints in the wrist and hand, ligament injuries are quite common. Sprains to the wrist (distal radial ulnar joint and carpal bones) often result from extending or flexing the wrist beyond its normal range of motion. Mechanisms include falling on an outstretched hand (hyperflexion and hyperextension), "jamming" the wrist during blocking or vaulting activities, and twisting maneuvers. Excessive radial or ulnar deviation may also injure the wrist ligaments. Signs and symptoms associated with wrist sprain include pain, swelling, and point tenderness over the injured joint consistent with the degree of injury. Pain will be experienced with both active and passive range of motion. Muscular weakness may result secondary to pain with resisted motions. In cases of third-degree sprains, there may be instability and joint deformity.

### Collateral Ligament Sprain

Collateral ligament sprains of the fingers are among the most common injuries resulting from physical activity. Collateral ligament injuries can occur at either the metacarpophalangeal (MCP) joint, the proximal interphalangeal (PIP) joint, or the distal interphalangeal (DIP) joint. A mechanism frequently associated with collateral ligament sprains is "jamming" the finger while catching a ball, sliding into base, or tackling, among other activities, which can force the joints beyond their normal range of motion and stretch the collateral ligaments (figure 6.1). Signs and symptoms associated with collateral ligament sprains include pain, swelling, point tenderness over the injured joint and ligament, increased pain with valgus/varus stress, and instability consistent with first-, second-, and third-degree classifications. It is not uncommon for pain and swelling to persist for a significant period of time. However, in some cases, chronic inflammation within the joint capsule (**capsulitis**) can ultimately result in adhesions and scarring that can deform the joint and permanently restrict range of motion. Therefore, even though collateral ligament injuries are often considered relatively minor, proper treatment and splinting are necessary to avoid permanent joint complications.

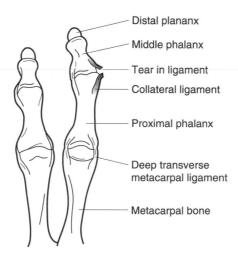

Distal plananx

Middle phalanx

Tear in ligament

Collateral ligament

Proximal phalanx

Deep transverse metacarpal ligament

Metacarpal bone

**❚ Figure 6.1**  Injury to the collateral ligament of the finger.

### Gamekeeper's or Skier's Thumb

A collateral ligament injury that can be particularly troublesome—known as "**gamekeeper's**" or "**skier's**" **thumb**—involves the ulnar (medial) collateral ligament (UCL) of the MCP joint of the thumb. The injury results from forced abduction and hyperextension of the thumb away from the hand, causing stretch and tearing of the UCL (figure 6.2). It has been termed skier's thumb because the mechanism and injury often occur in skiers when they fall on an outstretched hand while holding on to a ski pole. However, it is equally common in a variety of sports in which the thumb is vulnerable to direct contact with a ball or other object or with another person.

Signs and symptoms include pain, point tenderness over the medial aspect of the MCP joint of the thumb, swelling, and varying degrees of instability consistent with the degree of ligament injury. In cases of second- and third-degree sprains, pain and weakness with pinching between the thumb and index finger will also result from the lack of stability at the joint. A potential complication of UCL injury of the thumb is called a **Stener lesion**, in which the adductor aponeurosis comes between the ruptured ends of the ligament and prevents healing. Avulsion fractures may also result when the ligament is torn at the bony attachment.

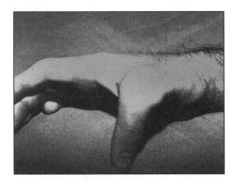

**▌Figure 6.2**   Gamekeeper's thumb.

*"Volar"* refers to the palmar aspect of the wrist or hand. Although "palmar" is the most widely accepted term for this surface, "volar" continues to be used to describe some injury conditions.

### Volar Plate Rupture

Hyperextension of the PIP joint can also result in rupture of the volar plate. Signs and symptoms of volar plate injury include pain, tenderness over the palmar aspect of the joint, swelling, and loss of function. If left unrecognized or untreated, volar instability can lead to either a flexion or extension deformity at the joint. When the volar plate is disrupted from its distal attachment, subluxation and permanent hyperextension of the joint can occur. This hyperextension deformity may subsequently cause hyperflexion at the DIP joint due to tensioning of the flexor tendons, resulting in a **swan-neck deformity** (figure 6.3a). Conversely, when the volar plate is disrupted from its proximal attachment, a flexion contracture or pseudoboutonniere deformity may result (figure 6.3b). Needless to say, proper management and treatment are imperative to prevent permanent joint deformity following a volar plate injury.

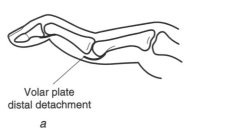
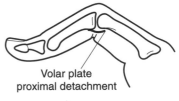

Volar plate
distal detachment

*a*

Volar plate
proximal detachment

*b*

**▌Figure 6.3**   (a) Swan-neck deformity and (b) pseudoboutonniere deformity.

### *Strains and Tendon Avulsions*

Tendon injuries to the fingers are also quite common in the physically active. Tendon injuries can result from a direct blow, but more often result from abrupt forces applied in the direction opposite to that in which a joint is contracting. This can create considerable tensioning of the tendon, causing it to tear away from its distal attachment.

#### Flexor Tendon Avulsion (Jersey Finger)

Flexor tendon avulsion injuries involve the flexor digitorum profundus tendon; they occur when the distal phalanx is forcefully extended while the finger is flexing. This injury is often called a **jersey finger** because it is frequently seen in athletes, such as football players, who get a finger caught while trying to grab and pull at an opponent's jersey. Signs and symptoms include immediate pain, swelling, and point tenderness at the attachment of the flexor tendon on the distal phalanx. With complete rupture (figure 6.4), the athlete will be unable to flex the distal phalanx while the proximal joint is held in extension. If the rupture is incomplete, pain and weakness will be noted with flexion.

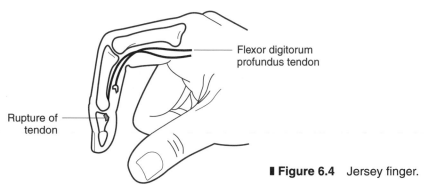

Flexor digitorum
profundus tendon

Rupture of
tendon

▮ **Figure 6.4**   Jersey finger.

#### Extensor Tendon Avulsion (Mallet Finger)

**Mallet finger**, or **baseball finger**, occurs when the extended distal phalanx is suddenly and forcefully flexed. A common example is seen when an athlete attempts to catch a ball and instead the ball makes contact with the tip of the extended finger. Rupture of the distal extensor tendon may or may not include avulsion of a bony fragment (figure 6.5). Signs and symptoms include pain, point tenderness over the distal attachment, flexion deformity of the distal phalanx, and an inability to actively extend the distal phalanx. Ruptures involving a bony avulsion have a greater chance of healing without surgical intervention if recognized early and treated with appropriate splinting.

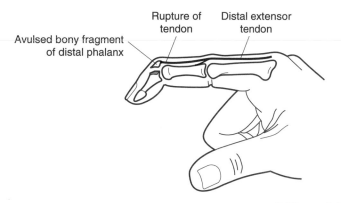

Rupture of      Distal extensor
tendon          tendon

Avulsed bony fragment
of distal phalanx

▮ **Figure 6.5**   Mallet finger.

### Extensor Tendon Rupture (Boutonniere Deformity)

A **boutonniere deformity** is characterized by flexion of the PIP joint and hyperextension of the DIP joint. This deformity most often results from injury to the central slip of the extensor digitorum tendon at its insertion at the base of the middle phalanx. Rupture of the extensor tendon at this location is most often a result of forced flexion of the PIP joint. Signs and symptoms include pain localized to the PIP joint, point tenderness near the tendon's insertion, swelling, and weakness with extension of the PIP joint. As a consequence of this injury, the surrounding retinacular tissues are also disrupted and the intact lateral bands of the extensor tendon, which extend to the distal joint, will begin to migrate toward the volar surface of the finger (figure 6.6). This migration changes the line of pull of the lateral bands to flexors of the PIP joint instead of extensors.

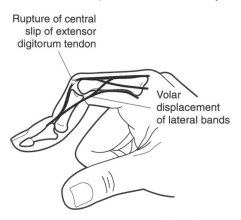

Rupture of central slip of extensor digitorum tendon

Volar displacement of lateral bands

■ **Figure 6.6**   Boutonniere deformity.

Additionally, the flexed PIP joint will protrude through the lateral bands like a "buttonhole," causing hyperextension of both the MCP and DIP joints.

## CHRONIC OR OVERUSE SOFT TISSUE INJURIES

Because of the repetitive nature of many hand movements, as well as the excessive use of the hands in many sport and occupational activities, chronic inflammatory conditions of the wrist, hand, and fingers are common. In addition, complications from unrecognized or untreated acute injuries can result in chronic and potentially disfiguring conditions.

### *Tendinitis and Tenosynovitis*

*Tenosynovitis is an inflammatory condition of the tendon and its synovial sheath that causes pain, crepitus with palpation and movement, and decreased range of motion.*

Inflammation of the tendon and/or its surrounding synovial sheath is common in physically active people. Overuse or repetitive motion, direct trauma, and continual use following tendon injury are all common mechanisms associated with tendinitis and tenosynovitis. Signs and symptoms include point tenderness over the involved tendon, swelling, palpable crepitus, pain with active and resistive motion, and pain with passive stretching of the tendon. With tenosynovitis, the tendon, the synovial sheath, or both can become inflamed. This inflammation will limit the tendon's ability to glide smoothly through the sheath, creating friction and discomfort. If the condition becomes chronic, the tissues can permanently thicken and limit motion. In severe chronic cases, contractures may result.

### De Quervain's Disease

**De Quervain's disease** is a tenosynovitis of the abductor pollicis longus and extensor pollicis brevis tendons and their sheaths on the radial side of the thumb (figure 6.7). Repetitive motions that combine gripping with the hand and ulnar deviation of the wrist can inflame these tendons as they pass through their osseofibrous tunnel, deep to the extensor retinaculum.

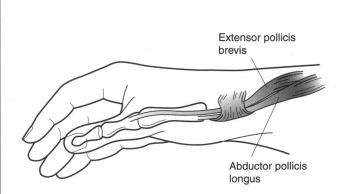

Extensor pollicis brevis

Abductor pollicis longus

■ **Figure 6.7**   Tenosynovitis of abductor pollicus longus and extensor pollicus brevis tendons (De Quervain's disease).

Signs and symptoms are consistent with a typical tenosynovitis. The athlete will complain of pain and crepitus at the base of the thumb, pain and weakness with active and resisted thumb extension/abduction, and increased pain when making a fist and deviating the wrist to the ulnar side (see Finkelstein test later in this chapter).

### Trigger Finger

**Trigger finger** is a condition associated with tenosynovitis of the flexor tendons, resulting from repetitive trauma to the flexor tendon sheath. Most commonly seen in the third and fourth digits, it results from thickening or nodules in the synovial sheath. This thickening decreases the space through which the tendon is able to glide (stenosis) and causes the tendon to "catch" and then "let go" as it moves through the sheath during finger flexion. As the condition worsens and the synovial tunnel becomes more **stenotic** (narrow), the finger may stick in a flexed position, requiring passive assistance to return to an extended position. The hallmark sign of a trigger finger is an observable "snapping" of the finger as it is actively flexed, much as in pulling a trigger. A snap or click may also be heard when this occurs. Depending on the state of the inflammatory response at the time of evaluation, signs and symptoms associated with tenosynovitis will also be noted.

*Stenosis is a stricture of any canal.*

### Dupuytren's Contracture

A flexion deformity more commonly seen in the older adult population is Dupuytren's contracture (figure 6.8). This condition of unknown etiology is characterized by a flexion contracture of the MCP and PIP joints, usually of the fourth or fifth digits, as a result of thickness and contracture of the palmar fascia and its eventual adherence to overlying skin (Harris 1983). In addition to the obvious deformity, thickening or nodules in the palmar fascia may be palpable. The tight palmar fascia will also appear as rigid bands underneath the skin when the fingers are extended.

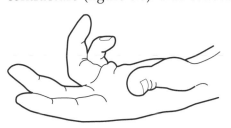

■ **Figure 6.8** Dupuytren's contracture deformity with thickening of palmar fascia.

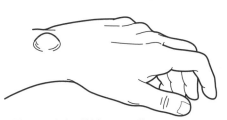

■ **Figure 6.9** Wrist ganglion.

### Wrist Ganglion

A wrist **ganglion**, or synovial cyst, is characterized by herniation of **synovial fluid** through the joint capsule or synovial sheath of a tendon. Minor sprains and strains often precipitate the formation of a wrist ganglion and are thought to weaken the capsule or synovial sheath, allowing fluid to escape and accumulate. Overuse mechanisms may also be an underlying cause of ganglion cysts. Wrist ganglions may form on either the dorsal or the volar aspect of the wrist, but are more common on the dorsal surface. Signs and symptoms include an observable and palpable localized mass over the wrist (figure 6.9). The mass may or may not be painful and may or may not restrict range of motion or impede function. However, there is typically some tenderness, and the athlete will experience mild to moderate pain and discomfort with wrist extension (dorsal ganglion). While some ganglion cysts can be quite small and others quite large, symptoms are not necessarily dependent on size. Symptoms may be more related to the location of the cyst and the motion restrictions it may create.

## BONY PATHOLOGY

Fractures and dislocations of the wrist and hand are among the most common in sport. The use of the hands for reaching, blocking, catching, and grabbing lends to their vulnerability to injury during sport activities.

### *Traumatic Fractures*

Traumatic fractures of the wrist and hand most often occur due to axial loading forces and falls on an outstretched hand.

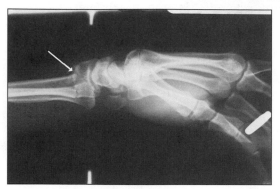

■ **Figure 6.10**   Colles's fracture with characteristic silver fork deformity.

### Colles's Fracture

A Colles's fracture of the distal radius and ulna is typically caused by a fall on an outstretched hand with the wrist extended. It is characterized by **silver fork deformity** or dorsal displacement of the distal fragments of the radius and ulna in relation to their proximal shafts (figure 6.10). Signs and symptoms include immediate wrist pain, rapid swelling, tenderness, and deformity. Loss of wrist and hand function may result both from an unwillingness to move the extremity because of pain and from restrictions caused by the displacement. Bony crepitus may also be noted over the fracture. The displaced proximal fragments may also injure the median nerve; when this happens, there may also be diminished sensation and loss of motor function over the median nerve distribution.

### Smith's Fracture

A Smith's fracture is the opposite of a Colles's fracture, with displacement of the distal radius and ulna being volar to the proximal fragment. The mechanism of injury is most often a fall onto the back of the hand, causing hyperflexion of the wrist joint. Signs and symptoms will be similar to those for Colles's fracture with the exception of their characteristic deformities.

### Bennett's Fracture

A Bennett's fracture, involving the base of the first metacarpal bone (thumb), is most often caused by striking an object with a closed fist, making contact specifically with the thumb. This axial loading of the metacarpal bone will cause a shear fracture at its base. While the proximal fragment will maintain its position with the carpal bones, the metacarpal will be displaced because of the pull of the abductor pollicis longus muscle (figure 6.11). Signs and symptoms include immediate pain, rapid swelling, tenderness, and crepitus at the MCP joint of the thumb, as well as loss of function. Deformity may also be present depending on the extent of metacarpal displacement. Because this fracture occurs so near the joint, there may be false joint motion with movement.

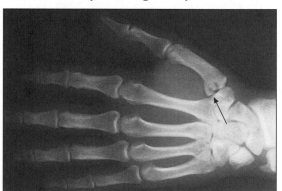

■ **Figure 6.11**   Bennett's fracture with MC displacement.

### Carpal Bones

Among the eight carpal bones, the navicular or scaphoid bone is the one most commonly fractured (figure 6.12). It can also be the most troublesome and slowest to heal. Navicular fractures typically occur when the bone is compressed against the radius during direct contact with the palm of the hand—for example, dur-

A hallmark sign of a navicular fracture is point tenderness specifically over the navicular on palpation in the anatomical snuffbox.

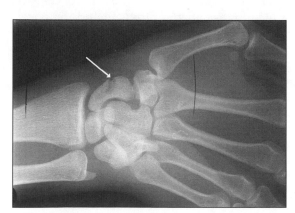

■ **Figure 6.12**   Navicular fracture.

ing blocking with the hands or in a fall in which the thumb and wrist are extended and the wrist is abducted. The athlete will complain of pain, swelling, and tenderness over the radial side of the wrist. A hallmark sign of a navicular fracture is point tenderness specifically over the navicular on palpation in the anatomical snuffbox. Crepitus and pain with wrist motion may also be noted. It is not uncommon for symptoms to be vague and for this injury to be missed on initial x-ray. Because of the poor vascular supply to the proximal portion of the bone, healing of fractures in the region may be difficult; early and adequate immobilization offers the optimal chance. Therefore, it is important to suspect and rule out fracture any time there is pain in the anatomical snuffbox.

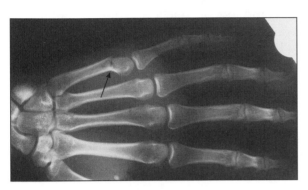

**Figure 6.13**    Boxer's fracture.

### Metacarpal Fractures

Fractures to the neck, shaft, and base of the metacarpal bones often result from axial loading of the metacarpal bone secondary to an indirect force such as striking an object with a closed fist. Other common causes are direct trauma or crushing injuries to the hand—for example, when the hand is stepped or landed on during sport activity. Signs and symptoms include pain, diffuse swelling over the dorsum of the hand, and tenderness over the metacarpal. Pain will likely increase with both longitudinal stress and axial compression or percussion of the metacarpal. Bony crepitus may also be noted. Deformity will also be noted if the bone is displaced. When the fracture specifically involves the neck of the fifth metatarsal, the injury is commonly referred to as a **boxer's fracture** (figure 6.13).

### Phalanges

Fractures of the phalanges can be caused by a variety of mechanisms. Direct contact, axial loading to the tip of the finger, torsion, and other indirect trauma are all common mechanisms. Fractures may also be associated with sprains and dislocations. Signs and symptoms include pain, swelling, and point tenderness over the fracture site. Loss of function, deformity, and crepitus may also result. If the fracture occurs near a joint and is displaced, there may be a false appearance of joint motion or dislocation. Fractures of the fingers are often missed or are dismissed as sprains without careful evaluation and x-ray. Because fractures through the joint have the potential for complications and permanent joint dysfunction, traumatic injuries to the phalangeal joints should be carefully evaluated by an orthopedist to rule out possible fracture.

## *Dislocation or Subluxation*

The same forces and mechanisms responsible for wrist and hand fractures may also result in joint dislocation or subluxation.

### Lunate Dislocation

In the wrist, the most commonly dislocated carpal bone is the lunate. Lunate dislocations can be caused by a fall on an outstretched hand or with hyperextension of the wrist. Through this mechanism, the lunate is displaced in a volar direction (figure 6.14). With volar displacement, the median nerve can sometimes be compressed. Signs and symptoms include pain,

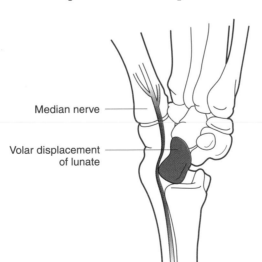

Median nerve

Volar displacement of lunate

**Figure 6.14**    Lunate dislocation.

swelling, and localized tenderness in the wrist. Deformity and loss of function may also be noted, with the lunate distinctly palpable on the volar aspect of the wrist. Numbness and tingling in the lateral palm and into the second and third fingers may also be present with medial nerve compression.

### Metacarpophalangeal and Interphalangeal Joint Dislocations

Dislocation of the MCP and interphalangeal (IP) joints is consistent with third-degree sprains in which the ligaments and joint capsule are stretched or torn sufficiently to allow joint displacement to occur. Unless the joint spontaneously reduces following injury, these injuries are quite obvious; the distal bone can be displaced in any direction, depending on the offending force. Signs and symptoms of dislocation include obvious deformity, pain, rapid swelling, and loss of function. Often, the athlete or coach will reduce the dislocation and not seek medical attention. However, all first-time dislocations should be evaluated by a physician to rule out any associated articular fractures or volar plate disruption.

## NERVE AND VASCULAR INJURIES

Most cases of neurovascular compromise at the wrist and hand are attributable to chronic inflammatory conditions resulting in compression of these structures. On occasion, severe fractures or dislocations can also result in secondary injury or compression of the nearby nerve or vascular structure.

### *Carpal Tunnel Syndrome (Median Nerve Compression)*

**Carpal tunnel syndrome** is a common condition of the wrist and hand characterized by compression of the median nerve as it passes through the carpal tunnel (figure 6.15). Compression of the median nerve within the tunnel can be caused by multiple factors, including overuse, bony protrusion into the tunnel, and fluid retention. Overuse conditions resulting from repetitive use of the wrist and finger flexors can cause tenosynovitis and inflammation within the tunnel. Fractures and dislocations at the wrist may also compress the nerve in the tunnel secondary to protrusion of bony fragments and resultant swelling. Finally, fluid retention, which can result from a number of medical conditions, can cause swelling of the tissues within the carpal tunnel.

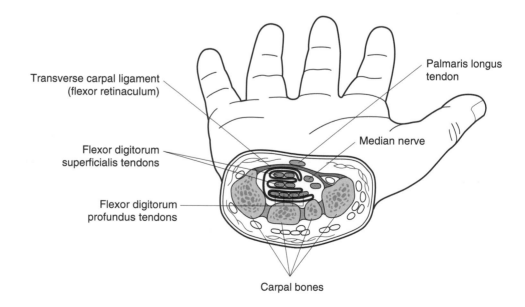

**Figure 6.15** Median nerve through the carpal tunnel.

Carpal tunnel occurs more often in mature adults than in other age groups, and more often in women than in men. It is less common in young adults but can occur in any sport involving repetitive wrist and finger flexion. Carpal tunnel syndrome may be unrelated to sport activity, as occupational and student activities such as excessive typing on a computer keyboard can be a causative factor. Signs and symptoms include pain, tenderness over the palmar aspect of the wrist, sensory changes, and motor weakness. Sensory changes may include tingling, numbness, and paresthesia over the median nerve distribution in the hand (palm and palmar aspect of the medial thumb and first and middle fingers). In severe or prolonged cases, muscle atrophy may be present in the thenar eminence; there may be weakness with flexion of the index and middle finger and with flexion, abduction, and opposition of the thumb. Pain and sensory changes are usually exacerbated with the offending activity or when the wrist is held in a flexed position for a prolonged period of time (i.e., during sleep). Tapping or percussion over the flexor retinaculum at the wrist may also reproduce symptoms of pain and paresthesia (i.e., Tinel's sign). Other causes of median nerve compression or injury include wrist fractures and dislocations as previously discussed. Median nerve palsy can also result from compression or injury at the elbow. In cases in which there is severe atrophy of the thenar eminence muscles, thumb opposition and flexion are lost. Additionally, secondary to pull of the extensor muscles, an **ape hand deformity** may result, characterized by extension of the thumb and alignment in the same plane as the fingers (figure 6.16).

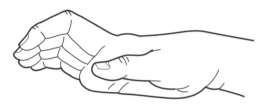

**▌Figure 6.16**   Ape hand deformity.

### Ulnar Nerve Compression

Compression injuries to the ulnar nerve can also occur at the wrist. Ulnar nerve palsy is commonly associated with cycling, as prolonged pressure of the handlebars over the hypothenar eminence causes irritation and compression of the ulnar nerve. Additionally, the nerve can be compressed in the tunnel of Guyon (figure 6.17) between the pisiform and hamate due to blunt trauma or fracture of the surrounding carpal bones. Signs and symptoms associated with ulnar nerve compression include pain, tingling, or numbness radiating into the ulnar distribution of the hand and fourth and fifth fingers. Motor weakness and atrophy may also be noted in the hypothenar, dorsal interossei, and fourth and fifth lumbricale muscles. Wasting of these muscles resulting from ulnar nerve palsy is known as a **bishop's**, or **benediction**, **deformity**.

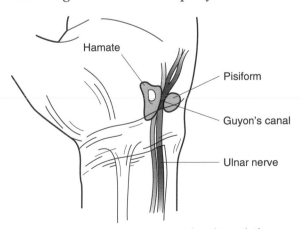

Hamate

Pisiform

Guyon's canal

Ulnar nerve

**▌Figure 6.17**   Ulnar nerve passing through the tunnel of Guyon.

### Radial Nerve Palsy

Wrist drop may also be noted at the wrist with upper-extremity injuries resulting in radial nerve palsy. If the radial nerve is severely traumatized or injured, there may be profound weakness or paralysis of the wrist and finger extensors. Because of an inability to extend the wrist, there will be a flexion deformity. This condition points to the importance of differential diagnosis in that pathology seen in the hand can originate anywhere in the upper extremity.

### *Claw Hand Deformity*

When both the median and ulnar nerves are injured, the consequent paralysis and wasting of all the interossei and lumbricale muscles of the hand result in a claw hand deformity. A claw hand is characterized by hyperextension of the MCP joint and flexion of the PIP and DIP joints. When intrinsic muscle function in the hand is lost, the ability to flex the MCP joint is subsequently lost and the joint hyperextends due to overpowering by the extrinsic finger extensors. This creates tension in the finger flexors, resulting in flexion of the IP joints. This claw hand deformity is often associated with a Volkmann's contracture (see figure 5.15, page 139).

## STRUCTURAL AND FUNCTIONAL ABNORMALITIES

The wrist and hand may show structural abnormalities of the joints, bones, and fingernails that indicate other medical conditions. Enlargement of the DIP joints (**Heberden's nodes**) and PIP joints (**Bouchard's nodes**) is often associated with arthritic conditions and disease. Severely concaved or spoon-shaped nails may be indicative of fungal infections. Nails that are clubbed, or large and convexed, can result from hypertrophy of the underlying soft tissue and may also be associated with respiratory and congenital heart disorders.

# INJURY ASSESSMENT

Because of its vital function in sport, the hand is the frequent site of injuries. Fortunately, most hand and wrist injuries sustained in sport are not serious, but because the hand is so vital to upper-extremity function, even relatively minor injuries can severely hamper performance. Moreover, seemingly insignificant injuries are often left untreated, and as you learned from the previous sections, these can lead to inadequate bone healing, capsulitis, contractures, and deformities. Therefore, accurate and prompt assessment is essential for successful treatment of the injury and restoration of full function.

## ON-FIELD ASSESSMENT

On-field assessment of wrist and hand injuries should be relatively brief in most cases, with the majority of the evaluation being deferred to the sidelines. However, a brief assessment is necessary to determine the extent and severity of the injury and the need for medical referral, as well as to ascertain whether immobilization is necessary before the athlete is moved.

As you approach the athlete, check the surroundings as well as the athlete's positioning and immediate response. Ask the athlete to describe the mechanism, the location of the injury, and any unusual sensations heard or felt. Understanding the mechanism will help you narrow down the potential structures involved. Observe bilaterally for obvious signs of severe bleeding, immediate swelling, discoloration, and deformity that would indicate a fracture or dislocation. If you note deformity, immediately assess for any neurovascular deficits. Because many wrist and hand injuries are distal to the palpation site of the radial or ulnar pulse, you can check circulation by squeezing the nail bed, looking for blanching and capillary return. If any signs of serious injury are present, immobilize and refer the athlete for appropriate medical care.

If there are no signs of serious injury, the on-field evaluation continues with palpation of the musculoskeletal structures. As you palpate, check for point tenderness, crepitus, swelling, deformity, or irregularities over the distal radius, ulnar, carpal bones, metacarpals, and phalanges. If you do not identify a potential fracture and the athlete's pain has subsided sufficiently to allow ambulation, the athlete can leave the field for further evaluation on the sideline.

## Checklist for On-Field Assessment of the Wrist and Hand

**Primary Survey**

✓ Airway, breathing, and circulation

✓ Severe bleeding

✓ Check for unusual positioning of the limb

✓ Assess for shock

**Secondary Survey**

History

✓ Mechanism of injury

✓ Location and severity of pain

✓ Unusual sensations heard or felt

✓ Information from bystanders

**Observation**

✓ Check for deformity, swelling, discoloration, pallor.

**Palpation**

✓ Check for bony tenderness, crepitus, and deformity along the following

✓ Distal radius and ulna, radiocarpal joint, carpal bones, CMC joints

✓ Metacarpals, MP joints, phalanges, PIP and DIP joints

Neurovascular assessment

✓ Sensory

✓ Motor

✓ Radial pulse and/or nail bed check

Gentle, active ROM

✓ Full finger extension?

✓ Full finger flexion?

If all tests are negative for serious injury, remove from field for continued evaluation on the sideline.

## SIDELINE ASSESSMENT

After the athlete has been assisted to the sideline, you can perform a more detailed evaluation to achieve a precise impression of the injury.

### History

With the athlete in a comfortable position and the distal upper extremity supported, ask him to provide a more detailed history of the injury and any prior injuries to the area. Ask about the position of the hand and wrist at impact and about the direction the impact came from. This is the time you will ask your usual questions regarding intensity, quality, and specific location of the pain. It is important to repeat questions regarding location and pain, because in many cases the athlete's symptoms will become more focalized after a few minutes once the immediate pain of the injury subsides. Be sure to check for any previous injuries to both the involved and uninvolved sides, as bony or soft tissue irregularities may have resulted from these injuries that are not consistent with the present injury.

### Observation

Observe the athlete's facial expression for signs of discomfort or pain. Also watch how the athlete supports and moves the wrist, hand, and fingers. Is he doing this guardedly, or does he use the hand freely to gesture as he speaks? Observe the injured area for signs of discoloration, skin interruptions and scars, deformity, finger alignment, nail appearance and color, and abnormal contours; and compare bilaterally. Check for skin creases in comparison to those on the other hand: are creases on the injured hand normal, or have they been diminished by swelling? Also check for equal skin coloration.

### Palpation

Palpation starts proximally and proceeds distally, moving to the area of injury last. Palpate the distal forearm for any musculotendinous or bony tenderness, crepitus, or irregularities. To palpate the dorsal hand, start at the radial styloid process and move just distal to the anatomical snuffbox. Palpate the scaphoid at the base of the

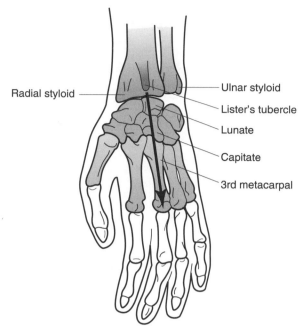

Radial styloid

Ulnar styloid

Lister's tubercle

Lunate

Capitate

3rd metacarpal

**▌ Figure 6.18** Lister's tubercle and surrounding bony anatomy.

snuffbox and the triquetrum at the top of the snuffbox. Tenderness here may be an indication of scaphoid fracture. The radial border of the snuffbox includes the abductor pollicis longus and extensor pollicis brevis, and the ulnar border is formed by the extensor pollicis longus. These tendons can be seen when the thumb is held in extension. Moving medially on the dorsal aspect, palpate Lister's tubercle; this should be in line with the lunate, capitate, and third metacarpal (figure 6.18). Directly adjacent and distal to Lister's tubercle is a slight depression in which the lunate lies. If the wrist is slightly flexed, you can palpate the lunate as it moves into your fingertip. Tenderness here may be an indication of lunate dislocation.

When the hand is held in a fist, you can see the carpi radialis longus and brevis and can palpate them as they insert on the base of the second and third metacarpals, respectively. The extensor indicis and extensor digiti minimi can be palpated as the index and little fingers are extended while the others are kept in flexion. The extensor digitorum communis is palpated with extension of all fingers.

Medial to the radius is the ulnar styloid process. Just distal to this process is the triquetrum. You can palpate it when the wrist is radially deviated. Rotating the hand so the palmar aspect can be palpated, locate the pisiform on top of the anterior surface of the triquetrum. Palpate the flexor carpi ulnaris at the pisiform where it first inserts. Moving distally at a 45° angle from the pisiform in a line lateral to the index finger, you can palpate the hook of the hamate. The pisiform and hook of the hamate form the medial and lateral borders, respectively, of Guyon's tunnel. You can palpate the ulnar nerve in Guyon's tunnel. Tenderness here because of nerve palpation is common, so be sure to compare tenderness bilaterally. The palmaris longus becomes prominent in the central palmar wrist area when the athlete opposes the thumb and little finger to one another. The flexor carpi radialis is just lateral to the palmaris longus and can be palpated in the wrist and distal forearm when the athlete flexes and radially deviates the wrist.

The metacarpals are more easily palpated on the dorsal aspect and can be palpated along their length. The metacarpal heads are located at the level of the distal palmar crease. The dorsal aspect has a groove through which the extensor tendons course that can be palpated. You can easily palpate the phalanges and IP joints for incongruity and tenderness. It is also easy to palpate the thenar and hypothenar eminences, which you should investigate for muscle spasm, tenderness, atrophy, or other contour abnormalities. Palpate the radial pulse and pinch the nail beds to ensure that circulation is intact, if this was not done on the field.

### Special Tests

Special tests for the wrist and hand include those for neurovascular compromise, presence of subtle fractures, tendon and muscle injury, and ligament stability.

### For Neurovascular Compromise

In addition to or as follow-up to the standard neurovascular assessment on the field, you can use special tests to evaluate further for neurovascular compromise. Both nerves and vessels can be compressed or compromised with hand and wrist injuries, so it is important to assess for these problems if the hand is cold, discolored, or tingling or if a radial pulse is diminished or absent.

### Tinel's Sign

This test assesses pathology of the median, ulnar, or radial nerve, depending on where it is administered. To test for the median nerve, tap the surface over the carpal tunnel (figure 6.19a). To test for the ulnar nerve, administer the tap over Guyon's tunnel (figure 6.19b). The radial nerve is tapped proximal to the radial styloid process (figure 6.20c). A positive sign is pain elicited with the tap.

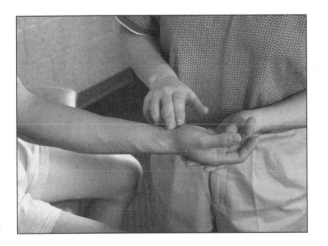

a

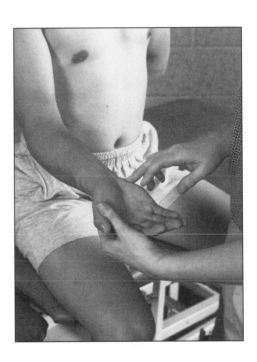

b

■ **Figure 6.19**  Tinel's location for the (a) median, (b) ulnar, and (c) radial nerve.

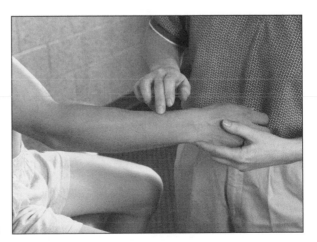

c

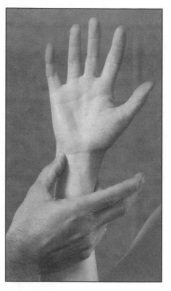

**■ Figure 6.20** Allen test.

## Allen Test

This test assesses the circulatory integrity of the hand. Instruct the athlete to open and close her hand rapidly several times and then keep a tightly closed fist; then apply pressure to the radial and ulnar arteries to compress them. While maintaining the pressure, instruct the athlete to relax the hand. Then release the pressure on one artery and observe the filling response (figure 6.20). Repeat the process with the other artery and compare between the two hands. If the filling response is uneven, the test is positive and is indicative of a restricted circulation flow into the hand.

### For Fractures

Since the wrist and hand bones are relatively close to the surface, most fractures in these areas are obvious. However, a fracture that is not displaced can be more difficult to identify except with radiographic examination. Wrist fractures such as Colles's fracture and Smith's fracture usually present with deformity so that the assessment is obvious. Phalangeal fractures are often obvious because the force of the tendons causes the bone fragments to become displaced. However, fractures within the joint may be difficult to differentiate from joint sprains—and both may in fact be present. Fractures of the carpals and metacarpals are sometimes less obvious. The following tests can be used to identify these fractures.

## Carpal and Metacarpal Fractures

It is common to observe isolated soft tissue swelling around the site of the fracture. For an easy confirmation test, have the athlete relax the fingers so the MCP joints are flexed to 90°. Then apply a compressive force to the end of the metacarpal (figure 6.21). If the athlete reports pain with this maneuver in either the metacarpal or its corresponding carpal, a fracture is likely present.

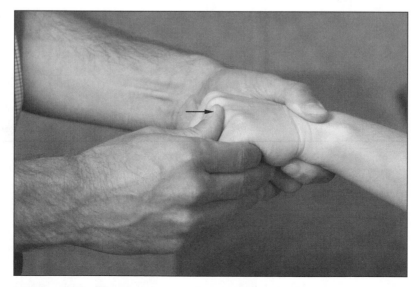

**■ Figure 6.21** Compression test for metacarpal fracture.

## Phalangeal Fractures

Phalangeal fractures can be tested either by an axial compressive force as described for the carpal and metacarpal fractures or by a vibration test. Apply the axial compressive force with the finger in full extension rather than flexed at the MCP joint as described earlier. Perform the vibration test with the athlete's hand supported and the fingers relaxed. Flick the end of the suspected finger to cause a vibration along the digit (figure 6.22). If the athlete reports significant pain, a fracture should be suspected.

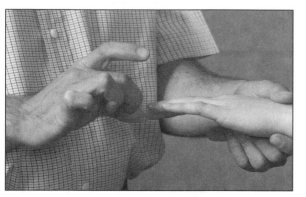

■ **Figure 6.22**  Vibration test for phalangeal fracture.

### For Tendons and Muscles

Usually it is acute injuries that are seen in a sideline assessment. For this reason, special tests for chronic or overuse injuries will be discussed in connection with the off-field assessment rather than here.

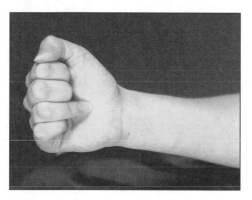

■ **Figure 6.23**  Jersey finger sign.

## Flexor Tendon Avulsion Test

This avulsion test is also called the jersey finger sign because the injury occurs when an athlete attempts to make a tackle by grabbing onto an opponent's jersey. Instruct the athlete to make a fist. The sign is positive if the finger with the ruptured flexor digitorum longus tendon does not fully flex into the palm (figure 6.23).

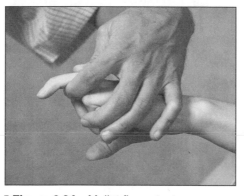

■ **Figure 6.24**  Mallet finger test.

## Extensor Tendon Avulsion Test

This test is also called the **mallet finger test** because the mechanism often involves an impact compression force with sudden flexion of the distal phalanx. Instruct the athlete to fully extend all the fingers. The distal phalanx of the injured finger will remain in partial flexion if an extensor tendon avulsion is present (figure 6.24).

### Ligament Stability Tests

You can assess joint integrity and instability due to ligament injury using various stress-testing techniques, depending on the location of the injury.

### Valgus and Varus Stress Tests

The valgus stress test assesses the integrity of the medial or ulnar collateral ligaments of the MCP and IP joints. The varus stress test assesses the integrity of the lateral or radial collateral ligaments of the MCP and IP joints. Each joint is assessed individually. Stabilize the proximal segment of the joint, and grasp the distal segment of the joint with your mobilizing hand. Then apply an ulnar (valgus) or radial (varus) force to the joint to stress the collateral ligaments (figure 6.25). Pain or laxity compared to what occurs in the opposite hand is a positive sign.

You can also apply a collateral stress test to the wrist. The radial collateral stress test assesses radial collateral ligament (RCL) integrity, and the ulnar collateral stress test assesses UCL integrity. Use one hand to stabilize the distal forearm and place your other hand over the athlete's metacarpals to apply the collateral stress. Move your hand toward the little finger side to stress the radial collateral ligament and toward the thumb side to stress the UCL (figure 6.26).

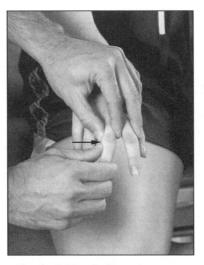

■ **Figure 6.25**   Collateral stress tests for phalangeal joints.

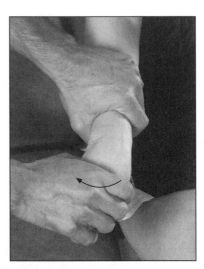

■ **Figure 6.26**   Radial collateral stress test for the wrist.

### Lunatotriquetral Ballottement Test

This test, also called **Reagan's test**, assesses the instability of the joint between the lunate and the triquetrum. The lunate is the most commonly dislocated carpal bone. Stabilize the triquetrum with the index finger of one of your hands on one side and the thumb on the other. With the other hand, grasp the lunate on the anterior and posterior surfaces as you did for the triquetrum. Keeping the triquetrum stable, move the lunate in an anterior-posterior direction to assess for pain, laxity, and crepitus, which are positive signs for this test (figure 6.27). Compare between the athlete's two hands.

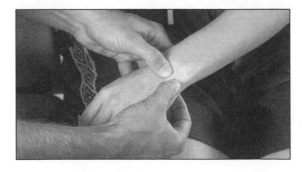

■ **Figure 6.27**   Lunatotriquetral ballottement (Reagan's) test.

### Glide Tests

The glide tests to follow are stress tests that will determine ligamentous integrity and stability at various wrist joints if the athlete reports pain or reduced active motion. They are used to assess joint laxity within the wrist, in either the carpal joints, the radiocarpal joint, the radioulnar joint, or a combination of these. The mobility of these joints will vary depending on the specific movement. Thus, injury to a specific joint may cause more restriction in one movement than in another, depending on how much mobility is required of that joint in order for the movement to occur. If the athlete has pain and limited wrist extension, the injury may be in the radiocarpal joints. Pain and restricted wrist flexion may be secondary to injury at the midcarpals. Look to the distal radioulnar joint if supination or pronation is restricted or painful.

The radiocarpal joints are tested in an anteroposterior glide test. Place your stabilizing hand around the athlete's distal forearm so that the hand is adjacent to the proximal carpal row. Place your mobilizing hand around the athlete's hand so that it touches your stabilizing hand. Perform an anterior-to-posterior glide with the mobilizing hand as you assess for joint mobility and pain (figure 6.28). Then, with your hands in the same position, perform a posterior-to-anterior glide. Compare between the athlete's two hands. A positive sign is present if the athlete reports pain, if crepitus is present, or if the area is either more or less mobile than its counterpart. These movements are also referred to as anterior and posterior glides, respectively.

A side glide test can be performed with the hands in the same position. The force applied is side to side rather than anterior to posterior.

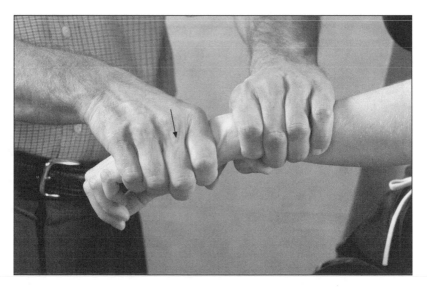

∎ **Figure 6.28**   Anterior-to-posterior glide test of radiocarpal joints.

### Range of Motion

Active range of motion is assessed prior to passive motion. A combined movement assessment includes making a fist and then opening the fist as wide as possible. This allows quick identification of any gross deficiencies. Observe for quality and quantity of movement of isolated joints and multiple joints. Isolated joint motions include forearm supination and pronation (figure 6.29a); wrist flexion and extension (figure 6.29b), radial deviation and ulnar deviation (figure 6.29c); MCP flexion, extension, abduction, and adduction (figure 6.29, d-e); and interphalangeal flexion and extension (figure 6.29f). The thumb has motions of flexion, extension, abduction, adduction, and circumduction (figure 6.29, g-i). The thumb and little finger also move in opposition to each other, and the thumb is able to oppose all the fingers (figure 6.29j).

Passive motion is performed to assess end feel of the joints and to help determine possible causes for any decreased range found during active motion testing. Most normal end-feel sensations for the wrist and hand are tissue stretch. The exceptions include a bony end feel in radial and ulnar deviation and, of course, tissue approximation with thumb and finger adduction.

Passive motion is performed either after each individual active motion has been performed or after all active motions have been completed.

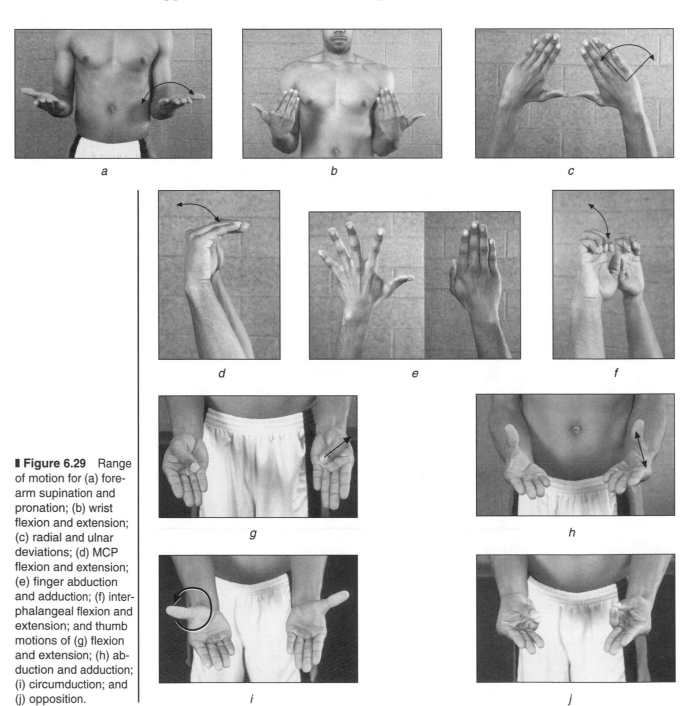

**Figure 6.29** Range of motion for (a) forearm supination and pronation; (b) wrist flexion and extension; (c) radial and ulnar deviations; (d) MCP flexion and extension; (e) finger abduction and adduction; (f) interphalangeal flexion and extension; and thumb motions of (g) flexion and extension; (h) abduction and adduction; (i) circumduction; and (j) opposition.

### Strength

On the sideline, the most convenient method of assessing strength is the manual muscle test. For each test, the hand should be positioned such that the muscle being tested is working against gravity, unless this position is too inconvenient or difficult. Always perform strength testing on the uninvolved side first and evaluate strength of the surrounding structures first, leaving the probable injured site for last. Be careful not to squeeze the athlete's injured hand too hard during the test. Position the segment to be tested in either neutral or slightly into the motion being tested. The fingers can be tested as a unit or individually. As an example, figure 6.30, a-b, demonstrates combined finger flexion resistance and individual finger resistance for the proximal and distal IP joints. If a finger is the injury site, individual finger strength tests are indicated. Manual muscle tests should be performed for all the motions of the wrist and fingers.

You can perform a grip strength test on the sideline as an assessment of general strength. Instruct the athlete to squeeze two to three fingers of your hand as hard as possible. Compare the involved to the uninvolved side by having the athlete perform the grip test on both your hands simultaneously.

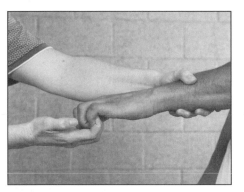 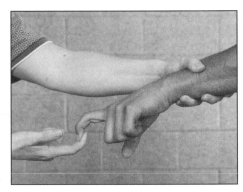

*a*  *b*

▌**Figure 6.30**   Testing strength of (a) combined finger flexion and (b) individual finger flexion at the proximal and distal IP joints.

### Neurological Tests

If you suspect a nerve injury on the basis of deficits or weakness found thus far in your exam, a complete neurological assessment is indicated.

#### Sensory Tests

Both light touch and pinprick methods are used to assess the sensation over the sensory distributions of the hand. The hand is divided into median, ulnar, and radial nerve distributions (see chapter 5, figure 5.27). Dermatomal distributions include C6, C7, and C8. C6 provides sensation to the thumb, index finger, and half of the middle finger and hand area; C7 supplies sensation to the middle finger and corresponding hand area; and C8 supplies sensation to the ring and little fingers and corresponding hand segment. The most sensitive and pure locations for assessment of each peripheral nerve are the dorsal web space (radial, C6); the distal, radial aspect of the second finger (median, C7); and the distal, ulnar aspect of the fifth finger (ulnar, C8).

#### Motor Tests

Motor supply to the hand was also discussed in chapter 5 (figure 5.28). Wrist extensors are innervated by C6; wrist flexors and finger and thumb extensors by C7; finger flexors and thumb adductors by C8; and finger adductors and abductors by T1. To assess wrist and hand injuries, manual muscle tests are performed for each peripheral nerve emanating from the brachial plexus. The radial nerve (C6-C7) is tested with wrist extension. The median nerve (C6-T1) is best tested with thumb opposition. The ulnar nerve (C8) is tested with finger abduction. If it is difficult to assess whether the athlete's weak response is due to a neurological or other soft tissue injury to these specific muscle groups, you should test other muscles innervated by the nerve that are away from the injured site. For example, if the athlete has a weak response to a wrist extensor strength test, try testing thumb extension, which is also innervated by the radial nerve. If you find no deficit in thumb extension upon comparison to the uninvolved side, the injury is likely not nerve related. If you are not sure whether the neurological deficit is localized to the wrist and hand rather than further up the chain, testing biceps strength may also be appropriate if there is a need to check integrity of the nerve root.

### Functional Tests

Because the hand serves so many functions, several different functional tests can be used in addition to sport-related functional tasks.

To test motion and coordination, have the athlete perform a rapid thumb-to-finger touch test. The athlete moves the thumb tip from the index finger to the middle, ring, and little finger, then back again to the starting position, as rapidly as possible. In another coordination test, the athlete supinates and pronates the injured segment as rapidly as possible while moving the opposite hand in opposing positions. For example, if her right wrist is injured, she begins with supination on the right and pronation on the left and then moves her hands in the opposite directions as rapidly as she can.

You can use more aggressive functional tests to assess strength and joint integrity. Weight bearing on the wrist in a push-up position with the palm flat on the floor, and then on the fingertips, will assess overall hand strength and integrity of the wrist and finger joints. Grip activities can also represent a variety of functional tests, since the hand normally uses a number of different grips. Examples of power grips are grasping an object such as a bat, tennis racket, hockey stick, or lacrosse stick and grasping, catching, and throwing a ball. Examples of precision grips, used for more finely tuned activities, are the chuck grip as in picking up a golf tee, the lateral pinch grip as in grasping a scorecard, and the pinch grip for fingertip prehension (i.e., tip to tip). Although the pinch grip is not often used in sport, it is vital for picking up very small objects such as a needle or a coin.

## OFF-FIELD ASSESSMENT

It is common for athletes to delay reporting wrist and hand injuries, so you may not have the opportunity to evaluate the injury until several days after it has occurred. As with other body segments, the wrist and hand can incur chronic or overuse injuries that athletes typically will not report until they interfere with performance.

### History

When obtaining a history from an athlete seeking assistance at some delay from the injury onset, get as much detailed information as possible regarding the history of the incident. Ask the same questions you would ask during a sideline assessment; but in addition, ask about the time of onset and the duration of symptoms for more chronic conditions. Determine whether the injury has worsened or improved over time and what activities tend to aggravate or ease symptoms, and to what extent. For chronic injuries, pay close attention to occupational or academic activities in addition to sport activities that may contribute to a repetitive stress injury. Ask the athlete if he notes any pain, weakness, or loss of motion with any daily activities such as gripping, typing, and opening doors. If so, find out which motions are most bothersome.

## Checklist for Sideline Assessment of the Wrist and Hand

### History

Ask questions pertaining to the following:

✓ Chief complaint

✓ Mechanism of injury

✓ Unusual sounds or sensations

✓ Type and location of pain or symptoms

✓ Previous injury

✓ Previous injury to opposite extremity for bilateral comparison

### Observation

✓ Check for visible facial expressions of pain.

✓ Check for swelling, deformity, abnormal contours, or discoloration.

✓ Check for skin creases, interruption, coloration, and scars.

✓ Check finger alignment, nail appearance and coloration.

✓ Check for use or guarding of the wrist and hand.

✓ Check muscle development—areas of muscular atrophy.

✓ Perform bilateral comparison.

### Palpation

Palpate for pain, tenderness, and deformity from proximal to distal over the following:

✓ Distal radius and ulna, Lister's tubercle, extensor tendons

✓ Carpal bones, anatomical snuffbox and tendon borders

✓ Flexor tendons, tunnel of Guyon

✓ CMC joints, metacarpals (base, shaft, head), MCP joints

✓ Phalanges, PIP and DIP joints

✓ Check radial pulse and look for nail bed blanching.

### Special Tests

✓ Neurovascular compromise (Tinel's sign, Allen test)

✓ Fractures (compression, vibration)

✓ Tendon and muscle (flexor and extensor tendon avulsion)

✓ Ligament stress tests (collateral, Reagan's, glide tests)

### Range of Motion

✓ Active ROM for the following:

  ✓ Forearm pronation/supination

  ✓ Wrist flexion, extension, radial and ulnar deviation

  ✓ MP flexion, extension, abduction, and adduction

  ✓ IP flexion, extension

  ✓ Thumb flexion, extension, abduction, adduction, and circumduction

✓ Passive ROM for same motions as for active ROM

✓ Bilateral comparison

### Strength Tests

✓ Grip strength

✓ Perform manual resistance against same motions as in active ROM.

✓ Check bilaterally and note any pain or weakness.

### Neurological Tests

✓ Sensory, motor, and reflex for radial, ulnar, and median nerve distributions.

✓ Sensory and motor for peripheral nerves: median, ulnar, musculocutaneous (sensory only), radial

### Functional Tests

### Observation

As with all injuries, begin your observation when the athlete enters the sport injury treatment facility. Observe for any guarding versus free movement of the wrist and hand. Check for signs of swelling, discoloration, deformity, and muscle atrophy, as well as skin coloration, and compare bilaterally. Check carefully for any areas of localized swelling or nodules (such as on the dorsum of the wrist, which may indicate a wrist ganglion). Check for equal and bilateral skin creases and angulation of the fingers.

### Differential Diagnosis

Because the cervical or upper thoracic spine, shoulder, and elbow can refer symptoms into the wrist and hand, you should assess these areas to eliminate them as possible sources of the athlete's complaints by performing range of motion movements with overpressure tests for each joint. The quadrant position for the cervical spine should be included as well. At the end of each active motion of each of the joints, apply an overpressure to move the joint to the maximum end range. If any of these movements reproduces the athlete's symptoms, you should evaluate that joint more closely before continuing.

Myofascial restriction can also cause pain and symptom referral into the wrist and hand. Travell and Simon (1983) showed that the most common sources of myofascial pain referral into the hand are the scalenes, infraspinatus, subscapularis, latissimus dorsi, coracobrachialis, brachialis, triceps, and forearm muscles. If pain is generalized and difficult to pinpoint, follows an atypical injury pattern, or radiates, you should perform soft tissue assessment for possible myofascial-related referrals.

For more information on guides to identifying particular pain patterns and the treatment of their release, refer to *Therapeutic Exercise for Athletic Injuries* (Houglum 2000), chapter 6.

If the athlete's pain follows a nerve pathway pattern or the athlete complains of tingling, burning, or shooting pain, neural pathology should be suspected. If nerve pathology seems to be involved, include a complete upper-extremity neurological assessment for motor and sensory integrity and specific special tests as part of the evaluation. Most of these tests were discussed in connection with the sideline assessment and in previous chapters. The neurological tests section later in this chapter will present some additional special tests.

### Range of Motion

Assessment of range of motion is consistent with that performed at the sideline. You can make a gross assessment of range of motion initially by having the athlete perform full active motions in all planes for the forearm, wrist, and fingers while you observe for smoothness and fullness of motion. If there is any discrepancy, make a more detailed assessment of the area. Forearm supination/pronation occurs primarily in the forearm with about 15° of movement taking place at the wrist, so if full supination/pronation is not possible, the forearm and wrist should be assessed as possible sources of deficient motion. Wrist flexion occurs primarily at the intercarpal joint margin between the proximal and distal carpal rows, while wrist extension occurs primarily at the radiocarpal joint. Radial deviation occurs mostly between the proximal and distal carpal rows, and ulnar deviation occurs primarily at the radiocarpal joint (Kapandji 1970). In the fingers, the greatest degrees of motion occur in the PIP joints, with about equal motion occurring in the MCP and DIP joints. The MCP joints have two degrees of freedom, while the IP joints have one. This allows for abduction/adduction and flexion/extension of the fingers at the MCP joints and only flexion/extension at the IP joints. Slight abduction and rotation are possible at the IP joints and rotation at the MCP joints. These movements are necessary for full function of the digits, but occur only passively. Since the thumb plays the most vital role in hand function, it has the greatest degree of freedom of movement and is the only digit of the hand that is innervated by all three nerves.

During your active range of motion assessment, check for capsular patterns in the wrist. The capsular pattern of the wrist is equal limitation of flexion and extension with mild limitation of supination and pronation at the distal radioulnar joint. The thumb's carpometacarpal (CMC) joint capsular pattern is more limited in abduction than in adduction, and the finger's MCP and IP joints are more limited in flexion than in extension. If this proportion of motion loss is noted on active range of motion, it is likely that capsular tightness is at least contributing to the athlete's limited motion.

**Passive Range of Motion**

Apply passive overpressure in the same manner as described for the sideline assessment. If the athlete's pain is reproduced during overpressure, investigate further for possible ligamentous or capsular injury. Ligament stress tests and capsular mobility tests should always be included in the evaluation if pain with overpressure occurs.

### *Strength*

Administer manual muscle tests in the same way as for the sideline assessment. In addition, you can perform more objective strength tests with various machines. Isokinetic assessment is possible for forearm and wrist supination/pronation and flexion/extension movements. Dynamometers can be used to assess grip strength and pinch strength (figure 6.31, a-b). The pinch dynamometer can be used to assess chuck, tip, and lateral pinch grips. The athlete performs the strength test with the uninvolved hand before attempting it with the involved hand.

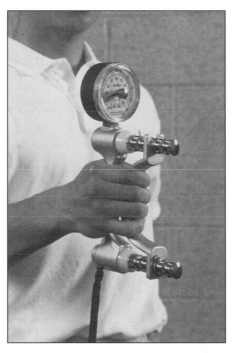
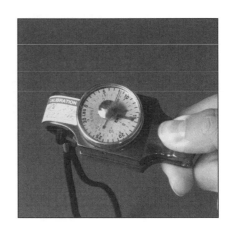

*a*    *b*

∎ **Figure 6.31**    (a) Grip and (b) pinch strength tests.

### *Neurological Tests*

The three components of the neurological assessment for the wrist and hand include sensory, motor, and other special tests. The sensory and motor tests were presented earlier in the discussion of the sideline assessment. In addition to standard sensory tests, you can use a two-point discrimination test.

### Two-Point Discrimination Test

Although this test can be performed on any aspect of the hand and wrist, it is used most commonly to assess two-point discrimination sensation in the fingertips. Use a paper clip, calipers, or a specifically designed two-point discriminator device to assess the athlete's ability to distinguish between one and two points. Normal sensation at the fingertips is discrimination to a 4 mm distance between the two points.

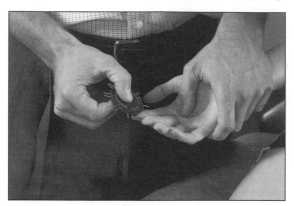

Place the ends of the device on the athlete's fingertips and ask the athlete—who keeps her eyes closed during the examination—if she feels one or two points (figure 6.32). The pressure should be light enough that it does not cause a blanching of the skin. If blanching occurs, the athlete will be able to rely on deep pressure sensation rather than light touch, and the test will not accurately assess the intended receptors. If the athlete is unable to detect two points, widen the distance between the points by 1 mm and retest until she can feel two points.

**■ Figure 6.32**   Two-point discrimination test.

### Special Tests

Any of the special tests described for the sideline assessment may be used in the off-field examination. You will select the tests on the basis of the athlete's history, your observations, and your objective findings up to this point. The following sections present some additional tests that identify more chronic, inflammatory-type conditions.

### Tests for Inflammatory Conditions

The following tests can confirm the presence of tendinitis or tenosynovitis in the wrist and hand.

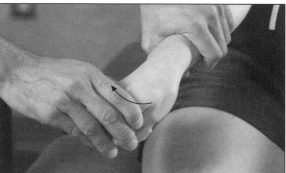

**■ Figure 6.33**   Finkelstein test.

### Finkelstein Test

Use this test to assess the presence of De Quervain's disease, a tenosynovitis of the extensor pollicis brevis and abductor pollicis longus tendons. The athlete places her thumb within her fist. Stabilize the forearm and move the wrist into ulnar deviation (figure 6.33). A positive sign is pain with the movement.

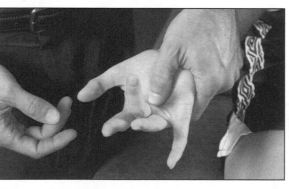

**■ Figure 6.34**   Trigger finger test.

### Trigger Finger Test

This test, which assesses the presence of flexor tenosynovitis, is used if the athlete complains that a finger "locks" in flexion when she attempts to extend it. The locking occurs because of the irregularity of the tendon's sheath that occurs with tendosynovitis, causing the tendon to catch in the retinaculum in the metacarpal area during movement. Palpate the location along the tendon where the athlete reports the locking. The athlete then flexes and extends the finger (figure 6.34). You can sometimes palpate a nodule, but the most common positive signs are pain with pressure over the area and a palpable clicking or snapping.

## Neurovascular Test

Phalen's test is used to assess for carpal tunnel syndrome.

### Phalen's Test

The athlete places the backs of the hands together with the wrists in full flexion. She then drops her elbows below the wrists and holds the position for about 1 min or until the symptoms are reproduced (figure 6.35). Pain in the wrist is not a positive sign, but numbness or tingling in the thumb, index, or middle finger is.

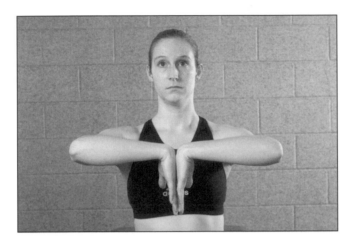

❚ **Figure 6.35**  Phalen's test.

## Ligamentous Tests

The tests presented next distinguish between tightness in the IP capsule and the collateral ligaments or intrinsic muscles.

### Bunnel-Littler Test

This test is used if the athlete demonstrates reduced flexion range of motion of the PIP joints. A passive test, it distinguishes between tightness of the joint capsule and tightness of the intrinsic muscles. Passively place the athlete's MCP joint in slight extension, and then flex the PIP joint (figure 6.36). If the PIP joint cannot be flexed in this position, maintain the PIP joint position and slightly flex the MCP joint. If the joint capsule is tight, the PIP joint will not fully flex with MCP joint flexion. If the intrinsic muscles are tight, the PIP joint will fully flex with MCP joint flexion.

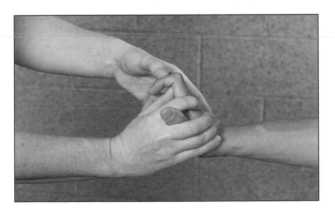

❚ **Figure 6.36**  Bunnel-Littler test.

## Retinacular Test

This passive test determines whether the cause of tightness in the PIP joint is the capsule or the retinacular (collateral) ligaments. Stabilize the PIP joint in neutral and then flex the DIP joint. If DIP movement is restricted, tightness may be present in either the capsule or collateral ligaments (figure 6.37). Then perform the test passively with the PIP joint in flexion to relax the collateral ligaments. If DIP movement is normal, the collateral ligaments are tight and the capsule is normal.

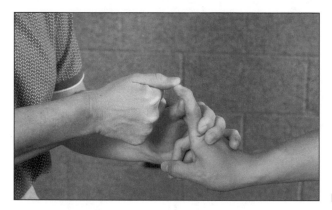

**▌Figure 6.37**    Retinacular test.

### *Joint Mobility*

Joint mobility tests, performed if there is a reduced range of motion, will help you determine whether the limited range of motion is caused by capsular restriction or other factors. If the athlete presents with a capsular pattern of movement for any joint, joint mobility assessment tests will help you ascertain where the capsule is restricted and will provide a basis for treatment. These tests are also used as treatment techniques.

For more information about joint mobility assessment tests, refer to *Therapeutic Exercise for Athletic Injuries* (Houglum 2000), chapter 6.

### Wrist—Radiocarpal Joint

Mobility of the radiocarpal joint can be assessed by means of the following mobilization techniques.

## Distraction

The distraction test assesses general joint mobility. Comparison to the uninvolved wrist joint shows whether laxity or restriction is present. With the athlete seated, the involved forearm resting in pronation, and the wrist over the end of a table, stabilize his forearm with your hand on the distal forearm adjacent to the wrist joint. Place your mobilizing hand around the distal carpal row. With the mobilizing hand, apply a longitudinal distracting force to the wrist (figure 6.38).

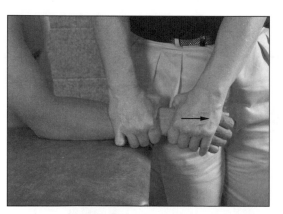

**▌Figure 6.38**    Radiocarpal joint distraction test.

## Glide Movements

The four glide tests for this joint are the dorsal (anterior-to-posterior) glide, to assess wrist flexion; the ventral (posterior-to-anterior) glide, to assess wrist extension; the

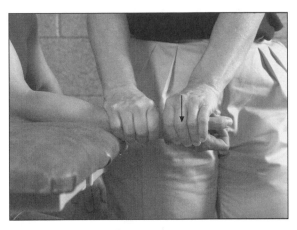

■ **Figure 6.39** Dorsal glide test.

radial glide, to assess ulnar deviation; and the ulnar glide, to assess radial deviation. Each movement is performed individually, but because hand placement is the same for all tests, they can be performed in sequence; that is, you can complete one test and then move to the next one. It is best to perform the tests on the uninvolved side first as a means of comparison. As with the distraction test, the athlete sits with his forearm on a table and his wrist and hand off the end of the table. Place your stabilizing hand on the distal forearm adjacent to the wrist joint and your mobilizing hand over the proximal carpal row.

Perform the dorsal glide with the athlete's forearm supine. Provide an anterior-to-posterior glide to the wrist joint (figure 6.39). For the ventral glide, performed with the athlete's forearm pronated, you will provide a downward glide in a posterior-to-anterior direction (figure 6.40). For the radial and ulnar glide tests, place the forearm in neutral with the thumb positioned up. For the ulnar glide, provide a downward glide force to move the wrist in an ulnar direction (figure 6.41); apply the radial glide force in an upward direction to move the wrist toward the radial aspect (figure 6.42).

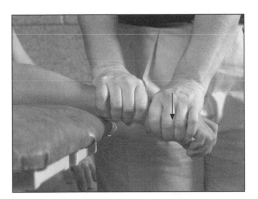

■ **Figure 6.40** Ventral glide test.

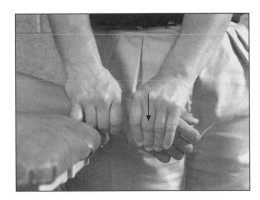

■ **Figure 6.41** Ulnar glide test.

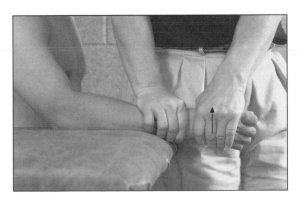

■ **Figure 6.42** Radial glide test.

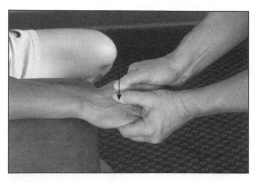

■ **Figure 6.43** #2-5 carpometacarpal ventral glide.

## Carpometacarpal Joints

### #2-5 Carpometacarpal Ventral Glide

The #2-5 carpometacarpal ventral glide test evaluates general metacarpal and intermetacarpal mobility. The athlete sits with the forearm pronated and supported on a table, and the hand and wrist off the table. Place the thumb of your stabilizing hand along the metacarpal that is being stabilized and your mobilizing thumb on the metacarpal that is being mobilized. Apply a downward mobilizing force to the metacarpal to assess its mobility (figure 6.43).

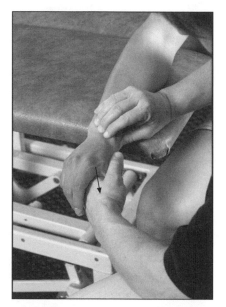

■ **Figure 6.44** #1 carpometacarpal distraction.

### #1 Carpometacarpal Distraction

This test assesses general mobility of the thumb CMC joint. The athlete is seated as for the other mobility tests. Using the thumb and index finger of your stabilizing hand, stabilize the scaphoid and trapezium bones; place the index finger and thumb of your mobilizing hand around the first metacarpal. Apply a longitudinal distraction force to the CMC joint (figure 6.44).

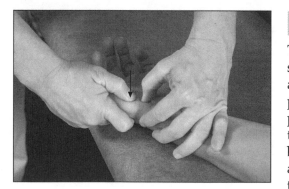

■ **Figure 6.45** #1 carpometacarpal dorsal glide.

### #1 Carpometacarpal Dorsal Glide

The #1 carpometacarpal dorsal glide assesses abduction of the thumb. With the athlete's forearm in supination and supported on a table as before, stabilize the proximal portion of the CMC joint with the thumb and index finger of your stabilizing hand. To assess joint mobility, apply a downward directed dorsal force to the joint with your thumb on top of the athlete's anterior first metacarpal (figure 6.45).

### Metacarpophalangeal and Interphalangeal Joint Mobility Tests

The MCP and IP joints are all tested in similar fashion; use the same stabilizing and mobilizing hand positions and apply the same test forces. The three test maneuvers are distraction for general mobility, a dorsal glide to assess limited joint extension, and a ventral glide to assess limited joint flexion. The athlete is positioned as for other wrist and hand mobility tests. The forearm is in pronation, with the wrist and hand over the end of a table. Stabilize the proximal arm of the joint being tested with the index finger and thumb of one of your hands, and apply the mobilizing force with the index finger and thumb of the opposite hand placed just distal to the joint (figure 6.46, a-b).

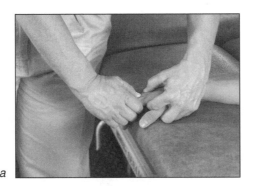 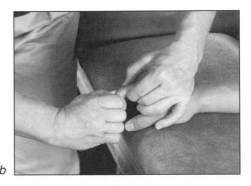

*a*                                          *b*

❚ **Figure 6.46**    (a) MCP and (b) IP joint mobility tests.

### *Palpation*

As with the sideline assessment, you will perform a methodical palpation of the distal forearm, wrist, hand, and fingers, moving from proximal to distal and from anterior to posterior. Carefully observe for areas of tenderness, deformity, spasm, swelling, crepitus, atrophy, nodules, and other abnormal contours. The forearm, thenar, and hypothenar areas may contain areas of myofascial restriction and should be inspected for pain that may cause referral to other regions. Palpate the area of the athlete's complaint last.

### *Functional Tests*

As discussed earlier, simple coordination exercises and activities such as push-ups and other strength maneuvers can be used along with sport-specific activities to determine the athlete's function and readiness to return to activity.

The athlete is ready to return to full participation if she can perform all the functional tests well, without hesitation; demonstrates balanced performance between the right and left upper extremities; appears to have no pain; and utilizes good motion, strength, endurance, power, agility, and control.

# Checklist for Off-Field Assessment of the Wrist and Hand

## History

Ask questions pertaining to the following:

- ✓ Chief complaint
- ✓ Mechanism of injury
- ✓ Unusual sounds or sensations
- ✓ Type, location, onset, and duration of pain or symptoms
- ✓ Previous injury
- ✓ Previous injury to opposite extremity for bilateral comparison

If chronic, ascertain:

- ✓ Aggravating and easing activities
- ✓ Training and daily activity history (repetitive stresses)
- ✓ Activity restrictions
- ✓ Treatment if any

## Observation

- ✓ Visible facial expressions of pain
- ✓ Swelling, deformity, abnormal contours, or discoloration
- ✓ Skin creases, interruption, coloration, and scars
- ✓ Finger alignment, nail appearance and coloration
- ✓ Use or guarding of the wrist and hand
- ✓ Muscle development—areas of muscular atrophy
- ✓ Presence of localized nodules
- ✓ Bilateral comparison

## Differential Diagnosis

- ✓ Clear cervical region with overpressure tests in straight planes and quadrant positions.
- ✓ Clear shoulder region with passive overpressures in all ranges.
- ✓ Clear elbow region with passive overpressures in all ranges.

## Range of Motion

- ✓ Active ROM for the following:
    - ✓ Forearm pronation/supination
    - ✓ Wrist flexion, extension, radial and ulnar deviation
    - ✓ MP flexion, extension, abduction, and adduction
    - ✓ IP flexion, extension
    - ✓ Thumb flexion, extension, abduction, adduction, and circumduction
    - ✓ Presence of capsular patterns

- ✓ Passive ROM for same motions as for active ROM
- ✓ Bilateral comparison

## Strength Tests

- ✓ Check grip strength.
- ✓ Perform manual resistance against same motions as in AROM.
- ✓ Check bilaterally and note any pain or weakness.
- ✓ Perform instrumented strength tests.

## Neurological Tests

- ✓ Sensory and motor for ulnar, radial, and median nerves
- ✓ Two-point discrimination test

## Special Tests

- ✓ Neurovascular compromise (Tinel's, Allen, Phalen's)
- ✓ Fractures (compression, vibration)
- ✓ Tendon and muscle (flexor and extensor tendon avulsion)
- ✓ Ligament stress tests (collateral, Reagan's, glide tests, Bunnel-Littler, retinacular)
- ✓ Tenosynovitis (Finkelstein, trigger finger)

## Joint Mobility Assessment

Note capsular restriction and end feel:

- ✓ Radiocarpal distraction and glide
- ✓ Carpometacarpal distraction and glide
- ✓ MCP and IP distraction and glide

## Palpation

- ✓ Palpate for pain, tenderness, and deformity over the following:
    - ✓ Distal radius and ulna, Lister's tubercle, extensor tendons
    - ✓ Carpal bones, anatomical snuffbox and tendon borders
    - ✓ Flexor tendons, tunnel of Guyon
    - ✓ CMC joints, metacarpals (base, shaft, head), MCP joints
    - ✓ Phalanges, PIP and DIP joints
- ✓ Check radial pulse and observe for nail bed blanching.

## Functional Tests

# SUMMARY

1. *Describe the general types and mechanisms of acute and chronic injuries of the wrist and hand that physically active people commonly experience.*

   The dexterity and precision required of the wrist and hand for fine motor control often leave these segments unprotected and vulnerable to injury during sport activity. Contact with the ground, an opponent, or balls and other sporting implements is the primary mechanism by which acute fractures, dislocations, sprains, and strains in the wrist and hand occur. The hand and wrist are also prone to repetitive stress injuries such as tendinitis, tenosynovitis, nerve compression syndromes, and capsulitis, as well as other chronic joint restrictions resulting from previous injury.

2. *Describe the potential complications and deformities that can result from seemingly simple sprains and strains.*

   Many times an athlete will sustain an injury to a finger that is painful but will dismiss it as a "simple sprain." However, these injuries may also represent fractures or injuries to the soft tissue structures that, if left unrecognized or untreated, will result in inadequate healing or a permanent restriction. These injuries include intra-articular fractures, volar plate ruptures, extensor tendon ruptures, and capsulitis. To avoid these conditions, all finger injuries should be thoroughly evaluated and referred if there is any question about their severity.

3. *Identify the common sites of nerve compression injuries, and the common signs and symptoms associated with each.*

   Nerve compression in the wrist and hand occurs primarily in the carpal tunnel (median) or the tunnel of Guyon (ulnar). Carpal tunnel syndrome can result from a variety of factors including repetitive stress and carpal fractures. Ulnar nerve compression is commonly seen in cyclists as a result of prolonged pressure that occurs as the heel of the hand rests on the handlebars. Signs and symptoms, which are consistent with other nerve compression injuries, include pain, paresthesia along the nerve distribution, and—in chronic cases—muscle weakness and atrophy.

4. *Discuss the common fractures that occur in the wrist and hand and their characteristic deformities, signs, and symptoms.*

   The small and fine bones of the wrist and hand are prone to fractures. Falling on an outstretched hand is a common mechanism for Colles's fracture and scaphoid fractures, whereas falling on the back of the hand will cause a Smith's fracture. While scaphoid fractures are often difficult to detect, Colles's and Smith's fractures each have a characteristic deformity. Both axial and longitudinal forces will fracture the metacarpals and phalanges, and displacement will be obvious because of the superficial nature of these bones. If any bony tenderness is noted, the athlete should be referred to a physician for x-ray.

5. *Perform an on-field assessment of the wrist and hand, being able to identify which conditions warrant immediate referral.*

   Most wrist and hand injuries are not severe enough to require immediate medical referral. When dealing with an on-field injury, the athletic trainer directs attention most immediately to any evidence of severe bleeding, potential fractures and dislocation, or neurovascular compromise. If any of these injuries are identified, immediate medical care and referral are required. If these conditions are not present, the athlete can be moved to the sideline for further evaluation.

6. *Perform a sideline assessment of the wrist and hand, including special tests used to evaluate acute conditions.*

Except in the case of serious injury, most hand and wrist injuries will be assessed on the sideline once the athlete has left the field. At the sideline a more detailed assessment is performed for active and passive range of motion, strength, ligamentous stability, musculotendinous injury, and neurovascular integrity. Vibration and compression tests are performed to detect less obvious fractures. A thorough knowledge of anatomy is required for accurate palpation and identification of the involved structures.

7. *Perform an off-field assessment of the wrist and hand, including evaluation techniques to assess injuries that are more chronic.*

The off-field assessment is similar to the sideline assessment for the wrist but includes additional tests to evaluate more chronic conditions such as nerve compression, tenosynovitis, and joint restrictions. With chronic conditions, it is important to gain a history of both sport and daily living activities, as these may equally expose the wrist and hand to repetitive stress injuries.

# REVIEW QUESTIONS

1. What characteristic joint postures are associated with the following deformities? What structural pathology is associated with each?
   - Boutonniere
   - Pseudoboutonniere
   - Silver fork
   - Ape hand
   - Benediction
   - Claw hand

2. What are the signs and symptoms of a volar plate rupture? How would you distinguish this injury from a collateral ligament sprain?

3. Name the sensory distributions and motor tests for each of the peripheral nerves. When would you include a neurological assessment in your evaluation of a wrist or hand injury?

4. Describe the etiology, signs, and symptoms of carpal tunnel syndrome. If you suspect that an individual has carpal tunnel syndrome, what special tests would you use to either rule out or confirm you impressions?

5. Now that you have studied the complete upper extremity, identify the joints and associated conditions that can refer pain to the wrist and hand. What specific differential tests would you use to rule out pathology in these other joints?

6. What is the purpose of Phalen's test? How is it performed, and what constitutes a positive test?

7. How do you determine whether tightness in a PIP joint is caused by capsular versus ligamentous versus muscle restrictions?

# CRITICAL THINKING QUESTIONS

1. Think back to the scenario at the beginning of the chapter. On the basis of the information you have learned, what would you do in this situation? Explain your rationale and discuss any evaluation procedures you would perform before making your decision.

2. A 20-year-old soccer player comes into the athletic training room holding her wrist. While playing soccer she lost her balance and put out her hand to break the fall. She complains of pain in her wrist, primarily on the palmar side. She reports no previous injury. On exam, you find some mild swelling on the palmar aspect of her wrist, but no immediate discoloration or deformity. On palpation, she is point tender over the same area but does not appear to have any bony crepitus, palpable deformity, or mass. You check for tenderness in the anatomical snuffbox, and it is mildly tender but similar bilaterally. On active motion, the athlete's pain intensifies with full wrist extension and is considerably less with flexion. On passive testing, the pain is considerable with wrist extension and nonpainful with wrist flexion, except at the extreme end range. She denies any referred pain into her hand. Given this history, what condition would you most likely suspect, and what specific tests would you use to (1) confirm your suspicions and (2) rule out other potential injuries?

3. An industrial worker on the company baseball team comes to you complaining of pain on the radial aspect of his wrist. He states that his pain has come on gradually over time; he notices it primarily during batting, especially when he "breaks" his wrists at the end of his swing. He has had no previous injury to this or his other hand. When you ask about his occupation, you find that he works on the assembly line in an automobile factory and that his job requires him to place about 100 radiator caps on radiators each day. Upon palpation, you notice tenderness and crepitus at the base of the thumb. You note pain and weakness with resisted thumb extension. On the basis of this history and these symptoms, what condition might you suspect, and how would you confirm your findings?

# CITED REFERENCES

Harris, R.B. 1983. *Textbook of disorders and injuries of the musculoskeletal system.* 2d ed. Baltimore: Williams & Wilkins.

Kapandji, I.A. 1970. *The physiology of the joints. Upper limb.* Vol. 1. New York: Churchill Livingstone.

Travell, J.G., and Simon, D.G. 1983. *Myofascial pain and dysfunction. The trigger point manual. The upper extremities.* Vol. 1. Baltimore: Williams & Wilkins.

# ADDITIONAL RESOURCE

Houglum, P.A. 2000. *Therapeutic exercise for athletic injuries.* Champaign, IL: Human Kinetics.

# CHAPTER SEVEN

# Lower Thoracic and Lumbar Spine

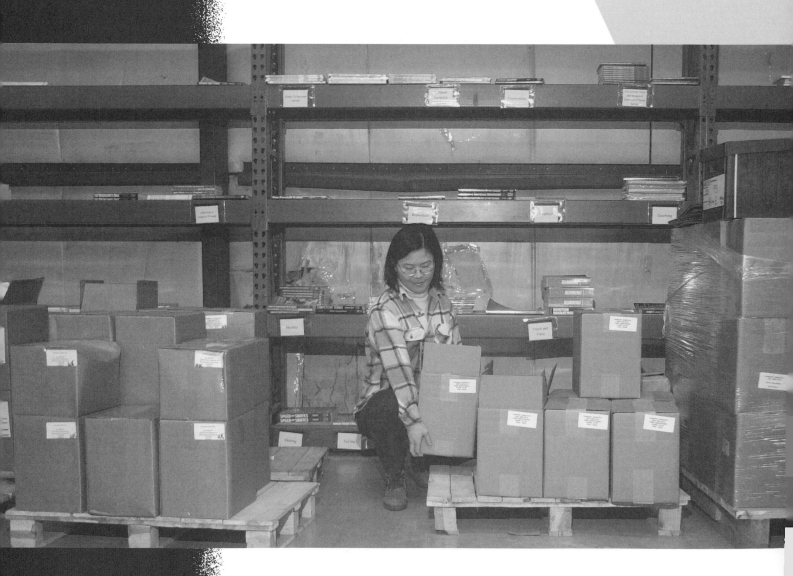

# OBJECTIVES

After finishing this chapter, readers will be able to do the following:

1. Describe the etiology, signs and symptoms, and potential complications associated with acute and chronic injuries of the thoracic and lumbar spine commonly encountered in the physically active

2. Describe the various congenital and degenerative conditions of the thoracic and lumbar spine

3. Describe the common causes, signs and symptoms, and indicative tests for nerve root compression in the lumbar spine

4. Identify the characteristics and potential contributing factors to functional and structural deformities in the thoracic and lumbar spine

5. Perform an on-field assessment of the lumbar spine, indicating criteria for immediate medical referral and transportation from the field

6. Perform a thorough and sequential sideline assessment of the lumbar spine

7. Perform a thorough and sequential off-field assessment of the lumbar and thoracic spine, noting considerations for differential diagnosis

Max had been working at UPS during the summers and holidays for the past three years to help put himself through school. He enjoyed his job, except for the fact that his supervisor was constantly on him about lifting properly when loading his truck. Max considered himself quite a strong specimen and a good athlete—he certainly didn't think lifting a few boxes was any big deal.

It was the Christmas holidays, and work at UPS was nuts! "Why is it that everyone waits until the last minute to send stuff!"—Max was tired and cranky. He bent over and reached for a box at his side; it was heavier than he had expected. Instead of turning around to get a better angle, he took a deep breath and lifted it hard and fast. At once, a searing pain shot through his back, and he dropped the box with a gasp. He could barely stand and needed assistance to get to the industrial clinic. There he encountered Ruth, a certified athletic trainer, who had recently been hired to head up the company's recreational sport program and to work in the clinic part time.

"Can you tell me what happened and where your pain is?" asked Ruth, taking his history.

"All I did was pick up a box. . . . It was heavy, but no heavier than a lot of the packages I lift."

"Can you tell me how you picked it up? What position were you in?" Ruth asked. When Max explained the mechanisms, Ruth had a pretty good idea why the injury had occurred. She continued with a thorough evaluation, including a neurological assessment to check for nerve root compression. Max showed no signs of neurological deficits but appeared to have a significant lumbar strain/sprain. However, because of his pain, she referred him to his physician for a secondary evaluation and possible medication.

After a couple of weeks of treatment in the clinic, Max was as good as new. "Hey, thanks for all your help, Ruth. I feel great!"

"I'm glad to hear it, Max. You know, you were lucky . . . lifting like that, your injury could have been a lot worse, and it may be next time. You really need to work on your lifting mechanics if you want to stay active in sports and not have a 70-year-old back by the time you're 30. Before you leave, let's work on it, okay?"

Max had a new appreciation for his supervisor's concern. "Yeah, okay, I think that would be a good idea."

The lumbar spine represents the strongest and thickest of all spinal vertebrae, providing both stability and mobility for the upper torso. The stability of the lumbar spine is achieved through large vertebral bodies anteriorly, strong anterior and posterior longitudinal ligaments, intervertebral discs, and broad musculature.

The functional unit of the lumbar spine comprises two adjacent vertebrae separated by a vertebral disc. The anterior segment (vertebral body and intervertebral disc) serves as the primary weight-bearing and shock-absorbing unit. Each intervertebral disc is composed of a nucleus pulposus surrounded by the thick annulus fibrosis. The fibers of the annulus fibrosis run obliquely to provide a strong attachment from one vertebra to the next. However, this oblique arrangement of fibers puts the disc under greatest tension in rotation; thus it is most often injured as a result of torsional movement.

The posterior segment, which is non-weight bearing except in extreme extension, serves as a protective structure for the spinal cord. The paired facet joints function to direct and limit movement of the unit and prevent forward slippage of one vertebra on another. These joints are often the site of inflammation and overstress types of injuries. Between the anterior body and the posterior facet joints is the intervertebral foramen that serves as the nerve root exit from the lumbar plexus to the lower extremity. When degenerative change or disc herniation occurs, this space can be compromised, causing compression of the nerve and neurological symptoms into the lower extremity.

Considerable mechanical and muscular forces are exerted on the thoracic and lumbar spines during jumping, twisting, bending, and lifting activities. The lumbar spine provides both mobility and stability for the upper-extremity and torso movements and effectively absorbs and transmits forces between the upper and lower extremities. Because of its greater mobility and load-bearing function in comparison to the thoracic and sacral spinal segments, the lumbar spine is particularly susceptible to episodes of pain and injury. This chapter will explore both the acute and chronic injuries that often occur in the lumbar spine and will provide the essential assessment techniques you will need to evaluate these conditions and make the appropriate judgments on treatment and referral.

# INJURIES TO THE THORACIC AND LUMBAR SPINE

Lumbar and thoracic pain is most often due to acute and chronic strains of the postural muscles supporting the lumbar region. Chronic strain may result from poor posture, poor mechanics, weakness, stiffness, and muscle restrictions. Occasionally low back pain is caused by congenital defects or degenerative changes. Traumatic injuries such as fractures may also occur, and the potential for a spinal cord injury and potential paralysis must always be considered with severe injuries.

## ACUTE AND CHRONIC SOFT TISSUE INJURIES

Soft tissue injuries comprise the majority of the injuries encountered in the lumbar spine. Those that physically active people most commonly experience include contusions, sprains, and strains.

### Contusions

The spinal structures vulnerable to direct contact and contusions are primarily the spinous processes and their overlying superficial ligaments. Contusions to these structures may result in point tenderness, localized swelling, and pain with flexion and extension movements. The surrounding musculature is also vulnerable to contusions resulting from direct contact with an opponent (football), a sport implement (baseball, lacrosse stick), or the ground. Contusions to the musculature may cause considerable muscle swelling, stiffness, and spasm resulting in loss of range of motion and function. Although these contusions are rarely serious or debilitating, athletes who have received significant direct trauma to the lower trunk and are complaining of severe or unrelenting low back pain should be thoroughly evaluated for possible kidney or other visceral trauma.

### Sprains

Sprains in the lumbar and thoracic region typically result from sudden loading or torsional movements. They can also result from direct or indirect trauma that forces the spinal segment(s) beyond their normal range of motion, as well as from compressive loading forces. The more common mechanism of injury to the lumbar region is a sudden extension movement with rotation. The lumbar spine depends heavily on the surrounding musculature to increase its stability during mechanical loading. If the spine is suddenly loaded and the muscles are unprepared, greater demands are placed on the ligament and capsular structures. Therefore, weak or poorly conditioned trunk and abdominal muscles may make one more susceptible to lumbar sprains. Sprains at the lumbosacral junction can result from this mechanism but may also result from a "jamming"-type mechanism, such as landing off balance on a straight leg, in which the spine absorbs most of the load.

Signs and symptoms of lumbar sprain include pain, swelling, muscle spasm, and decreased range of motion. If the spasm is severe, a lateral shift of the spinal column toward the spasm may be seen. Because of the muscular involvement, sprains will be painful with both active movement and passive stretching; consequently it is often difficult to distinguish a sprain from a strain.

### Strains

The mechanisms for muscular strains are similar to those for sprains, causing sudden contraction or stretching of the involved musculature. Sudden eccentric loading of an already contracting muscle is also a common cause of muscular strain. Strains can result from a single episode of muscle overload but also frequently from cumulative stress. Factors such as poor posture, muscular imbalance, poor conditioning, weak abdominal muscles, and inflexibility of the hamstrings, hip flexors, and/or back extensors can increase one's susceptibility to muscular strains. Signs and symptoms include pain, point tenderness, muscle spasm, and possible swelling in and around the involved musculature. With severe spasm, a lateral deviation in the spine may be noted. There will also be decreased range of motion and increased pain with active contraction and passive stretching of the involved muscle.

## BONE AND JOINT PATHOLOGIES

Bone and joint pathologies are less common than soft tissue injuries. Whereas traumatic fractures may occur in the lumbar and thoracic spine, the vast majority of bone and joint pathologies in this region are a result of congenital weakening, degenerative processes, or both.

### Traumatic Fractures of the Thoracic Spine

Because of the stability of the thoracic spine, fractures and dislocations are quite rare in athletics. Thoracic spine fractures typically involve compression of the vertebral body resulting from violent forward flexion or from axial loading in a forward flexed position. Axial loading forces can arise superiorly as a result of contact or of forces exerted through the head and shoulders, including heavy lifting techniques. Axial forces can also be transmitted inferiorly through the thoracic spine in a hard fall on the buttocks. Dislocation or instability is uncommon with these injuries, and neurological injury rarely results. Signs and symptoms include localized pain and discomfort, tenderness with palpation over the spinous process of the involved vertebra, muscle spasm and guarding, and increased pain with forward flexion and other movements of the thoracic spine. It is not uncommon for athletes with thoracic spine fractures to get up and walk off the field following injury. Therefore, it is important to carefully assess localized, central thoracic spine pain after a traumatic injury before allowing the athlete to return to activity.

### Traumatic Fractures of the Lumbar Spine

Traumatic fractures are relatively uncommon with sport-related activities, with the possible exception of high-speed impact sports. The structures most likely to be fractured secondary to acute trauma are the vertebral body, transverse processes, spinous processes, and pars articularis. Compression of the vertebral body will typically result from high compressive or axial loading forces to a partially flexed lumbar spine (figure 7.1). Because of the larger vertebral body size, designed to better withstand axial loading forces, com-

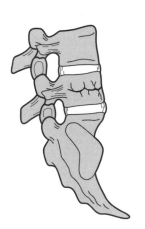

**Figure 7.1**    Compression of the vertebral body.

pression fractures in the lumbar spine are considerably less common than in the thoracic spine. However, skeletally immature athletes and athletes with diminished bone density secondary to aging, eating disorders, and amenorrhea may be more at risk for compression fractures in this area. Fractures of the transverse processes can result from direct trauma, violent torsional movements, or an avulsion of the psoas major muscle following a violent contraction (figure 7.2). Avulsion fractures of the transverse process can cause considerable pain and bleeding. Fractures of the relatively unprotected spinous processes are typically attributable to blunt trauma but may also result from forced hyperflexion of the lumbar spine. Pars interarticularis fractures are more commonly the result of stress reactions, but may also occur acutely with forced hyperextension or landing with the spine in hyperextension—particularly in individuals with underlying bony abnormalities or defects (figure 7.3).

Signs and symptoms associated with fracture include immediate pain, direct or indirect tenderness over the vertebral segment, crepitus, decreased range of motion, and an unwillingness to move. If the fracture encroaches on the spinal cord or nerve root, signs and symptoms of sensory or motor deficits associated with nerve compression or injury may also be present. Although unstable fractures with nerve involvement are rare in the lumbar spine, a thorough neurological assessment should be conducted whenever a spinal fracture is suspected following acute trauma.

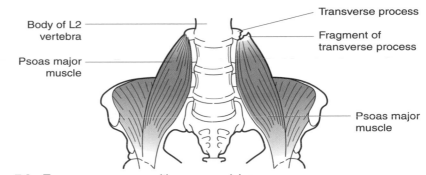

**Figure 7.2**   Transverse process with psoas avulsion.

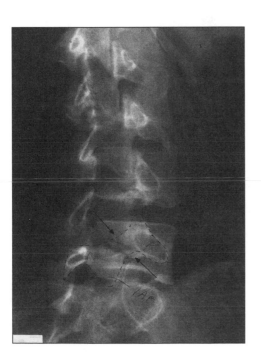

**Figure 7.3**   Pars fracture of the lumbar spine.

### Spondylolysis and Spondylolisthesis

A condition that is often attributed to a congenital abnormality, but may not manifest itself until the individual is physically active, is spondylolysis. **Spondylolysis** involves a fracture of **pars interarticularis**, located between the inferior and superior facets (see figure 7.3). It is typically thought to be a stress fracture secondary to a congenital weakening. Spina bifida occulta may also be a contributing factor in some individuals. These injuries occur most often in young, skeletally immature athletes and do not necessarily preclude physical activity except when the fracture is in an acute stage. When spondylolysis occurs bilaterally, a secondary condition known as spondylolisthesis may result.

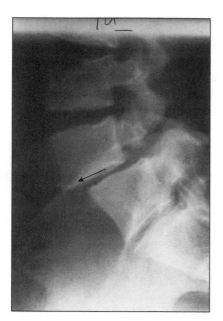

**Figure 7.4** Spondylolisthesis with forward slippage.

**Spondylolisthesis** is characterized by a forward subluxation of the involved vertebrae (figure 7.4). Because of the orientation of the facet joints, the spondylolytic vertebrae will displace anteriorly in relation to the vertebrae directly below. Spondylolisthesis is frequently found in gymnasts, weight lifters, and football linemen secondary to the repetitive flexion and hyperextension loading forces inherent in their activities. Progression of the forward slippage appears to be a concern in athletes only during their preadolescent and adolescent growth years; rarely does forward subluxation progress once the individual is an adult. In young athletes with this condition, the extent of forward subluxation should be evaluated regularly. The extent of subluxation of the vertebral body in relation to the vertebral body inferior to it is typically graded from stage I to stage IV. Athletes with stage I (<25% subluxation) and even stage II (<25-50%) may continue activity provided that pain and symptoms allow. Progression to stage III (50-75%) often requires removal from activity and surgical management for stabilization.

Signs and symptoms associated with spondylolysis and spondylolisthesis are centralized low back pain (possibly radiating into the buttocks and posterior thighs), swelling, muscle spasm, and a straightening of the lordotic curve. People with these conditions may exhibit decreased range of motion and increased pain with hyperextension. Standing on one leg (affected side) and extending the spine will also increase pain. A step deformity may be present in athletes with spondylolisthesis. Symptoms may mimic those of lumbar sprains and strains and usually require an x-ray for definitive identification.

### Facet Syndrome

Facet syndrome refers to an inflammation (**spondylitis**) of the facet joint and its surrounding capsule. Facet syndrome can result from both acute and chronic repetitive insult. Extension overload of the facet joint, particularly when combined with rotation, can compress and irritate the joint. Consequently, individuals with scoliosis are more susceptible than others to facet joint pain and dysfunction. Inflammation of the facet joint may also cause irritation of the nearby nerve root as it exits through the intervertebral foramen (figure 7.5). Because the facet joint is richly innervated, facet syndrome may be associated with considerable pain. Other signs and symptoms include localized swelling, paraspinal muscle spasm, tenderness upon palpation and movement of the facet joint, and increased pain with extension, compression, and rotation to the involved side. Pain referred down the leg may be present as well. There may also be a deviated posture (functional scoliosis) secondary to muscle spasm or as a consequence of an attempt to avoid pain due to joint compression.

### Degenerative Pathologies

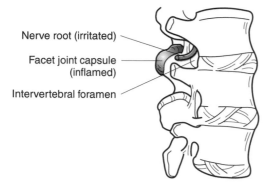

Nerve root (irritated)

Facet joint capsule (inflamed)

Intervertebral foramen

**Figure 7.5** Facet joint syndrome with nerve root irritation.

Whereas spondylolysis and spondylolisthesis may be the more common causes of bony pathology in the adolescent athlete, spondylitis and **spondylosis** (degenerative changes) of the vertebrae and disc are more frequently the cause of back pain in the physically active adult. As a person ages, the water content in the intervertebral disc decreases. This often will result in microtears and degeneration of the richly innervated annulus fibrosis, leading to low back pain and discomfort. Chronic joint inflammatory conditions resulting from cumulative and repetitive stress (i.e., spondylitis, facet syndrome) may also bring about degenerative changes such as osteophytes and capsular fibrosis. The L4/L5 and L5/S1 levels are particularly vulnerable to pain and degeneration because these joints are the most mobile, accounting for 80-90% of lumbar flexion. Moreover, the transition from the very mobile L5 vertebrae to the relatively stable S1 vertebrae also makes this joint prone to shear forces causing pain and injury. Poor posture, weak abdominal and back musculature, and inflexibility may contribute to the cumulative stresses placed on the spine and hasten degenerative changes.

Individuals with degenerative disc and joint disease will report decreased pain in the morning and increased pain throughout the day as the disc and joints are compressed with long standing and sitting. Other signs and symptoms include pain across the lower lumbar region and into the buttocks and decreased range of motion into flexion, extension, and/or rotation. As degenerative changes progress, nerve compression syndromes may result from narrowing of the intervertebral foramen (stenosis) secondary to encroachment by osteophytes or disc herniation.

Although degenerative joint disease may be a normal process of aging, symptoms can often be reduced and severe degeneration avoided through identification and correction of faulty posture and through proper training geared toward increasing flexibility, muscular strength, and spinal stability.

### Intervertebral Disc Herniation

Intervertebral disc **prolapse** (bulge) or herniation can be caused by both acute trauma and cumulative stress mechanisms. Faulty posture, faulty movement mechanics, weak musculature, and inflexibility can all contribute to repetitive microtrauma that weakens the annulus fibrosis and allows **protrusion,** prolapse, and possible extrusion or **sequestration** of the disc material (figure 7.6). Twisting and holding a heavy object away from the body while lifting is a frequent mechanism for acute lumbar disc herniation.

While the inner part of the disc is aneural and early protrusion will not cause pain, once the nucleus pulposus herniates through a tear in the annulus fibrosis, the extruded or sequestered portion of the disc will put pressure on adjacent structures that are richly innervated and compress the nearby spinal cord (posterior herniation) or nerve root (posterior-lateral herniation) (see figures 3.6 and 3.7).

Disc herniation can occur at any level, but most frequently occurs at L4/L5 and L5/S1. Posterolateral lesions are more common because of the strong posterior longitudinal ligament that stabilizes the spine and disc directly posteriorly. However, central herniations do occur and can place pressure on the **cauda equina**, which can result in a **cauda equina syndrome** and loss of bowel and bladder function. Signs and symptoms of disc herniation include centralized back pain, point tenderness over the spinal level, muscle spasm, and "sciatica," or referred pain along the nerve distribution. Signs and symptoms associated with nerve compression will also be noted; these will be covered in the next section.

## NERVE COMPRESSION INJURIES

Nerve compression injuries of the thoracic and lumbar spine most often involve the nerve roots of the sciatic nerve as they exit the intervertebral foramen of the lumbar vertebrae. Nerve compression can result from encroachment of a prolapsed or herniated intervertebral disc (see figure 7.6) or from degenerative osteophytes causing stenosis of

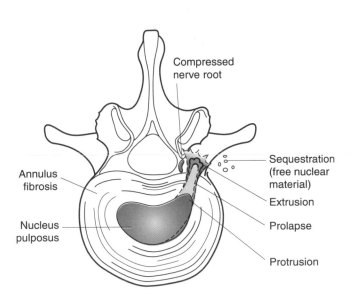

**▌Figure 7.6**  Four stages of disc herniation.

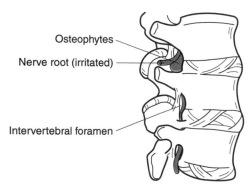

**Figure 7.7** Osteophytes and stenosis of intervertebral foramen causing nerve root compression.

If an athlete complains of changes in bowel or bladder function as a result of a back injury, this should be considered a medical emergency; immediate referral is required to prevent permanent dysfunction.

the intervertebral foramen (figure 7.7). In rare cases, nerve compression may result from excessive forward subluxation of the vertebral body in stage III or stage IV spondylolisthesis.

When injuries are associated with nerve compression, the athlete typically complains of sciatica, or radiating pain down the thigh, lower leg, and foot along the distribution of the sciatic nerve. The specific location and pattern of pain will depend on the lumbar level at which the nerve is compressed (figure 7.8). Coughing, sneezing, or straining (Valsalva maneuver) will significantly increase intrathecal pressure and increase pain. The athlete will list to one side, typically away from the side of nerve root compression. Side-bending and extension with rotation toward the involved side will close down the foraminal space and increase nerve compression and pain. Pain and increased symptoms with special tests including straight leg raise, well leg raise, Hoover, and Kernig tests are indicative of nerve compression. Paresthesia or numbness over the specific dermatome, motor weakness of the innervated muscles, and a diminished reflex may also be noted. Athletes exhibiting these neurological signs require immediate referral. If the athlete complains of bowel or bladder dysfunction, a cauda equina syndrome may be present, and this constitutes a medical emergency!

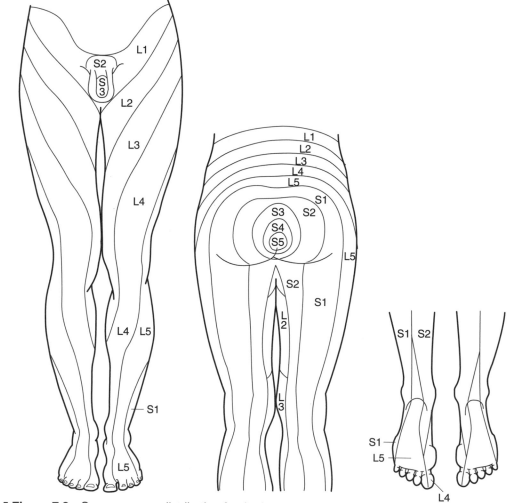

**Figure 7.8** Sensory nerve distribution for the lumbar plexus.

## STRUCTURAL AND FUNCTIONAL ABNORMALITIES

Other structural and functional abnormalities of the thoracic and lumbar spine are not necessarily symptomatic or associated with trauma. However, it is important to recognize these abnormalities, as they may be a contributing factor in cases of occasional or chronic low back pain. Although some of these abnormalities can be identified only through x-ray, others offer visible signs that are easily noted with careful observation.

### Cafe áu Lait Spots

Abnormalities in the appearance of the skin should be noted, as they may indicate underlying pathologies. Cafe áu lait spots, or darkened patches of skin, are indicative of collagen disease that is affecting the connective tissue.

### Spina Bifida Occulta

**Spina bifida occulta**, a congenital malformation of the lumbar spine, is characterized by incomplete closure of the posterior lamina at birth. The athletic population will include only those with mild cases, as more severe cases would likely preclude activity. Superficial signs that would indicate this underlying condition include a hairy patch (**faun's beard**), dimpling, and fatty deposits of the skin overlying the lumbar spine. Unless it has been problematic prior to athletic involvement, this condition is not likely to exhibit symptoms except for some occasional low back pain. However, those with spina bifida occulta are thought to be more prone than others to defects of the pars interarticularis (see discussion of spondylolysis).

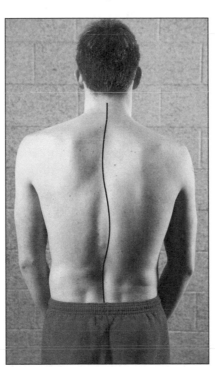

**∎ Figure 7.9**    Scoliosis.

### Scoliosis

**Scoliosis**, a deformity in which the spinal column has a lateral or "S" curvature (figure 7.9), may be either structural or functional. **Structural deformities** are characterized by permanent structural changes in the bone and are usually congenital. Structural or permanent changes may also result from mechanical dysfunction, ultimately leading to permanent degenerative changes that disrupt the normal contours and motions of the spine over time. With structural scoliosis, the vertebrae will be rotated with the anterior body toward the convex side. This rotation will cause the posterior ribs and posterior chest wall to be more prominent on the convex side and less prominent, or sunken in, on the concave side.

**Functional deformities** do not involve permanent bony changes and typically result from mechanical dysfunction due to poor posture, leg length discrepancy, joint inflammation, nerve root irritation, muscular imbalance, or a combination of these. These conditions are marked by observable postural deformity and loss of spinal range of motion. A distinguishing factor of functional versus structural curvatures is the disappearance of the functional curvature with forward flexion of the spine. Because of the muscular imbalance and compensatory changes created by these spinal curvatures, individuals with scoliosis often complain of pain, muscular fatigue, and spasm in the postural muscles. It is important to recognize functional scoliosis in the physically active and to correct the mechanical dysfunction in order to prevent irreversible structural changes over time.

### Kyphosis and Scheuermann's Disease

**Kyphosis** is an excessive posterior curvature of the upper and midthoracic spine (figure 7.10). The upper thoracic spine normally has a rounded contour, but this curve can be accentuated secondarily to congenital factors, compensatory changes, muscular imbalance, joint disease, compression fractures, osteoporosis in older adults, and Scheuermann's disease in youth. Scheuermann's disease is a growth disorder characterized by inflammation and osteochondritis of the thoracic vertebrae. This degenerative condition results in wedging or narrowing of the anterior vertebral body at three or more levels secondary to axial and flexion overload. When the condition is active, sport participation may be contraindicated and pain is often increased with activity and forward flexion movements. Athletes with a past history of Scheuermann's disease may complain of occasional pain, muscular fatigue, and spasm associated with the resulting increased kyphosis.

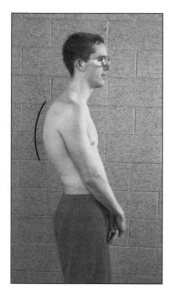

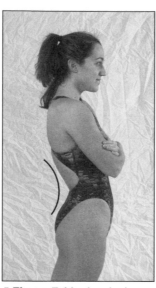

■ **Figure 7.10**   Kyphosis.          ■ **Figure 7.11**   Lordosis.

### Lordosis

**Lordosis**, the opposite of kyphosis, is an excessive anterior (forward) curvature of the lumbar spine (figure 7.11). An increased lordotic curve may be congenital, but may also be acquired secondary to muscle imbalances such as weak abdominals, tight hip flexors, and tight back extensors that cause the pelvis to rotate anteriorly. Increased lumbar lordosis can result in low back pain because of the increased stress placed on the musculature as well as the posterior, non-weight-bearing elements of the spine (facet joints).

### Lumbarization and Sacralization

Two other structural abnormalities that may contribute to low back pain are lumbarization and sacralization. In lumbarization, the S1 vertebral segment remains mobile and separate from the sacrum and will appear as a sixth lumbar vertebra on x-ray. Conversely, sacralization is a congenital fusion of the L5 vertebrae with S1. On x-ray, there will appear to be only four lumbar vertebrae. These abnormalities are often asymptomatic but may occasionally contribute to lower back pain in physically active individuals.

## INJURY ASSESSMENT

Back pain, a frequent complaint in the physically active, commonly results from acute traumatic episodes as well as from cumulative stress. Although not usual in sport, the most severe consequence of a back injury that you may encounter is paralysis. You must be able to quickly and effectively recognize the signs and symptoms of a serious back injury and manage accordingly to prevent further injury and neurological insult. However, the majority of your assessments will take place in the athletic treatment facility on athletes with postacute or chronic low back complaints. Even then, though, there is the potential for nerve root compression and neurological deficits, and you must recognize these symptoms early to ensure appropriate care and complete restoration.

Whenever assessing someone with back pain, it is important to remember that pain experienced in the thoracic and lumbar spine can also be referred from the viscera or can be a result of lower-extremity dysfunction. Conversely, lower-extremity pain can be caused by back pathology. It vital to consider these relationships when evaluating the low back.

## ON-FIELD ASSESSMENT

When approaching a downed athlete with a back injury on the field, observing his response and movement will provide immediate and important clues to the extent of the injury. If he is rolling around and trying to move, even though in pain, a spinal cord injury is of little concern. But if he is lying very still, you must consider the potential for a serious back injury and potential spinal cord injury.

Once at the athlete's side, perform a primary survey to assess his level of consciousness; airway, breathing, and circulation; severe bleeding; obvious signs of deformity or trauma; and the presence of shock. If he is unconscious, you must assume a serious spine injury and stabilize his head and neck. If he is conscious and not moving, determine why he is not moving. If the reason is that he can't move, or won't move because of pain or fear, you must consider a serious spine injury until you have proven otherwise.

Once you have confirmed that the athlete's vital signs are stable, begin your secondary survey by obtaining a brief history of what happened, whether or not you observed the injury. Knowing whether the injury was caused by a helmet directed at the small of the back, a tackle through the shoulder resulting in axial loading of the thoracic and lumbar spine, or a noncontact twisting motion will help you determine the nature of the injury. It is essential that you gain a clear picture from the athlete of the type and location of his pain and symptoms before moving or allowing him to move. Find out whether the pain is centralized over the spine or laterally over the musculature; also determine whether any unusual sensations of numbness, burning, or tingling were present at the time of injury and whether any are present now. Is the athlete able to wiggle his toes? If there are any signs of radiating pain, numbness, or inability to move the lower extremities, a serious spine injury should be suspected.

If these symptoms are negative, except for centralized back pain, perform a cursory sensory and motor neurological assessment before moving the athlete. Assess for sensation bilaterally with light touch on the upper thigh (L2), medial knee (L3), medial lower leg (L4), dorsum of the foot (L5), and lateral foot (S1). Since a spinal injury can affect both extremities equally, compare the sensation of light touch in the lower extremity to that in the upper extremity. For motor tests, have the athlete dorsiflex the foot and big toe and plantarflex the foot against your resistance, noting any change in symptoms or muscle weakness.

If you find no neurological deficits, palpate the lumbar spine for any tenderness along the spinous processes. Although this may be difficult if the athlete is lying supine, you can typically make the determination by reaching your hand under the small of his back without moving him. If pain is present over the spine, assume a serious spine injury. If there is no central spine pain and the pain is primarily in the surrounding musculature, ask the athlete to actively move his legs and assess for any changes in sensation. If your evaluation has shown that the athlete does not have a serious lumbar or lower thoracic spine injury, and the pain is not so severe that he is unable to ambulate, you can slowly move him from a lying-down position to sitting, and then to standing. If his condition remains unchanged during standing, assist him off the field to a location where you can perform a sideline assessment.

If at any time a serious spinal injury is suspected, emergency medical services should be notified and every precaution taken to transport the athlete according to the correct procedures. Fortunately, most lumbar injuries are not this extreme and include only temporarily painful but not life-changing signs and symptoms. The most immediate symptom with a back injury is often muscle spasm. If severe enough,

## Checklist for On-Field Assessment of the Lumbar and Thoracic Spine

**Primary Survey**

As you approach:

✓ Check surroundings and environment.

✓ Gain history from bystanders if you did not witness.

✓ Note position of body.

✓ Check level of consciousness, airway, breathing, and circulation.

✓ Check for severe bleeding.

✓ Check for movement of the extremities.

**Secondary Survey (Evaluate in the Position Found)**

✓ If athlete is unconscious, manage as a serious spinal injury.

✓ If conscious, assess the following:

  ✓ Presence and location of back pain

  ✓ Sensations of numbness, tingling, or burning

  ✓ Difficulty in moving extremities

✓ If any of these are positive, assume serious spine injury.

✓ If back pain only:

  ✓ Sensory testing over L2-S1 dermatomes

  ✓ Motor testing for dorsiflexion, big toe dorsiflexion, plantar flexion

  ✓ Palpation for tenderness and deformity

  ✓ If signs are positive, assume serious spine injury.

✓ If signs just listed are negative:

  ✓ Perform active range of motion of lower extremities

  ✓ Assess for sensory changes with motion

  ✓ If signs are positive, assume serious spine injury

  ✓ If negative, allow athlete to sit, then stand, then move to sideline for further assessment

✓ Continue to monitor vitals.

✓ Continue to check sensory and motor function in extremities.

---

this can cause immediate pain and disability that will not allow the athlete to ambulate unaided off the field. When performing an on-field assessment, therefore, you must find out how severe the injury is and whether the athlete needs passive transport off the field.

---

For discussion of procedures for transporting an athlete with a suspected spinal injury, refer to *Introduction to Athletic Training* (Hillman 2000), chapter 8.

---

## SIDELINE ASSESSMENT

You will perform a sideline assessment in the event that an athlete walks off the field with a low back injury or as a follow-up to any on-field evaluation. Since the postural muscles of the back and trunk are active in any position except lying down, the athlete may be most comfortable in a reclined position as you conduct the history portion of the assessment. If a table is not available at the sideline, it may be best to move the athlete into the athletic treatment facility if that is feasible, since getting up and down from the ground may be difficult for an athlete in acute pain and spasm. If a table is not available and a facility is not close by, you will need to use your best judgment as to whether the athlete can remain standing for early portions of the assessment.

### History

Once on the sideline, reassess the athlete's perception of the location, quality, and severity of her pain. Also ask again about any unusual sensations and about sensations of tingling, burning, or numbness in the lower extremities. This is also the time to obtain a history regarding any prior injuries to the lumbar or thoracic spine. If the athlete has a history of prior back pain, determine the number, severity, and duration of previous injury episodes, and find out about any treatment or evaluation procedures for these injuries.

## Observation

As usual, your observation should begin when the athlete comes off the field. Observe for freedom versus guarding of movement. When the athlete left the field, was she able to straighten up easily, or were her movements slow and painful? Athletes with acute low back injuries are often quite guarded, and this can make evaluation difficult. Observe the athlete's posture—is she holding herself in a different posture than normal? If you have the athlete recline on a table, note any difficulty or hesitancy as she gets onto the table, and observe how well she moves from side-lying to supine. As you prepare for your objective assessment, make the same observations as she gets off the table and returns to standing. Once the athlete is standing, note for any immediate signs of swelling, discoloration, deformities, unusual markings, or obvious muscle spasm or irregularities. Observe the lumbar spine for symmetry and correct alignment. From the side, check for presence or absence of a normal lumbar curve; when standing behind the athlete, check for soft tissue balance and straightness versus lateral curvature of the spine.

## Palpation

As with evaluation of other areas, palpation moves from superficial to deep structures. With the athlete comfortably positioned in prone, move systematically throughout the thoracic and lumbar spine regions. Checking first for temperature variations with the back of the hand, move your hand from left to right sides of the thoracic, lumbar, and sacral regions. Then palpate the spinal column and pelvis for signs of tenderness, crepitus, or subtle deformity. The spinous processes, interspaces, transverse processes, ribs and their interspaces, ilium, sacrum, sacroiliac joints, sacrotuberous ligament, and ischial tuberosities are all palpated for tenderness or abnormal structures. Superficial soft tissue mobility is then assessed from the thoracic region downward; this is followed by deeper soft tissue palpation of muscles. Spinal muscles are palpated first, then more lateral muscles. The paraspinals, quadratus lumborum, lateral abdominals, latissimus dorsi, lower trapezius, hip rotators (especially the piriformis), and gluteals should be included routinely. Muscles are assessed bilaterally for the presence of spasm, tenderness, and any restricted mobility.

## Special Tests

Special tests for the low back are used primarily to rule out or assess for neurological pathology or joint dysfunction.

### Neuropathy Tests
Neuropathy tests identify neurological dysfunctions such as disc herniations or any nerve irritation caused by nerve compression, inflammation of the nerve or its sheath, or restricted tissue mobility.

### Valsalva Maneuver

*Intrathecal describes a location within the spinal canal.*

The **Valsalva maneuver** is used to assess for a herniated disc or other space-occupying lesion within the spinal canal. To perform the test, have the athlete take a deep breath and hold it while bearing down (as if moving the bowels), or blow into a closed fist (chapter 3, figure 3.12). This technique causes an increase in intrathecal pressure and pain when pressure is applied to the spinal cord by the herniated disc material or other space-occupying lesion. A positive sign will elicit pain in the nerve root and along its sensory distribution (dermatome).

## Straight Leg Raise Test

This test assesses sciatic nerve root irritation, which can result from a disc hernia-tion, muscle spasm (especially in the piriformis), facet pathology, or sciatic nerve restriction or inflammation. When the test includes dorsiflexion and neck flexion, it is known as **Liségue's test**. It is performed passively with the athlete in supine. Posi-tion the athlete's hip in internal rotation and adduction with the knee in full exten-sion. Then, slowly flex the hip until the athlete reports pain in the back or leg or until you perceive tightness in the posterior thigh. Then reposition the leg in slightly less hip flexion so that the pain resolves. Next, passively dorsiflex the foot either with or without active neck flexion (figure 7.12). A positive result occurs if the athlete re-ports a return of the leg pain first noted with the straight leg raise.

Normal range of motion for a straight leg raise should be 80-90°. If disc involve-ment is present, the straight leg raise is limited to about 30°. Pain in the 50° to 70° range can indicate nerve irritation without disc herniation.

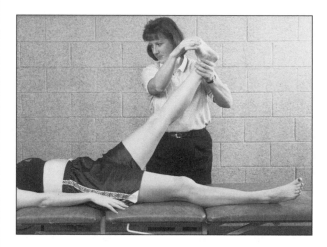

**❚ Figure 7.12**   Straight leg raise.

## Well Straight Leg Test

This test is used to identify a large disc lesion that protrudes medially to the nerve root. The straight leg test already described is performed on the uninvolved side. A positive sign occurs if the athlete reports pain on the involved side with the straight leg raise of the uninvolved leg.

## Kernig-Brudzinski Test

This active test is used to determine nerve root irritation, meningeal irritation, or dural irritation and is actually a combination of two separate tests, the **Kernig test** and the **Brudzinski test**. In the Kernig test, only the neck is flexed (figure 7.13); in the Brudzinski test, only the hip motion is per-formed to tension neural structures and elicit symptoms.

In the Kernig-Brudzinski test, the athlete lies supine with her hands clasped behind her head and her legs extended. The neck is flexed to bring the chin to the chest; then the hip is actively flexed with the knee extended until

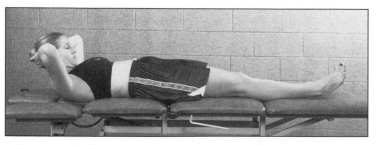

**❚ Figure 7.13**   Kernig test.

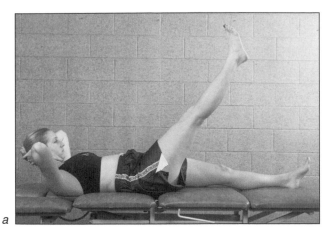
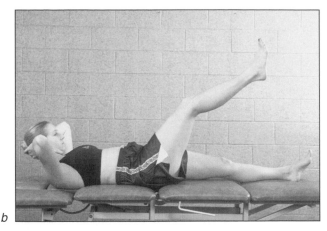

a              b

■ **Figure 7.14**    Kernig-Brudzinski test (a) extension and (b) flexion of the knee.

*Radicular describes pain referred into the extremity.*

pain is felt in the back or leg (figure 7.14a). Keeping the hip in the position where pain is first felt, flex the knee (figure 7.14b). The test is positive if the pain disappears.

### Bowstring Test

The bowstring, a modification of the straight leg test, is also called the **cram test**, or **popliteal pressure test**. It is used to identify compression or tension on the sciatic nerve. With the athlete in supine, move her leg into a straight leg raise until radicular pain is produced. Then flex the knee slightly (about 20°) to relieve the pain, and apply pressure to the popliteal fossa with your thumbs or fingers (figure 7.15). The test is positive if the athlete reports a return of the pain with popliteal pressure.

### Hoover Test

Use the Hoover test only when you feel it necessary to find out whether the athlete is **malingering** (pretending to be injured) or is truly unable to lift her leg. With the athlete supine, place one hand under each heel and lift both heels slightly off the table. Then instruct the athlete to try to lift one of her legs. If she is truly trying, you should feel a downward or counterpressure of the oppositive heel against the other hand (figure 7.16). If you do not feel any pressure on the other hand, the athlete is most likely not giving a full effort.

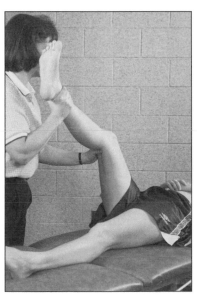

■ **Figure 7.15**    Bowstring test.

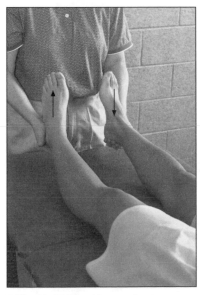

■ **Figure 7.16**    Hoover test.

## Babinski Test

The Babinski test identifies an upper motor neuron lesion. With the athlete relaxed, move a blunt object like a pen tip along the plantar aspect of the foot, from the heel toward the lateral aspect of the foot and over the ball of the foot (figure 7.17). A positive sign occurs if the great toe extends and the other toes abduct and plantarflex.

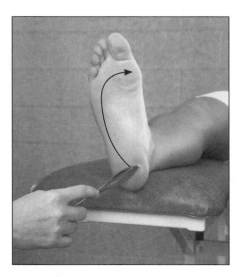

**▌Figure 7.17**   Babinski test.

## Oppenheim Test

This test also evaluates for the presence of an upper motor neuron lesion. Run your fingernail along the crest of the athlete's tibia. If the test is negative, the athlete will either have no reaction or will complain of pain. If the test is positive, you will see the same result as with a Babinski test: the great toe will extend and the other toes will abduct and plantarflex.

### Joint Dysfunction Tests

These tests of joint dysfunction are used to assess joint integrity of the lumbar spine or sacroilium. Pathology in these areas should be ruled out in cases of complaints of lower lumbar pain.

## Stork Standing Test

This active test is also referred to as the spondylolisthesis test. While balancing on one leg, the athlete extends the spine backward (figure 7.18). The test is repeated on the opposite side. If the test produces pain in the back, the athlete may have a pars fracture. If the pain occurs while the athlete is standing on one leg but not the other, the pars fracture may be unilateral. In the case of unilateral pain, pathology is typically present on the same side as the support leg.

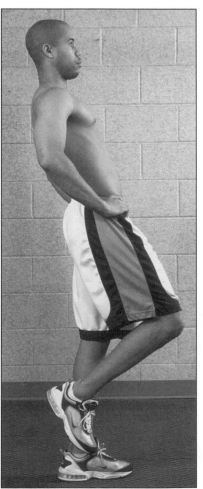

**▌Figure 7.18**   Stork standing test.

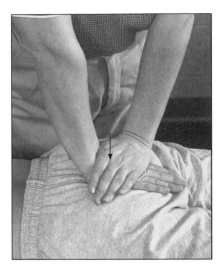

**Figure 7.19** Spring test.

### Spring Test

This passive test will determine whether or not the sacroiliac joint is the source of the athlete's pain. The athlete is in prone with a rolled towel under the anterior superior iliac spine (ASIS) bilaterally. Place the base of one of your hands over the apex of the athlete's sacrum, and place the other hand on top of the first hand. A shear stress between the sacrum and ilium occurs when a downward pressure is applied over the apex of the sacrum (figure 7.19). Pain is the positive sign. If there is pain or dysfunction in the sacroiliac region, perform other special tests for the sacroiliac joint as described in chapter 10.

### *Range of Motion*

If the athlete is able to stand, active range of motion of the trunk and lumbar spine should be attempted and assessed for quality and quantity of movement in all planes. There are various methods of measuring thoracolumbar range of motion; athletic trainers select a method that has proven reliable and consistent for them. Assess active range of motion first; if the movement is pain free, apply an overpressure force to assess passive motion and gross end feel. Since spine movement is a composite of motions of several vertebral levels, overpressure for each movement will provide only a gross estimate of end feel. Specific end feel of individual vertebral joints is most appropriately assessed through individual joint assessment techniques.

#### Active Range of Motion

It is easiest to observe forward **flexion** by having the athlete bend over to touch his toes. You should observe two factors: how far the athlete can reach to the floor, and the curvature of the thoracic and lumbar spines as he bends forward. Normal excursion allows the athlete to touch the fingers to the floor; if the motion is more limited, measure and document the distance between the fingertips and the floor for later comparison. A normal curve is smooth and continually rounded from the upper thoracic spine to the sacrum, with movement progressing from one vertebral level to the next as the athlete moves into full trunk flexion (figure 7.20). An abnormal curve is apparent when you observe flat sections or sharp angulations (figure 7.21). Remember, you cannot assume that forward flexion motion is normal

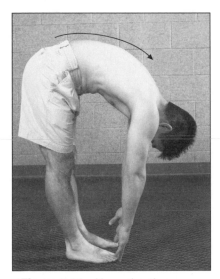

**Figure 7.20** Normal active forward flexion.

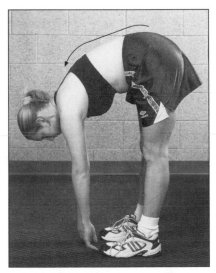

**Figure 7.21** Abnormal active forward flexion.

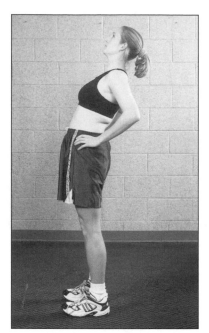

**Figure 7.22**    Active back extension.

solely on the basis of the athlete's ability to touch the floor. A straight spine with little segmental movement between the vertebrae can be compensated for by hip flexibility. This is why it is as important to note the curvature of the spine and the way the spine moves as to observe how far the athlete is able to reach.

The majority of **extension** motion occurs in the lumbar spine with minimal extension in the thoracic spine. The athlete should place her hands in the small of her back to provide stability during extension motion (figure 7.22). As she moves into extension, the thoracic curve should become straight and the lumbar curve more lordotic. Normal extension is approximately 30°.

Lateral flexion should be performed without compensatory lateral movement of the pelvis to the opposite side. To limit spinal rotation substitution, instruct the athlete to keep her hips square and to run her hand down the lateral thigh as she laterally flexes. As you observe lateral flexion, the thoracolumbar spine should move sequentially as it did during flexion and extension and should produce a smooth curve (figure 7.23). Normal lateral flexion should be equal on the two sides and is approximately 30° to 40° in each direction.

Rotation should be performed in sitting to eliminate hip and thigh movement. With her arms crossed and her hands on opposite shoulders, the athlete rotates to the left and to the right as far as possible (figure 7.24). Rotation occurs primarily in the thoracic spine with minimal contribution from the lumbar spine. Rotation is approximately 50° to 70°.

Assess costovertebral motion by measuring the difference between chest girth during maximum inspiration and maximum expiration. Place the tape measure around the athlete's chest just below the axilla (T4), and take measurements at the

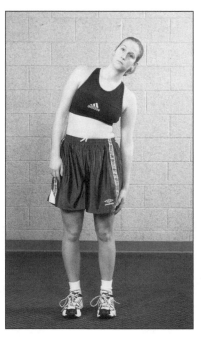

**Figure 7.23**    Active lateral flexion.

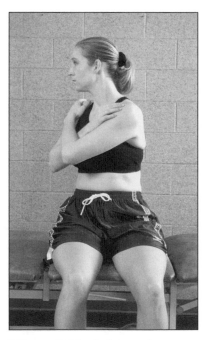

**Figure 7.24**    Active trunk rotation.

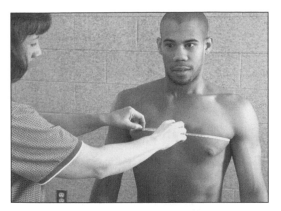

■ **Figure 7.25** Chest girth at maximum inspiration: costovertebral motion.

ends of inspiration and expiration (figure 7.25). Normal excursion is approximately 1 to 3 in., or 3 to 7.5 cm.

**Passive Motion**

If the athlete reports pain with any active motion, defer passive motion assessment. If no pain is reported, you can cautiously apply an overpressure at the end of the movement. All motions should produce an end feel that is a soft tissue stretch sensation, without a bony or hard end feel. Overpressure response is normally pain free.

### Strength

Strength is best evaluated with the trunk moving against gravity. Abdominals are tested in supine (figure 7.26a), lateral flexion in side-lying (figure 7.26b), and extensors in prone (figure 7.26c). Given the weight of the trunk, strength is usually assessed without resistance, as trunk weight alone provides considerable resistance and makes the movement quite challenging.

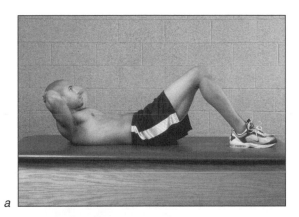

a

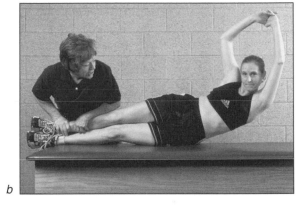

b

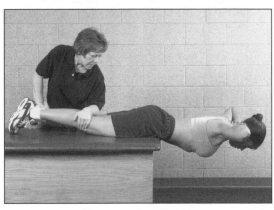

c

■ **Figure 7.26** Strength testing for (a) trunk flexion, (b) side-lying lateral trunk flexion, and (c) prone trunk extension.

### Neurological Tests

Perform neurological testing when the athlete reports weakness, referred pain, numbness, or tingling into the lower extremities. Neurological tests include motor, sensory, and reflex assessment. Both sensory and motor tests should be performed bilaterally, and simultaneously whenever possible, so that immediate comparisons can be made and more subtle differences identified.

Sensory testing for the lumbar plexus is performed with light touch or pinprick methods over the anterior thigh (L2), the medial aspect of the knee (L3), the medial lower leg (L4), the lateral lower leg and dorsum of the foot (L5), the lateral plantar foot (S1), and the posterior thigh (popliteal fossa) and posterior lateral heel (S2) (see figure 7.8).

Motor tests include manual resistance to hip flexion (L1-2), knee extension (L3-4), ankle dorsiflexion (L4), great toe extension (L5), ankle eversion or hip extension (S1), and knee flexion (S2) (figure 7.27, a-f).

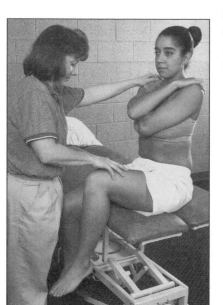

a

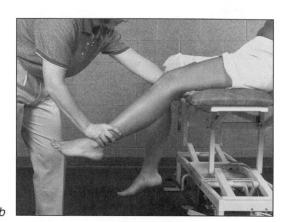

b

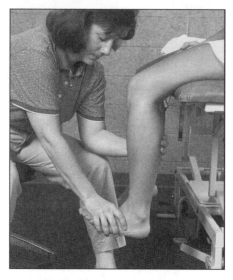

c

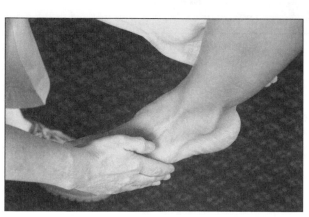

d

**▌Figure 7.27**
Motor tests for the lumbar plexus: (a) hip flexion, (b) knee extension, (c) ankle dorsiflexion, (d) great toe extension, (e) ankle eversion, and (f) knee flexion.

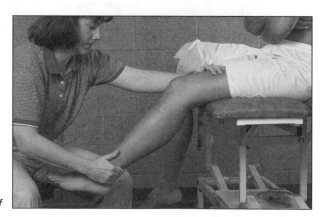

e

f

If you are having difficulty eliciting a reflex response, remember to use the Jendrassik maneuver to distract the athlete and increase the nervous system's sensitivity (see chapter 2, figure 2.1).

To assess deep tendon reflex and to differentiate between an upper and lower motor neuron lesion, perform a brisk patellar tendon tap (L3-4) (figure 7.28a) and Achilles tendon tap (S1-2) (figure 7.28b) with a reflex hammer (refer to page 36 for the grading scale). If a nerve root or peripheral nerve is involved, the reflex will be diminished, whereas a central nerve lesion may exhibit a hyperreflexivity.

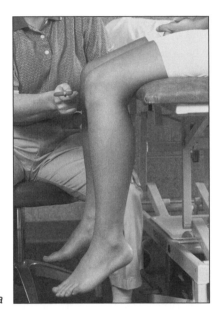
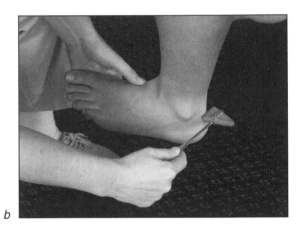

■ **Figure 7.28** Reflex testing for (a) patellar tendon and (b) Achilles tendon.

a

b

---

## Checklist for Sideline Assessment of the Lumbar and Thoracic Spine

### History

Ask questions pertaining to the following:

✓ Chief complaint

✓ Mechanism of injury

✓ Unusual sensations of numbness, tingling, burning pain into the lower extremities

✓ Type and location of pain or symptoms

✓ Previous injury (number of prior episodes and comparison with current episode)

### Observation

✓ Check for visible facial expressions of pain.

✓ Check for swelling, deformity, abnormal contours, or discoloration.

✓ Check for freedom of movement and ability to get on and off the table.

✓ Observe overall position, posture, and alignment.

✓ Check muscle development—areas of muscular spasm, atrophy.

### Palpation

Palpate for pain, temperature, tenderness, spasm, and restricted mobility.

✓ Bony palpation over spinous processes, interspaces and interspinous ligament, ilium, sacrum, sacroiliac joint, sacrotuberous ligament, ischial tuberosities

✓ Soft tissue (superficial to deep): paraspinals, quadratus lumborum, abdominals, latissimus dorsi, lower trapezius, hip rotators (piriformis), gluteals

### Special Tests

✓ Neuropathy tests (Valsalva, straight and well leg raise, Kernig-Brudzinski, bowstring)

✓ Joint dysfunction tests (stork, spring)

### Range of Motion

✓ Active ROM: forward flexion, extension, lateral flexion, and rotation

✓ Passive ROM for the same motions if nonpainful in active ROM

✓ Costovertebral motion

### Strength Tests

✓ Active ROM against gravity and weight of trunk for abdominals, lateral flexion, and extension

### Neurological Tests

✓ Sensory for L2-S1

✓ Motor for L2-S2

✓ Reflex (patellar and Achilles tendons)

### Functional Tests

### *Functional Tests*

Since functional tests are more typically a part of off-field assessment than of assessment at the sideline, they will be discussed in the next section.

## OFF-FIELD ASSESSMENT

It is common for athletes to report back injuries or back pain sometime after the onset of the pain. Because the back is complex, involving many structures that can be the source of pain, and because many of those structures can refer pain to the lower extremities, assessment of back injuries is a challenging task. It can be difficult to narrow down the cause of the pain and identify the source of the problem. A systematic approach that uses a thorough history to narrow the possibilities, along with a complete objective program that pinpoints and confirms your suspicions, is invaluable.

Many elements of the sideline assessment are used in the off-field assessment. Additional techniques are of value in the off-field assessment for identifying the structures that may be involved in the injury. The following discussion of assessment off the field refers only briefly to those components that were already described for the sideline assessment.

### *History*

In addition to taking the history as outlined for the sideline assessment, it is important to make further inquiries when assessing an athlete off the field. Since the injury is postacute or chronic at this point, other questions will help you obtain a better history of the nature, duration, and irritability of the athlete's symptoms.

**Nature**
When asking about unusual sensations such as numbness, tingling, or burning pain into the leg, include questions regarding any changes in or difficulty with coordination (e.g., tripping), urination, or bowel movements. If the athlete complains of urinary or bowel dysfunction, immediate referral to a physician is indicated. Try to get a good sense of the quality and nature of the pain—whether it is superficial or deep, localized or radiating, central over the spine or lateral in the musculature. Ask about aggravating symptoms, such as any increased pain with coughing, sneezing, or laughing, that may indicate a disc lesion. Determine whether the pain changes with activity or during the course of the day. Pain with activity may be related to disc pathology, whereas arthritic-based pain will be worse in the morning and will ease with some activity. If pain is activity related, what motions cause the most pain? Does the pain increase or decrease with activities such as sitting, standing, walking, or getting up from a chair? Standing and walking are extension activities, while sitting is a flexion activity; mechanical dysfunctions can be related to these activities.

**Duration**
To determine the duration of symptoms, ask the athlete when and where she first felt pain. Determine whether the pain has been intermittent or constant and whether it has improved or gotten worse over time. Most pain will be intermittent and will normally change over time. Rarely is it constant or consistent over time, and athletes with this type of pain may have psychological overlay.

**Irritability**
To get a sense of the irritability of a condition, ask how intense the pain is when it occurs and how long it lasts. Very irritable injuries will become painful easily and will persist, while less irritable conditions may exhibit delayed pain into or after an activity, with shorter durations. Disruption of sleep patterns also provides clues regarding the irritability.

### Previous Injury History

Obtain from the athlete a history of any prior injury to the back, including information about the number and frequency of earlier episodes and a specific account of the most recent episode, treatments and their success or failure, medications received, evaluations performed, and prior identification of the injury. If the athlete is taking medications, find out what they are, as some medications may mask the pain or aid in relieving inflammation, perhaps clouding the picture.

### *Observation*

Your observation begins from the moment you see the athlete and continues through the history-taking portion of the examination. Does the athlete sit and move comfortably or does he hesitate? Does he maintain a position without difficulty or does he need to change positions frequently? Does he avoid certain positions, such as standing or sitting? Is his gait normal?

You should perform a posture evaluation as outlined earlier in this chapter before conducting any other portion of the objective assessment. Consider posture from anterior, lateral, and posterior views. A simple checklist is provided on page 222.

For further discussion on posture assessment, refer to *Therapeutic Exercise for Athletic Injuries* (Houglum 2000), chapter 12.

### *Differential Diagnosis*

Since the spine can refer into the lower extremities and present symptoms similar to those of many other injuries, differential diagnosis to rule out injuries within the extremities and sacroiliac regions is necessary.

A quick test for the lower extremities is a full squat test. Ask the athlete to go into a full squat while you observe for quality and quantity of motion. The athlete should be able to fully flex his hips and knees while keeping his heels on the floor, and should be able to maneuver easily into full flexion and then into full standing. If he hesitates or is unable to complete the exercise, further assessment of the lower extremities is in order.

Sacroiliac dysfunction is quickly identified with the athlete in standing and the athletic trainer positioned behind him. Place one thumb on a posterior superior iliac spine (PSIS) and the other thumb on the sacral spinous process. The athlete then flexes the hip of the palpated PSIS (figure 7.29a). The thumb on the PSIS should move caudally; the test is abnormal if the PSIS moves upward. Repeat the test on the other side with one thumb on the opposite PSIS and the other on the sacral spinous process. Next, place one thumb on an ischial tuberosity and the other on the central apex. When the athlete flexes the ipsilateral hip, the ischial tuberosity should move laterally; the result is abnormal if it moves upward (figure 7.29b). Repeat this test on the opposite side. If these tests are positive, the sacroiliac joint will require further investigation.

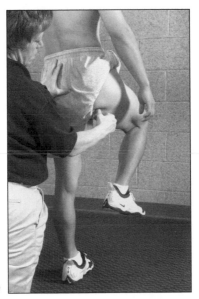

*a*　　　　　*b*

**Figure 7.29** Sacroiliac dysfunction tests: (a) upward movement of PSIS and (b) upward movement of the ischial tuberosity are considered abnormal.

## Checklist for Postural Assessment of the Lower Thoracic and Lumbar Spine

**Anterior**

Check for the following:

✓ Head straight on shoulders
✓ Nose in line with manubrium and umbilicus
✓ Shoulders and clavicles level and equal (dominant may be slightly lower)
✓ Waist angles equal (heights of the iliac crests should be equal—check leg length if not)
✓ Equal levels of ASIS
✓ Patella pointing straight ahead
✓ Feet angling out equally

**Lateral**

Look for the following:

✓ Earlobe in line with acromion process and high point of iliac crest

✓ Each segment of spine has normal curve (look for exaggerated or decreased curve)
✓ Rounded shoulders or forward head

**Posterior**

Check for the following:

✓ Level of shoulders, spines of scapulae, inferior angles of scapulae
✓ Lateral spinal curve (scoliosis)
✓ Equal waist angles
✓ Level of PSIS
✓ Gluteal folds and knee joint crease of equal height

### Range of Motion

Active and passive movements are consistent with those described for assessment at the sideline.

### Strength

Manual resistance strength tests are also consistent with those described for the sideline assessment. Additionally, isokinetic strength assessment can be used to identify specific weaknesses. The trunk flexors are not as strong as the trunk extensors. If the athlete reports any possible nerve root or referred pain symptoms, rotation tests should be avoided and aggressive machine testing should be performed with caution to avoid aggravation of the injury.

### Neurological Tests

Neurological testing was outlined in connection with the sideline assessment. A variety of sensory tests, such as temperature, deep pressure, or vibration, can further identify other sensory deficiencies; use the same dermatome patterns as previously described to identify levels of involvement (see figure 7.8).

If no neurological deficiencies with symptoms distal to the gluteal fold are evident, the neurological examination can be deferred. You would anticipate that in the absence of symptoms, the examination would be negative.

### Special Tests

The same tests that were described for the sideline assessment can be used off-field. Although many other special tests are available to assess the low back for neuropathology and joint dysfunction, those presented in this chapter are most commonly used for athletic injuries.

### Joint Mobility

End feel is the primary reason to perform joint mobility assessment of the thoracolumbar spine. Pain and joint play are evaluated along with joint mobility. For all the procedures described here, the athlete is prone. It may be necessary to position a pillow under the abdomen for improved comfort.

Prior to joint mobility assessment, the spinous processes of the middle and lower thoracic and lumbar vertebrae are palpated for alignment and tenderness. T7 is at the level of the inferior angle of the scapula, and L4-5 interspace is at the level of the crest of the ilium. Each spinous process is palpated either from caudal to cephalad or the reverse. Posteroanterior (PA) vertebral pressure can be applied centrally and unilaterally. Apply a central PA pressure over each spinous process, directing pressure from your shoulders through your thumbs (figure 7.30). Apply the force slowly and precisely in order to determine end-feel movement, excursion, and quality.

Unilateral PA force is also applied with the thumbs through a vertical force from the shoulders, but it is applied lateral to the spinous process over the transverse process of each vertebra. Compare the left and right sides of each level. The degree of movement and end feel should be the same and should be pain free bilaterally.

*Caudal means away from the head.*

*Cephalad means toward the head.*

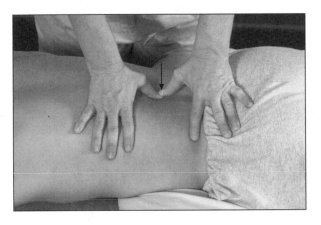

**▌Figure 7.30**   Assessment of central posteroanterior (PA) mobility over spinous process.

### Palpation

Palpation as described for the sideline assessment should be an integral part of assessment off the field. Soft tissue with areas of tenderness and limited mobility can be a common source of pain in athletes with a history of prior injuries and in older athletes.

### Functional Tests

Functional tests are performed only if the athlete has minimal symptoms and has full, unrestricted mobility.

While the athlete is performing these tests, observe closely for any hesitation; lack of normal movement, power, and flexibility; inability to bend, cut, turn, twist, or make contact with opponents; reduced quality in stride, throw, or stroke; diminished effort; or lack of confidence. You should assess the athlete's condition after the functional tests, since it is common for postactivity pain or spasm to occur if a back injury is not completely resolved.

If the athlete executes all tests well, has no pain nor muscle spasm, displays confidence in skill execution, and has normal range of motion, strength, agility, and performance, he is able to return to full sport participation.

## Checklist for Off-Field Assessment of the Lumbar and Thoracic Spine

### History

Ask questions pertaining to the following:

- ✓ Chief complaint
- ✓ Mechanism of injury
- ✓ Unusual sensations of numbness, tingling, burning pain into the lower extremities
- ✓ Bowel or bladder dysfunction
- ✓ Type, quality, and location of pain or symptoms
- ✓ Previous injury (number of prior episodes and comparison with current episode)

If chronic:

- ✓ Onset and duration of symptoms and pain patterns over time
- ✓ Irritability of symptoms

### Observation

- ✓ Check for visible facial expressions of pain.
- ✓ Check for swelling, deformity, abnormal contours, or discoloration.
- ✓ Check ability to sit, stand comfortably; freedom of movement versus guarding.
- ✓ Observe overall position, posture, and alignment.
- ✓ Check muscle development—areas of muscular spasm, atrophy (compare bilaterally).

### Differential Diagnosis

- ✓ Squat test
- ✓ Sacroiliac dysfunction

### Range of Motion

- ✓ Active ROM for forward flexion, extension, lateral flexion, and rotation
- ✓ Passive ROM for same motions if nonpainful in active ROM
- ✓ Costovertebral motion

### Strength Tests

- ✓ Active ROM against gravity and weight of trunk for trunk flexion (abdominals), lateral flexion, and extension

### Neurological Tests (If Pain or Symptoms Below the Gluteal Fold)

- ✓ Sensory for L2-S1
- ✓ Motor for L2-S2
- ✓ Reflex (patellar and Achilles tendons)

### Special Tests

- ✓ Neuropathy tests (Valsalva, straight and well leg raise, Kernig-Brudzinski, bowstring)
- ✓ Joint dysfunction tests (stork, spring)

### Joint Mobility Assessment

- ✓ Central PAs over spinous processes
- ✓ Unilateral PAs over transverse processes

### Palpation

Palpate for increased temperature, pain, tenderness, spasm, and restricted mobility.

- ✓ Bony palpation over spinous processes, interspaces and interspinous ligament, ilium, sacrum, sacroiliac joint, sacrotuberous ligament, ischial tuberosities
- ✓ Soft tissue (superficial to deep): paraspinals, quadratus lumborum, abdominals, latissimus dorsi, lower trapezius, hip rotators (piriformis), gluteals

### Functional Tests

- ✓ Check for normal and unrestricted movement.
- ✓ Check ability to bend, turn out, cut, twist, run, stride.
- ✓ Check for postactivity pain and spasm.

# SUMMARY

1. *Describe the etiology, signs and symptoms, and potential complications associated with acute and chronic injuries of the thoracic and lumbar spine commonly encountered in the physically active.*

Tremendous mechanical loads are placed on the lumbar spine during physical activity, making it susceptible to injury. Lumbar and thoracic pain is most often due to acute and chronic strains of the postural muscles supporting the lumbar region. Chronic strain may result from poor posture, poor mechanics, weakness, stiffness, and muscle restrictions. Occasionally low back pain is caused by congenital defects or degenerative changes. Traumatic injuries such as fractures may also occur, and the potential for a spinal cord injury and potential paralysis must always be considered with severe injuries.

2. *Describe the various congenital and degenerative conditions of the thoracic and lumbar spine.*

   On occasion, low back pain will be caused by a congenital weakness or by degenerative changes with repetitive stress over time. Spondylolysis is thought to result from congenital weakness of the pars interarticularis. These injuries are most often seen in young and skeletally immature athletes. If the defect is bilateral, spondylolisthesis, or forward slippage of the vertebrae, may result. In older adults, degenerative changes may be the culprit with respect to back pain and can range from chronic inflammatory conditions to degenerative disc changes to osteophyte formation. Poor posture, weak abdominals and back musculature, and poor mechanics often contribute to the mechanical stress placed on the spine.

3. *Describe the common causes, signs and symptoms, and indicative tests for nerve root compression in the lumbar spine.*

   Nerve root compression can be caused by any space-occupying lesion that impinges on the spinal cord or nerve root. Lumbar disc lesions are often the cause of nerve root compression due to herniation of the disc into the central or intervertebral foramen. Osteophytes resulting from degenerative changes may also narrow the intervertebral foramen and put pressure on the nerve. The signs and symptoms of a nerve root compression are pain into the lower extremity along the distribution of the involved nerve root. Paresthesia along the dermatome, motor weakness, and diminished reflex may also be present. Special tests that tension the nerve root and increase intrathecal pressure will elicit pain and an increase in symptoms. Signs and symptoms of bladder and bowel dysfunction can occur with compression of the cauda equina, which constitutes a medical emergency.

4. *Identify the characteristics and potential contributing factors to functional and structural deformities in the thoracic and lumbar spine.*

   Structural and functional deformities of the lumbar spine are not uncommon; they include lumbarization of the spine, spina bifida occulta, scoliosis, and excessive kyphosis and lordosis. Whereas structural deformities are characterized by a permanent structural change that is often congenital, functional deformities are usually caused by mechanical stress, muscle imbalance, and dysfunction. However, a functional deformity can ultimately become a structural deformity if it leads to degenerative and permanent changes in the spine.

5. *Perform an on-field assessment of the lumbar spine, indicating criteria for immediate medical referral and transportation from the field.*

   Although severe life-changing injuries to the lumbar spine are uncommon in sport, the athletic trainer must be constantly aware that they are a possibility and must rule them out before the athlete is removed from the playing field. If there is any evidence of sensory or motor deficits, or centralized spine pain, the athlete should be immobilized and transported on a spine board for further medical evaluation. In addition to ruling out catastrophic spinal cord injury, the immediate assessment must include an accurate evaluation of the athlete's alertness and respiratory and cardiovascular status; and the athletic trainer must be aware of any signs of bleeding, fractures, dislocations, or shock. Only then should the athletic trainer determine the appropriate method of transportation.

6. *Perform a thorough and sequential sideline assessment of the lumbar spine.*

   Once the athlete is on the sideline, a more thorough assessment of the injury can be made. The athletic trainer obtains a more detailed history and performs an objective assessment that includes observation, palpation, special tests, active and passive range of motion and strength. Neurological tests are also performed if the athlete reports any symptoms below the gluteal fold. Although many special tests for spine injuries are available, only those most commonly used were presented in this chapter—including the Valsalva maneuver, straight leg raise test, well straight leg raise test, Babinski test, Oppenheim test, Kernig-Brudzinski test, bowstring test, Hoover test, stork standing test, and spring test.

7. *Perform a thorough and sequential off-field assessment of the lumbar and thoracic spine, noting considerations for differential diagnosis.*

   If the athlete does not report the injury immediately, the athletic trainer sees the spine injury in the athletic treatment facility at some interval after it occurred. In this case the athletic trainer must obtain a more detailed history and pain profile and must perform tests that will provide a differential diagnosis, eliminating other potential causes of the athlete's complaints. Most of the tests used in the sideline assessment are also used in the off-field assessment. In addition, joint mobility tests will further define the injury, and functional tests will evaluate the athlete for safe and appropriate return to sport participation.

# REVIEW QUESTIONS

1. What are the common mechanisms of sprains and strains? What are some of the causative factors of these injuries, and what preventive measures can be taken to avoid these injuries?

2. Discuss some of the locations where spinal fracture can occur and the potential complications that may be associated with each.

3. What is the difference between spondylolysis, spondylolisthesis, spondylosis, and spondylitis? What, if any, are the differential signs and symptoms of each, and what implications do these conditions have for physical activity?

4. Discuss the causes, pathology, and signs and symptoms associated with a lumbar intervertebral disc herniation. What are some of the special tests you would use to confirm a lesion?

5. What is the difference between the straight leg and the well leg raise test?

6. What tests are used to assess for low back pain caused by sacroiliac dysfunction?

# CRITICAL THINKING QUESTIONS

1. A basketball player comes to you complaining of pain in his lower lumbar region that travels down his left buttock and into his lateral lower leg. On exam, you note some spasm and guarding. During your objective assessment, you find increased pain with active extension, and with lateral flexion and rotation to the left side. On neurological testing, you note paresthesia on the lateral leg and dorsum of the foot and mild weakness with extension of the

great toe. The athlete denies pain with coughing, sneezing, or laughing, and the Valsalva maneuver is negative. Straight leg raise is positive. On the basis of these findings, what injury or condition do you suspect, and at what level?

2. You have a young, female gymnast who comes to you complaining of central lower back pain. She describes a strip of pain that runs across her back at the level of the iliac crests. She describes the pain as a deep, aching pain that travels into both buttocks, but she denies any pain down her leg. On observation, you note an increased lordotic curve. Although she does not complain of pain in forward flexion, you note that the spinous process at L4 does not seem to be as apparent as at L3 and L5. Her pain is increased on active extension. What condition(s) and level might you suspect, and what test(s) would you use to confirm your suspicions?

3. You are invited to speak at an educational workshop for industrial workers on the prevention of back pain and injury. Based on the knowledge you have gained in this chapter, what information do you think would be important to share with the audience, and what prevention strategies could you offer?

# ADDITIONAL RESOURCES

Hillman, S.K. 2000. *Introduction to athletic injuries.* Champaign, IL: Human Kinetics.

Houglum, P.A. 2000. *Therapeutic exercise for athletic injuries.* Champaign, IL: Human Kinetics.

# CHAPTER EIGHT

# Leg, Ankle, and Foot

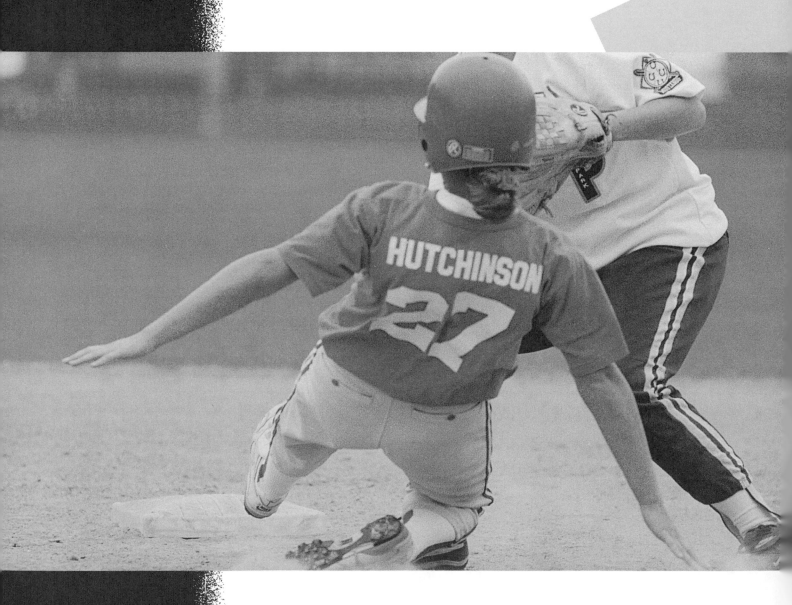

# OBJECTIVES

After completing this chapter, the reader will be able to do the following:

1. Describe the etiology, signs and symptoms, and potential complications associated with acute injuries of the foot, ankle, and lower leg commonly encountered in the physically active

2. Describe the etiology, signs and symptoms, and potential complications associated with chronic or overuse injuries of the foot, ankle, and lower leg commonly encountered in the physically active

3. Identify the signs and symptoms of neurovascular injury at the foot and ankle and differentiate those that indicate a medical emergency

4. Identify the common functional and structural abnormalities of the foot and their potential effects on lower-extremity mechanics and injury

5. Perform an on-field assessment of the foot, ankle, and lower leg, noting criteria for medical referral and mode of transportation from the field

6. Perform a sideline assessment of the foot, ankle, and lower leg, including differential diagnosis of referring lumbar, hip, and knee pathologies

7. Perform an off-field assessment of the foot, ankle, and lower leg, including functional tests for return to activity

Bill was covering baseball practice at Monrovia University when Eddie got hit in the shin with a line drive while pitching batting practice.

"Hey, Eddie, looks like you took a pretty good shot! Where did it hit you?" Bill asked as he approached.

"It hit me right in the muscle," Eddie said in a great deal of pain.

As Bill looked, he could see the swelling and discoloration already begin to form over the belly of Eddie's anterior tibialis. It was pretty obvious what had happened, so rather than waste any time, Bill got an ice bag and wrapped it on Eddie's shin to try to control the bleeding and the pain. Twenty minutes later, Eddie was still pretty restless.

"Man, Bill, this really hurts . . . I've been hit in the shin before, but this is out-of-control pain. I'm also getting some numbness in my foot. Do you think this Ace wrap is too tight?"

"Maybe, let's loosen it up a bit and see if that relieves the pressure," Bill offered. As he took off the Ace wrap, he noticed that the leg was even more swollen than before.

After another 20 minutes, Eddie called Bill over again. "Hey Bill, you gotta do something about this—this isn't feeling any better. I can't even move my foot, it hurts so bad."

Bill came and took a look. It was apparent that the whole anterior compartment was now swollen and the skin was taking on a whitish, glossy appearance. "Eddie, can you feel when I touch you here?" Bill asked as he did a sensory check over the dorsum of the foot.

"No, I can't!"

"How about trying to bring your toes up toward your shin—can you try that for me?" Bill was getting a little concerned at this point. Eddie tried to lift his foot, but he couldn't. Bill palpated for a pedal pulse and felt one, but it felt faint compared to the one in the other leg. "Eddie, I think you have a little more than a contusion here—I think we better get you to the emergency room right away." Bill called emergency medical services and within 5 minutes they were there.

About an hour later, Bill saw Doc Rogers, Monrovia's team physician. "Hi, Doc, how's Eddie?"

"Hi, Bill, Eddie's on his way to surgery. He developed an acute anterior tibial compartment syndrome from the hemorrhage resulting from the contusion. He was lucky that you were there and recognized the signs and symptoms. . . ."

Actually, Bill was wishing to himself that he hadn't used that Ace wrap and had recognized the signs a little sooner.

---

The lower leg, ankle, and foot represent a complex relationship of 28 bones (tibia, fibula, 7 tarsals, 5 metatarsals, and 14 phalanges), multiple ligaments, and both intrinsic and extrinsic muscles that function together to provide stability, adaptability, and shock absorption for optimal support and locomotion of the entire body. The lower leg complex is often referred to in three segments, the hindfoot, midfoot, and forefoot (figure 8.1). Although movement at any one joint may be minimal, in combination the joints of the foot and ankle offer a great deal of flexibility and adaptability.

The majority of physiological movement occurs in the hindfoot, at the talocrural and subtalar joints. Two motions of the subtalar joint that you will read about throughout this chapter are pronation and supination. These are not "true" motions but rather represent a composite of three motions occurring at the joint. In the open chain, **pronation** results from eversion, dorsiflexion, and abduction of the foot; **supination** results from inversion, plantar flexion, and adduction of the foot. In the closed chain, however, pronation is a result of eversion, plantar flexion, and abduc-

*Open chain* refers to a segment where the distal end is not fixed or in contact with the ground.

*Closed chain* refers to a segment that has the distal end fixed or in contact with the ground.

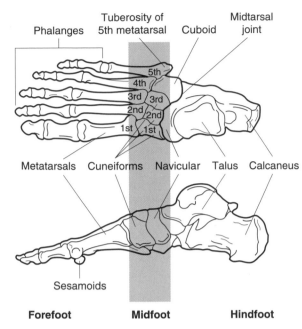

Phalanges
Tuberosity of 5th metatarsal
Cuboid
Midtarsal joint

Metatarsals — Cuneiforms — Navicular — Talus — Calcaneus

Sesamoids

**Forefoot** **Midfoot** **Hindfoot**

**▌Figure 8.1** Bony anatomy of the foot, identifying the hindfoot, midfoot, and forefoot.

tion, whereas supination is a result of inversion, dorsiflexion, and adduction. It is important to understand and appreciate these composite motions, as they play a major role in lower-extremity function and mechanics.

The primary functions of the lower leg, ankle, and foot are to provide both a rigid lever for propulsion and a stable, but adaptable structure to support the body's weight during gait. In the stance phase of gait, the foot begins to pronate immediately after heel strike. This unlocks the midtarsal joints and increases **flexibility** and adaptability in the forefoot to absorb the shock of heel strike and to adapt to the ground surface. During midstance, the foot begins to supinate. Supination acts to lock the midtarsal joints to provide maximum **stability** of the forefoot, making the foot rigid for maximal propulsion during push-off. Appreciating the balance between mobility and stability at the foot and ankle is essential, as changes in joint function resulting from injury and functional and structural abnormalities can have a tremendous influence on this balance, and thus on lower-extremity mechanics, stress, and future injury.

For a more complete discussion on gait, refer to *Therapeutic Exercise for Athletic Injuries* (Houglum 2000), chapter 12.

# INJURIES TO THE LOWER LEG, ANKLE, AND FOOT

The majority of the active population will experience some lower leg and foot problems sometime in their lives. Tremendous forces, both compressive and rotational, are transmitted through the weight-bearing structures of the foot, ankle, and lower leg. Consequently, both traumatic and chronic injuries to this region are frequent. Even seemingly minor injuries can be quite debilitating given the need for strength and stability of the foot and ankle structures for daily weight-bearing activities, let alone sport activities. Additionally, lower leg and foot problems can alter gait or lower-body mechanics, resulting in increased stress and compensatory problems up the kinetic chain in the knee, hip, or lower back.

## ACUTE SOFT TISSUE INJURIES

The lower leg complex relies on the integrity of both active and passive soft tissue structures for both stability and propulsion. Just consider the tremendous loads and demands that dynamic sport activity places on the foot and ankle. Soft tissue injuries commonly occur as a result of direct contact and intrinsic or extrinsic forces acting on the foot, ankle, and lower leg.

### Contusions

Severe contusions to a muscular compartment should be closely monitored for excessive swelling and neurovascular compromise.

The lower leg, ankle, and foot are quite vulnerable to direct trauma in sport activity. Making contact with the ground or an opponent, kicking an unyielding object, being hit in the shin by a baseball, and being stepped on or kicked by another player are all common injury mechanisms resulting in soft tissue and periosteal contusions. Signs and symptoms include pain, swelling, and discoloration. Direct contact to the superficial and unprotected anterior medial border of the tibia can result in localized inflammation (**periostitis**) and hematoma formation under the periosteum, which can take considerable time for the body to absorb. Disability and loss of function are usually more severe with muscle contusions due to tenderness, swelling, and spasm within the muscle tissue. Decreased range of motion and strength will also be present and will vary according to the degree of tissue injury. Although contusions to muscle rarely result in serious injury, complications can arise from severe contusions and excessive bleeding within the enclosed anterior tibial compartment of the lower leg (see discussion of anterior compartment syndrome later in this chapter). Therefore, severe contusions to a muscular compartment should be closely monitored for neurovascular compromise.

A heel contusion, or **stone bruise**, can be particularly problematic. A heel bruise can result from landing hard on the heel during jumping activities or stepping on an uneven surface or a stone at heel strike with little or no footwear protection. A contusion to the fat pad of the heel can cause considerable pain and point tenderness, making it difficult to bear weight or walk with a normal gait. Discoloration and swelling may or may not be evident, depending on severity.

### Sprains

The foot and ankle comprise multiple joints and ligaments that provide stability during weight-bearing activities. Given the tremendous forces exerted on these structures with landing, cutting, and running, the ligaments are prone to injury when the joint is forced beyond its normal range of motion. Sprains occur most often at the **hindfoot**, which is composed of the distal tibiofibular (syndesmosis), talocrural (tibia, fibula, and talus), and subtalar (talus, calcaneus, navicular) joints. Ligamentous support is essential for stability of the hindfoot, particularly when the ankle is plantarflexed. Stability is provided laterally by the anterior talofibular, calcaneofibular, and posterior talofibular ligaments and medially by the deltoid ligament complex. The distal tibiofibular joint is stabilized by the interosseous membrane and the anterior and posterior tibiofibular ligaments. Although sprains occur most often at the hindfoot, sprains in the **midfoot** (talocalcaneonavicular, cuneonavicular, intercuneiform, and calcaneocuboid joints) and **forefoot** (tarsometatarsal, intermetatarsal, metatarsophalangeal, and interphalangeal joints) regions are not uncommon. Which joint structures are involved will be determined by the injury mechanism.

### Lateral Ankle Sprains

The most common mechanism of ankle injury involving the lateral ligament complex is inversion with or without plantar flexion. In typical scenarios, a basketball player comes down on an opponent's foot or lands awkwardly on the outside of her own foot, causing her ankle to turn in (inversion mechanism). The athlete will complain of immediate pain upon injury and may hear a "pop." The anterior talofibular ligament is almost always involved (figure 8.2). The calcaneofibular and, less often, the posterior talofibular ligaments may also be involved. Signs and symptoms are consistent with first- through third-degree ligament sprains. With second- and third-degree sprains, there may also be injury to the medial structures of the ankle due to compression from the inversion force. Dislocation of the ankle mortise rarely results with third-degree ligament injuries, but associated avulsion and/or push-off fractures of the lateral and medial malleolus, respectively, are not uncommon with more severe ankle sprains.

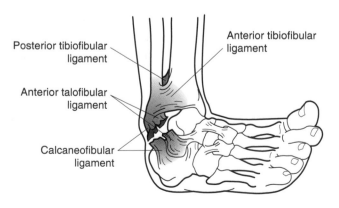

Posterior tibiofibular ligament

Anterior tibiofibular ligament

Anterior talofibular ligament

Calcaneofibular ligament

**▋ Figure 8.2** Lateral ligaments of the ankle.

> The distal fibula should be carefully palpated for possible fracture with all serious eversion injuries.

### Medial Ankle Sprains

Medial ankle sprains resulting from eversion forces are considerably less common, representing less than 5% of all ankle sprains. A primary reason for this lower incidence is the greater stability of the medial ankle, a consequence of the thickness and strength of the deltoid ligament complex as well as the longer lateral malleolus, which prevents excessive eversion range (figure 8.3). As a result, the distal fibula should be palpated for possible fracture with severe eversion injuries. Signs and symptoms are consistent with first-, second-, and third-degree sprains. However, disability and recovery may be prolonged with medial ankle sprains, given the support the deltoid ligament provides to the medial longitudinal arch of the foot. As a consequence, even simple weight bearing will stress the injured structures. Furthermore, pes planus and excessive pronation may also result from chronic medial instability.

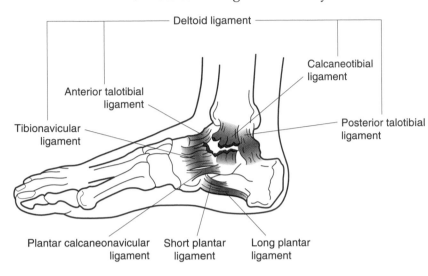

**■ Figure 8.3**   Medial ligaments of the ankle.

### Syndesmosis Sprains

Syndesmotic, or high, ankle sprains involve disruption of the tibiofibular ligaments and distal interosseous membrane, causing instability of the tibiofibular joint and widening of the ankle mortise (figure 8.4). Although less frequent than lateral ankle sprains, this injury can result in prolonged disability and recovery when not identified and managed properly. Syndesmotic ankle sprains are typically caused by forced hyperdorsiflexion or external rotation of the foot, resulting in forced separation of the tibiofibular joint. These injuries are most often seen in contact sports, such as football, in which the foot is planted and externally rotated and contact is made to the lateral aspect of the lower leg. Signs and symptoms include pain and swelling anterior to the ankle joint. Pain in the anterolateral aspect of the ankle with weight bearing, with passive external rotation of the foot, or with forced dorsiflexion is also indicative of injury to the syndesmosis.

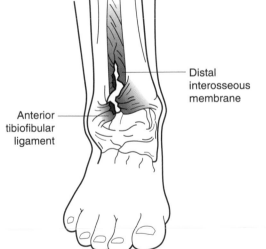

**■ Figure 8.4**   Syndesmosis sprain of the tibiofibular joint.

### Foot Sprains

Given the number of bony articulations and ligaments in the foot, myriad foot sprains can result from both direct and indirect forces. Because of the stability of the foot, sprains to the mid- and forefoot are less common than sprains to the ankle joint. Sprains to the metatarsal and long arch can result from both chronic overuse and acute traumatic forces that stretch the supporting ligamentous structures, causing a fallen arch. Signs and symptoms of foot and arch sprains include pain, point tenderness over the involved structure(s), swelling, discoloration, and difficulty with weight bearing. Because it is often difficult to distinguish bony from ligamentous injury in the foot given the smaller structures, evaluation by a physician and radiographic examination are often necessary to rule out fracture.

### Toe Sprains

Toe sprains most often result from direct contact at the end of the toe, such as "stubbing" or "jamming" the toe while kicking a nonyielding object. However, any direct or indirect mechanism that causes the joint to go beyond its normal range can result in sprains. Most problematic are sprains to the great toe, also known as **turf toe**. Turf toe can result from extreme dorsiflexion of the first metatarsophalangeal joint during push-off, extreme plantar flexion or axial compression while kicking an unyielding object, or quick stops that cause the foot to slide forward in the shoe. Signs and symptoms of toe sprains include pain, swelling, and ecchymosis. Decreased range of motion and pain with passive and active movements will also be noted. There may be joint instability with second- and third-degree classifications. Pain will be particularly apparent with push-off, making normal gait and running difficult.

### Strains

Numerous muscles originating from and contained within the lower leg are responsible for a variety of ankle and foot motions. Given the large mechanical forces associated with running, jumping, and cutting, muscle strains commonly result from overstretch and muscular overload mechanisms. Strains of the lateral peroneal muscles can result from forced and rapid eversion forces or overstretching with excessive inversion motions. Strains of the triceps surae muscles and common Achilles (calcaneal) tendon typically result from forceful and rapid plantar flexion movements during sport activities. Acute strains to the posterior tibial and toe flexor muscle/tendons can also occur with forceful plantar flexion and inversion, although repetitive stress and chronic tractioning with a valgus foot are more frequent causes. Signs and symptoms of muscle and tendinous strains include pain with active and resistive movement, pain with passive stretch, muscle spasm, swelling, and point tenderness over the area of injury. A palpable defect may be noted with second- and third-degree muscle injuries. While the degree of symptoms and disability will vary according to the severity, even first-degree (mild) strains can be debilitating given the constant demands placed on these structures during everyday walking and weight-bearing activities.

Muscle spasms are also common, particularly in the calf muscles. Muscular fatigue, dehydration and electrolyte imbalance, and direct blows are typical predisposing factors. Signs and symptoms include immediate pain, observable spasm, and loss of function. If spasm is severe and prolonged, signs and symptoms consistent with a first-degree strain may be present the following day.

### Rupture of the Achilles (Calcaneal) Tendon

Rupture of the Achilles tendon (figure 8.5) can result from a sudden, violent plantar flexion movement during eccentric loading in full weight-bearing activity. A rapid "punch" in gymnastics and the push-off in tennis are common mechanisms. The athlete will complain of immediate pain and disability and often will report a feeling of being "kicked" or "shot" in the calf. Considerable swelling and discoloration will also occur. There will be an observable defect in the contour of the Achilles tendon, and the athlete will be unable to actively plantarflex her foot. A Thompson test will be positive.

### Rupture of the Plantaris Muscle

The plantaris muscle can also rupture with forceful contraction or stretch at its musculotendinous unit during running, jumping, and rapid change of direction. The athlete will complain of a sudden, sharp pain felt deep in the posterior lower leg with push-off that may also resemble a feeling of being kicked or shot in the back of the leg. Pain, spasm, and possible loss of function may be present, and there may be swelling and discoloration around the ankle the next day. Tenderness may be noted deep to the belly of the gastrocnemius, and pain may increase with passive dorsiflexion. Given the relatively insignificant function of the plantaris muscle, pain and disability after the initial acute stages of injury are usually minimal.

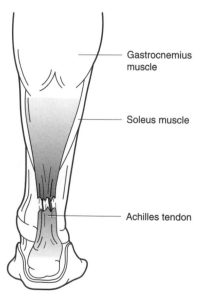

Gastrocnemius muscle

Soleus muscle

Achilles tendon

**Figure 8.5**   Achilles tendon rupture.

*Fibular and fibularis are synonymous with "peroneal" and "peroneus." Although some of the newer anatomical texts use "fibular" and "fibularis" with reference to specific muscles and nerves of the lower extremity, we have elected to use the more familiar terms "peroneal" and "peroneus" throughout this text.*

### Rupture of Peroneal Retinaculum

The peroneal (fibular) retinaculum, which tethers the peroneus longus and brevis tendons behind the lateral malleolus, can be strained or ruptured via a direct blow, by forceful eversion or plantar flexion forces, or with inversion ankle injuries (figure 8.6). When the peroneal retinaculum is disrupted, the peroneal tendons are allowed to sublux and "snap" over the lateral malleolus when the foot is moved into eversion and plantar flexion. Other signs and symptoms include pain, swelling, and inflammation of the tendons with repetitive subluxation.

## CHRONIC AND OVERUSE SOFT TISSUE INJURIES

Chronic soft tissue injuries are a frequent complaint in physically active people as a consequence of repetitive microtrauma resulting from abnormal friction, traction, structural mechanics, or some combination of these. As you will note in this section, excessive pronation is associated with a number of chronic overuse conditions. When pronation is excessive and continues past midstance, there is increased stress on the medial long arch and soft tissue structures that can cause abnormal stresses to be transmitted further up the lower-extremity chain.

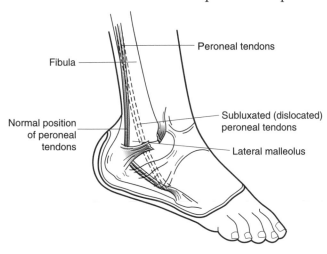

**Figure 8.6** Ruptured peroneal retinaculum, allowing the peroneal tendons to dislocate.

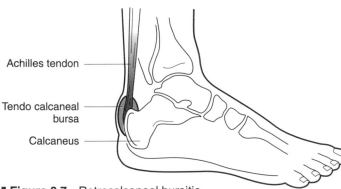

**Figure 8.7** Retrocalcaneal bursitis.

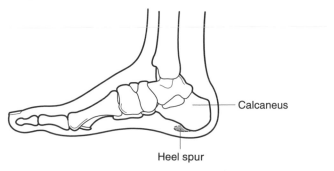

**Figure 8.8** Heel spur resulting from chronic tractioning of a tight plantar fascia.

### Retrocalcaneal Bursitis

The tendo calcaneal bursa lies between the calcaneus and the distal insertion of the Achilles tendon (figure 8.7). Inflammation and swelling of this bursa can result from repetitive overuse with running, direct pressure, or friction from poorly fitting footwear. Signs and symptoms include localized swelling, redness, and point tenderness near and around the calcaneal attachment of the Achilles tendon. Pain with active or resistive plantar flexion may also be noted. Thickening of the bursa and eventual calcium formation may occur in chronic cases.

### Plantar Fasciitis

Inflammation of the plantar fascia is seen most often in individuals with abnormal foot alignment and is precipitated by overuse, poor footwear or playing surface, or improper conditioning. The athlete's history is the primary evaluative tool. The athlete will typically complain of a gradual onset of pain and stiffness on the plantar surface of the foot, extending from the heel to the metatarsal heads. If the condition is prolonged, a **heel spur** may develop at the proximal calcaneal attachment (figure 8.8). It is important to note that the heel spur is not the cause of plantar fasciitis, but a result.

### Tendinitis and Tenosynovitis

Tendinitis and chronic strain of the peroneal, posterior tibial, and Achilles tendons are common in the athletic population. In all cases, injury results from repetitive overuse, friction, or tractioning of the tendon. Improper mechanics and abnormal foot alignment are often predisposing factors. Tendinitis may also occur in the toe extensor tendons where they cross superficially on the dorsum of the foot. Typically, inflammation of these tendons results from shoe pressure or friction or from shoelaces that are too tight. Signs and symptoms associated with tendinitis include pain, point tenderness, and crepitus over the inflamed tendon, decreased range of motion, and swelling. Pain with passive stretch or active/resistive movement of the involved muscle/tendon will be present as well. Inflammation and irritation of the Achilles tendon may also involve the synovial sheath (tenosynovitis), with swelling and snowball crepitus that are more pronounced than with simple tendinitis. Chronic thickening of the tendon may occur with prolonged inflammation.

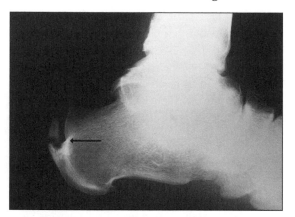

**Figure 8.9**  Calcaneal apophysitis (Sever's disease).

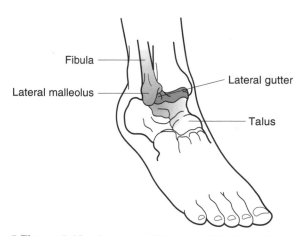

**Figure 8.10**  Anatomical location of the lateral gutter and area of impingement.

*Pes cavus is an abnormally high or excessive arch.*
*Pes planus is a "flat" foot that has lost the normal concavity on its plantar surface.*

### Calcaneal Apophysitis (Sever's Disease)

In young, skeletally immature athletes, the calcaneal apophysis can become inflamed secondary to repetitive traction stress of the Achilles tendon (figure 8.9). Common signs and symptoms include posterior inferior heel pain, point tenderness, and increased pain with weight-bearing, running, or jumping activities. Decreased dorsiflexion range secondary to tightness of the Achilles tendon during rapid growth phases is likely a predisposing factor.

### Anterolateral Impingement

Chronic anterolateral ankle pain can result from synovitis and scar tissue thickening following lateral ankle injuries (Ferkel et al. 1991). Specifically, anterolateral impingement is caused by chronic inflammation and impingement of hypertrophic scar tissue between the talus and fibula in the lateral gutter (figure 8.10). Signs and symptoms include persistent pain over the anterolateral aspect of the ankle for weeks and even months following a lateral ankle sprain. Athletes with persistent anterior lateral ankle pain who do not respond to conservative treatment and rest should be referred to a physician for further evaluation.

### Tibial Stress Syndrome

Tibial stress syndrome, commonly referred to as **shinsplints**, is usually an inflammation of the long toe or ankle flexors at or near their insertion to the posterior medial tibial border. There are a number of predisposing factors. Excessive pronation, inflexibility of the calf muscle, Achilles tendon, or long toe flexors (posterior tibialis and flexor hallucis longus), dorsiflexion weakness or fatigue, and foot conditions such as pes cavus and pes planus can alter the shock-absorbing or decelerating capabilities of the lower leg, resulting in transmission of increased stress to the shin and lower leg muscles. Medial tibial stress syndrome is characterized by diffuse pain, point tenderness, and inflammation along the medial border of the tibia. Usually with tibial stress syndrome, the pain is diffuse along a broad area of the medial

> **!** If medial shin pain becomes localized or if percussion of the bone causes pain, a tibial stress fracture should be suspected and the athlete referred to a physician.

tibial surface. However, if the pain becomes localized or if percussion of the bone causes pain, a tibial stress fracture should be suspected and the athlete should be referred to a physician.

# TRAUMATIC FRACTURES

Traumatic fractures can result from the same mechanisms that cause ankle and foot sprains. In fact, it is not uncommon for both fracture and ligament injury to be present with traumatic ankle injuries.

### Tibia and Fibula

Traumatic fractures of the tibia and fibula can result from a direct blow or indirect torsional stress or in association with inversion and eversion ankle injuries.

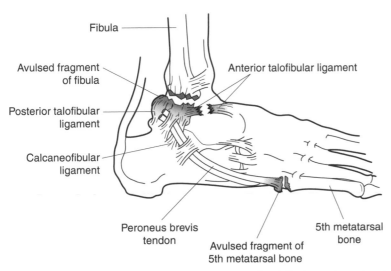

Fractures to the shaft of the fibula can result from a direct blow to the lateral aspect of the leg or from a severe eversion/external rotation stress. Fractures to the tibial shaft, which are less common, require much greater forces; but they can occur in contact sports such as football with a direct blow to the shin, or in skiing with a severe torsional stress. Fractures involving the epiphyseal plate of the distal tibial typically result from either compressive or torsional forces in skeletally immature athletes. Avulsion fractures of the distal fibula (lateral malleolus) occur secondary to an inversion stress (figure 8.11), while push-off fractures are caused by eversion mechanisms when the everted calcaneus butts up against the distal fibula. Fractures to the medial malleolus

**Figure 8.11** Avulsion fractures of both the distal fibula and proximal 5th metatarsal.

of the tibia similarly result from severe eversion (avulsion) or inversion (push-off secondary to contact with the talus) forces. Bi-malleolar fractures can also result from these mechanisms. A **Pott's fracture** occurs when the foot is forcibly everted, causing an avulsion fraction of the medial malleolus and a shear fracture of the lateral malleolus or distal fibula. Fractures through the articulating surface of the tibia (chondral and osteochondral fractures) may also occur with forcible compression of the ankle joint into excessive inversion/plantar flexion or eversion/dorsiflexion.

General signs and symptoms of fracture include immediate pain, swelling, and possible deformity if the fragments are displaced. Tenderness will be noted over and around the fracture site. Muscle splinting and spasm may also occur. Other indicative signs of fracture include pain with bony percussion or with transverse stress such as that produced when the tibia and fibula are squeezed together. False joint motion and/or crepitus may also be noted with manipulation of the bone. While a fracture of the tibia will result in an inability or unwillingness to bear weight, this may not be the case in the non-weight-bearing fibula. However, pain with active or resisted eversion will be apparent.

> **!** The ability of an athlete to bear weight on an injured ankle does not rule out the possibility of a fracture.

### Foot

Traumatic fractures in the foot typically involve the metatarsals and phalanges. The mechanisms associated with toe sprains also apply here. Traumatic fractures of the metatarsal shaft(s) most often result from direct trauma, for example when an athlete is stepped on by another player or when a weight is dropped on the foot. Pain associated with longitudinal stress applied to the plantar surface of the foot, axial stress to the bone, or with torsional stress applied through twisting the toe, is often indicative of metatarsal fractures. Fracture at the base of the fifth metatarsal (**Jones' fracture**) is usually caused by indirect loading of the bone with plantar flexion and eversion stress. Avulsion fractures of the proximal fifth metatarsal may also occur at the insertion of the peroneus brevis tendon with inversion stress injuries (see figure 8.11). Whenever there is point tenderness over the base of the fifth metatarsal or pain with resisted eversion, fracture should be suspected.

Although less common, fractures of the calcaneus and talus can also occur secondary to athletic activity. The most frequent cause of fractures of the calcaneus is direct trauma from falling or landing on the heel from a height. Talar dome fractures are typically associated with compressive ankle injuries. General signs and symptoms of foot fractures are consistent with those previously mentioned.

## BONY DEFECTS AND ABNORMALITIES SECONDARY TO REPETITIVE STRESS

The bone is also susceptible to chronic stress injuries secondary to repetitive tractioning or compressive forces. Stress injuries to the bone include stress fractures, bone spurs, and degenerative changes.

### Stress Fractures

*Amenorrhea is the absence or cessation of menses.*

The tibia and metatarsals are the most common sites of stress fractures in the lower leg, which result from repetitive stress associated with running and jumping activities. Stress fractures of the fifth metatarsal and fibula are also common secondary to repetitive tractioning of the peroneal muscles with eversion/plantar flexion forces. Tibial stress fractures most often occur in the distal one-third of the tibia, and metatarsal stress fractures most often involve the second or third metatarsal shafts. Athletes with excessive pronation or impaired shock absorption capabilities due to an immobile pes cavus, a hypermobile pes planus, muscle weakness, or muscular fatigue are especially susceptible to tibial and metatarsal stress fractures. Female athletes with compromised bone density associated with secondary amenorrhea are also thought to be at increased risk.

*Sequelae refers to the progressive course of a pathological condition.*

Typical sequelae of a developing stress fracture include an insidious onset of pain that initially occurs only during activity and subsides with rest. If the repetitive stress continues, the athlete will also begin to complain of continued pain after activity and into the night. Eventually, if the stressful activity is not curtailed, he will experience pain throughout the day. Typically the athlete will report no history of trauma, but training history will likely indicate recent high-intensity training or an abrupt change in training practices, surface, or equipment (footwear). Other signs and symptoms may include localized tenderness over the bone, pain with axial and transverse stress, and swelling.

### Exostosis

Excessive calcification or **bone spurs**, identified by radiographic examination, can develop at various locations of the foot and ankle secondary to repetitive stress and contact. Repetitive contact between the head of the talus and distal tibia with extreme dorsiflexion can result in an anterior **talotibial exostosis**. The athlete will experience anterior ankle pain, palpable tenderness over the anterior talar dome, pain and limited range of motion into dorsiflexion, and pain with push-off. Similarly, repetitive extreme plantar flexion will cause spurring of the posterior talus and calcaneus. Pain deep in the posterior aspect of the heel and pain with forced plantar flexion are hallmark symptoms. A posterior **calcaneal exostosis**, or **pump bump**, can result from chronic irritation at the attachment of the Achilles tendon. Individuals with an already prominent posterior calcaneal tuberosity are more susceptible to irritation, for which chronic friction and pressure from ill-fitting shoes are usually responsible. Signs and symptoms in addition to the bony prominence include pain, localized swelling, and redness. Inflammation and irritation associated with a calcaneal exostosis may also involve the retrocalcaneal bursa and distal Achilles tendon.

### Osteochondritis Dissecans

*Avascular necrosis (osteochondritis dissecans) is tissue death resulting from lack of blood supply (ischemia).*

The talar dome is the most common site of osteochondritis dissecans in the lower leg and foot. Although rare, compression mechanism associated with inversion, eversion, and dorsiflexion can impinge on and injure the articular surface of the talus, resulting in avascular necrosis of the subchondral bone. Signs and symptoms may resemble those of an ankle sprain. The athlete will typically complain of nonspecific ankle joint pain and swelling that worsen with activity. Locking, clicking, and decreased range of motion may also be noticeable if there is a loose fragment in the joint. Athletes complaining of prolonged ankle pain that does not respond to conservative treatment should be referred to a physician for further evaluation.

## DISLOCATION AND SUBLUXATION

As with any dislocation or fracture, distal pulses and neurological checks should be performed to rule out associated vascular or nerve injury.

Dislocations of the ankle, hindfoot, and midfoot joints are relatively uncommon. Tremendous forces are required to cause them; thus when these dislocations occur, they are almost always associated with fracture. Dislocation of the phalanges commonly results from the same mechanisms as for sprains and fractures. Dislocations are readily apparent secondary to joint deformity. Immediate pain, swelling, and loss of function will also be present.

## NERVE AND VASCULAR INJURIES

Because of the compartments and tunnels that the nerves and vessels of the lower extremity must pass through on their way to the foot, neurovascular compromise is not uncommon. Neurovascular compromise can result from both acute and chronic compression mechanisms; acute conditions usually represent more serious injury. It is important that you be able to distinguish between these conditions and know which signs and symptoms represent a medical emergency.

### Tarsal Tunnel Syndrome

Tarsal tunnel syndrome is characterized by compression of the tibial nerve in the tarsal tunnel. The tarsal tunnel is a fibroosseous, inelastic tunnel composed of the talus, calcaneus, tibialis posterior, flexor digitorum longus, and flexor hallucis longus (forming the floor) and the flexor retinaculum (roof) (figure 8.12) (Jackson and Haglund 1991). Because of the tunnel's inelasticity and fixed space, the tibial nerve can become entrapped by surrounding structures when the normal spatial relationships are disrupted. Although the nerve within the tunnel can be compressed or tractioned as a consequence of direct trauma, acute fractures, or dislocation, the condition is most often seen in athletes with abnormal foot and ankle mechanics resulting in chronic eversion and excessive pronation.

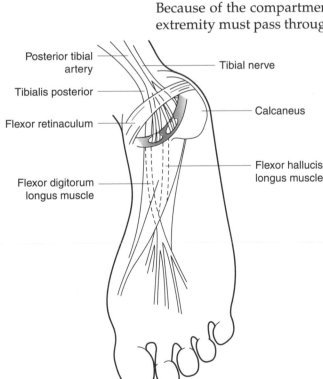

Posterior tibial artery
Tibial nerve
Tibialis posterior
Flexor retinaculum
Calcaneus
Flexor digitorum longus muscle
Flexor hallucis longus muscle

■ **Figure 8.12** Tarsal tunnel boundaries and contents.

Symptoms of tarsal tunnel syndrome include pain and numbness in the foot's arch that can radiate upward into the medial ankle region. Running activities and ankle dorsiflexion will often increase the discomfort. Pain may also be worse at night. Foot fatigue, numbness, and burning may also be noted on the plantar surface and into the toes (Jackson and Haglund 1991). Weakness of the foot intrinsics and toe flexors may also be present if the condition is prolonged.

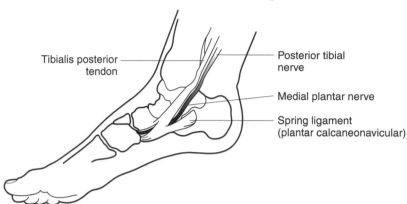

**Figure 8.13**  Medial plantar nerve where it passes under the spring ligament.

### Medial Plantar Nerve Compression Syndrome

The medial plantar nerve is a distal branch of the posterior tibial nerve. It can become entrapped in the longitudinal arch as it passes under the spring ligament (figure 8.13). This occurs most often in runners who have rearfoot valgus. The athlete will report symptoms of burning in the arch that can extend in the sole from the heel to the great toe.

### Morton's Neuroma

Also referred to as **metatarsalgia**, Morton's neuroma usually occurs at the bifurcation of the digital nerves as they angle sharply and branch off between the third and fourth metatarsal heads (figure 8.14). This is a prime area of pressure and friction that can cause formation of a fibrous tumor or tissue buildup around the nerve. Pain with weight bearing and tight-fitting shoes, burning, numbness, and shooting pain are common complaints.

### Peroneal Nerve Palsy

The peroneal nerve is susceptible to injury with inversion ankle injuries. Since this nerve has a significant sensory branch, the athlete will complain of sensory changes along its dermatome along the lateral lower leg and dorsum of the foot. Eversion weakness thought to be due to lateral muscle weakness, as well as pain associated with the ankle sprain, may in fact be the result of superficial peroneal nerve injury. When weakness is prolonged or is accompanied by sensory changes, peroneal nerve injury should be suspected. Sensory disturbances will often be exacerbated with plantar flexion and inversion of the ankle.

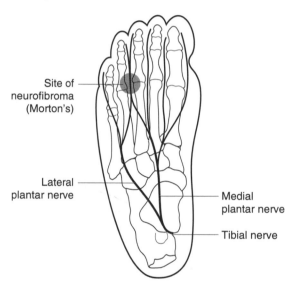

**Figure 8.14**  Location of Morton's neuroma between the 3rd and 4th metatarsal heads.

### Compartment Syndrome

In a compartment syndrome, pressure within a muscle compartment increases to the point that it causes neurovascular compromise. There are four muscular compartments in the lower leg (anterior, lateral, deep posterior, and superficial posterior) (figure 8.15). Each is bound by a thick, elastic fascial sheath that limits the expansion of the compartment when there is significant swelling. Although any compartment can be affected, the most common site of compartment syndrome is the anterior tibial compartment, which houses the anterior tibialis, extensor hallucis longus and extensor digitorum longus muscles, the anterior tibial artery and vein, and the deep peroneal nerve. These structures are surrounded and enclosed by the fibula,

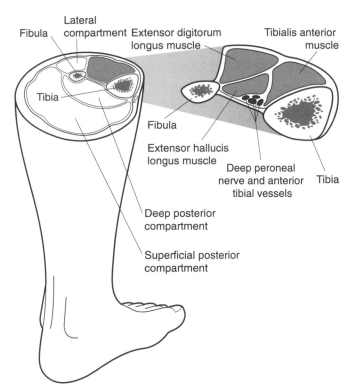

**Figure 8.15** Location of the leg's muscular compartments. The anterior compartment and its contents are shown in blue.

tibia, intermuscular septum, and the crural fascia. A compartment syndrome can be classified as either chronic (exertional) or acute.

### Chronic (Exertional) Compartment Syndrome

Chronic or exertional compartment syndrome usually results from excessive muscle hypertrophy during exercise. During activity, the tissue pressure remains high during contractions, impeding blood flow and causing muscle ischemia. This transient ischemia will cause the athlete to stop or slow activity secondary to symptoms of pain, muscular fatigue, a feeling of heaviness within the compartment, and reduced dorsiflexion muscle function. Pain will be exacerbated with passive plantar flexion. Once activity ceases, interstitial volume and blood flow will return to normal and symptoms will subside. In exertional compartment syndromes, pressure is usually not high enough to cause vascular collapse and rarely results in a medical emergency. It is not uncommon to see fascial defects and herniation of the muscle through the fascia resulting from increased intracompartmental pressure. Athletes who experience exertional compartment syndromes often undergo a surgical fasciotomy to remove the fascial restriction and allow sufficient room for muscle hypertrophy during activity.

### Acute Compartment Syndrome

The acute compartment syndrome represents a medical emergency and typically results from acute trauma such as a fracture, a kick to the leg, or other direct trauma. Intensive exercise can be a causative factor, although this is rarely the case. As a result of the acute trauma, vasodilatation and bleeding within the compartment will increase compartmental pressure and cause venous compromise and eventual collapse. Given the higher pressure of the anterior tibial artery as compared to the veins, blood will continue to flow into the compartment even after venous collapse has occurred, thus further contributing to the rising pressure. If the condition is left untreated, muscle ischemia and tissue necrosis will occur within 6-12 h. Therefore immediate recognition and medical referral are imperative. Signs and symptoms of an impending acute compartment syndrome include pain out of proportion to the injury that is greatly intensified with plantar flexion of the ankle. The compartment will be warm to the touch, and the overlying skin will be tense, glossy, and pale. Sensory and motor loss will be noted over the distribution of the deep peroneal nerve, with motor deficits ranging from weakness of great toe extension and dorsiflexion to eventual foot drop. If any of these signs are apparent, the athlete should be referred immediately for medical attention. In addition, compression and elevation are contraindicated as they can create further pressure and vascular compromise.

### *Deep Vein Thrombophlebitis*

Deep vein thrombophlebitis is the inflammation of a deep vein and may be associated with a **thrombus,** or blood clot. The lower leg, particularly the calf, is the most frequent site for these conditions. Venous inflammation or clotting in athletes may result from direct trauma such as the impact of a batted ball or a hard kick to the calf.

If an acute compartment syndrome is left untreated, muscle ischemia and tissue necrosis will occur within 6-12 h. Immediate recognition and medical referral are imperative.

Compression and elevation are contraindicated with a suspected compartment syndrome, as they can cause a further increase in pressure and vascular compromise.

Watch for the 5 P's of an impending compartment syndrome: **P**ain, **P**aresthesia, **P**allor, **P**ulselessness, **P**aralysis.

! A potential complication of a thrombus is a pulmonary embolism, which occurs when a clot breaks loose and travels to and obstructs a pulmonary artery.

Signs and symptoms may include a vague, dull ache in the posterior calf, swelling, pallor, diminished or absent pedal pulse, and a positive Homan's sign (see special tests section later in this chapter). A potential complication of a thrombus is a **pulmonary embolism**, which occurs if the clot were to break loose and travel to and obstruct the pulmonary artery or one of its branches.

## STRUCTURAL AND FUNCTIONAL ABNORMALITIES

Collectively, the joints of the midfoot and forefoot are positioned so as to form structural arches that provide spring and shock absorption both lengthwise and crosswise. The four arches of the foot that contribute to both its stability and its shock absorption capabilities are the medial longitudinal, lateral longitudinal, and transverse and metatarsal arches (figure 8.16). Structural or functional abnormalities in the foot may alter these supportive arches, leading to decreased stability or shock absorption capabilities or both. Changes resulting from these structural and functional abnormalities can have a tremendous influence on gait, lower-extremity alignment, and mechanics, leading to a host of chronic stress and compensatory problems not only in the foot and ankle, but also up into the knee, hip, or low back.

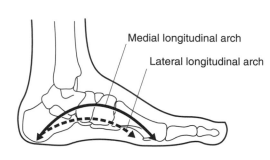
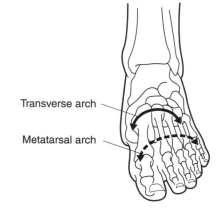

**Figure 8.16**  Arches of the foot.

## Characteristics of a Normal Foot in Neutral Position

**Anatomic Contour in Neutral Position:**

a. Metatarsal heads will be in the same plane as the ground and in the same plane with each other.

b. Calcaneus is centrally located below the leg and perpendicular to the floor.

   • Both condyles should be flat on the ground.

c. Talus is in neutral.

d. Medial border of the foot should lie in a straight line from heel to big toe.

e. Each toe should be flexible and in straight alignment.

f. Medial longitudinal arch should be visible and should form a gentle, smooth curve.

g. Normal range of motion should be available at the ankle (−10° to 65°).

h. Muscles should have good tone and strength.

i. Weight is distributed between heel and ball of foot with all metatarsal heads on the floor.

j. Foot should be asymptomatic.

## *Forefoot-to-Rearfoot Relationships*

The relationship between the forefoot and rearfoot is defined by alignment of the metatarsal heads (forefoot) and plantar surface of the calcaneus (rearfoot). In a normal or neutral foot, the plane of the metatarsal heads is perpendicular to a line bisecting the calcaneus in the frontal plane. However, a number of structural deformities result in a deviation from this neutral alignment.

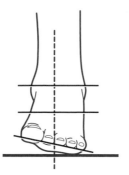

### Forefoot Varus

Forefoot varus is characterized by inversion of the forefoot relative to the rearfoot secondary to inadequate rotation of the talus medially. Consequently the medial side of the foot is raised (figure 8.17). In an effort to bring the first metatarsal into contact with the ground for push-off, the athlete will pronate the foot excessively; this adaptation resembles a pes planus foot. Excessive pronation can precipitate a host of lower-extremity complaints including posterior tibial and Achilles tendinitis, patellofemoral disorders, and hip or low back pain.

**▌ Figure 8.17** Forefoot varus.

### Forefoot Valgus

Conversely, forefoot valgus is an eversion of the forefoot relative to the rearfoot. Because of excessive medial rotation of the talus, the plane of the metatarsals is everted, with the lateral border of the forefoot riding higher than the medial side. To compensate, the athlete will supinate at the midfoot to bring the lateral border of the foot into contact with the ground. Common lower-extremity complaints associated with a forefoot valgus may include increased susceptibility to inversion ankle sprains and lateral knee pain.

### Rearfoot (Hindfoot) Varus

Rearfoot varus, the most common structural foot deformity (Tiberio 1988), is characterized by an inverted calcaneus that causes the medial condyle of the calcaneus to lose contact with the ground (figure 8.18). Either **tibial varum** or **genu varum** may also be present and may contribute to a rearfoot varus. The result is that initial contact is on the lateral aspect of the foot and there is compensatory plantar flexion of the first ray or subtalar pronation to bring the medial calcaneal condyle and forefoot into contact with the ground. Chronic injuries that may ensue include plantar fasciitis, metatarsalgia and/or stress fracture of the second ray, hallux valgus (see figure 8.22), posterior tibialis tendinitis, and medial tibial stress syndrome (Tiberio 1988).

### Rearfoot Valgus

Hindfoot valgus is caused by eversion of the calcaneus (figure 8.19). This may result in a hypermobile foot and excessive subtalar pronation. Hindfoot valgus is typically less problematic than a rearfoot varus.

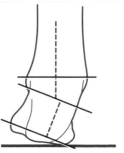

**▌ Figure 8.18** Rearfoot varus.

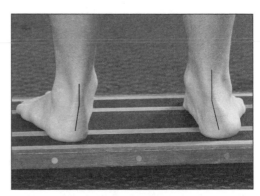

**▌ Figure 8.19** Rearfoot valgus.

### Pes Planus

**Pes planus**, or **flatfoot**, is caused by hypermobility resulting from increased ligament laxity and muscle weakness on the plantar surface of the foot (figure 8.20). It can also result from trauma such as severe medial ankle and arch sprains. Athletes with a pes planus foot may have greater and more prolonged subtalar pronation during gait secondary to the hypermobility, resulting in medial stress injuries at the ankle, lower leg, and knee. They may also complain of medial arch pain and fatigue with activity. However, many active individuals with a pes planus foot have no complaints of pain.

### Pes Cavus

A **pes cavus** foot is characterized by an abnormally high and rigid arch, contracture of plantar soft tissue structures, prominent metatarsal heads, and elevation of toes off the ground (figure 8.21). The plane of the metatarsals is plantarflexed in relation to the calcaneus. The pes cavus foot is typically hypomobile and therefore has poor shock-absorbing capabilities. Callus formation, plantar fasciitis, Achilles tendon tightness, and stress injuries are frequent complaints in individuals with a pes cavus foot.

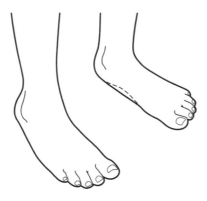

**∎ Figure 8.20**  Pes planus foot.

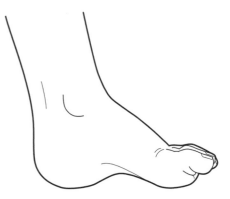

**∎ Figure 8.21**  Pes cavus foot.

### Plantarflexed First Ray

Plantar flexion of the first ray relative to the rest of the metatarsal plane can be attributable to either a structural or a functional deformity. As mentioned previously, plantar flexion of the first ray may occur as a compensatory motion for a rearfoot varus. A structural deformity is often present in association with a congenitally pes cavus foot. A rigid plantarflexed first ray will compromise normal mechanics at the first metatarsophalangeal joint during gait and may result in joint rigidity (Tiberio 1988). Callus formation under the first metatarsal head will usually be more pronounced than normal.

### Equinus Deformity

Equinus deformity refers to a limitation in dorsiflexion range at the ankle. It can be caused by a structural forefoot equinus, in which the forefoot is plantarflexed relative to the rearfoot, or by a rigid forefoot varus or abnormal tightness in the calf or Achilles. The consequence is midtarsal hypermobility and excessive pronation to compensate for the lack of dorsiflexion range at push-off.

### Toe Deformities

Toe deformities may be congenital or may be acquired as a consequence of other forefoot and rearfoot deformity or dysfunction.

#### Hallux Valgus and Bunions

Hallux valgus is a valgus deformity at the first metatarsophalangeal joint characterized by a medial deviation of the joint and lateral angulation of the phalanx (figure 8.22). It may be congenital or may result from trauma or ill-fitting shoes.

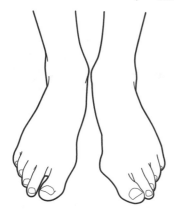

**∎ Figure 8.22**  Hallux valgus.

As a result of the angulation, the extensor and flexor hallucis longus tendons will deviate laterally and compromise joint function. The prominent medially deviated metatarsophalangeal (MP) joint will be subject to increased pressure and friction from footwear. A bunion will develop secondary to callus formation, bursal thickening, and excessive bone formation.

### Hallux Rigidus

Degenerative or arthritic changes resulting from joint dysfunction or pathomechanics may lead to fusion and rigidity at the first metatarsophalangeal joint. Signs and symptoms include decreased active and passive range of motion and palpable tenderness. Because of the inability to fully extend the toe, the athlete will experience pain with push-off and demonstrate an altered gait.

### Claw Toes

Claw toes are often found in conjunction with a pes cavus foot and are characterized by hyperextension of the metatarsophalangeal joint and flexion of the distal and proximal interphalangeal joints (figure 8.23). They can also result from neurological problems, dysfunction of the lumbricals and interosseous muscles, or both.

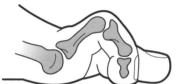

▮ **Figure 8.23**   Claw toes.

### Hammertoes

Similar to claw toes, hammertoes are characterized hyperextension of the metatarsophalangeal joint and a flexion contracture of the proximal interphalangeal joint. However, the distal interphalangeal joint may be flexed, hyperextended, or neutral (figure 8.24). A callus is frequently noted over the flexed and prominent proximal interphalangeal joint due to contact and friction with the top of the shoe. This deformity may be congenital or may result from poorly fitting shoes or intrinsic muscle dysfunction. Insufficiency of the intrinsics will result in an inability to hold neutral or to flex the metatarsophalangeal joint, and consequently a hyperextension deformity due to overpowering by the extrinsic toe extensors. This hyperextension in turn creates tension in the toe flexors, resulting in a flexion deformity of the proximal interphalangeal joint.

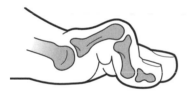

▮ **Figure 8.24**   Hammertoes.

### Mallet Toe

Mallet toe, which is similar to mallet finger, is a flexion of the distal phalanx of the toe. As a consequence of a mallet toe, a callus may form over the dorsal aspect of the distal joint. This deformity is fairly benign and causes little or no joint dysfunction or compensatory motion.

### Morton's Toe

With Morton's toe, the second toe extends distally beyond the first toe and therefore the second metatarsal is subjected to greater-than-normal stress at push-off. This may alter the function and mobility of the first metatarsophalangeal joint and increase the risk of stress fracture in the second metatarsal.

## INJURY ASSESSMENT

By now you should appreciate the variety of conditions, both acute and chronic, that you may encounter when evaluating the foot and ankle. To be able to evaluate and differentiate these injuries, you will need both a sound knowledge of injury pathology and a good understanding of normal foot alignment and mechanics. The following assessment techniques will provide the additional tools you will need to accurately determine the stage, irritability, nature, and severity of the injury.

As with any on-field evaluation, assess first for presence of airway, breathing, and circulation, severe bleeding, and shock.

# ON-FIELD ASSESSMENT

Although injuries to the lower leg, ankle, and foot are rarely life threatening, severe injuries to these areas demand accurate and rapid assessment and efficient and effective transport and care. The athletic trainer therefore should be aware of the signs and symptoms of acute injuries that occur in these areas and be ready to treat them appropriately.

When the athlete suffers an injury to this lower segment and is unable to stand, it is obvious that either the injury is significant or the athlete's tolerance may be limited. In any case, you must be able to quickly assess the nature and severity of the injury and determine the method of transport off the playing surface. As you approach the downed athlete, observe her for movement and reaction to the injury. Check the position of the injured leg and observe whether the athlete is willing to move the injured area.

## History

Injury to the foot and ankle can be very painful, and your first responsibility may be to calm the athlete before you can get an adequate history. Once the athlete is calm, obtain a history regarding the mechanism of injury, the location and severity of the pain, and any unusual sensations heard or felt at the time of injury. This should help you quickly focus on the area of injury. Athletes with Achilles tendon rupture commonly report a sensation of having been "kicked in the calf." For second- and third-degree ankle sprains, it is not unusual for athletes to state that they heard a pop at the time of injury. However, this sign may also be indicative of a fracture and must be carefully assessed before the athlete is moved.

## Observation

Observe the area for immediate signs of swelling, deformity, or discoloration. Depending on the severity of the injury, this may require taking time on the field to carefully remove the shoe and sock. You should also remove the shoe and sock on the uninvolved side to allow bilateral comparison. This will enable you to observe skin and nail coloration to monitor any circulatory impairment as well.

## Palpation

Palpate the area to determine any tenderness, crepitus, or abnormal configurations that may not be obvious upon observation; to identify the structure(s) involved; and to rule out any potential fracture or dislocation. Your palpation of the injured area should be brief, but thorough, including the distal tibia, tip of the medial malleolus, deltoid ligament, distal fibula, lateral malleolus, lateral ligament complex, anterior tibiofibular joint, Achilles tendon, tarsals, metatarsals (including the base of the fifth), and phalanges. If you suspect fracture or dislocation, palpate the pedal pulse and perform a quick sensory check along the lateral and medial borders of the foot to rule out neurovascular compromise.

## Special Tests

Dislocations are usually obvious in the lower leg, foot, and ankle, but fractures may not be, even after palpation. The Potts compression test (see page 248) can be used to quickly assess the potential presence of a fracture of the distal lower leg. If you suspect an ankle sprain, an anterior drawer test (see page 249) to determine severity of the injury is in order.

If bony deformity, tenderness, or crepitus is present, the limb should be immobilized and the athlete removed from the field by passive transport. Passive transport is also necessary when the injury is painful or severe enough to prevent weight bearing. Even if the athlete is willing to stand and ambulate with assistance, a two-person support should be used to move the athlete off the field and avoid weight bearing on the injured segment pending a more detailed evaluation on the sideline.

For more details on passive transport and two-person support, refer to *Introduction to Athletic Training* (Hillman 2000), chapter 8.

## SIDELINE ASSESSMENT

When an athlete is removed from the field because of an ankle or foot injury, a thorough sideline assessment is performed to determine more precisely the nature and severity of the injury and the athlete's playing status.

### *History*

Obtain a thorough history of the mechanism of injury and location, type, and severity of symptoms. With ankle injuries, try to determine whether the mechanism resulted in inversion, eversion, or rotation of the ankle. Determine whether the foot was planted and ascertain the direction of the applied force. Ask the athlete what activity he was engaged in at the time of the injury: was he pushing off, jumping, landing, cutting, or pivoting? Be sure to ask about previous injuries to both the involved and uninvolved side, as this may influence your findings. For example, a severe injury to the opposite ankle may have resulted in laxity from ligament damage or restricted mobility from scar tissue, leaving a poor comparison for the injured side that may not reflect what should be "normal."

### *Observation*

If the athlete was able to walk off the field, observe for normal gait, weight bearing, stride, and swing-through. Does the athlete exhibit a full range of motion when walking, or does she avoid toe-off or full dorsiflexion? If you did not do so on the field, remove the socks and shoes on both sides. Observe closely, and compare bilaterally, for signs of local or diffuse swelling, discoloration, and deformity. Note the "attitude"

---

### Checklist for On-Field Assessment of the Lower Leg, Ankle, and Foot

**History**
- ✓ Mechanism, location, and severity of pain
- ✓ Unusual sounds and sensations
- ✓ Information from bystanders

**Observation**
- ✓ Deformity, swelling, discoloration
- ✓ Unusual positioning of the limb
- ✓ Skin coloration

**Palpation for Tenderness, Crepitus, or Deformity**
- ✓ Distal tibia, medial malleolus, deltoid ligament
- ✓ Distal fibula, lateral malleolus, lateral ligaments
- ✓ Anterior tibiofibular ligament, anterior talar dome
- ✓ Achilles tendon
- ✓ Tarsals, metatarsals, phalanges

**Neurovascular Assessment**
- ✓ Pedal pulse
- ✓ Sensory over dorsum of foot, lateral border of foot, posterior calcaneus

**Special Tests**
- ✓ Potts compression test
- ✓ Anterior drawer test

**Active Range of Motion**

If all tests are negative, assist from field and have athlete avoid weight bearing until complete assessment is performed on the sideline.

of the foot and observe whether the foot rests in a more inverted position in comparison to the uninvolved side; this may indicate second- or third-degree injury to the lateral ligament complex. Also check at this time for any scars or indications of previous injury that the athlete may have forgotten to mention when giving the history.

### Palpation

Develop a routine so that your palpation of the lower leg, ankle, and foot is systematic and methodical; this will help you avoid inadvertently omitting a structure. Remember to palpate both sides, and focus on the area of pain last.

Anterior structures of the lower leg and ankle include the tibial crest, anterior tibiofibular ligament, anterior dome of the talus, anterior tibialis muscle and tendon, and extensor tendons as they cross the anterior ankle joint. Distal into the foot the anterior structures include the extensor hallucis longus tendon, extensor digitorum longus and brevis tendons, dorsal pedal pulse, cuneiforms, metatarsals, and toes. Lateral structures of the lower leg, ankle, and foot include the fibula, peroneal muscles and tendons, lateral malleolus, anterior and posterior talofibular ligaments, calcaneofibular ligament, sinus tarsus, cuboid, and base of the fifth metatarsal. Posterior lower leg and ankle structures include the gastrocnemius and soleus muscles, Achilles tendon, and calcaneus. Plantar structures include the plantar aponeurosis, metatarsal heads, and toes. The medial lower leg and foot structures consist of the tibial shaft; medial malleolus; deltoid ligament; the three tendons as they pass posteriorly to the medial malleolus (tibialis posterior tendon, flexor digitorum longus tendon, and flexor hallucis longus tendon); posterior tibial artery; navicular tuberosity; medial cuneiform; first metatarsal base, shaft, and head; and first toe.

Palpate the bony prominences and joints for tenderness, swelling, crepitus, lack of conformity, and other signs of pathology. Palpate the muscles for areas of tenderness, swelling, myofascial restriction, herniation and nodules, and incongruity compared left and right. Palpate the tendons for tenderness, nodules, and crepitus during both active and passive movement.

### Special Tests

Special tests for on-field and sideline assessment of the lower leg, ankle, and foot are primarily stress tests to evaluate the integrity of a bone, ligament, or tendon. Always compare bilaterally, testing the uninvolved side first.

#### Potts Compression Test

It is a misconception that an athlete is unable to walk if a bone is fractured. Traumatic injury with torsion or impact forces can produce fractures of the lower leg and foot. Although an x-ray is the definitive means for diagnosing a fracture, the athletic trainer can tentatively identify a fracture with a commonly used test.

A Pott's fracture occurs in the distal lower leg, but if the bones are not displaced it may be difficult to detect. The following test will often enable you to identify a Pott's fracture.

Place your hands around the upper aspect of the lower leg with the pad of one hand just distal to the fibular head and the pad of the other hand at the same level on the medial tibia. Then push your hands toward one another to squeeze the tibia and fibula together (figure 8.25). A positive sign occurs if the athlete reports increased pain in the distal fibula or tibia.

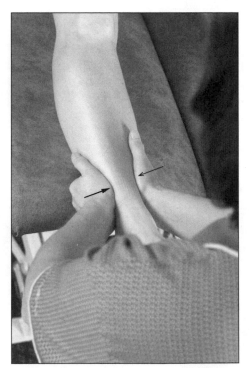
**Figure 8.25** Potts compression test.

## Thompson Test

The Thompson test assesses the integrity of the Achilles tendon. The athlete lies prone with her foot over the end of the table. With the athlete relaxed, squeeze her calf. Normal response is foot movement into plantar flexion (figure 8.26). A lack of movement of the foot is a positive sign, indicative of an Achilles tendon rupture. When you don't have access to a table on the sidelines, you can also perform this test as the athlete kneels with the foot unencumbered.

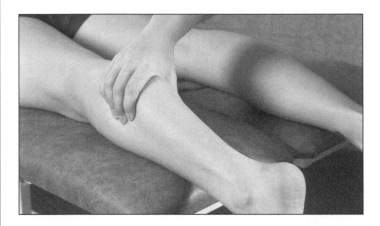

∎ **Figure 8.26**
Thompson test.

### Ligamentous Stability Tests
To evaluate the integrity of the medial, lateral, and tibiofibular ligaments of the ankle, perform the following tests.

## Anterior Drawer Test

This test assesses the integrity of the anterior talofibular ligament and the calcaneofibular ligament. A positive sign can occur with a tear of only the talofibular ligament, but laxity will be greater when both ligaments are injured.

With the athlete in either a sitting or a supine position and the knee slightly flexed to relax the gastrocnemius, passively position her ankle in about 20° plantar flexion and stabilize the lower leg. Pull the foot forward by grasping the calcaneus (figure 8.27). A positive result occurs if this produces pain and laxity. It is common to see a dimple in the skin over the site of the anterior talofibular ligament during this test. In an alternate testing position, the athlete is prone with her foot hanging off the edge of the table. Place one hand under the distal anterior surface of the tibia, and apply an anteriorly directed force to the calcaneus.

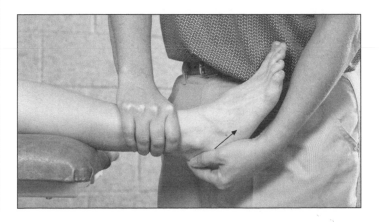

∎ **Figure 8.27**
Anterior drawer test.

## Talar Tilt

This test is used to determine the integrity of the calcaneofibular and deltoid ligaments. The athlete can be positioned supine, sitting, or side-lying. Place the ankle in the anatomic position and support it with both of your hands. Then adduct the foot into a varus position to test the calcaneofibular ligament. Test the deltoid ligament with the foot abducted into a valgus position. Pain or laxity with end-range varus (figure 8.28a) is positive for calcaneofibular ligament injury, and pain or laxity with end-range valgus (figure 8.28b) is a positive sign for deltoid ligament injury.

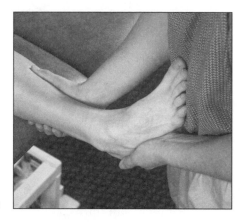
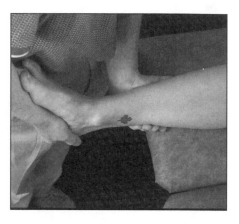

a  b

**▌Figure 8.28** Talar tilt tests at (a) end range varus to stress lateral ligaments and (b) end range valgus to stress medial ligaments.

## Kleiger Test

This test assesses the integrity of the deltoid ligament. With the athlete sitting, the knee flexed to 90°, and the foot relaxed and non-weight bearing, grasp the foot and rotate it laterally (figure 8.29). A positive test occurs with medial and lateral ankle pain with or without palpated displacement of the talus.

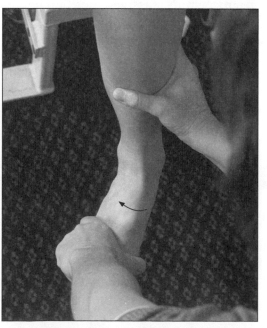

**▌Figure 8.29** Kleiger test.

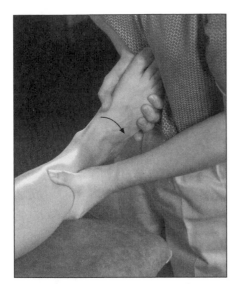

**Figure 8.30**   Stress test for the syndesmosis.

## Syndesmosis Separation

To evaluate the integrity of the anterior tibiofibular ligament and syndesmosis, fully dorsiflex the ankle to end range, forcing the dome of the talus to stress the tibiofibular joint. You can further stress the joint by externally rotating the foot when it is in this dorsiflexed position (figure 8.30). Pain over the anterior distal tibiofibular joint is considered a positive test.

### *Range of Motion*

Follow the standard guidelines for range of motion testing: test and compare bilaterally each movement of the lower legs, ankles, and feet, using the uninvolved side as a guide for what is normal for the individual. Perform painful movements last, and follow active movements by passive overpressure if the athlete can tolerate it.

### Active Motion

The athlete can perform bilateral non-weight-bearing movements simultaneously for easy comparison of left and right. Ankle dorsiflexion (figure 8.31a), plantar flexion (figure 8.31b), inversion (figure 8.31c), and eversion (figure 8.31d), as well as toe extension (figure 8.31e), flexion (figure 8.31f), and abduction, are performed with the ankles over the end of the bench or

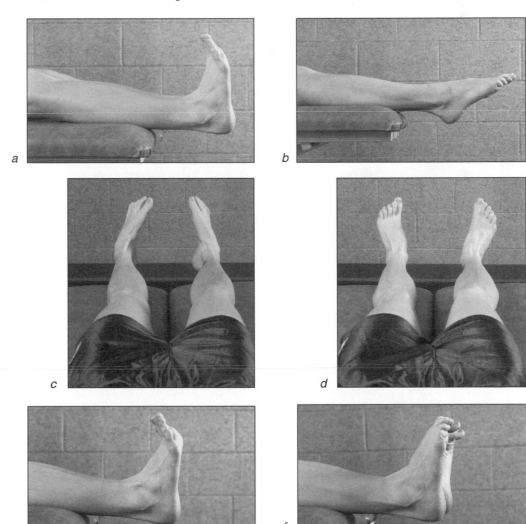

**Figure 8.31**   Active ROM movements for ankle (a) dorsiflexion, (b) plantar flexion, (c) inversion, (d) eversion, and for toe (e) extension and (f) flexion.

table. In weight bearing, the movements can also be performed with the two feet simultaneously. The movements should include ankle plantar flexion, dorsiflexion, inversion, and eversion and also toe flexion and extension. Observe for differences in total range for each motion and indications of pain or hesitancy with any of the movements.

**Passive Motion**

Passive motion can immediately follow active motion in the non-weight-bearing position. Passively move the ankle and foot into full dorsiflexion, plantar flexion, rearfoot inversion, rearfoot eversion, forefoot inversion, and forefoot eversion, as well as toe flexion and extension.

## Strength

Strength assessment for most of the lower leg, ankle, and foot muscle groups can be performed in a non-weight-bearing position. Apply manual resistance to ankle dorsiflexion, inversion, and eversion and toe flexors and extensors, with the joint positioned at midrange of the motion you are testing. If calf strength is difficult to resist manually, plantar flexion may be more accurately assessed in weight bearing. The athlete stands on only the involved leg and raises the heel off the floor for 20 repetitions. Observe for control of movement throughout the range of motion and for heel height for all repetitions. Test the uninvolved leg first for comparison.

## Neurovascular Tests

With suspected neurological injury at the knee or below, peripheral sensory nerve assessment should include the deep peroneal nerve in the dorsal web space, the superficial peroneal nerve on the dorsum of the foot and lateral, lower leg, the tibial nerve over the posteriomedial plantar heel, and the medial plantar nerve over the medial plantar surface of the foot. If any result is abnormal, a more detailed sensory examination is warranted. For myotome assessment the posterior tibial nerve innervates the muscles in the posterior compartment and is assessed with plantar flexion and toe flexion. The superficial peroneal nerve innervates the lateral compartment muscles and is tested with eversion. The deep peroneal nerve innervates the muscles in the anterior compartment and can be tested with dorsiflexion and great toe extension.

For symptoms below the knee, you can elicit a deep tendon reflex from the Achilles tendon (S1-S2). Place the ankle in slight dorsiflexion and lightly tap the Achilles tendon with a reflex hammer. If there is no response or the response is diminished, ensure that the athlete is not inhibiting the response by having him close his eyes, hook the fingertips of each hand over the other, and pull his hands in oppposite directions (see Jendrassik's maneuver, chapter 2, figure 2.1). You can also test the posterior tibialis tendon (L4-5) on the medial aspect of the ankle for reflex response, but this is not a commonly used site. If vascular compromise is suspected, palpate the dorsalis pedis and posterior tibial arteries for presence and strength of pulse and compare bilaterally.

## Functional Tests

Some ankle sprains may be mild enough to warrant return to participation immediately after the sideline assessment, with or without external support. To determine the appropriateness of return to full participation, you must first assess the athlete and the athlete's ankle for readiness.

The functional tests for the ankle include both general and specific tests for strength, power, flexibility, and agility. The general tests may or may not be sport specific but will evaluate the ankle's general mobility, strength, and response to mechanical stresses. These activities include change of direction with circle-8 runs; forward-to-backward running; side-to-side movements such as cariocas and side shuffles; forward and lateral jumps; and sudden stop-and-start maneuvers such as

## Checklist for Sideline Assessment of the Lower Leg, Ankle, and Foot

### History
Ask questions pertaining to the following:

✓ Chief complaint

✓ Mechanism of injury and position of the limb when injured

✓ Unusual sounds or sensations

✓ Type and location of pain or symptoms

✓ Previous injury

✓ Previous injury to opposite extremity for bilateral comparison

### Observation

✓ Check for visible facial expressions of pain.

✓ Check for swelling, deformity, abnormal contours, or discoloration.

✓ Observe gait, willingness to bear weight, range of ankle motion.

✓ Observe overall posture and alignment of lower leg, ankle, and foot.

✓ Make bilateral comparison.

### Palpation
Palpate for pain, tenderness, crepitus, defects, and deformity over the following:

✓ Tibial crest, anterior tibiofibular ligament, anterior dome of talus, anterior tibialis muscle and tendon, extensor digitorum and hallucis tendons, extensor digitorum brevis, dorsalis pedis pulse, cuneiforms, metatarsals, and phalanges

✓ Fibula, peroneal muscle and tendons, lateral malleolus, anterior and posterior talofibular ligaments, calcaneofibular ligament, sinus tarsus, cuboid, base of fifth metatarsal

✓ Gastrocnemius, soleus, Achilles tendon, calcaneus

✓ Plantar fascia, metatarsal heads

✓ Tibial shaft, medial malleolus, deltoid ligament, tibialis posterior tendon, flexor digitorum tendon, flexor hallucis longus tendon, tibial nerve and tibial artery, navicular tubercle, medial cuneiform, and first metatarsal (base, shaft, and head)

### Special Tests

✓ Potts compression test

✓ Thompson test

✓ Ligament laxity tests (anterior drawer, talar tilt, Kleiger, syndesmosis)

✓ Bilateral comparison

### Range of Motion

✓ Active ROM for plantar flexion, dorsiflexion, inversion, eversion, toe flexion and extension

✓ Passive ROM for plantar flexion, dorsiflexion, rearfoot inversion and eversion, forefoot inversion and eversion, toe flexion and extension

✓ Bilateral comparison

### Strength Tests

✓ Perform manual resistance against same motions as in active ROM.

✓ Check bilaterally and note any pain or weakness.

### Neurovascular Tests

✓ Sensory over dorsum of the foot (deep peroneal), lateral border of the foot (superficial peroneal), posterior heel (posterior tibial)

✓ Motor for dorsiflexion (deep peroneal), eversion (superficial peroneal), and plantar flexion (posterior tibial)

✓ Pedal and posterior tibial pulses

### Functional Tests

cutting, stop jumps, and zigzag running. These functional tests should first be performed at half speed, using large sweeping arcs of movement, and progress to faster speeds, tighter circles, and sharper cuts.

Specific functional tests that mimic a particular sport activity are performed using the same progression. For example, you may have a basketball player run, jump, and land on one foot as in a layup maneuver. A volleyball player may run and stop with a two-footed jump and land with immediate lateral movement, or may perform jump-squat maneuvers and backward and lateral runs.

To pass these functional tests, the athlete must be able to perform these movements without hesitation and without favoring the injured ankle; she must also demonstrate adequate strength, flexibility, and agility without an increase in or recurrence of pain and without compensatory movements. You should weigh any questionable performance with other determining factors before allowing the athlete to return to full participation.

# OFF-FIELD ASSESSMENT

Most acute lower leg, ankle, and foot injuries that occur during practice or competition will be first evaluated on the field or sideline. However, on occasion, lesser injuries will not be immediately reported as significant pain and swelling may not appear until the following day. These types of acute injury, as well as chronic and overuse injuries, are more commonly seen in the athletic injury treatment facility.

The foot and ankle are equally prone to overuse conditions, but unfortunately the cause will not always be obvious. Therefore the off-field assessment uses a number of tools to help identify the nature and severity of the condition, as well as potential predisposing factors that may have contributed to the injury. Many of the assessment tools discussed here will also become important when you are evaluating chronic conditions further up the chain, as their origin may lie in structural or functional abnormalities in the foot.

## History

In addition to asking the questions discussed in relation to the sideline assessment, you must obtain a thorough history regarding the athlete's training and activity history. First establish the onset and duration of symptoms to determine the stage of the injury. Assess aggravating and easing factors to determine the level of irritability and also to obtain information regarding the potential structures involved. Whereas stress fractures are more painful with activity and will ease with rest, tendon and muscle injuries may warm up with activity and be more painful at rest. Inflammatory conditions will usually be stiff in the morning and loosen as the day progresses, with a return of pain from fatigue and overuse toward the end of the day. Ascertain the nature of the injury further through careful questioning about the athlete's training practices including changes in mileage, training frequency, training surface, shoes, or orthotics. Sudden changes in workout intensity or terrain are frequent culprits in overstress injuries.

Thoroughly investigate any prior injuries, the dates and number of previous incidents, the method and effectiveness of the treatments provided, and the duration of disability for each occurrence—especially the most recent. If the current injury is a repeat of a previous overuse injury, the underlying cause may still be present, and you must identify and account for this in your objective assessment. If the athlete has suffered prior ankle sprains, find out when the last episode was and compare the severity of the previous and the present injuries. There may be scar tissue that either restricts mobility or is weaker than normal tissue, making the ankle susceptible to chronic inflammatory or impingement conditions. If the athlete's leg was casted for a prior injury, there may be weakness or tightness within the calf muscle that reduce ankle dorsiflexion and make the gastrocnemius vulnerable to strains. Also obtain information regarding injuries to other segments of the lower extremities, as these may impact the current injury. For example, immobilization of the knee may result in secondary weakness, reduced flexibility, and soft tissue restriction in the ankle and lower leg.

## Observation

As the athlete comes toward you, observe whether his gait is normal, whether he is favoring the limb, and whether the ankle exhibits reduced range of motion. Note whether his weight bearing is equal or whether he is shifting weight to avoid putting pressure on the injured joint. Is he cautious when removing his shoe and sock?

Observe for any deformity, ecchymosis, muscle atrophy, or swelling in the lower leg, ankle, or foot. Localized swelling and discoloration are common around the lateral malleolus with postacute inversion ankle sprains. Note any scars, calluses, blisters, or bony structural changes that would indicate previous injury or areas of increased pressure or friction. What are the structure and position of the lower leg, ankle, and foot in weight bearing and non-weight bearing? Compare their structure and alignment to what you would expect for a healthy foot as outlined previously in this chapter. How does the relationship of these structures change when the athlete moves from weight bearing to non-weight bearing? Does the height of the longitudinal arch or angle of the Achilles tendon change? Check the alignment of the toes and feet in relation to the lower leg, as well as the alignment of the knees and hips and any influence they might have on the lower leg, foot, and ankle.

Your observation should also include inspection of the athlete's footwear. Note the type of shoes, excessive or abnormal wear patterns, differences in wear patterns left to right, and the amount of breakdown.

### Differential Diagnosis

Since you did not witness the injury, you must eliminate potential injuries from other regions that may refer pain to the lower leg, ankle, and foot before proceeding with your objective assessment. The back, hip, and knee can refer pain into the lower leg and ankle. You can quickly eliminate the back as a source of lower leg and foot pain by having the athlete perform trunk range of motion with overpressure. Eliminate the hip and knee as sources of pain into the lower leg, foot, and ankle in the same manner using active range of motion and overpressures for the range of motion for each joint. The hip and knee motions are best performed with the athlete in supine.

If no other joint motions reproduce the athlete's pain, proceed to the specific objective examination for the lower leg, ankle, and foot. If, on the other hand, any motion does reproduce the athlete's complaint, investigate that joint further before examining the lower leg and foot.

### Range of Motion

The active motions performed in the off-field assessment are the same as those for assessment at the sideline. In addition, you will perform passive movements of the ankle and foot joints, noting end feel and presence of pain. Passive movement of the ankle into dorsiflexion and plantar flexion with the rearfoot in and out of neutral, movement of the rearfoot into supination and pronation, and movement of the first ray are all assessed for laxity or restriction of movement. If inflammation of the extensor and flexor digitorum longus tendons is suspected, toe flexion and extension with and without ankle plantar flexion and dorsiflexion are also performed.

### Strength

Strength is assessed in the same way as at the sideline. More precise objective measures can also be obtained from isokinetic devices. Dorsiflexion, plantar flexion, inversion, and eversion can all be assessed for strength, endurance, and power on most isokinetic and instrumented ankle devices.

### Neurological Tests

Neurological testing takes place when one suspects that the athlete's symptoms stem from a back or neurological injury. Neurological testing is also routine when the source of the athlete's symptoms is unknown; when the athlete reports numbness, burning, tingling, or weakness; or when objective findings indicate weakness in the leg. Neurological tests include assessment of motor, sensory, and deep tendon reflexes.

Sensory testing should be performed for the lumbosacral plexus. Although several sensory nerves can be assessed, the most commonly evaluated sensation is light touch. You can also test sharp-dull sensation, temperature, deep touch, and joint position if the light touch assessment results are abnormal. You can perform a sensory scanning examination with rapid assessment of L2-L3 in the anterior thigh, L3-L4 in the anteromedial lower leg, L5 in the lateral lower leg and dorsum of the foot, S1 in the lateral plantar foot and in the central and posterior lateral lower leg, and S2 in the posteriolateral plantar heel (see chapter 7, figure 7.8). With suspected injury at the knee or below, peripheral nerve sensation should also be assessed as previously described in sideline assessment.

Myotome assessment is performed with manual muscle tests of those lumbosacral levels innervating the lower extremity. As with the sensory examination, the motor assessment is a scanning evaluation. If you observe any discrepancy, you should complete a more specific motor assessment examination. As mentioned in chapter 7 and chapter 2 (table 2.2), L4 is tested with resisted ankle dorsiflexion, L5 with great toe extension, S1 with ankle plantar flexion and eversion, and S2 with flexor hallucis longus. For injuries isolated to the lower extremity, you should also assess integrity of the peripheral nerves.

### Special Tests

All the sideline tests discussed earlier are appropriate for the off-field assessment. In addition, tests for malalignment, chronic, and inflammatory conditions are included here.

For further discussion on assessing posture, gait, and lower-extremity alignment, refer to *Therapeutic Exercise for Athletic Injuries* (Houglum 2000), chapters 11 and 12.

#### Alignment Tests

If the results of one or more of the following tests are positive, malalignment may be the cause of the athlete's injury and pain, particularly if the condition is either chronic or recurring. Correction of the malalignment is a necessary part of the treatment for complete resolution of the injury.

#### Calcaneal-Tibial Alignment

This alignment identifies the presence of a rearfoot valgus or varus and is a reliable determinant of rearfoot supination or pronation. The athlete lies prone with her foot over the end of the table; the opposite leg is flexed, and the ankle on that leg is crossed over the knee of the leg being investigated (figure 8.32a). This position stabilizes the pelvis and prevents unwanted movement of the lower extremity. Palpate the calcaneus and draw a line from the medial to the lateral calcaneal process. Then, palpate and mark the center of the calcaneus near the insertion of the Achilles tendon. Next draw a perpendicular line from the midcalcaneal mark to the horizontal line. Mark the medial-lateral midpoint of the distal third of the tibial shaft, and draw a line to connect this point with the midcalcaneal point. After marking the leg, place the rearfoot in neutral by palpating the talus medially and laterally while moving the forefoot with your hand over the distal lateral fourth and fifth metatarsal heads (figure 8.32b). The rearfoot is in neutral when the talus is palpated equally on its medial and lateral aspects. It is important that the athlete remain relaxed during this process so that you can obtain an accurate position and alignment. In this position, the alignment of the two vertical lines should be straight or in slight varus, no more than approximately 5-8°. If the inversion angle is greater than 8°, the rearfoot is in varus. If the heel is angled in eversion, the rearfoot is in valgus.

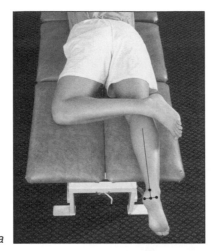

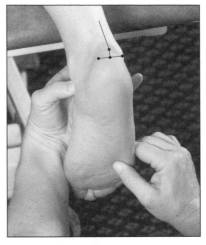

*a*

*b*

**▌Figure 8.32**   (a) Position for calcaneal-tibial alignment test and (b) athlete's foot in neutral alignment and with reference lines marked.

## Forefoot-Rearfoot Alignment

This test is used to determine the alignment relationship between the rearfoot and forefoot. The athlete is positioned as in the calcaneal-tibial alignment assessment, prone in

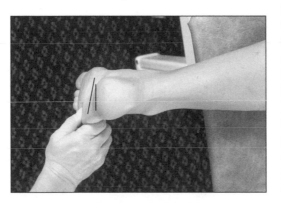

a figure-4 position. Place the rearfoot in neutral as described earlier, and then visually assess the relationship between the rearfoot angle and the forefoot angle. In the normal foot, the plantar surface of the heel and the metatarsal heads are parallel in the same plane. If the metatarsal head of the great toe is higher than that of the little toe, the forefoot is in varus (figure 8.33). If the first metatarsal head is lower than the fifth metatarsal head, the forefoot is in valgus.

**▌Figure 8.33**   Forefoot-rearfoot alignment test showing forefoot varus.

## Feiss Line

The Feiss line is used to assess navicular drop, and navicular drop in turn can be used to determine rearfoot-to-forefoot alignment. Draw a line from the inferior aspect of

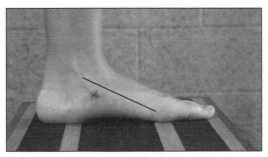

the medial malleolus to the plantar aspect of the metatarsophalangeal joint of the great toe. With the athlete in normal relaxed standing with his feet about 6 in. (15 cm) apart, determine the position of the navicular tuberosity. It should lie on the line. If the navicular tuberosity is below the line, the foot is considered pes planus with a low longitudinal arch (figure 8.34). If the navicular tuberosity lies above the line, the foot is considered an equinus foot with a high arch.

**▌Figure 8.34**   Feiss line. Note that the navicular tuberosity is below the line, indicating a pes planus foot.

### Fracture Tests

#### Morton's Test

The metatarsals are the most frequent site of stress fractures in the lower quarter. To test for this, have the athlete in supine, and grasp the midfoot region and squeeze the metatarsal heads together (figure 8.35). If the test produces pain, there may be a stress fracture. You can also use this test in suspected cases of Morton's neuroma. If the result is positive, refer the athlete to the physician for further evaluation.

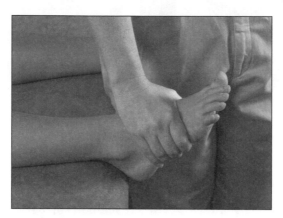

■ **Figure 8.35**  Morton's test for metatarsal stress fractures and Morton's neuroma.

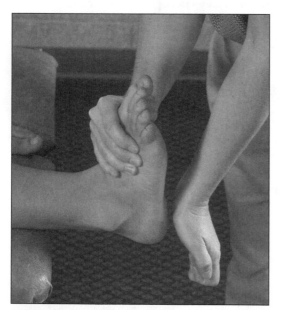

■ **Figure 8.36**  Heel percussion for tibial stress fracture.

#### Percussion Test

Another way to identify fractures is with vibration or percussion. To differentiate a tibial stress fracture from medial tibial stress syndrome, apply a percussive force to the plantar surface of the heel (figure 8.36). If there is localized pain near the suspected fracture site, the test is considered positive. You can also apply a percussion test to the metatarsals by stabilizing the toe in neutral and tapping the end of the toe to create a vibration down the shaft of the metatarsal.

#### Hoffa's Test

This test is used to rule out a calcaneal fracture. With the athlete prone and the injured foot over the end of the table, instruct the athlete to plantar- and dorsiflex the ankle while you palpate the Achilles tendon. A positive sign occurs if the Achilles tendon on the injured side is less taut during movement than the uninjured one; in this case, refer the athlete to the physician for further testing.

### Special Neurovascular Tests

Special neurovascular testing is used to determine peripheral nerve injuries or circulatory problems of the lower leg and ankle. Whereas both nerve and vascular injuries can occasionally result from acute trauma, nerve compression injuries more often result from overuse and chronic inflammatory conditions. Any complaint of numbness, burning, or tingling along a specific nerve pathway should be assessed for possible nerve compression or injury. In nontraumatic cases, the athletic trainer should look to structural malformations or malalignments as possible causes for nerve compression.

## Homan's Sign

Homan's sign is used to identify deep vein thrombophlebitis. With the athlete in a relaxed position, passively extend the knee while the ankle is passively dorsiflexed. Pain in the calf is a positive sign. Palpation of the calf can also elicit complaints of tenderness.

## Deep Peroneal Nerve Compression Tests

The deep peroneal nerve runs through the anterior compartment and into the dorsum of the foot; both of these are sites for compression secondary to acute trauma, or to increased volume within the lower leg compartment after prolonged activity. (High arches or tight shoelaces can also lead to compression of the anterior tibial branch of the deep peroneal nerve as it passes superficially along the dorsum of the foot.) The sensory loss is often less than the motor loss, since the deep peroneal nerve primarily supplies the anterior foot muscles. Loss of dorsiflexion, reduced ankle control, and pain or burning during plantar flexion are the primary complaints. Forceful passive plantar flexion will reproduce the athlete's pain, especially after activity. Strength of toe extension or ankle dorsiflexion will be reduced in comparison to that for the uninvolved extremity. An athlete who demonstrates positive test results should be referred to a physician for additional assessment.

## Superficial Peroneal Nerve

The superficial peroneal nerve can be injured during ankle sprains. Since this nerve has a significant sensory branch, the athlete will complain of sensory changes along its dermatome along the lateral lower leg and dorsum of the foot. Eversion weakness that may be masked by weakness of the lateral muscles in an ankle sprain may be the result of superficial peroneal nerve injury—especially if the weakness is accompanied by sensory changes. Sensory disturbances will occur when the nerve is placed on stretch with plantar flexion and inversion of the ankle.

## Tinel's Sign

This is also called the percussion test and is used to identify nerve pathology, usually compression or entrapment. There are two places in the ankle where a Tinel's sign can be used to assess nerve compromise. One is on the dorsum of the proximal foot over the anterior ankle where the anterior tibial branch of the deep peroneal nerve emerges. The other is just behind the medial malleolus where the posterior tibial nerve passes (figure 8.37). A tapping or percussion of the nerve should not produce any sign; if it produces a paresthesia or tingling, this is a positive sign for nerve dysfunction.

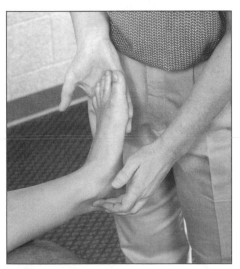

∎ **Figure 8.37** Tinel's sign for posterior tibial nerve pathology at the ankle.

## Morton's Test

Morton's test is used to identify the presence of a Morton's neuroma. Passive extension of the toes with pressure over the neuroma site will reproduce the athlete's pain. The Morton's test for stress fracture previously mentioned (i.e., squeezing of the metatarsal heads) may also compress the nerve and reproduce the athlete's pain (see figure 8.35).

## Overuse Tests

### Plantar Fasciitis

The athlete's history is the primary assessment tool for plantar fasciitis. The athlete will report a gradual onset of pain; the pain will occur especially in the morning upon arising and also after prolonged sitting, and will improve after the individual takes a few steps. The hallmark sign of plantar fasciitis is significant pain with direct, point pressure to the calcaneal tuberosity on the plantar surface of the anterior aspect of the heel.

### *Joint Mobility*

Accessory movements of the lower leg, ankle, and foot are complex because of the numerous joints in this segment of the lower extremity. A few of the commonly used techniques will be discussed here. These techniques determine hypomobility or hypermobility of the joints in this lower-extremity segment. They can also be used to treat hypomobile areas.

> For treatment techniques, refer to *Therapeutic Exercise for Athletic Injuries* (Houglum 2000), chapter 6.

### Distal Tibiofibular Joint

### Ventral Glide

If foot pronation is limited, the ventral glide will be restricted. The athlete is prone, with her foot over the end of the table and a padded wedge under the distal lower leg. Place your stabilizing hand over the distal tibia just above the medial malleolus, and place the thenar eminence of your mobilizing hand over the posterior distal fibula just above the lateral malleolus. With the mobilizing hand, apply a posterior-to-anterior (PA) force to take up the slack of the joint, and then apply an additional force to assess the amount of movement available (figure 8.38).

### Dorsal Glide

If supination is limited, the dorsal glide will be restricted. The athlete lies supine with her heel off the end of the table. Apply your stabilizing hand to the distal tibia just above the malleolus, and the thenar eminence of your mobilizing hand on the anterior distal fibula just above the lateral malleolus (figure 8.39). Apply an anterior-to-posterior (AP) force to the fibula to assess the amount of play and movement available.

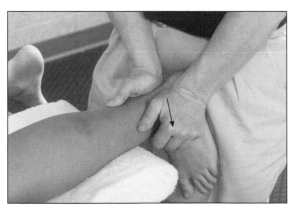
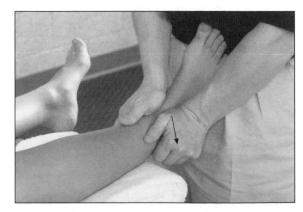

**▌Figure 8.38**   Distal tibiofibular ventral glide test.     **▌Figure 8.39**   Distal tibiofibular dorsal glide test.

## Talocrural Joint

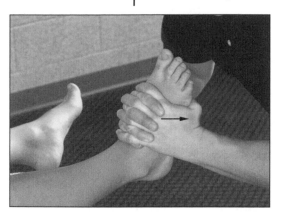

**■ Figure 8.40**   Talocrural joint distraction test.

### Distraction

Use distraction to assess general mobility of the talocrural joint. The athlete lies supine with her foot just off the table and her lower leg strapped to the table. With the ankle in about 10° of plantar flexion and neutral inversion/eversion, place your hands around the athlete's foot with the ulnar borders close to the talus and apply a distraction force to the foot, primarily from the medial aspects of your hands (figure 8.40).

### Dorsal Talar Glide

This technique is used to assess AP movement of the talus. If dorsiflexion is limited, this movement is likely to be restricted. The athlete is supine with her foot over the end of the table. Place your stabilizing hand on the distal lower leg while your mobilizing hand grasps the talus and midfoot to maintain the joint in a loose-packed position (figure 8.41). Apply an AP force to the talus perpendicular to the tibia's long axis as you assess the amount and quality of movement and end feel.

### Ventral Talar Glide

This maneuver is used to assess PA movement of the talus. If plantar flexion is limited, this movement will be restricted if the capsule is restricted. The athlete lies prone, with her foot over the end of the table and a pad placed under her distal lower leg. Place your stabilizing hand over the distal lower leg, and place your mobilizing hand around the calcaneus and talus (figure 8.42). Apply a downward PA force to assess the amount and quality of movement and end feel.

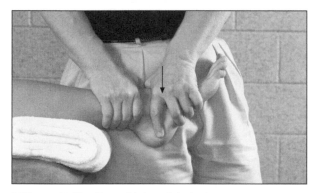

**■ Figure 8.41**   Dorsal talar glide test.

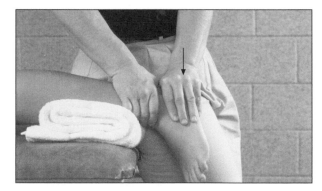

**■ Figure 8.42**   Ventral talar glide test.

## Other Glide Tests

### Subtalar Joint Medial-Lateral Glide

This is a test of lateral motion within the subtalar joint. Restriction of inversion or eversion will limit the amount of medial-lateral glide in this movement. The athlete is side-lying with his foot over the end of the table and a pad under his distal lower leg. Place your stabilizing hand on the distal lower leg and your mobilizing hand around the calcaneus. Use your thigh to maintain the athlete's foot in neutral (figure 8.43). Apply a downward force in the same plane as the subtalar joint. The opposite glide can be assessed in two ways: either apply the force in an upward direction to the calcaneus with the athlete in the same position or rotate the athlete to the opposite side and apply a downward force to the joint in the opposite direction.

### Midtarsal Joint Anterior-to-Posterior and Posterior-to-Anterior Glides

These movements will be restricted if abduction/adduction of the foot is limited by capsular adhesions of these joints. With the athlete supine and the foot supported either on the table or on your thigh, use the index finger and thumb of your stabilizing hand to secure one tarsal bone while the index finger and thumb of the mobilizing hand are placed around the adjacent tarsal bone (figure 8.44). Apply an AP and a PA force parallel to the joint's surface.

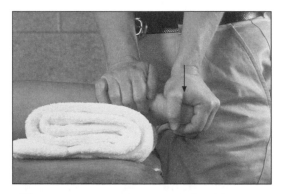

**Figure 8.43**   Medial-to-lateral glide of subtalar joint.

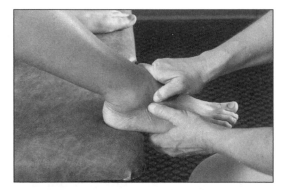

**Figure 8.44**   Midtarsal joint anterior-to-posterior and posterior-to-anterior glides.

### Tarsometatarsal Joint Anterior-to-Posterior Glide

These movements are used to assess the mobility between each distal tarsal and metatarsal. With the athlete in supine and her hip and knee flexed so that the heel is supported on the end of the table, grasp the distal tarsal row with your stabilizing hand and the metatarsal with your mobilizing hand (figure 8.45). Apply an AP glide to each tarsometatarsal joint to assess accessory movement excursion, quality, and end feel.

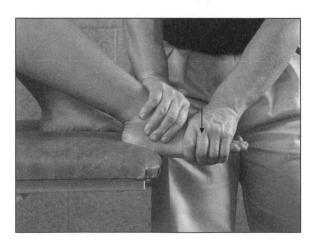

**Figure 8.45**   Tarsometatarsal joints anterior-to-posterior glide.

## Metatarsophalangeal and Interphalangeal Joints

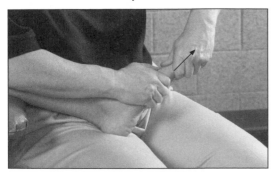

**■ Figure 8.46** Metatarsophalangeal and interphalangeal joints distraction.

### Distraction

This movement is used to assess general joint mobility. With the athlete comfortably supine and his foot on your thigh, stabilize the proximal joint end with one hand and grasp the distal joint end with the mobilizing hand (figure 8.46). Apply a traction force to separate the joint as you assess it for mobility and end feel.

### Rotation

Rotation provides an assessment of general joint mobility and end feel. The athlete's foot is positioned on your thigh as for the distraction movement. Grasp the proximal end of the joint with your stabilizing hand and the distal end with your mobilizing hand (figure 8.47). Apply a rotational force with the mobilizing hand in a clockwise and then in a counterclockwise direction.

### Dorsal and Ventral Glides

Dorsal (PA) glides, used to assess extension mobility, will be restricted if the capsule is preventing full extension. Ventral or plantar (AP) glides, which are used to assess flexion mobility, will be restricted if the capsule prevents full flexion of the joint. With the athlete's heel anchored on the table or your thigh, grasp the proximal segment of the joint with your stabilizing hand, and grasp the distal segment of the joint with the index finger and thumb of your mobilizing hand (figure 8.48). Apply PA and AP glides parallel to the joint surface.

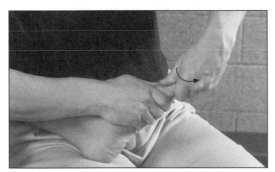

**■ Figure 8.47** Metatarsophalangeal and interphalangeal joint rotation.

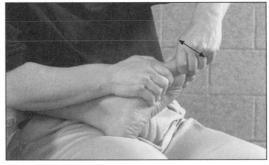

**■ Figure 8.48** Dorsal and ventral glide tests of the metatarsophalangeal and interphalangeal joints.

### *Palpation*

Palpation, as outlined for the sideline assessment, should proceed systematically: start at one location and gradually cover all tissue within the lower leg, ankle, and foot. Pay particular attention to any tenderness and restriction along the medial border of the tibia, which may indicate a medial tibial stress syndrome. Also be sure to palpate the calcaneal tubercle on the anterior, plantar aspect of the heel at the insertion of the plantar fascia. Refer back to the sideline assessment for detailed description of all other palpation points.

### *Functional Tests*

Proprioception, agility, and balance are all important functional qualities of athletic performance; they are particularly important in the lower extremity to ensure

# Checklist for Off-Field Assessment of the Lower Leg, Ankle, and Foot

## History

Ask questions pertaining to the following:

- ✓ Chief complaint
- ✓ Mechanism of injury
- ✓ Unusual sounds or sensations
- ✓ Type and location of pain or symptoms
- ✓ Previous injury
- ✓ Previous injury to opposite extremity for bilateral comparison

If chronic, ascertain:

- ✓ Onset and duration of symptoms
- ✓ Aggravating and easing factors
- ✓ Training history (change in practice intensity, duration, frequency, training surface, footwear, orthotics)

## Observation

- ✓ Check for swelling, deformity, abnormal contours, discoloration, scars, calluses, blisters, exostoses.
- ✓ Observe gait, weight bearing, ankle motion.
- ✓ Observe overall position, posture, and alignment of foot, ankle, and lower extremity.
- ✓ Check muscle development—areas of muscular atrophy.
- ✓ Inspect shoes bilaterally for abnormal, uneven, or excessive wear.
- ✓ Make bilateral comparison.

## Differential Diagnosis

- ✓ Clear low back, hip, and knee with active ROM and overpressure tests.

## Range of Motion

- ✓ Active ROM for plantar flexion, dorsiflexion inversion, eversion, and toe flexion and extension
- ✓ Passive ROM for plantar flexion, dorsiflexion, rearfoot inversion and eversion, forefoot inversion and eversion, and toe flexion and extension
- ✓ Bilateral comparison

## Strength Tests

- ✓ Perform manual resistance against same motions as in active ROM.

- ✓ Check bilaterally and note any pain or weakness.

## Neurovascular Tests

- ✓ Sensory over anterior thigh (L2, L3), anteromedial lower leg (L3, L4), lateral lower leg and dorsum of foot (L5), lateral plantar foot (S1), plantar, posterolateral plantar heel (S1, S2)
- ✓ Peripheral sensory assessment over dorsal web space (deep peroneal), dorsum of foot and lateral lower leg (superficial peroneal), posteromedial plantar heel (posterior tibial)
- ✓ Assessment of myotomes with ankle dorsiflexion (L4), great toe extension (L5), ankle plantar flexion and eversion (S1), great toe flexion (S2)
- ✓ Peripheral motor assessment with ankle dorsiflexion (deep peroneal) and plantar flexion and toe flexion (posterior tibial) and eversion (superficial peroneal)
- ✓ Reflex—Achilles tendon (S1, S2)

## Special Tests

- ✓ Potts compression test
- ✓ Thompson test
- ✓ Ligament laxity tests (anterior drawer, talar tilt, Kleiger, syndesmosis)
- ✓ Alignment tests (calcaneal-tibial, forefoot-rearfoot, Feiss line)
- ✓ Stress fracture tests (Morton's, percussion, Hoffa's)
- ✓ Neurovascular (Homan's, deep and superficial peroneal nerve compression, Tinel's, Morton's)
- ✓ Bilateral comparison

## Joint Mobility Assessment

- ✓ Distal tibiofibular (ventral and dorsal glides)
- ✓ Talocrural (distraction and glides)
- ✓ Subtalar (medial-lateral glides)
- ✓ Midtarsals (AP and PA glides)
- ✓ Tarsometatarsals (AP glides)
- ✓ Metatarsophalangeal and interphalangeal (distraction, rotation, and AP/PA glides)

**Palpation**

Palpate for pain, tenderness, crepitus, defects, and deformity over the following:

✓ Tibial crest, anterior tibiofibular ligament, anterior dome of talus, anterior tibialis muscle and tendon, extensor digitorum and hallucis tendons, extensor digitorum brevis, dorsalis pedis pulse, cuneiforms, metatarsals, and phalanges

✓ Fibula, peroneal muscle and tendons, lateral malleolus, anterior and posterior talofibular ligaments, calcaneofibular ligament, sinus tarsus, cuboid, base of fifth metatarsal.

✓ Gastrocnemius, soleus, Achilles tendon, calcaneus

✓ Plantar fascia, metatarsal heads

✓ Tibial shaft, medial malleolus, deltoid ligament, tibialis posterior tendon, flexor digitorum tendon, flexor hallucis longus tendon, posterior tibial artery and nerve, navicular tubercle, medial cuneiform, and first metatarsal (base, shaft, and head)

✓ Medial border of the tibia

✓ Calcaneal tuberosity and insertion of the plantar fascia

**Functional Tests**

safe participation and prevent secondary injury due to compensatory motions. As mentioned in relation to the sideline assessment, functional activities include running, jumping, lateral movements, rapid acceleration and deceleration movements, and combined upper- and lower-extremity movements. Specific activities to use in testing depend on the athlete's specific sport and position within the sport.

# SUMMARY

1. *Describe the etiology, signs and symptoms, and potential complications associated with acute injuries of the foot, ankle, and lower leg commonly encountered in the physically active.*

The lower leg, ankle, and foot represent the most frequently injured region in the body. The foot and ankle undergo tremendous stress during sporting activities because of their propulsive and weight-bearing functions. Acute injuries often result when the forces exerted on the ankle and foot exceed the tensile strength of the soft tissue or exceed the allowable range of motion. Lateral ankle sprains, the most common injury in the lower leg, typically result from inversion mechanisms. Medial ankle sprains are less common because of the anatomical makeup of the joint and the strength of the deltoid ligaments. Dislocations are rare, but fractures are common; these can result from the same mechanisms that produce sprains. Contusions and muscle strains also occur frequently.

2. *Describe the etiology, signs and symptoms, and potential complications associated with chronic or overuse injuries of the foot, ankle, and lower leg commonly encountered in the physically active.*

Also because of their weight-bearing and propulsive functions, the lower leg, ankle, and foot are equally prone to chronic and overstress injuries as a result of repetitive stress. Many times, these injuries are precipitated by structural or functional abnormalities that compromise the stability and shock absorption capabilities of the foot and ankle. Chronic stress injuries that occur commonly in the lower leg complex include retrocalcaneal bursitis, plantar fasciitis, tendinitis and tenosynovitis, anterolateral impingement, and tibial stress syndrome.

3. *Identify the signs and symptoms of neurovascular injury at the foot and ankle and differentiate those that indicate a medical emergency.*

Neurovascular compromise can result from both acute and chronic conditions. An acute anterior compartment syndrome, which represents a medical emergency, occurs when pressure within one of the muscular compartments of the leg exceeds the pressure of the vessels, causing vascular collapse. If the syndrome is not recognized and treated immediately, avascular necrosis and irreversible nerve damage will result. A more transient ischemia can occur with an exertional compartment syndrome but usually does not cause vascular collapse. Nerve compression syndromes can also result from chronic narrowing of a space or tunnel through which a nerve is traveling. It is important that you be able to differentiate the signs and symptoms of acute versus chronic neurovascular compromise and identify those that indicate a medical emergency.

4. *Identify the common functional and structural abnormalities of the foot and their potential effects on lower-extremity mechanics and injury.*

   The ability to recognize foot malalignments is an essential tool in the assessment process. Many deformities can affect lower-extremity alignment and mechanics sufficiently to cause abnormal stress and a host of lower-extremity injuries including tendinitis, medial tibial stress syndrome, plantar fasciitis, and stress fractures. Depending on the structural abnormality, shock absorption or stability of the foot structures may be compromised.

5. *Perform an on-field assessment of the foot, ankle, and lower leg, noting criteria for medical referral and mode of transportation from the field.*

   The goal of the on-field assessment is to quickly determine the presence of severe trauma, including any potential fracture or dislocation that would warrant immobilization and medical referral before the athlete is transported from the field. Your on-field evaluation should include a brief history to determine the mechanism and location of injury; careful observation for immediate signs of swelling, discoloration, or deformity; assessment for neurovascular compromise if fracture or dislocation is suspected; a brief but thorough palpation of bony and soft tissue structures to identify any defects, deformities, or crepitus; and stress tests for bone and ligament integrity. Once it is clear that there are no signs of severe trauma, the athlete is assisted off the field and prevented from weight bearing pending a more thorough assessment on the sideline.

6. *Perform a sideline assessment of the foot, ankle, and lower leg, including differential diagnosis of referring lumbar, hip, and knee pathologies.*

   Assessment at the sideline includes a complete investigation of current and past injury history and a more thorough observation and palpation assessment. A clear picture of the mechanism of injury will help greatly in the process of defining the potential structures involved. Additional stress tests, as well as active, passive, and resistive range of motion, are performed to assess ligamentous and muscle integrity. Motions to be tested include plantar flexion, dorsiflexion, inversion, eversion, and toe flexion and extension. Before the athlete returns to activity, all tests should be negative and pain should be sufficiently controlled to allow full, unrestricted participation without hesitation or compensation.

7. *Perform an off-field assessment of the foot, ankle, and lower leg, including functional tests for return to activity.*

   If the first time the athlete is seen is in the athletic injury treatment facility, the injury may be the result of an acute trauma that has worsened over the first 24-48 h following injury or may be the result of overuse. Many of the assessment procedures are the same as for the sideline assessment. Additional tests assess alignment and structural faults that may contribute to lower-extremity pain and dysfunction, stress fractures, nerve compression syndromes, and joint mobility.

# REVIEW QUESTIONS

1. What are the two primary functions of the lower leg and foot? What role do pronation and supination of the foot play in these functions?
2. Describe the mechanisms that result in lateral, medial, and syndesmosis ankle sprains. What tests would you use to evaluate ligament integrity?

3. What is Sever's disease? How is this condition different from retrocalcaneal bursitis and Achilles tendinitis?

4. Describe the mechanisms of injury associated with the following fractures:
   - Push-off fracture of the lateral malleolus
   - Avulsion fracture of the lateral malleolus
   - Jones' fracture
   - Stress fractures of the tibia and metatarsals

5. What is the difference between an acute and a chronic anterior tibial compartment syndrome? Describe the hallmark signs and symptoms of each and identify the symptoms that indicate a medical emergency.

6. Describe the normal alignment characteristics of the foot. How do the following structural abnormalities deviate from this normal alignment?
   - Rearfoot varus
   - Rearfoot valgus
   - Equinus deformity
   - Hallux valgus

7. What is the purpose of the Thompson test? If the test is positive, what condition is indicated, and what are the other signs and symptoms associated with this injury?

# CRITICAL THINKING QUESTIONS

1. A 26-year-old female runner comes to you complaining of "shinsplints" along the medial border of the tibia. Describe how you would differentiate in your evaluation between medial tibial stress syndrome, posterior tibial tendinitis, and a tibial stress fracture. What specific questions would you ask in the history, and what clues could the athlete provide to help differentiate these conditions?

2. Syndesmotic and medial ankle sprains, less common in sport than lateral ankle sprains, often result in prolonged disability due to difficulty with weight bearing. On the basis of the structures involved, discuss why weight bearing would be difficult and why weight bearing too soon after injury may prolong healing.

3. A basketball player complains of occasional sensations of pain, numbness, and tingling along the posteriomedial ankle and into the medial arch. She states that when she runs, her symptoms get worse and she gets an aching, burning sensation on the bottom of her foot. You have noted in the past when she runs down the court that she appears to pronate excessively. What nerve compression syndrome might you suspect, and what special tests might you use to identify this condition? What structural or functional abnormalities may contribute to this condition, and how would you assess for these in your evaluation?

# CITED REFERENCES

Ferkel, R.D., Karzel, R.P., Del Pizzo, W., Friedman, M.J., and Fischer, S.P. 1991. Arthroscopic treatment of anterolateral impingement of the ankle. *Am J Sports Med* 19(5):440-470.

Jackson, D.L., and Haglund, B. 1991. Tarsal tunnel syndrome in athletes. *Am J Sports Med* 19(1):61-65.

Tiberio, D. 1988. Pathomechanics of structural foot deformities. *Phys Ther* 68(12):1840-1849.

# ADDITIONAL RESOURCES

Hillman, S.K. 2000. *Introduction to athletic training*. Champaign, IL: Human Kinetics.

Houglum, P.A. 2000. *Therapeutic exercise for athletic injuries*. Champaign, IL: Human Kinetics.

# CHAPTER NINE

# Knee and Thigh

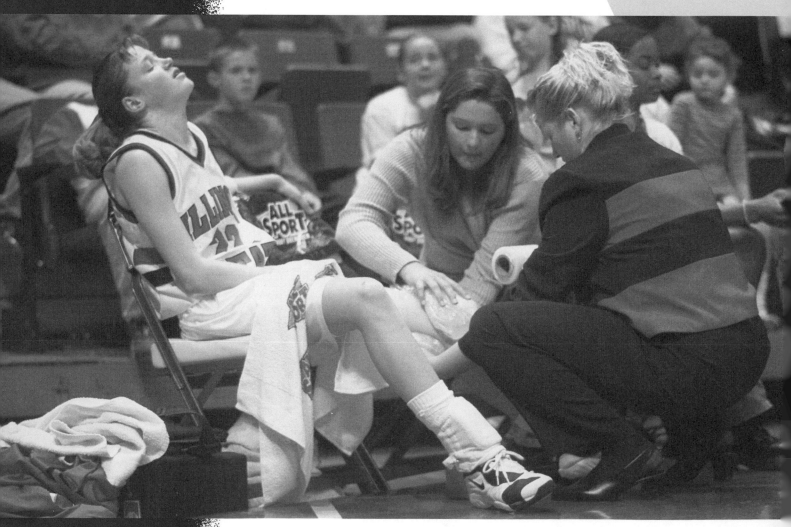

# *OBJECTIVES*

At the completion of this chapter, the reader will be able to do the following:

1. Describe the etiology, signs and symptoms, and potential complications associated with acute and chronic injuries of the knee frequently encountered in the physically active

2. Describe the etiology and signs and symptoms, including predisposing structural and biomechanical factors, associated with chronic patellofemoral pathologies

3. Describe and perform the various stress tests for assessing internal derangement of the knee joint

4. Describe and perform various special tests for assessing patellofemoral dysfunction

5. Perform an on-field assessment of the knee, indicating criteria for immediate medical referral and mode of transportation from the field

6. Perform a sideline assessment of the knee, including functional criteria for return to activity

7. Perform an off-field assessment of the knee, including assessment of lower-extremity alignment and considerations for differential diagnosis of referring pathologies from the back, hip, foot, and ankle

Connie was enjoying the break from the athletic training room while covering women's basketball practice at Virginia State University. About 30 minutes into practice, Molly, the point guard, was running down the court and quickly changed directions to go around a defender. Connie saw her knee buckle, and Molly went down in a heap, holding her knee. Just from watching the injury occur, Connie already had a good sense of what had happened.

"I felt my knee give out and I heard a pop," Molly said in obvious pain.

Connie did not observe any immediate swelling, deformity, or discoloration and found no palpable tenderness along the joint line, bony prominences, or surrounding soft tissue. Given the mechanism of injury, Connie performed a Lachman test to assess the integrity of Molly's anterior cruciate ligament, first on her uninjured and then on her injured leg. There was an obvious difference, and Connie could feel no end point on the injured leg.

"Let's help you off the court and get some ice on this right away. The doc will be in the athletic training room in a couple of hours and we will have him take a look."

Four hours later, as Connie was attending to another athlete, Dr. Steve came out of the exam room to talk to Connie about Molly. "Molly is very sore, swollen, and apprehensive. . . . It was difficult to get a good evaluation. What did you find when you assessed her immediately after injury, Connie?"

"She clearly had a positive Lachman and had no previous injury to either knee. Her joint swelling developed within about two hours. I saw her go down, and her mechanism was consistent with an ACL tear."

"That's what I suspected as well. . . . The information you gained in your initial assessment immediately after injury is very helpful—let's get her scheduled for an MRI to confirm. Good call, Connie!"

The knee is a complex joint that absorbs and transmits forces through the lower extremity in weight bearing and that provides mobility for locomotion. Although the knee can easily withstand three to four times its body weight in compressive loads, because of its bony configuration it has a much lower tolerance to shear and rotational loads. As the link between the femur and tibia, the knee experiences considerable torques through these long levers during physical activity. These factors make the knee quite vulnerable to injury.

The knee comprises three joints: the tibiofemoral, patellofemoral, and proximal tibiofibular joint. The tibiofemoral joint, the primary weight-bearing joint, is the largest joint in the body. It is characterized as a modified hinge joint that allows a large flexion/extension range, limited rotation, and minimal abduction and adduction. The congruency of the tibiofemoral articulation is improved by the medial and lateral menisci, which attach to the periphery of the tibial plateaus. The menisci help to stabilize the joint by deepening the articular surface, improving weight distribution, and increasing contact area between the tibia and the femur. They also serve as shock absorbers to decrease the loading stress placed on the joint during weight-bearing activities. When injury to these structures occurs, joint stability and biomechanical function are affected.

Except in the case of axial loading forces, the knee joint relies primarily on ligament, capsular, and muscular support, since there are no bony limitations in the transverse plane. The primary stabilizing ligaments of the knee (anterior cruciate, posterior cruciate, medial collateral, lateral collateral) provide the principal support system to limit excessive motion between the tibia and the femur. Secondary support is provided by the capsule and menisci and through dynamic muscular activation of thigh and lower leg muscles that cross the knee joint. When mechanical loads are placed on the joint, the primary stabilizing ligaments are most often injured.

The patellofemoral joint, also susceptible to injury, is formed by the articulation of the patella with the anterior surface of the femur in the intracondylar groove. The patella, the largest sesamoid in the body, is completely contained within the quadriceps tendon; it functions to protect the anterior knee joint and improve the mechanical advantage of the quadriceps with knee extension activities. As the knee moves from flexion to extension, the surface and area of joint contact will vary considerably, as will the compressive loads. This is a common area for overstress injuries, particularly when structural malalignments in the lower extremity (including ankle and hip) alter the position of the patella in the intracondylar groove, resulting in abnormal joint contact and compressive loads.

Biomechanically, the knee relies on the coordination between muscular control and the static constraints to guide skeletal motion through its full range of motion. This coordinative movement represents a combination of roll, slide, and glide movements at the joint surfaces as the knee moves between full flexion and extension to allow unrestricted motion and optimal joint efficiency. If any of the structures contributing to joint control are damaged due to injury, the normal mechanics of the knee will be disrupted, resulting in either joint restriction or instability that can severely hamper physical activity and sport performance. The various knee joint injury pathologies, the impact they have on knee joint function, and the assessment tools used to identify them will be the focus of this chapter.

# INJURIES TO THE KNEE AND THIGH

The knee joint is one of the most frequently injured joints in physically active people. It is particularly susceptible to injury because of its lack of bony stability, its reliance on soft tissue structures for stability, and the large mechanical forces imposed on it during sport activity. Compressive, varus/valgus, anterior/posterior shear, and rotational forces are constantly applied to the knee joint during sport activities, particularly those that require running, jumping, cutting, and rapid change of directions. When intrinsic or extrinsic forces exceed the structural integrity of the supporting tissues, injury will result.

## ACUTE SOFT TISSUE INJURIES

Because the knee relies so heavily on the soft tissue structures for stability, injuries to these structures are most common. Acute soft tissue injuries can result from both contact and noncontact mechanisms, with or without the foot in contact with the ground.

### Contusions

To allow full, unrestricted motion, the knee and thigh are often unprotected during sport activity, leaving the area vulnerable to direct contact with a sport implement, another player, or the ground. Because of the mobility required at the knee, contusions around the joint can be particularly bothersome. Signs and symptoms include pain, swelling, point tenderness, and discoloration. Range of motion and function may also be limited secondary to pain and swelling.

### Contusion of the Infrapatellar Fat Pad

With knee hyperextension injuries, it is not uncommon for the infrapatellar (I-P) fat pad to get impinged between the tibia and femur, resulting in a contusion (figure 9.1). Signs and symptoms of a fat pad contusion include pain, swelling, and point tenderness deep to and on either side of the

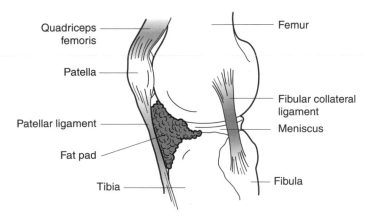

**Figure 9.1** Location and inflammation of the I-P fat pad.

patellar tendon. Range of motion will be limited in knee extension, and the athlete will be apprehensive about fully extending the knee because of increased pain. The athlete may also complain of the knee giving out with activity as a result of an unconscious avoidance of pain into extension.

### Quadriceps Contusion

Muscle contusions in the thigh, particularly the quadriceps, can be quite troublesome and can result in prolonged disability. Quadriceps contusions occur most often when direct contact is made while the muscle is in a contracted rather than relaxed state. Significant pain, spasm, and loss of function will be noted immediately following injury. Range of motion into flexion will be limited secondary to pain and spasm, but gentle stretching and ice may afford relief. With severe contusions in the muscle belly, considerable hemorrhage and swelling can occur over the 24-48 h following injury. Discoloration and a palpable hematoma may also be noted. An increase in leg circumference of 1 in. (2.5 cm) or more is indicative of significant hemorrhage. Depending on severity, the athlete may be unable to fully contract the quadriceps or achieve end-range extension. Knee flexion range may also be severely limited secondary to hemorrhage and spasm.

### Myositis Ossificans

A potential consequence of a quadriceps muscle contusion is **myositis ossificans**, which occurs when the body's inflammatory response during absorption of the hematoma causes calcification or bony deposits to form in the muscle. Calcification most often occurs secondary to severe hemorrhage, repetitive insult, or a too aggressive or too early return to activity following a severe contusion. The calcification may occur solely within the muscle belly or may appear as a bony stalk off the femur that extends into the muscle; this is typically more restrictive because of the muscle's attachment to the bone (figure 9.2). Signs and symptoms include a history of severe or repetitive insult to the quadriceps, pain, a palpable mass within the muscle belly, decreased knee flexion range, decreased quadriceps strength, and evidence on radiograph within three to four weeks after injury.

### Traumatic Bursitis

Direct contact over one of the superficial bursae of the knee may cause traumatic bursitis. Falling on the knee and making knee-to-knee contact with another player are the most common mechanisms. Those bursae most prone to traumatic injury include the prepatellar, suprapatellar, infrapatellar, and pes anserine (figure 9.3).

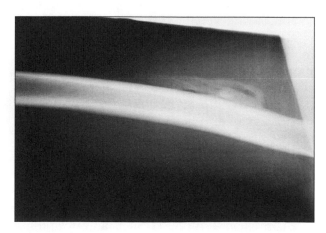

**■ Figure 9.2**   Myositis ossificans in the quadriceps.

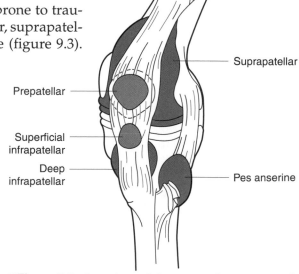

**■ Figure 9.3**   Locations of the prepatellar, suprapatellar, infrapatellar, and pes anserine bursae.

Signs and symptoms include immediate observable bursal swelling, redness, and mild pain. The area will be warm to the touch, and a soft fluid-filled pouch will be palpable. Range of motion will be limited with flexion resultant from the swelling and increased pressure in the bursa as the skin tightens over the knee during flexion.

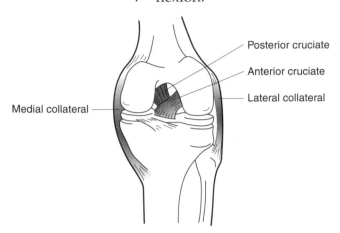

■ **Figure 9.4** Primary stabilizing ligaments of the knee.

### Sprains

The cruciate (anterior, posterior) and collateral (medial, lateral) ligaments act as the primary stabilizers of the knee joint (figure 9.4). Injury to these ligaments often occurs during athletic activities and may cause considerable instability and activity restriction. Although each ligament injury will be discussed separately, it is not uncommon for more than one structure to be injured, particularly with contact mechanisms. Injuries to more than one ligament, or associated injury of the capsule or meniscus, can result in rotatory or multiplanar instabilities at the knee.

#### Anterior Cruciate Ligament

The anterior cruciate ligament (ACL) originates from the intercondylar eminence of the tibia and runs in a posterior, lateral, and superior direction to attach on the posterior medial aspect of the lateral epicondyle of the femur. It consists of three bundles arranged such that some portion of the ligament is taut throughout the range. The ACL is tightest in extension and most lax in 45° of flexion. Its primary functions are to limit extension, forward translation (glide), internal rotation, and extreme external rotation of the tibia relative to the femur and to act as a guide wire for the femur as it rolls from flexion into extension.

Anterior cruciate ligament sprains have become the most prevalent third-degree ligament injury at the knee. The ACL can be injured in both contact and noncontact mechanisms. In a contact mechanism, the foot is firmly planted and externally rotated when a valgus force is applied to the lateral aspect of the leg with the knee slightly flexed. Noncontact mechanisms account for the majority of ACL injuries, particularly in females. In fact, females are two to five times more likely to injure their ACL than males, depending on the sport. With noncontact mechanisms, injury is usually associated with a sudden deceleration or change of direction. Thus it is not surprising that the majority of these noncontact injuries occur in sports such as basketball, gymnastics, lacrosse, and soccer. The knee is typically at or near full extension at the time of injury, and the athlete will complain of the knee's "buckling" or "giving way" during a sudden stop or landing from a jump, or during cutting or pivoting. Landing off balance with the center of body mass lateral and posterior to the landing leg can also injure the ACL secondary to excessive valgus and rotary forces at the knee upon ground contact.

Signs and symptoms include immediate pain and unwillingness to move the knee. The athlete may also hear a "pop" at the time of injury. Immediate symptoms usually subside sufficiently within a few minutes to allow a full knee evaluation. A large joint effusion and loss of motion usually result within 24 h. Therefore, it is important to assess the knee shortly after injury; examination becomes much more difficult once pain, swelling, and muscle guarding have set in. The athlete will initially be unwilling to bear weight or will have a sense of weakness or instability with weight bearing. Anterior and rotatory instability with stress tests will be noted with second- and third-degree sprains.

### Posterior Cruciate Ligament

The posterior cruciate ligament (PCL), which has a wide attachment on the anterior surface of the medial femoral condyle, expands posteriorly under the ACL to attach to the posterolateral tibial plateau. Much shorter than the ACL, it acts to limit extension, posterior translation, and internal rotation of the tibia on the femur. It is most taut in flexion and most lax in 45° of flexion; but because of its length, it is fairly taut throughout the full range of motion. It also functions biomechanically to limit the amount of forward roll of the femur and to cause the femur to pivot as the knee moves from flexion into extension.

The PCL is most often injured secondary to a direct blow to the anterior tibia that drives it posteriorly on the fixed femur. Common scenarios are making contact with the dashboard during a traffic collision and falling on the anterior tibia with the knee flexed and the foot and ankle plantarflexed. Additionally, any hyperflexion or hyperextension mechanism that forces the tibia posteriorly in relation to the femur can result in stretching or tearing of the PCL and posterior joint capsule. Signs and symptoms include pain, joint effusion, and limited range of motion into full flexion and extension. With complete rupture there may be an audible pop. With more serious second-degree as well as third-degree injuries, the examiner will observe a "posterior sag" of the tibia when the quadriceps are relaxed and will note posterior instability with posterior stress tests. Athletes who have good quadriceps and hamstring muscle strength may not complain of feelings of instability with weight bearing, so these injuries are sometimes missed. Athletes with PCL tears often do well following rehabilitation and are able to return to full activity without surgical intervention.

### Medial (Tibial) Collateral Ligament

The medial collateral ligament (MCL) is a broad, fan-shaped ligament that consists of two layers. The superficial layer runs outside the joint capsule, from the medial femoral condyle to well below the joint line on the tibial flare, distal to the adductor tubercle. The deep layer dives into the capsule and attaches to the medial meniscus. The MCL functions to limit abduction of the tibia on the femur and also assists in limiting extension and external rotation of the tibia. In addition, the deep fibers function to stabilize the medial meniscus.

A straight valgus stress can result in an isolated MCL injury. Typically the foot will be planted in neutral or external rotation, and contact will be made to the lateral aspect of the abducted leg, resulting in a valgus stress to the medial joint structures. With severe valgus injuries, it is not uncommon for the ACL and medial meniscus to be injured also (i.e., **unhappy triad**) if the valgus force continues once the MCL fails. Signs and symptoms of MCL injury include pain, mild to moderate swelling, discoloration, and point tenderness in the midsubstance of the MCL or near its femoral or tibial attachment. Pain may also be present at the medial joint line if the deep portion of the ligament and/or its attachment to the medial meniscus is torn. Since the ligament is primarily located outside of the joint capsule, there is usually no joint effusion with an isolated MCL sprain. The athlete will experience increased pain when the ligament is taut during full knee flexion and extension, as well as with an applied valgus stress. Instability will be noted during valgus stress with second- and third-degree injuries.

### Lateral (Fibular) Collateral Ligament

The lateral collateral ligament (LCL) runs from the lateral epicondyle of the femur to its attachment on the fibular head. It is completely separate from the capsule and does not attach to the lateral meniscus. It functions to limit knee extension and adduction of the tibia relative to the femur. It also assists in limiting external rotation of the tibia when the knee is extended.

The LCL is injured less frequently than the other knee ligaments. The mechanism responsible for injuries to the LCL is a varus force applied to the medial aspect of the knee. The LCL is most vulnerable when the varus force is applied while the leg is adducted and the tibia internally rotated. Injuries to the LCL most often occur in contact sports such as football, soccer, and wrestling when one player falls into or makes contact against the medial side of another player's leg, the foot of which is planted. Signs and symptoms include pain, lateral knee swelling, ecchymosis, and point tenderness over the fibular collateral ligament. The athlete may hear or feel a pop with complete rupture and will note varus instability with second- and third-degree injuries. He will experience increased pain when the ligament is put on tension during full knee flexion, extension, and varus stress. Pain and swelling will also cause limited range of motion. As with the MCL, the LCL lies outside of the joint capsule, and a joint effusion with this injury typically indicates associated injury to the capsule or meniscus. Injury to the posterolateral capsule commonly occurs with an LCL sprain.

### Rotary and Multiplanar Instabilities

It is not uncommon for the mechanisms described to cause injury to more than one structure. In addition to the primary ligament involved, the capsule, secondary ligament restraints, and muscular insertions can also be disrupted, leading to instability in more than one direction or plane. The presence of rotary instabilities usually denotes a serious injury, resulting in considerable instability. Rotary instabilities can be anteromedial, anterolateral, posterolateral, and posteromedial. Understanding the structures and mechanisms involved in these rotary instabilities will help you in your objective assessment of knee ligament injuries and in interpretation of your findings.

- **Anteromedial Rotary Instability.** Anteromedial rotary instability, the most common type of instability, occurs when the medial tibial plateau subluxes on the femur. It results when the ACL, MCL, medial capsule, and possibly the medial meniscus are torn. The posterior medial capsule and posterior oblique ligament may also be involved. The typical mechanism for this injury is external rotation of the tibia with valgus stress.

- **Anterolateral Rotary Instability.** Anterolateral rotary instability results from injury to the ACL, LCL, and lateral capsule. It is characterized by subluxation of the lateral tibial plateau with anterior translation and internal rotation of the tibia on the femur.

- **Posterolateral Rotary Instability.** Posterolateral rotary instability allows posterior subluxation of the lateral tibial plateau. It is caused by injury to the posterolateral compartment, PCL deficiency, or both. Posterior lateral structures usually include the LCL and popliteus tendon; they sometimes may also include the biceps femoris and lateral head of the gastrocnemius. Posterolateral rotary instability most often results from an anterior blow to the tibia with the foot externally rotated and the knee under varus stress.

- **Posteromedial Rotary Instability.** Posteromedial rotary instability results from combined injury to the PCL, MCL, and medial joint capsule. The typical mechanism is an anterior blow to the tibia with the knee partially flexed and under valgus stress and the foot externally rotated. Instability will be noted with valgus stress, posterior translation, and internal rotation of the tibia.

### Meniscal Injuries

The menisci are two semilunar cartilages that sit on the tibial plateau, attaching only at their peripheral margins (figure 9.5). They are thickest at their peripheral borders and thin toward the center. They move with the tibia during flexion and extension, and with the femur during rotation. They possess no nerves, and their vascular supply is primarily along the periphery. The primary functions of the menisci are to (1) help stabilize the joint by deepening the tibial condyles, (2) absorb the shock of weight bearing and decrease loading stress, (3) lubricate the joint and reduce friction during movement, and (4) make joint surfaces more congruent and improve weight distribution by increasing the contact area between the tibia and femur.

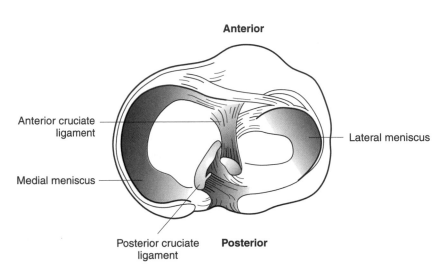

**Anterior**

Anterior cruciate ligament

Lateral meniscus

Medial meniscus

Posterior cruciate ligament    **Posterior**

■ **Figure 9.5**    Medial and lateral menisci at their attachments on the tibial plateau.

Tearing of the medial or lateral meniscus typically occurs as a consequence of compression and rotation of the femur on the fixed tibia. Cutting and pivoting with the joint in full weight bearing can pinch the menisci between the femur and tibia and cause it to tear as the femur rotates on the joint surface. Tears to the posterior horn of the menisci can also occur with hyperflexion and compression mechanisms. In addition, the menisci can be torn in association with ligament injuries when there are axial compression and excessive translation of the femur on the tibia as the ligament fails. Because the medial meniscus has a broader attachment to the tibial surface and is attached to the MCL and semimembranosus, it is less mobile and more frequently injured than the lateral meniscus. Older athletes are more prone to injuries of the menisci as these structures becomes less compliant and degenerate with age.

The athlete may or may not recall the specific injury occurrence. Signs and symptoms include pain, swelling, and joint line tenderness. Because there is virtually no pain sensation in the menisci themselves, the pain typically results from surrounding inflammation and synovial irritation. Delayed or persistent joint effusion may also occur with meniscal injuries. If the torn portion of the meniscus is displaced or detached, it may become impinged as the joint moves through its range of motion, resulting in symptoms of clicking, catching, or locking of the joint. The athlete may have complaints of pain, instability, or "giving way" during cutting or pivoting as well. If the tear is in the posterior horn, the athlete will complain of posterior knee pain and pain with deep squatting. Special tests involving compression and rotation of the joint (see McMurray's, Apley's tests, page 295) will also elicit symptoms.

### Strains

Muscular strains typically stem from forceful contraction of the muscle during eccentric loading or from overstretching. Inflexibility, fatigue, weakness, muscular imbalance, and inadequate warm-up may increase an athlete's susceptibility to thigh muscle strains. Recurrent strains are a common problem, as the symptoms often subside and the athlete returns to activity before adequate healing has occurred.

#### Quadriceps Strain

The quadriceps muscle is most often overloaded during sudden acceleration or deceleration. Therefore injuries most often occur during sprinting, kicking, and weight-lifting activities. Injury typically involves the rectus femoris muscle. The athlete will usually complain of immediate pain, spasm, and loss of function. However, with some first-degree strains, the athlete may find that initial pain quickly subsides, allowing return to activity, only to have pain return and remain the next day. The athlete will experience pain with passive stretch into knee flexion with the hip extended. Pain and weakness with active/resistive extension will be consistent with the degree of injury. The athlete will be palpably tender over the injured area, and a defect may be present with second- and third-degree injuries. Second- and third-degree injuries may also result in observable swelling, ecchymosis, and a quadriceps avoidance gait.

### Hamstring Strain

Hamstring strains—more common than quadriceps strains—occur most often with sprinting activities. Injury can occur in the midbelly of the muscle, at the distal myotendon junction, or at the proximal insertion at the ischial tuberosity. Proximal strains near the ischial attachment typically result from overstretching or hyperflexion of the hip with the knee extended. Unfortunately, proximal injuries heal very slowly, and disability can be prolonged. Tearing in the midbelly or myotendon junction most often results when the quadriceps are forcefully contracted while the hamstring is eccentrically contracting. Asynchronous muscle timing, inflexibility, and muscular imbalance (excessive quad:ham strength ratio) appear to be contributing factors to this mechanism. At the time of injury, the athlete will typically "pull up" or shorten her stride on the involved leg and grab her thigh while trying to decelerate.

Signs and symptoms include an immediate sharp or burning pain in the hamstring at the time of injury. With some first-degree sprains, though, pain and stiffness may be delayed until the next day. Palpable tenderness and spasm will be noted over and around the injured fibers. The athlete will experience pain with passive stretching and active/resistive knee flexion. There may be a palpable defect with second- and third-degree injuries. The athlete may also exhibit a shortened stride during gait on the involved side to avoid fully extending the knee and placing the muscle on stretch. Delayed swelling and ecchymosis often occur within 24-48 h following second- and third-degree strains.

### Patellar Tendon Rupture

A violent, rapid quadriceps contraction can result in a midsubstance rupture of either the infrapatellar or suprapatellar tendon. Patellar tendon ruptures, which are infrequent, can occur in a healthy tendon as a result of an acute, one-time mechanism; more often the tear is precipitated by episodes of chronic tendinitis or inflammation that weaken the structure. At the time of injury the athlete will complain of immediate, severe pain and loss of active knee extension. He may also hear or feel a pop as the tendon ruptures. The patella will appear to sit more superiorly with an infrapatellar tendon rupture, and there will be a palpable gap between the inferior pole of the patella and tibial tuberosity. With suprapatellar tendon ruptures, the defect will be superior to the patella. Considerable swelling and ecchymosis will likely result within 24 h following injury. Ruptures in the midsubstance of the tendon are less common in young athletes, with failure typically occurring at the tibial apophysis where the tendon attaches (figure 9.6) (see also discussion of Osgood-Schlatter disease later in this chapter).

## CHRONIC AND OVERUSE SOFT TISSUE INJURIES

The soft tissue structures of the knee are also prone to chronic inflammatory conditions caused by repetitive friction and overuse. The soft

**❚ Figure 9.6** Avulsion fracture of the tibial apophysis.

tissues most prone to overuse are the numerous tendons that cross and attach at the knee joint, and the bursae that function to reduce friction and allow free movement of the tendons. Repetitive kneeling, jumping, and flexion/extension movements are common mechanisms associated with inflammation of these structures. Inflammation of a tendon or bursa can cause considerable discomfort and have a significant impact on performance.

### Bursitis

Carpet layers, roofers, tilers, wrestlers, distance runners, and other individuals involved in activities that result in repetitive trauma or friction over a bursa can experience episodes of chronic bursitis. Numerous bursae have been identified around the knee; they are typically present between tendons and other joint structures to prevent friction during knee movement. Those most prone to irritation and inflammation are the pes anserine, infrapatellar, prepatellar, and suprapatellar bursae (see figure 9.3). The suprapatellar, prepatellar, and superficial infrapatellar bursae are prone to friction and irritation with frequent kneeling or bending. Because the suprapatellar bursa is continuous with the synovium, irritation or inflammation affecting one will affect the other. The deep infrapatellar bursa lies deep to the infrapatellar tendon and anterior to the infrapatellar fat pad and the anterior surface of the tibia. It also is prone to irritation with frequent kneeling, but subsequent swelling is more obscured and will appear on either side of the patellar tendon when the leg is extended. Chronic irritation of the pes anserine bursa, which lies between the pes anserine tendons and the MCL, is typically caused by overuse and repetitive valgus loading in distance runners and cyclists.

Signs and symptoms of chronic bursitis include pain, redness, and localized swelling. The area will be tender to palpation and warm to the touch. Crepitus and bogginess, or thickening of the bursal fluid, will also occur with chronic bursitis. Flexion of the knee may be painful or limited with patellar bursitis secondary to increased pressure over the bursa as the skin tightens into flexion. Extension may also be limited with suprapatellar and deep infrapatellar bursal swelling. Pes anserine bursitis is painful with knee flexion and extension and internal tibial rotation. In prolonged cases of bursitis, permanent thickening of the bursal wall may occur, and calcium deposits may also form within the bursa.

### Popliteal Cyst (Baker's Cyst)

A popliteal cyst typically results from a herniation of the synovial cavity and accumulation of fluid in the popliteal space (figure 9.7). Fluid accumulation may also result from distension of either the popliteal, semimembranosus, or subtendinous bursa, all of which also communicate with the synovial cavity. Signs and symptoms include a palpable, fluid-filled cyst in the inferomedial popliteal fossa. The cyst may or may not be tender and typically in and of itself does not restrict activity. However, significant swelling may cause discomfort and restriction of knee flexion. Because popliteal cysts are commonly associated with meniscal tears and arthritic conditions, you

> Because popliteal cysts are commonly associated with meniscal tears and arthritic conditions, be suspicious of internal derangement or other intra-articular pathology when the athlete presents with a posterior cyst as the primary complaint.

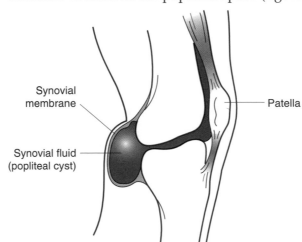

Synovial membrane

Synovial fluid (popliteal cyst)

Patella

**▌Figure 9.7**    Baker's cyst.

should be suspicious of internal derangement or other intra-articular pathology when the athlete presents with the posterior cyst as the primary complaint.

### *Tendinitis and Strains*

Given the many tendons that cross and attach at the knee, tendinitis resulting from repetitive or overuse mechanisms is a frequent complaint in the physically active. As with most tendinitis conditions, the athlete will present with an insidious onset of pain and a history of repetitive activity or significant increase in training over the past few days or weeks. Initially he may feel pain only after activity and cool-down; he may also experience pain at the beginning of activity but note that it improves with warm-up. As symptoms worsen, he will complain of pain throughout activity as well as during the day.

### Patellar Tendinitis (Jumper's Knee)

Patellar tendinitis frequently occurs from overuse as a consequence of repetitive jumping (basketball, volleyball, long jump, triple jump), running, or weight-lifting exercises (leg extension, squats, lunges). Overloading of the extensor mechanism can cause microtearing and inflammation of either the suprapatellar or infrapatellar tendons. Patellar tendinitis is characterized by symptoms of pain, inflammation, and mild swelling either superior or inferior to the patella. Palpable tenderness and crepitus are often present over the inflamed tendon. The athlete will complain of pain with passive stretching of the tendon and active or resisted knee extension. In prolonged, chronic cases, degeneration and scarring within the tendon can weaken its structure and increase susceptibility to patellar tendon rupture.

### Iliotibial Band Friction Syndrome

Iliotibial band friction syndrome is an overuse injury most typically seen in runners and cyclists. It is caused by excessive friction between the iliotibial (IT) band and the lateral femoral epicondyle. At approximately 30° of flexion, the IT band changes from a knee extensor to a knee flexor (figure 9.8, a-b). When the knee is flexed less than 30°, the IT band lies anteriorly to the lateral epicondyle and assists with knee extension. As the knee is flexed, the IT band will ride over the epicondyle at about 25-30° of flexion and then sit posteriorly past 30° of flexion, assisting with knee flexion. Irritation occurs with repetitive activity at the transitional range if there is excessive friction or snapping of the IT band as it passes over the epicondyle. Athletes with increased genu valgum, excessive quadriceps angle, excessive pronation, or leg length discrepancy are more prone than others to IT band friction syndrome. Tightness in the IT band (see Ober's test, page 338 in chapter 10), training errors, downhill running, and running on a slanted surface may also be predisposing factors.

Signs and symptoms include pain and point tenderness over the lateral femoral condyle just proximal to the lateral joint line. Pain may also radiate up and down the IT band to its insertion at Gerdy's tubercle. As with other inflammatory conditions, pain is often first noted only after activity and does not restrict activity initially. As

*Genu valgum (valgus) is excessive lateral angulation of the tibia relative to the femur. See table 9.1 and figure 9.33.*

*Quadriceps angle is the angle created by a line from the anterior superior iliac spine through the midpoint of the patella and a line from the tibial tubercle through the midpoint of the patella. See table 9.1 and figure 9.40.*

**▌ Figure 9.8** (a) At less than 30° the IT band is anterior to the lateral epicondyle and acts as an extensor. (b) As the leg moves to more than 30°, the IT band passes posteriorly to the lateral epicondyle to act as a flexor.

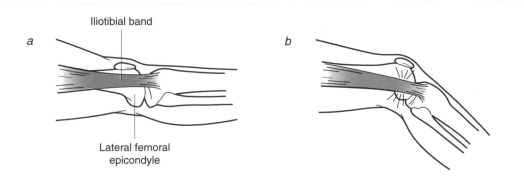

inflammation and irritation increase, pain will gradually appear during running and if left untreated will eventually restrict activity. Pain and snapping may also be noted with walking down stairs or squatting, or with flexion and extension movements of the knee around 30° of flexion.

### Hamstring Tendinitis

Hamstring tendinitis can occur in both the proximal and distal tendons. Proximal hamstring tendinitis near the insertion to the ischial tuberosity is less common, but can result either from repetitive friction and pressure over the tendon and tuberosity—as in cycling when the seat is improperly adjusted—or from overstretching or tensioning of the proximal attachment with straight-leg hip flexion. Because of poor vascularization of the proximal tendon, healing is quite slow and symptoms often persist for a prolonged period of time. Signs and symptoms include an achy pain just below the gluteal fold and deep palpable tenderness just distal to the ischial tuberosity. Pain is often exacerbated by passive stretching into straight-knee hip flexion, resisted straight-knee hip extension, and long striding.

Distal hamstring tendinitis most often results from repetitive flexion and overuse during running and weight-lifting activities. Signs and symptoms include an insidious onset of pain, palpable tenderness, mild swelling, and crepitus in the inflamed tendon. With medial hamstring tendinitis, the athlete may complain of snapping or clicking behind the knee with knee flexion that occurs when the inflamed tendons ride over adjacent structures. Pain may also be noted with passive knee extension and active/resistive knee flexion.

### Pes Anserine Tendinitis

The same mechanisms that result in bursitis of the pes anserine can also cause inflammation and irritation of the tendons near their attachment on the medial tibial plateau. Pes anserine tendinitis is most often seen in runners and cyclists. Anteroinferior medial knee pain, palpable tenderness over the anteromedial tibial plateau, crepitus, and local swelling are typical signs and symptoms. Pain will also be noted with active knee flexion, with passive knee extension, and possibly with valgus stress.

### *Plica Syndrome*

Plica syndrome is an anomaly or fold in the synovial membrane on the anterior aspect of the knee that runs from the lateral femoral condyle, superior and medial to the patella, and down toward the fat pad (figure 9.9). While a synovial fold can occur anywhere around the knee, the most typical location is along the superior medial border of the patella. Although a plica is often asymptomatic, it can become a problem if the area becomes inflamed or taut, resulting in a snapping, clicking, or "jumping" of the patella as the knee moves into flexion. Other signs and symptoms include pain along the medial border of the patella, swelling, and a possible locking sensation. One can often palpate the snapping or clicking of the patella by placing a finger on the patella during flexion and extension of the knee.

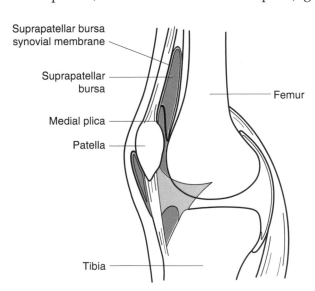

Suprapatellar bursa synovial membrane

Suprapatellar bursa

Medial plica

Patella

Femur

Tibia

**▌Figure 9.9**   Medial plica.

# TRAUMATIC FRACTURES

Traumatic fractures occur less frequently at the knee than at other joints because the ligaments and soft tissues provide most of the stability to the knee joint and thus are more likely to fail. As is typical for other body regions, fractures of the knee and thigh are more commonly seen in young, skeletally immature athletes. When fracture is suspected, the extremity should be immobilized and the athlete immediately referred to a physician.

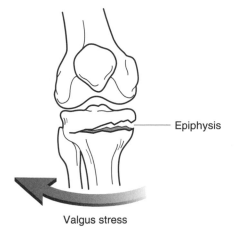

Epiphysis

Valgus stress

**▌Figure 9.10** Epiphyseal plate injury at the proximal tibia and false joint motion with valgus testing.

### Epiphyseal Fractures

Fractures through the proximal tibial epiphysis, and less often the distal femoral epiphysis, can result from rotational and shearing forces at the knee joint. Twisting, varus, or valgus forces directed at the knee with the foot firmly planted are the more common mechanisms in the adolescent athlete. Signs and symptoms include immediate pain, tenderness along the bone, swelling, loss of function, and possible deformity. The athlete may report hearing a pop or snap at the joint. Crepitus may be observable with joint motion, but the athlete will typically be unwilling to move the extremity. False joint motion, or opening of the epiphyseal joint with varus and valgus testing, may make it difficult to distinguish an epiphyseal fracture from a collateral ligament injury (figure 9.10). Therefore as an athletic trainer you should have a high index of suspicion when evaluating varus/valgus injuries in the adolescent. A potential complication of epiphyseal fractures is disruption and premature closing of the growth plate, which may ultimately result in a true leg length discrepancy.

### Tibial Plateau Fracture

Tibial plateau fractures can also result from severe varus, valgus, or rotational forces in combination with axial compression when the foot is firmly planted. The athlete will complain of severe and immediate pain and be unwilling to move the knee joint. Other signs and symptoms include swelling, tenderness over the proximal tibia, pain with percussion, crepitus, and possible deformity.

### Patella

Fractures of the patella can be caused by direct contact, as in a fall directly on the patella with the knee flexed, or by indirect forces, such as severe tractioning produced by a forceful quadriceps contraction. The athlete will complain of sudden and severe pain in the kneecap and will be unwilling to contract the quadriceps or extend the knee—or is unable to do so without considerable pain. Immediate tenderness, rapid swelling, and crepitus will also be observable over the patella. Patellar fractures can often result in considerable and prolonged disability. Inhibition or inability to contract the quadriceps for an extended period of time can result in severe atrophy and delayed rehabilitation. Fractures through the articular surface of the patella are particularly troublesome, as they create an uneven or roughened articular surface that may cause chronic pain and symptoms similar to those associated with chondromalacia patella.

### Femur

Femoral shaft fractures resulting from athletic activity are quite rare because of the relative strength of the femur. When femoral fractures do occur, the frequency is greatest in contact sports such as football as a result of a severe, direct blow to the midthigh; but such fractures may also occur secondary to severe torsional

Because of the potential for arterial injury, hemorrhage, and shock, femoral fractures constitute a medical emergency.

forces. Femoral shaft fractures are readily apparent. Signs and symptoms include immediate and severe pain, muscle spasm, and inability to move the extremity. Considerable hemorrhage may occur, resulting in shock. Complete fractures are usually displaced because of the strength and resultant spasm of the surrounding musculature. The characteristic deformity is typically a shortened, externally rotated thigh.

### Chondral and Osteochondral Fractures

Chondral fractures (fractures of the articular cartilage) and **osteochondral** fractures (fractures extending through the articular cartilage and into the bone) of the femoral condyle may occur in isolation or at the same time as a ligament injury, as a result of similar mechanisms. Joint compression combined with a varus, valgus, or rotational shearing force can contuse the articular surface and cause a compression or avulsion fracture (figure 9.11), resulting in loose fragments (**joint mice**) that can produce irritation, locking, and clicking within the joint.

Signs and symptoms of chondral or osteochondral fracture include pain, immediate or delayed swelling, locking or clicking, and pain with joint compression or weight bearing. Depending on the extent of injury, the athlete may be unable to bear weight or move the knee. When the fracture extends into the underlying bone, considerable bleeding and joint effusion may result. Palpable tenderness and crepitus may also be present near the joint line and femoral condyle. Pain will increase with manual joint compression combined with knee flexion, extension, or rotation.

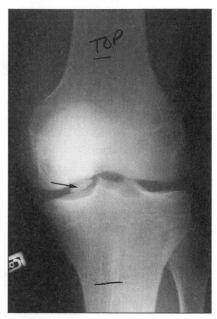

**Figure 9.11**  Osteochondral fracture of the femoral condyle.

## DISLOCATION AND SUBLUXATION

Of the three joints that comprise the knee complex, the patellofemoral joint is most prone to subluxation and dislocation. Although dislocation of the tibiofemoral joint is less common, it represents a much more serious and potentially limb-threatening injury.

### Patellofemoral Subluxation and Dislocation

*Patella alta is a patella that sits abnormally high in the femoral groove. See table 9.1.*

Patellar dislocations, which can result from either direct or indirect forces, typically occur lateral to the femoral groove secondary to the more lateral angular pull of the quadriceps and the lesser height of the lateral femoral condyle in relation to the medial femoral condyle. A direct blow to the medial patella, and indirect forces applied by the quadriceps during cutting maneuvers with the tibia externally rotated, can force the patella to displace over the lateral femoral condyle. Athletes with an abnormally shallow femoral groove, excessive Q-angle (see table 9.1), hypermobile patella, weak medial quadriceps, or patella alta are more prone than others to recurrent patellar dislocations. Consequently patellar dislocations occur more frequently in females than males secondary to a larger Q-angle and greater propensity for lateral tracking problems.

When the patella subluxates or dislocates, the athlete will complain of a sharp pain and pop in the anterior knee and a feeling of the knee giving way at the time of injury. If the patella remains displaced, the deformity is quite obvious. However, often the patella will spontaneously reduce so that the injury is more difficult to identify. The athlete will be palpably tender along the medial border of the patella and soft tissue structures. The lateral femoral condyle may also be tender. Considerable anterior knee swelling will be noted, particularly in first-time dislocations, shortly after injury. The athlete will be apprehensive when the patella is moved laterally. First-time dislocations or subluxations, especially those resulting from direct trauma, should be evaluated by a physician, and x-rays should be obtained to rule out any associated chip fractures of the patella or lateral femoral condyle.

### *Tibiofemoral*

A total knee dislocation of the tibia and the femur is a very serious and potentially limb-threatening injury that fortunately occurs rarely in sports. Knee dislocations due to indirect forces are extremely unusual; the majority of cases are caused by large mechanical forces that force the joint to go well beyond its normal range of motion. Given that the ligaments act as the primary stabilizers of the knee joint, multiple ligaments—including both cruciate ligaments and at least one of the collateral ligaments—must be torn in order for the joint to dislocate. In addition to the significant soft tissue damage that occurs, the risk of neurovascular injury is high, particularly with posterior dislocations (figure 9.12). Knee dislocations require immediate neurovascular assessment and medical referral.

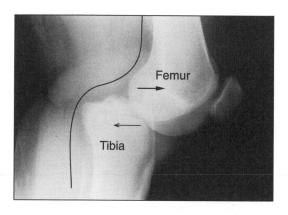

**▌Figure 9.12**  Posterior dislocation of the knee. The location of the posterior tibial artery has been drawn in to illustrate the potential for neuro-vascular injury.

## BONY AND ARTICULAR DEFECTS SECONDARY TO REPETITIVE STRESS

The articular surfaces of the tibiofemoral and patellofemoral joints are subject to considerable compressive forces during physical activity. The patellofemoral joint is most often affected, particularly in athletes with faulty alignment. There are additional concerns when the athlete is an adolescent.

### *Patellofemoral Pain Syndrome*

Patellofemoral pain syndrome, also known as **miserable malalignment syndrome**, is a general term used to describe anterior knee pain. Anterior knee pain can be caused by a variety of factors that result in patellar malalignment, increased patellofemoral compression, and/or poor patellofemoral tracking. These include anatomical and biomechanical abnormalities, muscular weakness and imbalance, and training errors. Anatomical and biomechanical abnormalities that can alter lower-extremity limb alignment include subtalar pronation, external tibial torsion, genu valgum, increased Q-angle, hip anteversion, and patella alta (see table 9.1). Weakness in the vastus medialis muscles as compared to the lateral quadriceps, and tightness in the lateral retinaculum and IT band, can also pull the patella laterally, as shown by the arrow in figure 9.13. An abrupt change in training activity, surface, intensity, or duration that substantially increases the

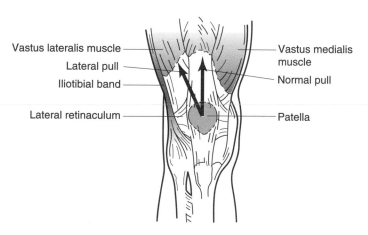

**▌Figure 9.13**  Attachments to the patella and lateral pulling of the patella secondary to tightness in these structures.

load on the patellofemoral joint may also cause symptoms. Regardless of the causative factor or factors, the result is the same in each case: pain and irritation consequent to increased patellofemoral compression and pressure.

Signs and symptoms of patellofemoral pain syndrome include poorly localized anterior knee pain that is exacerbated by activity, squatting, going up and down stairs, or ambulation after prolonged sitting (**theater sign**). Most of the time there is little or no observable swelling. The athlete may be palpably tender under the lateral border of the patella. There is usually no history of specific onset; instead the pain appears gradually. However, sudden changes in the training regime may initiate symptoms. Patellofemoral pain syndrome is often difficult to manage; success in decreasing the athlete's symptoms depends on both the identification and the correction of predisposing factors. A rehabilitation program designed to increase mobility of lateral soft tissue structures and improve lower-extremity limb alignment and muscle function is usually indicated.

For more information on the management of patellofemoral syndromes, refer to *Therapeutic Exercise for Athletic Injuries* (Houglum 2000), chapter 21.

### Chondromalacia Patella

While chondromalacia patella fits within the general category of patellofemoral pain syndrome, it is a specific condition characterized by softening, roughening, and eventual degeneration and defects of the articular surface of the patella. The articular facet is the one most commonly affected. Chondromalacia patella can be caused by direct and repetitive trauma, patellar malalignment, or previous trauma such as a patella dislocation or a fracture that extends through the articular surface. Patellar malalignment, or abnormal tracking of the patella within the femoral grove, can result from a variety of predisposing factors, including tight lateral soft tissue structures, increased quadriceps angle, excessive hip anteversion, excessive pronation, or other structural and functional abnormalities of the lower extremity. These abnormalities lead to increased compression and friction of one or more of the articular facets within the femoral groove. Signs and symptoms include general anterior knee pain, crepitus, minor swelling, and increased pain with patellofemoral compression in activities such as deep knee bending, knee extension exercises, or walking up and down stairs. Palpable tenderness may be noted under the medial or lateral border of the patella.

### Apophysitis (Osgood-Schlatter Disease)

In young athletes, the apophysis of the tibial tubercle can be subjected to considerable stress due to repetitive tractioning by the patellar tendon. During adolescence, the epiphyseal line is weaker than the quadriceps muscle and tendon. Muscle tightness, repetitive jumping, and running during significant growth spurts can cause excessive tractioning of the apophysis leading to irritation, inflammation, and partial avulsion (figure 9.14). Signs and symptoms include focused anterior knee pain, swelling and tenderness over the tibial tuberosity, and increased prominence of the tibial tuberosity. The athlete will complain of increased pain with knee extension exercises, squatting, kneeling, and jumping.

### Osteochondritis Dissecans

Osteochondritis dissecans, or avascular necrosis of the osteochondral surface of the knee, usually involves the femoral condyle and occurs

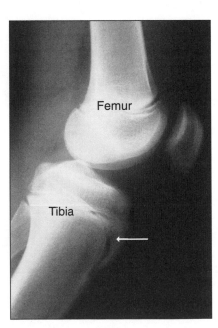

Femur

Tibia

■ **Figure 9.14**   Osgood-Schlatter disease (traction tibial apophysitis).

most often in adolescent athletes. The cause is often unknown but may be repetitive insult. Signs and symptoms include a gradual onset of pain and periodic swelling after activity. The athlete may complain of occasional clicking or catching in the joint if there is a loose fragment. Palpable tenderness may be present on the femoral condyle near the joint line.

## NERVE AND VASCULAR INJURIES

The neurovascular structures are well protected at the knee as they pass through the popliteal space. Only with severe joint disruption are these structures at risk. One exception, however, is the common peroneal nerve as it courses superficially around the proximal fibula.

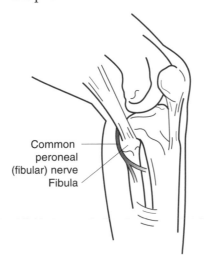

Common peroneal (fibular) nerve
Fibula

■ **Figure 9.15** Location of common peroneal nerve where it courses superficially around the head of the fibula.

### *Peroneal Nerve Palsy*

The common peroneal nerve is vulnerable to injury where it wraps superficially around the head of the fibula (figure 9.15). The nerve can be traumatized secondary to a direct blow (contusion), severe cold (ice bag application), or tractioning (varus injury force). Signs and symptoms of nerve palsy include pain and tenderness over the distal fibula; numbness, burning, or tingling along the lateral aspect of the lower leg and into the dorsum of the foot; and motor weakness of the dorsiflexors, everters, and toe extensors. A foot drop may be noted immediately with severe trauma or may appear progressively over the next day secondary to delayed swelling.

### *Popliteal Artery or Nerve Injury*

The popliteal vessels and nerves are well protected in the popliteal space. Injury to these structures, although rare, can result from a severe fracture or total knee (tibiofemoral) dislocation. Distal pulses and sensory checks should be conducted to assess nerve and vessel integrity with any severe knee trauma.

!  Distal pulses and sensory checks should be conducted to assess nerve and vessel integrity with any severe knee trauma.

## STRUCTURAL AND FUNCTIONAL ABNORMALITIES

Structural abnormalities at the knee have been implicated as predisposing factors in a variety of lower-extremity ailments. The athletic trainer must be able to recognize these abnormalities in order to fully evaluate chronic conditions at the knee. The reference point for the structural abnormalities listed in table 9.1 (see next page) is with the athlete standing with feet straight ahead and knees fully extended. Unless the abnormality is a functional deformity resulting from some pathology, it will typically be noted bilaterally.

# INJURY ASSESSMENT

An injury to the knee is often quite debilitating and can seriously jeopardize an athlete's career in sport. Therefore, accurate assessment, appropriate care, and applicable rehabilitation are absolutely necessary. Since the accurate assessment guides the care and rehabilitation, your initial assessment of the injury is crucial to the athlete's outcome.

## Table 9.1   Structural Abnormalities at the Knee

| Abnormality | Characteristics |
| --- | --- |
| Genu recurvatum | Excessive knee hyperextension; normal knee extension may include a few degrees past neutral; females tend to have greater knee laxity and incidence of knee recurvatum than males; see figure 9.34, page 299 |
| Genu valgus | Excessive valgus (lateral) angulation at the tibia relative to the femur; may be caused by hip anteversion or external tibial torsion; commonly referred to as "knock-kneed"; see figure 9.33, page 299 |
| Genu varus | Decreased valgus or actual varus (medial) angulation at the tibia relative to the femur; may be caused by hip retroversion or internal tibial torsion; commonly referred to as "bowlegged"; see figure 9.31, page 299 |
| Patella alta | The patella sits abnormally high in the femoral groove; indicated by a lengthened infrapatellar tendon relative to the height of the patella |
| Patella baja | The patella sits inferiorly in the femoral groove; indicated by a shortened infrapatellar tendon relative to the height of the patella |
| Quadriceps angle | Excessive angulation (>18-20°) of the quadriceps line (from the anterior superior iliac spine) and the infrapatellar tendon line (from the tibial tubercle) at their bisection through the midpoint of the patella; often associated with genu valgus, hip anteversion, or external tibial torsion; Q-angles are normally higher for females than males; see figure 9.40, page 303 |
| Squinting patella | Medially rotated or inward-facing patellae; may be caused by hip anteversion or external tibial torsion |
| Tibial torsion | Rotation of the tibia such that when the medial and lateral condyles are in the frontal plane, the foot is angled either out or in; external tibial torsion will cause the feet to point outward excessively (slight outward angulation is normal); internal tibial torsion will cause the feet to angle in toward each other ("pigeon-toed"); see figure 9.32, page 299 |

## ON-FIELD ASSESSMENT

Other than the rare occasion when a knee injury includes occlusion of the popliteal artery, this is not an area in which consequences typically threaten life or limb. However, because that rare occasion does exist, you must always be alert in your on-field assessment to immediate signs and symptoms that would indicate a medical emergency.

As you approach the athlete, note the position of the limb and his response. Often the athlete will be holding the injured muscle or joint. If he is holding a flexed knee, the injury is likely to be a knee sprain. A position in which the knee is locked out straight is more indicative of a fracture or dislocation. Upon arriving at the athlete's side, you should include in your primary survey the assessment for obvious deformities indicating fracture or dislocation, severe bleeding, and signs and symptoms of shock. If you note severe deformity, immediately assess neurovascular status by palpating for a posterior tibial or pedal pulse, and perform a cursory sensory assessment over the distribution of the tibial and peroneal nerves. If you note any of the signs and symptoms just mentioned, treat the injury as a medical emergency. If all findings are negative, proceed with your on-field assessment.

Obtain a brief history from the athlete to ascertain the chief complaint, mechanism of injury, type and location of symptoms, and any unusual sounds or sensa-

## Checklist for On-Field Assessment of the Knee and Thigh

### Primary Survey

Observe immediately upon approaching the athlete for the following:

✓ Airway, breathing, and circulation

✓ Position of the limb and athlete's response to injury

✓ Obvious deformity indicative of severe fracture or dislocation

    ✓ If deformity, immediately check neurovascular status

✓ Severe bleeding

✓ Signs and symptoms of shock

If any of the signs listed are positive, treat as a medical emergency. If all of the signs are negative, proceed with your on-field assessment.

### History

Quickly ascertain the following:

✓ Chief complaint

✓ Mechanism of injury

✓ Unusual sounds or sensations

✓ Type and location of pain or symptoms

### Observation

✓ Note immediate swelling, deformity, discoloration.

✓ Note willingness to move the limb or position holding the limb.

### Cursory Palpation to Identify the Following:

✓ Bony tenderness, abnormal contours, or subtle deformities

✓ Soft tissue tenderness, defects or bulges, muscle spasm/guarding

### Special Tests

✓ Perform ligament stress test if sprain suspected.

✓ Perform active ROM if strain suspected.

✓ Compare bilaterally.

If all tests are negative, remove athlete from field with assistance as needed pending more thorough evaluation on the sideline.

---

tions noticed at the time of injury. Since time is of the essence on the field, you need to focus in quickly on the area of injury. Observe the area for immediate signs of swelling, discoloration, or deformity.

Palpate the injured area to determine any areas of bony tenderness or deformity, soft tissue tenderness, defects, or spasm. If a sprain is suspected, whenever possible you should perform a stress test of the ligament immediately after injury to determine the severity or degree of ligament injury. The stress tests will be discussed in detail in connection with the sideline assessment. With a suspected strain, you should perform an active range of motion test. If the motion is weak and painless, you should suspect a rupture; but if the athlete reports pain with movement or resistance, a first- or second-degree strain is likely. Once you have enough information to determine the nature and severity of the injury, you will decide on the mode of transportation from the field. If you have any doubt about the nature of the injury or the athlete's ability to ambulate off the field, use either a passive or an assistive carry to avoid weight bearing pending a more thorough assessment.

## SIDELINE ASSESSMENT

Once the athlete is on the sideline, you can assess the injury further in order to determine more precisely its nature and severity, to decide whether the athlete can return to participation, and to select appropriate immediate treatment.

### History

With the athlete on the sideline and in a calmer state, find out more about her recollection of the injury. If the mechanism was one of contact, note whether the pain is on the same side or on the opposite side of the limb. Pain on the opposite side tends to be indicative of a sprain, and pain on the same side is more indicative of a contusion. If the mechanism was one of noncontact, determine whether the athlete was bearing weight, rotating with the foot planted, or both. See if she can recall whether the knee was flexed, extended, or hyperextended at the time. Was she accelerating (possible meniscus injury) or decelerating (possible cruciate ligament injury)? At this time ask again about any unusual sounds or sensations, current location and type of pain, and any radiation of pain to other areas. Note whether the pain has changed much from the time of injury. Isolated meniscal injuries may cause pain when they occur, but the pain can quickly subside and then return later; in contrast, the pain of a musculotendinous injury does not subside. Ligamentous injuries are not always predictable. It is not uncommon for a third-degree ACL injury to hurt immediately, for the pain to then quickly subside, and for considerable pain to return a few hours or a day later once swelling begins to set in. It is important to take full advantage of this time window and obtain a thorough and accurate evaluation on the sideline, since evaluation will be much more difficult once secondary pain and swelling set in.

Your history should also include questions regarding previous injuries to the lower extremity. Previous ligament or meniscal injuries are particularly important, as they may result in residual laxity or other positive signs that may confound your findings regarding the current injury. And although prior history of injury to the knee is a primary concern, you should also be interested in other lower-extremity injuries. For example, a fractured ankle that was immobilized, requiring the athlete to ambulate on crutches, may have left the knee muscles weak and atrophied and thus susceptible to injury.

### Observation

By this time you have been able to observe how the athlete is responding to the injury, how he moves and protects the injured part, how he stands and walks, and how he transfers from sitting to standing or moves onto the bench, evaluation table, or to the ground. Note any hesitation, evidence of guarding, unequal weight distribution, or favoring of the injured limb with standing and walking. It is important to remember that in some cases an athlete is able to ambulate fairly well following a meniscal or ligament injury. So be careful not to underestimate the injury based on observation alone.

When inspecting the knee itself, observe again for any signs of swelling, discoloration, or deformities. Check the contour and muscle tone of the thigh and lower leg for equal appearance bilaterally. Note any scars that would indicate previous injury. Observe the alignment and relationship of the femur, tibia, and patella.

### Palpation

For palpation the leg is comfortably positioned in slight flexion. Begin palpation with superficial structures and move to deeper tissue, palpating the injured area last. Note any temperature differences, tenderness, swelling, crepitus, incongruency, and differences in soft tissue mobility throughout the palpation process. Although your palpation can follow any systematic routine you desire, the approach described here is a regional one.

Anterior palpation includes the quadriceps muscle group, suprapatellar tendon, suprapatellar pouch, patella, infrapatellar tendon, tibial tuberosity, patellar retinaculum, superficial bursa, and evidence of a plica. The quadriceps and oblique fibers of the vastus medialis (VMO) in particular are palpated for muscle spasm, myofascial restriction, and tenderness. The suprapatellar pouch lies between the superior patella and the muscle belly of the quadriceps. Note the presence of any tenderness, nodules, thickening, or soft tissue restriction in this area. Palpate the patella for areas of tenderness and irregularity, and follow around its medial and lateral borders

When obtaining a history of previous injuries, be sure to ask about both the involved and uninvolved extremities, since you will use the uninvolved knee as your reference for what is "normal" for that individual.

When asking about previous injuries, determine the nature and severity of the injury, the time of onset and duration of the injury and disability, any treatment or surgical interventions, and final outcome.

The results of sideline observations help the athletic trainer create a full picture of the injury's severity, the way the athlete regards the injury, and the amount of disability the athlete has with the injury.

to its apex. You can palpate the medial and lateral articular surfaces of the patella by moving the patella medially and laterally, respectively, and feeling under its rim. Tenderness and roughness may be present if the athlete has a history of patellofemoral dysfunction. From the patella, palpation follows the patellar tendon and tibial tuberosity. Palpate bursae around the anterior knee, in locations superficial and deep to the patellar tendon and over the patella, for tenderness, texture, and swelling. Palpate the patellar retinaculum superiorly, medially, and laterally to the patella for tenderness and restriction of normal tissue mobility. If plica is present, you can palpate it medial to the patella as a thickened ridge running toward the patella either horizontally or at a slight angle.

On the medial aspect of the knee, palpate the medial femoral condyle and epicondyle, and the MCL from its origin on the femoral epicondyle to its insertion just below the joint line on the tibial flare. Palpate the adductor tubercle and pes anserine insertion, medial joint line and tibial plateau, and medial hamstring and gastrocnemius tendons for tenderness and swelling. The pes anserine is located distal to the knee joint medial to the tibial tuberosity. Laterally, palpate the lateral femoral condyle, epicondyle, LCL (lateral epicondyle to fibular head), fibular head, IT band to its insertion on Gerdy's tubercle, lateral joint line, and biceps femoris and gastrocnemius tendons. The LCL is easily palpated if the athlete crosses the ankle of the palpated leg onto the opposite knee. With your fingertips on the lateral joint margin, you should feel the ligament pop into the fingertips as the leg is crossed. The IT band inserts on and just proximal to the fibular head on the tibial condyle and can be followed superiorly toward the tensor fascia lata. Normally a thick, broad band of connective tissue, it should be smooth and not tender.

The medial and lateral joint lines can be more easily palpated with the knee in flexion; they are palpated anteriorly on either side of the patella's apex for tenderness and irregularity. Follow the joint margins around toward the posterior knee as far as possible. As your palpation approaches the posterior joint, the joint margin will be too difficult to palpate. Medially rotating the lower leg allows palpation of the rim of the medial meniscus, and lateral rotation of the lower leg permits palpation of the rim of the lateral meniscus. The tibial and femoral plateaus can also be palpated inferiorly and superiorly to the menisci respectively.

Posteriorly, palpate the hamstrings and gastrocnemius muscle bellies and tendons, as well as the soft tissue structures in the popliteal fossa. Note areas of tenderness, nodules, spasm, and swelling. The pulse of the deep popliteal artery can sometimes be palpated in the posterior center of the knee. The biceps femoris tendon, lateral gastrocnemius tendon, popliteal muscle, and occasionally the posterior aspect of the lateral meniscus and joint margin can be palpated on the posterolateral aspect of the knee. The posteromedial compartment palpation includes identification of the flat semimembranosus tendon and the chordlike semitendinosus tendon that you can follow as it traverses medially and anteriorly into the pes anserine, the medial gastrocnemius, and occasionally the medial meniscus.

### Special Tests

As already mentioned, acute knee injuries often involve ligament, capsular, or meniscal structures and are best assessed immediately following injury. The special tests described here include those tests used to identify and quantify the severity of acute injuries. Other special tests for assessing overuse and alignment injuries will be presented later in connection with the off-field assessment.

## Acute Patella Injury Test—Apprehension Test

It is common for a dislocated patella to spontaneously reduce before you have the opportunity to evaluate the athlete. Although the athlete may or may not be able to describe the injury, he will recall the sensation of the dislocation. If he feels the same sensation during this test, he will contract the quadriceps or stop the test to prevent the patella from dislocating again. This is often referred to as an **apprehension sign**.

With the athlete supine and the quadriceps relaxed, the knee is positioned in 20-30° flexion. Carefully and slowly glide the patella laterally (figure 9.16). A positive test result occurs if the athlete prevents the maneuver or stops the test in anticipation of dislocation of the patella.

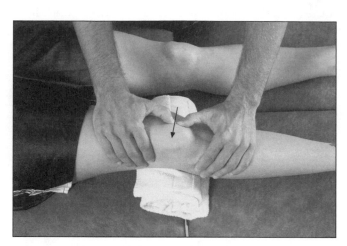

■ **Figure 9.16** Patellar apprehension test.

### Uniplanar Ligament Stress Tests

When applying stress tests, always assess the uninvolved extremity first. To ensure muscular relaxation during the test, instruct the athlete to relax prior to the stress test application, and also monitor the muscles during the test. The stress needs to be gentle but forceful enough to produce an accurate result.

Signs and symptoms of severity will be consistent with those generally described for first-, second-, and third-degree sprains in chapter 1. It is important to remember that pain will likely occur during stress tests on new sprains. Therefore it is important that you practice and become proficient at these skills to avoid having to test the knee three to four times to get a good result.

It is important to use the stress tests relatively soon after the injury, before muscle spasm, guarding, and swelling occur, as these can cause inaccurate test results.

When applying stress tests, always assess the uninvolved extremity first. This gives the athlete an understanding of the test to be performed and gives you the information you need in order to make a comparison.

## Valgus Stress Test

The valgus stress test, also known as the abduction or medial instability stress test, is used to assess the integrity of the inert and active structures providing medial joint stability. The athlete is in a supine position with the injured leg relaxed. Place one of your hands around the distal medial lower leg, and position the other hand on the lateral side of the knee. The hand on the lateral knee acts as a fulcrum while the hand on lower leg applies a lateral force to the lower leg to gap the medial joint (figure 9.17). This test is performed with the knee in full extension and in 20-30° flexion. With the knee in extension, the primary structures stressed include the MCL and posteromedial capsule. Other structures, including the posterior and anterior cruci-

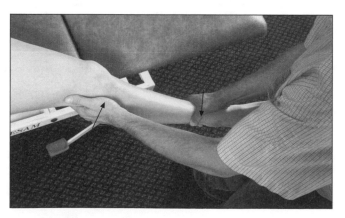

■ **Figure 9.17** Valgus stress test.

ate ligaments, posterior oblique ligament, medial quadriceps muscle, and semimembranosus muscle are also stressed. When the knee is in slight flexion, the primary structure tested is the MCL, since the capsule becomes relaxed; but the medial capsule and other structures including the posterior oblique ligament and PCL can also be stressed. Placing the tibia in external rotation during the stress test in knee flexion will reduce the stress on the PCL; and if the tibia is internally rotated, the stress increases to the cruciate ligaments and decreases to the MCL. If the maneuver causes pain or gapping of the joint in extension, the injury is more severe than is the case if the positive results occur with the knee in partial flexion. You must take care to avoid hip rotation during the stress test so that the force application is appropriate.

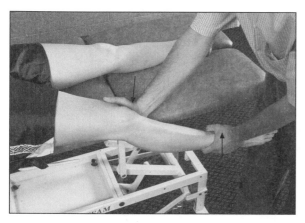

**■ Figure 9.18**  Varus stress test.

### Varus Stress Test

In the varus stress test, also known as the adduction or lateral instability stress test, the athlete is supine with the leg relaxed. Place one hand on the athlete's distal lateral lower leg and the other on the medial aspect of the knee. Using the hand on the knee as a fulcrum, apply a varus force to the knee with the hand on the lower leg (figure 9.18). As with the valgus stress test, perform the test first with the knee in full extension, and then in 20-30° of flexion. Pain or gapping on the lateral joint margin is a positive sign. A positive sign in extension indicates serious instability of the lateral knee. Although the primary structures stressed with the knee in full extension are the LCL and posterolateral capsule, other structures may also be involved, including the arcuate complex, anterior and posterior cruciate ligaments, biceps femoris tendon, IT band, and lateral gastrocnemius. With the knee in slight flexion, the capsule is more lax, so the primary structure involved when the test is positive is the LCL; but other structures such as the posterolateral capsule, arcuate complex, biceps femoris tendon, and IT band may also be involved. If the tibia is externally rotated during this test with the knee in flexion, additional stress will be applied to the LCL. It is important to take care to avoid hip rotation during these stress tests.

### Lachman Test

This one-plane instability test assesses the integrity of the ACL. Also known as the **Ritchie test**, **Lachman-Trillat test**, or **Trillat test**, it has become the test of choice for evaluating anterior cruciate sufficiency. With the athlete supine, grasp her distal thigh with one hand and grasp the medial proximal tibia just below the knee joint with the other hand. The knee is placed in approximately 20-30° flexion, which

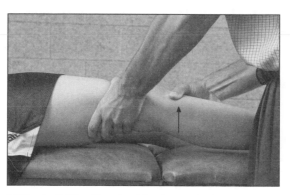

**■ Figure 9.19**  Standard Lachman test.

is the resting position of the joint (loose-packed) and which isolates the anterior cruciate as the primary restraint to anterior tibial translation. With the tibia in slight external rotation to clear the posterior meniscal horns from the femoral condyles, apply a posteromedial-to-anterolateral translational force to the tibia while stabilizing the thigh (figure 9.19). The result is positive if the tibia translates forward more than on the contralateral knee.

For examiners with small hands who are testing an athlete with a large thigh, there are a number of alternative positions for a Lachman test. Two common positions are shown in figures 9.20 and 9.21. In figure 9.20, the tibia is held between the examiner's thigh and the side of the table so that the limb is better stabilized in 20-30° of flexion while the examiner pulls forward on the tibia. In figure 9.21, the examiner's knee is under the athlete's distal thigh. This allows the hand on the thigh to simply stabilize the thigh against the knee while the other hand is used to translate the tibia anteriorly.

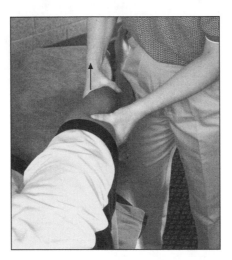

**Figure 9.20**   Modified Lachman test with the thigh stabilized between the examiner's leg and the side of the table.

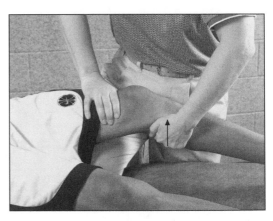

**Figure 9.21**   Modified Lachman test with the thigh stabilized between the examiner's knee and hand.

### Anterior Drawer Test

This test, which also assesses the integrity of the ACL, was the primary assessment tool for ACL instability until the Lachman test appeared. Although many still use the anterior drawer test, it is not as reliable as the Lachman, primarily because of the knee flexion angles it uses. Whereas the Lachman test uses limited knee flexion, the anterior drawer test is performed at 90° of flexion. In a more flexed knee position, other capsular and ligamentous structures are also taut, and the hamstrings are in an optimal position to oppose anterior tibial translation when contracted or in spasm. Because of these potential secondary restraints, an isolated tear of the ACL may produce a false-negative test result.

For the anterior drawer test, the athlete lies supine with the hip flexed about 45° and the knee flexed 90° so that the foot is positioned flat on a table or the ground. Place your hands around the proximal tibia with your thumbs over the joint margins anteriorly. The athlete's foot is in a neutral position and anchored by your thigh. With your hands in contact with the hamstring tendons to monitor their relaxation, pull the tibia forward (figure 9.22). Normal excursion is about 4-6 mm. Motion greater than that or greater than the uninvolved side indicates possible injury to the ACL, as well as possible involvement of the posterior capsule, MCL, IT band, posterior oblique ligament, and arcuate complex.

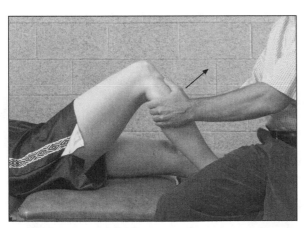

**Figure 9.22**   Anterior drawer test.

## Posterior Drawer Test

This test is used to identify instability of the PCL. The position and hand placements are the same as for the anterior drawer test. The tibia is then pushed posteriorly on the femur (figure 9.23). Since structures other than the posterior cruciate provide posterior stability, including the posterior oblique ligament, arcuate complex, and ACL, they are also stressed in this test. If they are intact but the PCL is damaged, the test may be negative or may demonstrate only moderate instability.

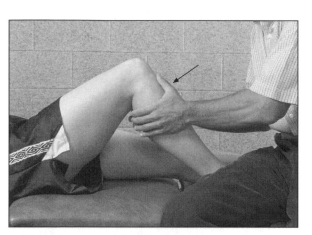

**I Figure 9.23**   Posterior drawer test.

## Posterior Sag Sign

This test is also referred to as the gravity drawer test or the drop back sign. It is used to identify instability of the PCL and related injury of the ACL, posterior capsule, and arcuate complex. A positive sign can also indicate injury to the IT band and LCL. Place the athlete's lower extremity in the drawer test position with the hip flexed to 45°, the knee flexed to 90-110°, and the foot flat on the table. A positive sign occurs if the tibia sags posteriorly on the femur in comparison to the uninvolved side (figure 9.24). For this test the quadriceps should be completely relaxed, as contraction of the quadriceps can pull the tibia forward and make the tibial position appear normal.

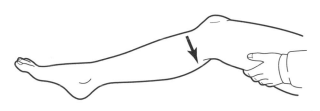

**I Figure 9.24**   Posterior sag sign.

### Multiplanar Stress Tests

These tests incorporate the use of rotatory forces to the ligaments to aid in assessing joint stability. Generally, positive results indicate a severe injury to the cruciate ligaments and joint capsule. Other structures such as the arcuate complex, collateral ligaments, and tendons may also be affected.

## Slocum Test

The Slocum test evaluates medial and lateral anterior rotary instabilities. The athlete lies supine on the table with the involved hip flexed to 45°, the knee at 90° flexion, and the foot flat on the table (i.e., drawer position). To test anterolateral rotary instability, the lower leg is rotated so that the foot is placed at 30° internal rotation. Anchor the foot with your thigh, and place both hands behind the proximal tibia with your thumbs on the joint margins as for the anterior drawer test. Then translate the tibia forward. If anterolateral rotary instability is present, the lateral side of the tibia moves forward more than on the uninvolved knee. Involved structures may include the ACL, posterolateral capsule, arcuate complex, LCL, PCL, and IT.

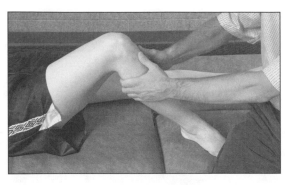

∎ **Figure 9.25**   Starting position of the Slocum test for anteromedial rotary instability. Note the external rotation of the tibia.

For assessment of anteromedial rotary instability, the foot is positioned in 15° of external rotation (figure 9.25). The positions are otherwise the same as those just described except for the tibial rotation component. Assess anterior translation of the tibia as just described; excessive movement will occur primarily on the medial side if instability is present, indicating injury to the ACL, posteromedial capsule, MCL, posterior oblique ligament, or more than one of these.

## Lateral Pivot Shift Maneuver

This test, also known as the **McIntosh test**, assesses anterolateral instability. It is used primarily to identify anterior cruciate ruptures, but positive results also indicate possible injury to the posterolateral capsule, arcuate complex, LCL, and IT.

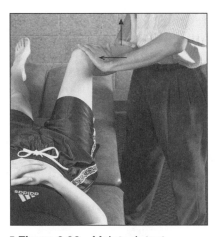

∎ **Figure 9.26**   McIntosh test.

With the athlete in supine, position the hip of the involved extremity in 30° abduction, 30° flexion, and about 20° internal rotation. Use one hand to place the knee in about 5-10° of flexion by putting the heel of the hand behind the fibula, over the lateral gastrocnemius muscle. With the other hand, grasp the ankle and hold the leg in slight internal rotation. Attempt to sublux the tibia anteriorly with a shift maneuver by applying a valgus stress to the knee while maintaining internal rotation of the tibia and moving the knee into extension (figure 9.26). If the test is positive and the IT band is intact, at 20-40° the tibia "slips" backward as the IT band's line of pull changes from that of a knee extensor to that of a knee flexor as the knee is moved into flexion.

## Hughston's Test

∎ **Figure 9.27**   Hughston's test.

This test is also referred to as the jerk test of Hughston and, similarly to the lateral pivot shift test, is used to assess anterolateral instability of the knee. With the athlete in supine, the hip is flexed to 45° and the knee to 90°. While maintaining the lower leg in internal rotation, apply valgus stress and simultaneous knee extension (figure 9.27). If the test is positive, at 20-30° of knee flexion the lateral tibia jerks forward as the lateral tibial plateau subluxes.

## Meniscal Tears

As with ligament instability, several assessment tests for meniscal injuries are available. Because the menisci are primarily aneural, these tests are not always reliable; pain is often considered the positive sign, but may not be present unless surrounding structures are also irritated or inflamed. The most commonly used tests will be presented here.

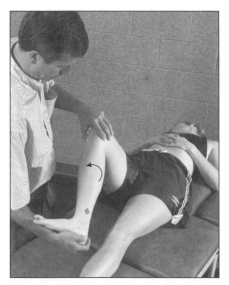

**Figure 9.28** McMurray test for medial meniscus.

### McMurray Test

With the athlete in supine, place one hand on top of the knee and the other hand around the heel. Move the leg passively into full flexion. Rotate the tibia externally and move it into extension to stress the medial meniscus (figure 9.28). To stress the lateral meniscus, reposition the leg into full flexion and internally rotate the tibia before moving it into extension. Joint line pain or an audible click is considered a positive sign.

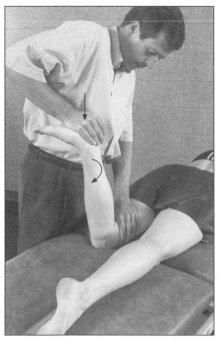

**Figure 9.29** Compression and external rotation of tibia with the Apley test.

### Apley Test

With the athlete in prone, stabilize her thigh with your knee and passively flex the involved knee to 90°. Rotate the tibia into internal and external rotation while applying traction to the knee. Then repeat the rotation movements while compressing the knee joint (figure 9.29). If the athlete reports pain with distraction, the injury is likely ligamentous; but if she reports pain with compression, the injury more probably involves the meniscus.

### *Range of Motion*

Active range of motion testing at the knee should include flexion (~135°) and extension (~0°), and internal (10-20°) and external (20-30°) tibial rotation (figure 9.30, a-d) (see next page). Active extension and flexion are best evaluated with the athlete supine; internal and external tibial rotation are best performed with the athlete seated and the lower leg hanging off the edge of a table or bench. As the athlete moves the knee through the range of motion, observe for equal and full movement bilaterally, noting any hesitation, pain, or audible clicks during motion. Active knee hyperextension (i.e., –5-10°) is not uncommon but should be equal bilaterally and pain free.

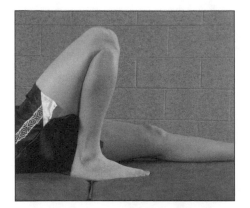
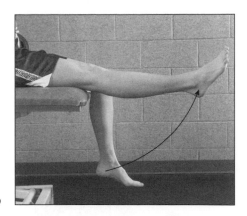

a

b

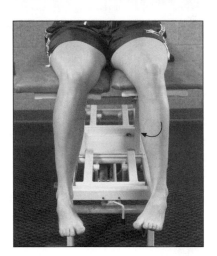

c                                    d

**▌ Figure 9.30**  Range of motion of the knee, including (a) flexion, (b) extension, (c) internal tibial rotation, and (d) external tibial rotation.

Passive motion will be slightly greater than active motion moving into flexion. Overpressure in flexion should be a soft tissue end feel as the calf moves against the posterior thigh. Overpressure in extension and internal and external tibial rotation is a firmer end feel as the soft tissue is stretched at the end of the motion. Range of motion and motion extremes should be pain free for all motions.

You can also assess passive patellar motion on the sideline with medial, lateral, inferior, and superior glide motions using the thumb and index fingers. Medial and lateral glide excursion can occur up to half the width of the patella in each direction.

### Strength

Isometric strength assessment is performed at multiple knee positions for the quadriceps and hamstrings. Quadriceps resistance can be applied at 0°, 30°, 60°, and 90°. Hamstring resistance can be applied with the knee at 90° and the tibia in neutral, internal rotation, and external rotation. Hip flexion and ankle plantar flexion strength should be assessed with the knee extended, since muscles producing these motions also cross the knee joint.

### Neurovascular Tests

With a blow to the lateral aspect of the knee, the common fibular nerve can be contused, and the athlete may complain of pain, tingling, or numbness referred down the lateral aspect of the lower leg and top of the foot. If you think the nerve may be involved, perform sensory and motor testing over the distribution of the common fibular nerve. The sensory component is evaluated over the lateral aspect of the leg

## Checklist for Sideline Assessment of the Knee and Thigh

### History

Ask questions pertaining to the following:

✓ Chief complaint

✓ Mechanism of injury (contact vs. noncontact)

✓ Position of the knee/foot at time of injury

✓ Unusual sounds or sensations

✓ Type and location of pain or symptoms

✓ Previous injury to involved and uninvolved extremities

### Observation

✓ Check for visible facial expressions and response to injury.

✓ Check for swelling, deformity, abnormal contours, or discoloration.

✓ Note gait, willingness to bear weight.

✓ Observe overall position, posture, and alignment of lower extremity.

✓ Compare bilaterally.

### Palpation

Palpate for pain, tenderness, crepitus, defects, and deformity over the following:

✓ Quadriceps muscle (including VMO), suprapatellar tendon, suprapatellar pouch, patella, infrapatellar tendon, tibial tuberosity, patellar retinaculum, superficial bursae

✓ Evidence of plica

✓ Medial femoral condyle and epicondyle, MCL, adductor tubercle, pes anserine insertion, medial joint line and tibial plateau, medial hamstring and gastrocnemius tendons

✓ Lateral femoral condyle and epicondyle, LCL, fibular head, IT band, Gerdy's tubercle, lateral joint line and tibial plateau, biceps femoris and gastrocnemius tendons

✓ Hamstring and gastrocnemius muscle bellies and tendons, popliteal fossa

### Special Tests

✓ Patellar apprehension

✓ Uniplanar ligament stress tests (valgus, varus, Lachman test, anterior drawer, posterior drawer, and sag)

✓ Multiplanar ligament stress tests (Slocum, lateral pivot shift, Hughston's)

✓ Meniscal tests (McMurray's, Apley's)

✓ Bilateral comparison

### Range of Motion

✓ Active ROM for knee flexion and extension, internal and external tibial rotation

✓ Passive ROM for the same motions

✓ Passive ROM for medial, lateral, inferior, and superior patellar glide

✓ Bilateral comparison

### Strength Tests

✓ Perform manual resistance against knee flexion and extension, hip flexion and extension, ankle plantar flexion.

✓ Check bilaterally and note any pain or weakness.

### Neurovascular Tests (If Warranted)

✓ Sensory, motor (common fibular nerve)

✓ Popliteal, posterior tibial, and pedal pulses

✓ Sensory, motor, and reflex of lumbar plexus

### Functional Tests

---

(superficial peroneal) and the dorsum of the foot in the first web space (deep peroneal). Motor testing is performed for ankle dorsiflexion and eversion. If the neuropraxia is severe, a foot drop may be observable. Tibial nerve injury is very uncommon, as this nerve is well protected in the popliteal fossa. Integrity of the tibial nerve is tested for sensation over the posterior medial plantar heel, and motor function with plantar flexion and toe flexion. If neurological involvement proximal to the knee is suspected, dermatome and myotome assessment of the lumbar plexus is also warranted (see chapter 7 and table 2.2). If the injury may result in vascular compromise, pulses should be palpated at the popliteal fossa (popliteal/tibial artery), posterior medial ankle (posterior tibial artery), and dorsum of the foot (dorsalis pedis artery).

### Functional Tests

As mentioned previously, it is important to consider both your subjective and objective findings when determining whether or not the athlete can return to sport participation. For example, consider a meniscal injury profile, which often includes immediate pain that quickly subsides and does not return until later. If you rely only on subjective reports of no pain by the athlete following injury, you may allow her to return prematurely—and with that decision expose her to the potential of a more serious injury. In addition to subjective assessment, you must be confident in your objective assessment in order to make the best determination about participation status. If ever in doubt, the safer approach is to defer the functional assessment and restrict participation for the remainder of the day, to see how the knee responds.

If you are confident that the knee injury is minor and that it may be appropriate for the athlete to return to participation, you will perform a functional assessment before making a final decision. Since the ankle, knee, and hip encounter the same stresses during sport participation, the functional tests are similar to those discussed for ankle injuries (see chapter 8).

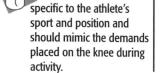
Functional tests should be specific to the athlete's sport and position and should mimic the demands placed on the knee during activity.

## OFF-FIELD ASSESSMENT

Athletes often do not report an injury until the next day, as pain and swelling are frequently delayed. The assessment procedures for these injuries are similar to those at the sideline, but include a more in-depth history and differential diagnostic tests to rule out involvement of other joints. Unfortunately, these injuries are often more difficult to evaluate once pain, swelling, and muscle guarding have set in; so in this situation you must rely more heavily on the history before proceeding with the evaluation. You will also see many chronic and overuse injuries in the athletic training facility. These warrant investigation in other realms, including structural and postural assessment of the entire lower-extremity chain, joint mobility assessment, and soft tissue assessment, since these factors often contribute to these types of injuries.

### History

After determining the initial onset and mechanism of injury, duration of symptoms, and immediate response to the injury, investigate the athlete's current complaints and symptoms. Find out how the knee pain has changed since the initial injury and what activities aggravate the symptoms. Ask the athlete to describe his pain. Sharp pain may indicate a mechanical problem; an aching pain accompanied by stiffness often indicates inflammation. Generalized pain may point to partial musculotendinous tears, large joint effusions, or contusions. Knee pain with ankle movement may indicate tibiofibular joint dysfunction.

Determine whether the athlete is experiencing any grating, clicking, locking, or giving out of the knee. Grating in the anterior aspect of the knee is common with degenerative patellofemoral disorders. Clicking and snapping are common complaints when inflamed tendons, such as the IT band and hamstring tendons, ride over other structures. Locking can be a sign that either a loose body or a meniscal tear is interfering with normal joint motion. Giving out can be a sign of instability, meniscal injury, and patellar subluxation, or it may simply occur secondary to pain and muscle weakness. Pain that affects daily activities such as stair climbing, squatting, standing, or prolonged sitting often relates to patellofemoral dysfunction.

Asking about the swelling behavior of the knee will also yield important clues. Find out whether the swelling occurred immediately after injury or later. Swelling that occurs within 2-3 h following injury is most often the result of blood extravasation. Swelling that occurs 8-24 h after injury or irritation is usually the result of synovial irritation. If the swelling is chronic, see if you can determine what activities cause the knee to swell. When the swelling does occur, is it localized (i.e., bursa) or diffuse?

As with chronic injuries at other joints, always consider the athlete's training history and type of footwear. Training on hills (particularly downhill) and training on slanted surfaces are common factors associated with patellofemoral pain and IT band friction syndrome. Any abrupt change in training intensity, duration, surface, or type of training is often a predisposing factor to chronic inflammatory conditions. By the time you have completed the history portion of the assessment, you should have a good sense of the stage, irritability, nature, and severity of the injury, as well as of how aggressive you can be in the objective portion of the assessment. You should also be aware of any previous injuries to either lower extremity, as well as any previous occurrences of the current complaint.

### Observation

In addition to making the observations outlined for the sideline assessment, inspect for structural and biomechanical abnormalities that may be contributing or causative factors in chronic or overuse injuries (see table 9.1). Posture and alignment of the lower extremities must be observed from anterior, posterior, and lateral views. Hip and ankle alignment, which can also impact the knee, must also be evaluated for their potential influence.

*Genu varum (varus) is a decrease in the normal valgus angle or a medial angulation of the tibial relative to the femur. See also table 9.1.*

*Genu recurvatum is excessive hyperextension of the tibiofemoral joint. See also table 9.1.*

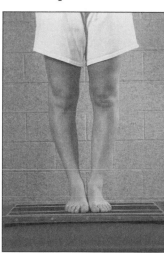

■ **Figure 9.31** Genu varum (varus).

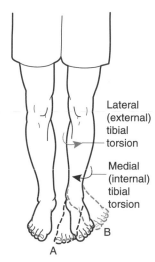

■ **Figure 9.32** Lateral tibial torsion (A) and medial tibial torsion (B). The arrows show the direction of rotation.

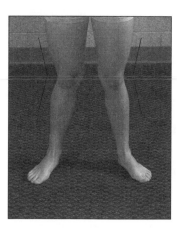

■ **Figure 9.33** Genu valgus.

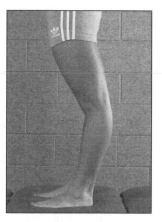

■ **Figure 9.34** Genu recurvatum.

Any abnormal alignment of the lower extremity or pelvis can cause compensatory changes at the knee and place increased stress on its supporting structures. For example, genu varus (figure 9.31) can be related to pes cavus, internal tibial rotation (figure 9.32), hip abduction, or excessive external hip rotation. Genu valgus (figure 9.33) can be secondary to pes planus, external tibial rotation (figure 9.32), hip adduction, or excessive internal hip rotation. Genu recurvatum (figure 9.34) can be related to excessive internal hip rotation with pes planus or to tightness of the ankle or gastrocnemius restricting dorsiflexion. Therefore, it is important to focus on the overall alignment of the lower extremity and then assess the collective impact at the knee.

Symmetry of the lower extremities in weight distribution, position, alignment, size, color, and definition should be assessed. Observe for any swelling, atrophy, bruising, scars, or protuberances. In young athletes with anterior knee pain, be sure to note any increased prominence of the tibial tubercle, which may indicate apophysitis or Osgood-Schlatter disease. As part of your general observation you should also note patellar alignment and location relative to the anterior knee and femur. Compare the patellar tilt and rotation left to right. Normal alignment is with the patella facing straight ahead, with no tilt or rotation, and with its inferior pole at the level of the joint margin.

Observe gait with the athlete in shoes and also barefoot. Assess normal gait cadence first. If there are no abnormalities and the athlete is pain free with normal ambulation, you can assess increased speed on a treadmill. You should be familiar with normal gait assessment for walking and running. Perform this evaluation, as for standing, from anterior, lateral, and posterior views. Stride length, swing-through, and weight bearing should be equal left to right. The athlete should move smoothly from heel strike to foot flat to toe-off without hesitation or imbalances from one side to the other. Shortened stride length, less weight-bearing time on the involved leg with a reduced swing through time on the uninvolved leg, rapid foot flat, limited toe-off, and a dropping of the contralateral hip (Trendelenburg gait, chapter 10) are all indications of a reluctance to bear weight on the involved extremity because of pain, weakness, or limited motion.

For more explicit information on techniques for assessing posture and ambulation, refer to *Therapeutic Exercise for Athletic Injuries* (Houglum 2000), chapters 11 and 12.

### Differential Diagnosis

Because the back, hip, and ankle can all refer symptoms to the knee, you must eliminate each of these areas as possible causes of the athlete's complaints before proceeding to a full knee assessment. A scanning examination is used to rule out causes for knee symptoms other than knee structures.

For ruling out the back as a source of knee pain, standing range of motion with overpressure is the most widely recognized technique. The athlete stands and goes into full trunk flexion, extension, and side-bending, all with overpressure. In sitting, trunk rotation with overpressure is performed. The hip is ruled out with the athlete in supine. The athlete performs active hip flexion, abduction, and rotation; and overpressure techniques are applied at the end of each motion. The ankle is ruled out in similar fashion with both active motion and passive overpressures to each motion. You should further evaluate any pain caused by these tests that refers to the knee before continuing with your knee assessment.

### Range of Motion

Range of motion assessment of the knee is performed actively and passively as discussed for the sideline assessment. Provide overpressure if the athlete reports no pain with active motion. If pain does occur with active motion, there is no need to apply overpressure, since active motion has accomplished the goal of reproducing the athlete's symptoms. Overpressure will also cause undue stress to the knee and should be avoided when pain on active motion occurs.

You should pay careful attention to the presence of an **extensor lag**. With this condition the athlete is unable to fully extend the knee during active motion, but full passive motion is present. An extensor lag is usually the result of quadriceps weakness or inhibition secondary to pain or chronic swelling. It is important that the athlete regain this active motion before returning to activity.

### Strength

Manual resistance is the most efficient method of strength assessment off the field and is consistent with that for the sideline assessment. Often the athlete with patellofemoral pain will tolerate a series of isometric tests at varying angles better than she will tolerate resistance applied through a full range of motion. Isometric tests at incremental angles will also help you identify the point in the range of motion at which the pain or compression may be occurring.

Manual resistance should also include assessment of the ankle (chapter 8) and hip muscles (chapter 10), since prolonged disability secondary to chronic or overuse pain can result in disuse atrophy, muscle imbalance, an antalgic (abnormal) gait, or some combination of these. You must find out about deficiencies in any lower-extremity muscle group so that they can be corrected during the rehabilitation program.

Mechanical assessment of strength through the use of weight machines and isokinetic equipment is more objective than manual muscle testing. One must be cautious, however, in deciding to use machine and isokinetic equipment because of the additional stress these devices can impose on the knee. For example, the applied forces these machines create can aggravate patellofemoral dysfunction and exacerbate symptoms. Moreover, when pain is present with these tests, muscle strength results will be inaccurate because of the pain withdrawal reflex that occurs. In these instances, mechanical and even manual strength assessment may have to be deferred until later.

### Neurological Tests

When the athlete reports symptoms of tingling, numbness, shooting pain, burning, or weakness, a neurological assessment is performed. This may begin as a scanning evaluation followed by a more detailed neurological evaluation if positive findings are noted.

The sensory examination includes either a light touch or pinprick assessment of the dermatomes within the lower extremity. The assessment is the same as that discussed for the lumbar region. Readers may refer to back to chapter 7, figure 7.8, for the dermatome and peripheral nerve (chapter 8) sensory distribution of the lower extremity.

Motor assessment incorporates manual muscle tests to evaluate any weakness associated with a particular nerve root. Motor tests include isometric manual resistance to hip flexion (L1-2), knee extension (L3-4), ankle dorsiflexion (L4), great toe extension (L5), ankle eversion or hip extension (S1), and knee flexion (S2). (See also chapter 7, figure 7.27.) Motor tests for peripheral nerves include plantar flexion and toe flexion (posterior tibial), eversion (superficial peroneal) and dorsiflexion and great toe extension (deep peroneal) (figure 9.35).

Deep tendon reflex assessment is most often performed on the quadriceps tendon (L3-L4), but it can be performed on any lower-extremity tendon, including the Achilles tendon (S1-S2) and hamstring tendon (L5-S1) (see chapter 2, table 2.2, and chapter 7).

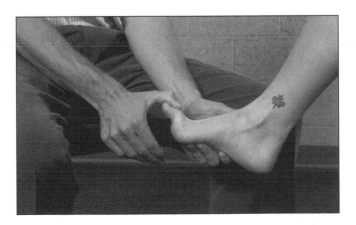

❙ **Figure 9.35**  Motor assessment of great toe extension.

### *Special Tests*

The special tests presented for the sideline assessment are also used in assessment off the field. Tests for overuse injuries are included if chronic symptoms are indicated by the athlete's history and previous objective tests.

**Tests for Swelling**

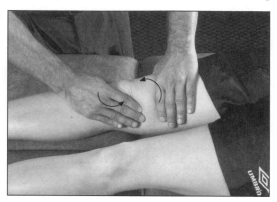

■ **Figure 9.36**  Sweep test.

#### Sweep Test

This test, also known as the brush test, stroke test, or wipe test, detects minimal joint effusion. With the knee relaxed in full extension, stroke the medial aspect of the knee from distal to the joint margin upward into the suprapatellar pouch in a sweeping motion toward the hip. With the other hand, stroke downward on the lateral side of the patella toward the little toe (figure 9.36). If there is any excess fluid in the knee, a small bulge or wave on the medial aspect of the knee just inferior to the patella will be noticeable within 1 to 2 s.

#### Ballotable Patella Test

This test, also referred to as the patellar tap test or the dancing patella sign, assesses moderate to severe effusion. With the knee in a comfortable position near full extension, apply light pressure or a tap to the top of the patella (figure 9.37). The test is positive if the patella bounces or seems to "float" or "bob."

**Tests for Patellofemoral Dysfunction**

#### Grind Test

The grind test evaluates the integrity of the articulating surface of the patellofemoral joint. With the thigh relaxed and the knee in full extension, place the web of one of your hands just proximal to the superior pole of the patella. Push down on the thigh and instruct the athlete to contract the quadriceps (figure 9.38). A positive test occurs if the athlete reports pain. This test can produce a positive sign on almost everyone if administered incorrectly. Be cautious about the amount of force you apply, as well as the location. The force should be applied in a gradual fashion, immediately superior to the patella, not directly over it. The test should be repeated three to four times, each time with application of a greater force. It is also repeated in different knee flexion positions to coincide with the various patellofemoral articular contacts: 30°, 60°, and 90°.

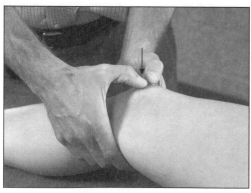

■ **Figure 9.37**
Ballotable patella
test.

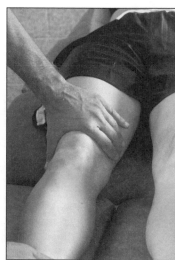

■ **Figure 9.38**
Grind test.

## Lateral Glide Test

This test identifies a tightness of the lateral thigh structures or muscle imbalance of the quadriceps that contributes to patellofemoral pain syndrome. The athlete lies supine with her legs in extension and the thigh muscles relaxed. Instruct the athlete to contract the quadriceps, and observe the patellar movement. Normally the patella will move to an equal extent superiorly and laterally (figure 9.39). A positive sign is present if the patella moves laterally an excessive amount. The athlete can also perform this test in a straddle squat, with the involved leg in front and the uninvolved leg behind, for assessment of lateral glide during weight bearing.

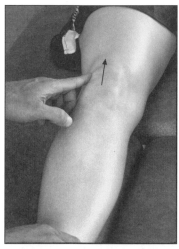

■ **Figure 9.39** Active lateral glide test.

## Patellofemoral (Quadriceps) Angle

This test, also called the quadriceps or Q-angle, measures the angle between the quadriceps muscle and the patellar tendon. With the athlete supine, the leg in full extension, and the hip and foot in neutral positions, draw a line from the anterior superior iliac spine to the midpoint of the superior patella. Draw another line from the tibial tuberosity to the midpoint of the patella (figure 9.40). Normal patellofemoral angle for men is approximately 10-12° and for women is approximately 15-18°. Angles less than 10° or more than 18° are abnormal, and can be a contributing factor to patellofemoral pain syndrome.

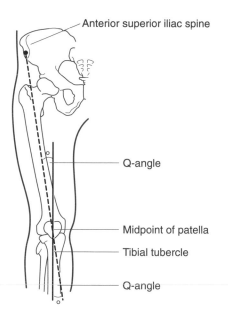
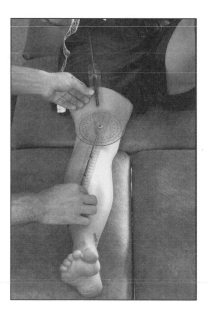

Anterior superior iliac spine

Q-angle

Midpoint of patella

Tibial tubercle

Q-angle

■ **Figure 9.40** Measurement of Q-angle as shown in both the line drawing and photo.

## Other Special Tests

### Wilson Test

The Wilson test assesses the presence of osteochondritis dissecans if the location of injury is the classic site near the intercondylar notch on the medial aspect of the medial femoral condyle. With the athlete sitting and her lower legs over the end of

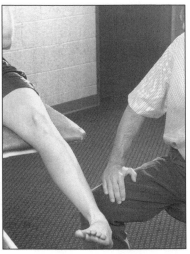

**■ Figure 9.41**    Wilson test.

the table, the knee is actively extended with the lower leg in internal rotation (figure 9.41). If the test is positive, the athlete will report pain in the knee at about 30° from full extension and a resolution of the pain if the lower leg is externally rotated.

### Noble Compression Test

This test is used to assess the presence of IT band friction syndrome. The athlete is in supine, and the involved knee is passively flexed to 90° and the hip to at least 45°. Apply and maintain pressure just proximal to the lateral femoral condyle while the knee is passively or actively extended (figure 9.42). The test is positive if the athlete reports pain over the lateral femoral condyle when the knee is approximately 30° from full extension as the IT band passes over the femoral condyle.

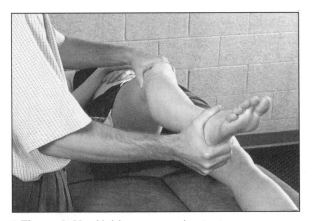

**■ Figure 9.42**    Noble compression test.

### Joint Mobility

The knee's capsular pattern is more limited in flexion than in extension. If this is the range of motion profile of the athlete with reduced range of motion, you should perform joint mobility assessment to determine the specific capsular restrictions limiting normal motion. Assess joint accessory movements of the patellofemoral, tibiofemoral, and tibiofibular joints. Always compare with the contralateral joint to determine normal mobility for the athlete. A positive sign for each of these tests is pain and restricted mobility in comparison to the opposite side.

### Patellofemoral Joint—Patellar Glides

This maneuver assesses patellar mobility. If patellar mobility is restricted, knee flexion may be limited. The athlete is supine with the knee extended and the muscles relaxed. Place the flat part of your thumbs against the lateral patella and glide it medially; then use the flat part of the fingers on the medial patella to move it laterally (figure 9.43). Inferior and superior glides should also be assessed. It is not uncommon for patellar glide restrictions to be bilateral. For this reason, comparison to the uninvolved side may tell you that the range is normal for that person but may not indicate that mobility

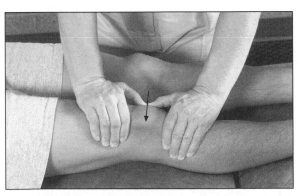

**■ Figure 9.43**    Lateral patellar glide.

is sufficient. Therefore it is helpful to practice your assessment techniques on multiple individuals to get a better sense of what may be considered restricted versus normal mobility.

### Tibiofemoral Joint—Dorsal Tibial Glide

This movement is used to assess joint mobility and end feel of the knee joint. If flexion is limited, mobility in the maneuver will be restricted compared to that for the opposite knee. The athlete is supine, with a towel roll under the distal femur and the knee muscles relaxed. Place one hand over the other for leverage over the proximal tibia just distal to the knee joint (figure 9.44). Apply an anterior-to-posterior force parallel to the joint surface.

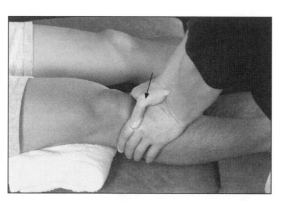

**▌Figure 9.44** Dorsal tibial glide.

### Tibiofemoral Joint—Ventral Tibial Glide

This test is for tibiofemoral joint mobility, which will be limited if the athlete has restricted knee extension range of motion. The athlete lies supine with his hip and knee flexed so that his foot rests comfortably on the table. Place both hands around the proximal tibia as close to the joint margin as possible (figure 9.45). Instruct the athlete to relax the leg muscles, and apply a posterior-to-anterior force parallel to the joint surface.

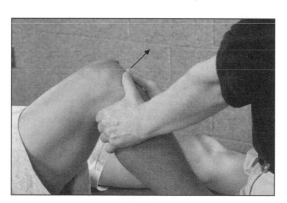

**▌Figure 9.45** Ventral tibial glide.

### Anteroposterior Fibular Glide

This maneuver assesses the mobility and end feel of the superior tibiofibular joint. Restriction of the joint, which can result from knee or ankle injuries, can influence ankle mobility. With the athlete supine and his hip and knee flexed so that his foot is flat on the top of the table, grasp the fibular head with your mobilizing hand and place your stabilizing hand around the superior tibia (figure 9.46). Perform a glide motion from anterior to posterior and then from posterior to anterior to assess mobility and end feel.

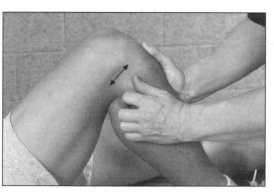

**▌Figure 9.46** Anteroposterior fibular glide.

# Checklist for Off-Field Assessment of the Knee and Thigh

## History

Ask questions pertaining to the following:

- ✓ Chief complaint
- ✓ Mechanism of injury
- ✓ Unusual sounds or sensations (grating, clicking, locking, giving out, referred pain)
- ✓ Type, quality, and location of pain or symptoms
- ✓ Previous injury
- ✓ Previous injury to opposite extremity for bilateral comparison
- ✓ Previous injury to involved and uninvolved lower extremities

If chronic, ascertain:

- ✓ Onset and duration of symptoms
- ✓ Aggravating and easing activities
- ✓ Training history
- ✓ Footwear

## Observation

- ✓ Check for visible facial expressions of pain.
- ✓ Check for swelling, deformity, abnormal contours, scars, or discoloration.
- ✓ Check muscle tone and atrophy.
- ✓ Note gait, willingness to bear weight.
- ✓ Check for structural or biomechanical abnormalities of the knee (genu varus, valgus, and recurvatum; Q-angle; patella alta and baja; squinting patellas).
- ✓ Observe overall position, posture, and alignment of lower extremity.
- ✓ Compare bilaterally.

## Differential Diagnosis

- ✓ Clear low back, hip, and ankle with active ROM and overpressure tests.

## Range of Motion

- ✓ Perform active ROM for knee flexion and extension, internal and external tibial rotation.
- ✓ Check for extensor lag.
- ✓ Perform passive ROM for same motions as for active ROM.
- ✓ Perform passive ROM for medial, lateral, inferior, and superior patellar glide.
- ✓ Make bilateral comparison.

## Strength Tests

- ✓ Perform manual resistance against knee flexion and extension, as well as hip flexion, hip extension, and ankle plantar flexion with knee extended.
- ✓ Perform isometrics at incremental angles for patellofemoral disorders.
- ✓ Compare bilaterally and note any pain or weakness.

## Neurovascular Tests

- ✓ Sensory (L1-S2, peripheral)
- ✓ Motor (L1-S2, peripheral)
- ✓ Distal pulse (popliteal, posterior tibial, and dorsalis pedis)

## Special Tests

- ✓ Patellofemoral tests (apprehension, ballotable patella, grind, lateral glide, Q-angle)
- ✓ Uniplanar ligament stress tests (valgus, varus, Lachman, anterior drawer, posterior drawer, and sag)
- ✓ Multiplanar ligament stress tests (Slocum, lateral pivot shift, Hughston's)
- ✓ Meniscal tests (McMurray's, Apley's)
- ✓ Wilson test
- ✓ Noble compression test
- ✓ Compare bilaterally

## Joint Mobility Assessment

- ✓ Tibiofemoral glides (dorsal, ventral)
- ✓ Patellofemoral glides (medial, lateral, superior, inferior)
- ✓ Tibiofibular glides
- ✓ Bilateral comparison

## Palpation

Palpate for pain, tenderness, crepitus, defects, and deformity over the following:

- ✓ Quadriceps muscle (including VMO), suprapatellar tendon, suprapatellar pouch, patella, infrapatellar tendon, tibial tuberosity, patellar retinaculum, superficial bursae
- ✓ Evidence of plica

### Palpation

Palpation is consistent with that performed at the sideline. For optimal palpation, the knee should be palpated in both extension and in flexion to relax and tighten tissues as necessary. Remember that for palpation of the joint line and surfaces adjacent to the joint margin, the knee is best positioned in about 90° of flexion.

### Functional Tests

As mentioned in relation to the sideline assessment, the functional tests for the knee are the same as those for the ankle. Specific skill tests will be dictated by the athlete's sport.

## SUMMARY

1. *Describe the etiology, signs and symptoms, and potential complications associated with acute and chronic injuries of the knee frequently encountered in the physically active.*

   The knee joint is one of the most frequently injured joints in physically active people. It is particularly susceptible to injury because of its lack of bony stability, its reliance on soft tissue structures for stability, and the large mechanical forces imposed on the knee during sport activity. Compressive, varus/valgus, and anterior/posterior shear and rotational forces are constantly applied to the knee joint during sport activities, particularly those that require running, jumping, cutting, and rapid change of directions. When intrinsic or extrinsic forces exceed the structural integrity of the supporting tissues, injury will result. The soft tissue structures of the knee are also prone to chronic inflammatory conditions caused by repetitive friction and overuse. Repetitive kneeling, jumping, and flexion/extension movements are common mechanisms associated with tendinitis and bursitis conditions of the knee. Lower-extremity malalignments can also contribute to overstress injuries of the knee.

2. *Describe the etiology and signs and symptoms, including predisposing structural and biomechanical factors, associated with chronic patellofemoral pathologies.*

   Patellofemoral pain syndrome is a general term used to describe anterior knee pain. Patellofemoral pain can result from a variety of factors that cause patellar malalignment, increased patellofemoral joint compression, and/or poor patellofemoral tracking. These factors include anatomical and biomechanical abnormalities, muscle weakness or imbalance, and training errors. Regardless of the cause, the result is pain, irritation, and sometimes degeneration of the articular surfaces consequent to decreased patellofemoral contact area and increased patellofemoral pressure.

3. *Describe and perform the various stress tests for assessing internal derangement of the knee joint.*

   A variety of stress tests are available to evaluate structural integrity of the knee joint. Tests for uniplanar instability are designed to evaluate the primary and secondary stabilizing structures in a varus, valgus, anterior, or posterior direction. Multiplanar stress tests incorporate rotational forces to check for the presence of rotary instabilities that indicate an injury to one or more of the cruciate ligaments, the joint capsule, and possibly other ligamentous and muscular constraints. Compression tests are used to identify whether the menisci are involved. All stress tests should be performed bilaterally and compared for end feel. Proper positioning and stabilization of the proximal and distal segments are essential for accurate results, and mastering the technique for each test requires practice.

4. *Describe and perform various special tests for assessing patellofemoral dysfunction.*

   The patellofemoral joint is prone to chronic inflammatory and degenerative conditions, and pain in this region is a frequent complaint in the athlete. Special tests for swelling, degeneration, and mobility help determine the nature and severity of the injury. The difficulty is not so much in identifying the nature of problem as in understanding the potential contributing or causative factors. Therefore careful assessment of lower-extremity alignment and structural abnormalities at the knee in standing, walking, and running is an integral part of evaluation.

5. *Perform an on-field assessment of the knee, indicating criteria for immediate medical referral and mode of transportation from the field.*

   Most knee injuries are not life threatening; but before the athlete is moved off the playing field, the athletic trainer must assess for signs and symptoms that could indicate serious injury. Signs of shock, severe bleeding, dislocation, fractures, and compromised neurovascular supply all necessitate precise, deliberate, and efficient management and transportation. The majority of acute injuries will involve the soft tissue structures of the knee. If ligament injury is suspected, a stress test should be performed on the field for best results, before swelling and muscle guarding set in.

6. *Perform a sideline assessment of the knee, including functional criteria for return to activity.*

   Once the athlete is on the sideline, a complete evaluation can determine more precisely the nature and extent of the injury. Important clues to the nature of the injury come from a thorough history of the mechanism and from information about contact versus noncontact. All joint line and soft tissue structures should be palpated at this time, and stress tests for patellofemoral and tibiofemoral joint stability are performed to assess ligament, meniscal, and capsular integrity. Although there may be multiple tests for a particular ligament structure, not all need to be performed; the athletic trainer should choose those tests that best isolate the structure and, in some cases, accommodate the athletic trainer's hand size. Degrees of injury severity for sprains and strains of the knee are consistent with those described in chapter 1.

7. *Perform an off-field assessment of the knee, including assessment of lower-extremity alignment and considerations for differential diagnosis of referring pathologies from the back, hip, foot, and ankle.*

   When an injured athlete is seen for the first time in the athletic injury treatment facility, additional assessment tools are often necessary to determine the nature, severity, irritability, and stage of the injury for postacute and chronic conditions. In the off-field assessment, the athletic trainer must rule out the possibility of referring pathologies from the ankle, hip, and low back through differential diagnostic tests. Joint mobility should be assessed if the athlete has a capsular pattern of reduced range of motion of the knee. Postural and lower-extremity alignment should be assessed for possible abnormalities that may act as contributing or causative factors for chronic, overuse-type injuries. Functional tests for dynamic lower-extremity movements required in the athlete's sport always take place before the athlete is permitted to return to full sport participation.

## REVIEW QUESTIONS

1. What is a potential complication of a severe quadriceps contusion? What causes this complication, and what signs and symptoms would you look for?

2. Discuss the different mechanisms associated with isolated injuries to the four major stabilizing ligaments of the knee. Which structures are involved in an "unhappy triad," and what is a common mechanism for this type of injury?

3. Describe the etiology and signs and symptoms of a meniscus injury. Why are these injuries sometimes difficult to detect, and what special tests would you use to identify injury to these structures?

4. What is the difference between the Lachman test and the anterior drawer test? Which is the preferred test for assessing an isolated ACL injury? Explain your answer.

5. What tendon structures around the knee are most susceptible to chronic inflammatory conditions? Describe the repetitive mechanisms most often associated with each.

6. What are the predisposing factors that may make an individual more prone than others to patellar dislocations? If you suspect that an athlete has suffered a dislocation that has spontaneously reduced, what signs and symptoms would you look for? Include any special tests you would use to confirm your suspicions.

7. Describe the tests you would use to assess rotary instabilities of the knee. For each test, discuss what structures may be involved if the test is positive.

## CRITICAL THINKING QUESTIONS

1. You are evaluating a 14-year-old athlete who was playing soccer. Observing the injury, you noted that his foot was firmly planted and that he appeared to "twist" his knee while an opponent made contact against the lateral aspect of his knee. You note immediate swelling, and the athlete is complaining of severe pain and tenderness along the proximal tibia. He also reported hearing a pop at the time of injury. Given the mechanism observed and these initial findings, what injuries might you suspect, and how would you proceed with your evaluation?

2. What is the difference between patellofemoral pain syndrome and chondromalacia patella? In your evaluation, how might you differentiate chondromalacia patella from other causes of anterior knee pain?

3. A female runner comes to you complaining of anterior knee pain. She reports that she has just returned to training after taking six weeks off because of a tibial stress fracture. She also reports that she has had recurrent anterior knee pain for the past five years and does not seem to know what causes it when it occurs. Given her history of previous injury and her current complaint, describe your observational assessment of this athlete and explain what specifically you would look for to obtain clues to contributing factors. Include any special tests or measurements you would use to confirm your observational findings.

## ADDITIONAL RESOURCES

Hartley, A. 1990. Knee assessment. In *Practical joint assessment: A sports medicine manual* (chapter 8, pp. 464-543). St. Louis: Mosby Year Book.

Hillman, S.K. 2000. *Introduction to athletic training*. Champaign, IL: Human Kinetics.

Houglum, P.A. 2000. *Therapeutic exercise for athletic injuries*. Champaign, IL: Human Kinetics.

# CHAPTER TEN

# Hip, Pelvis, and Groin

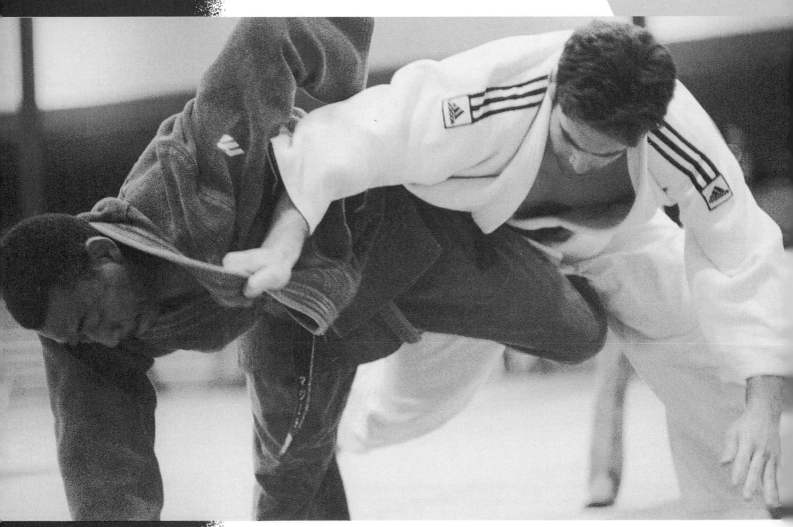

# OBJECTIVES

After finishing this chapter, the reader will be able to do the following:

1. Describe the etiology, signs and symptoms, and potential complications associated with acute and chronic injuries of the hip, pelvis, and groin commonly encountered in the physically active

2. Identify conditions and concerns specific to the pediatric athlete

3. Identify common structural and functional abnormalities of the hip and pelvis

4. Perform an on-field assessment of the hip, pelvis, and groin, noting criteria for immediate medical referral and mode of transportation from the field

5. Perform a thorough and sequential sideline assessment of the hip, pelvis, and groin

6. Perform a thorough and sequential off-field assessment of the hip, pelvis, and groin, including differential diagnosis of referring back and lower-extremity pathologies

7. Describe and differentiate potential causes and conditions of groin pain

Donna was a dual-certified athletic trainer and strength and conditioning specialist working at Silver's Gym in Manhattan Beach. She noticed that Nancy, one of her clients, appeared to be limping when she came into the gym. "Hey Nancy, how are you doing today? You got a bit of a limp there?" Donna asked.

"Hi Donna! . . . yeah, I've had this nagging groin strain for about four weeks now and I'm getting kind of sick of it."

"How do you know it's a groin strain? How did you hurt it?" Donna asked—she was not quite so ready to dismiss the pain as Nancy was.

"I guess I must have slipped or something while running one day, but I can't say I really remember when. I just noticed it starting to hurt one day," Nancy said, trying to remember when it really did start.

"You're a pretty avid runner, right? What did you say you were running, 25-30 miles a week?" Donna tried to recall.

"Yes, that's about right . . . only thing that keeps my sanity!" Nancy said.

"Is there any other activity that makes it hurt?" Donna continued with her questions.

"You know, that's what's interesting about this strain. It hurts while I'm running, but it never bothers me while I'm lifting."

"Nancy, from what you're saying, it may not be a groin strain. . . . It could be a number of things, maybe even a stress fracture from what you are telling me," Donna cautioned.

"A what? A stress fracture . . . no way!"

"I'm not saying it is for sure—I am just saying we should take a closer look and evaluate what is causing your pain. You know, a number of injuries can refer to the groin area. In addition to stress fractures, bursitis and problems from your low back and sacroiliac joints can also cause groin pain. Let's evaluate it and see if we can find out where this pain is coming from. If we can figure that out, we can come up with the right treatment plan to get you better and back to running pain free . . . deal?"

"I'd appreciate that, Donna, thanks."

The hip and pelvis are among the strongest and most stable joints in the body. The pelvic girdle is made up of three joints, the hip joint (acetabular femoral), the sacroiliac joint, and the pubic symphysis, which work in unison to provide both mobility for locomotion and stability to support the upper torso (figure 10.1).

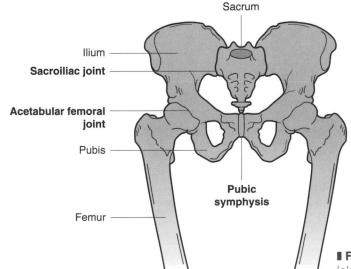

**Figure 10.1** Bony anatomy and joints of the hip and pelvis.

Mobility is provided primarily by the hip joint, which is the only movable joint of the three. The hip is a multiaxial ball-and-socket joint in which the head of the femur fits well into the deep concavity of the acetabulum. The acetabular labrum functions to further deepen the acetabular cavity and embrace the head of the femur. The joint is further strengthened by the articular capsule and the broad ligamentous support provided by the iliofemoral ("Y"), pubofemoral, and ischiofemoral ligaments (figure 10.2). As such, the hip represents the strongest joint in the body; tremendous forces are required to disrupt the integrity of the joint and cause injury. When injury does occur at this joint, long-term complications from avascular necrosis can result if the blood supply to the head of the femur is disrupted.

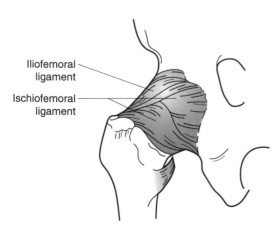

Iliofemoral ligament

Ischiofemoral ligament

**❚ Figure 10.2** Posterior view of the ligamentous support of the hip joint. The pubofemoral ligament can only be seen in the anterior view.

The pelvis or pelvic girdle forms the base of the trunk, which functions to support the abdominal contents and to provide a link between the lumbar spine and the lower extremities. It consists of two innominate bones—each comprising three parts, the ilium, pubis, and ischium—that fuse together between 12 and 16 years of age. Anteriorly, the two innominate bones articulate with each other to form the symphysis pubis; posteriorly, they articulate with the sacrum to form the sacroiliac joints. Very little movement occurs at these joints, lending to their primary function of stability. However, these joints can become irritated or inflamed due to mechanical forces or repetitive stress caused by weight-bearing activity and muscular tension.

The strong muscular support provided to the hip and pelvis lends to their strength, stability, and mobility. The hip and pelvis serve as attachment sites for muscles of the trunk as well as the lower extremity, allowing the transfer of forces between the lower extremity and upper torso. Therefore, the muscles about the hip and pelvis play a major role in locomotion and postural stability; and when muscle injury occurs, weight-bearing and locomotor functions are usually affected.

Given the functional anatomy of the hip and pelvis and the tremendous forces that can be exerted on these structures during sport activity, injuries in this region may range from minor strains and irritations to severe joint disruptions. It is important to appreciate the types of injuries that you may encounter in the physically active and to be able to adequately assess and differentiate these injuries for proper referral and care. The information in this chapter will provide you with both the injury knowledge and the assessment techniques that you will need to identify and differentiate common injuries in the hip and pelvis.

# INJURIES TO THE HIP, PELVIS, AND GROIN

Considerable forces can be transmitted through the hip and pelvis during weight-bearing activities. Primarily because of the strength and stability of the hip and pelvis, injuries to this region are less common than those to the knee and ankle. However, when injuries do occur, even those that are minor can be quite painful and debilitating because of the role these structures play in weight bearing and locomotion.

## ACUTE SOFT TISSUE INJURIES

The most common types of acute injury are contusions, muscle strain (particularly in the groin), and sprains. Traumatic fractures and dislocations are rare, with stress fractures of the femoral neck and avulsion fractures being more common. In children, acute apophysitis and epiphyseal injuries are also a concern.

### Contusions

Because of their many superficial bony prominences, the hip and pelvis are prone to contusions. Most vulnerable to injury are the lateral hip, iliac crest, and coccyx. Contusions to these areas can cause considerable pain and disability, particularly when they occur near a muscular attachment.

Direct contact to the lateral hip can contuse the soft tissue and bursa overlying the greater trochanter. Signs and symptoms include localized pain, swelling, and ecchymosis. The athlete will be point tender over the greater trochanter, and the inflamed bursa may be palpable. Because the greater trochanter serves as the attachment site for the gluteus medius and minimus and the hip rotators, pain and weakness may be present with hip abduction and internal rotation.

Even more disabling is a contusion to the iliac crest, commonly known as a **hip pointer** (figure 10.3). A direct blow can cause considerable pain and hemorrhage along the superficial crest. The athlete will complain of exquisite tenderness at the point of contact and in the surrounding area. Swelling and ecchymosis will be easily observable. Because of the broad attachment of the abdominal muscles along the crest, trunk flexion and rotation, as well as sneezing and coughing, will cause considerable pain. Often the athlete will lean the trunk to the side of injury in an effort to avoid muscular tension at its insertion. Single-leg weight bearing may also be painful on the side of injury. It is not uncommon for a hip pointer to severely restrict an athlete's activity until pain and inflammation subside. Proper padding can protect the area from further insult.

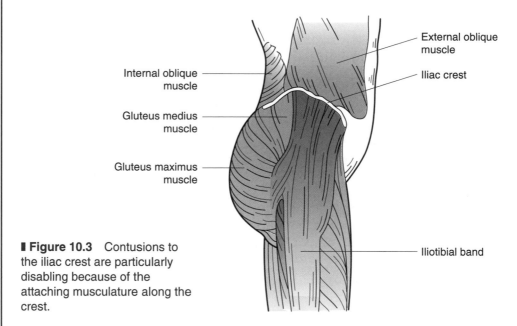

**▌Figure 10.3**  Contusions to the iliac crest are particularly disabling because of the attaching musculature along the crest.

Landing or sitting hard on the "tailbone" can contuse the coccyx. The athlete will complain of pain and difficulty with sitting, particularly when leaning back or slouching. Point tenderness, swelling, and possible discoloration will be observable. If pain persists for an extended period of time, the athlete should be referred to a physician to rule out fracture.

### Sprains

Because of the relative stability of the hip and sacroiliac joints and the strength of the surrounding ligaments, sprains to this region are less common compared to other lower extremity joints. However, when they do occur, physical activity will most likely be limited.

### Sacroiliac Joint

Sacroiliac sprains most often result from "jamming"-type mechanisms—for example, when a basketball player comes down from a rebound and lands off balance on a single leg with the leg straight and the back extended. This can result in the transmission of sizable forces through the lumbosacral and sacroiliac regions, causing joint contusion and possible ligament disruption. Signs and symptoms associated with sprains to this area include pain, swelling, and tenderness over the affected joint and ligaments. Pain may be localized to the involved area but may also be felt as a deep ache or radiating pain into the buttock and thigh. Unilateral or bilateral hip flexion and unilateral leg stance often increase pain. Pain with pelvic rock or Faber's tests (see special tests section) is also a common finding. An "upslip" of the pelvis on the affected side may also be noted.

### Hip Joint

Direct and indirect forces that cause excessive rotation or abduction, or that drive the femur posteriorly when the hip is flexed, can stretch or tear the surrounding ligaments of the hip joint. Extreme rotation at the trunk and hip with the foot planted on the ground is one example. A third-degree sprain that results in hip dislocation is a serious injury that can present considerable complications (see section on dislocations and neurovascular disorders later in this chapter). Signs and symptoms of a hip joint sprain are pain deep in the joint and difficulty with weight bearing. Because the ligaments are covered by the surrounding soft tissue and muscle, it is difficult to palpate them. The athlete will complain of pain with passive movement of the hip as the ligaments become taut. Pain with passive extension and external rotation will tension both the iliofemoral "Y" and the ischiofemoral ligaments (see figure 10.2). Abduction will stress the pubofemoral ligament. Decreased range of motion and pain with active movement will also be noted.

### *Strains*

Muscular strains about the hip are relatively common, resulting from overstretching or from a rapid, forceful contraction of the muscle. Explosive starts and slipping of the foot during cutting are common mechanisms for hip flexor and adductor strains. Abductor strains occur less frequently but can result from quick and forceful movements such as cutting away from the side of the plant leg. Improper warm-up, muscle fatigue, and weakness will increase an athlete's risk for muscle strain; thus these injuries frequently occur during the beginning of practice and preseason training. Signs and symptoms may include pain and a burning or tearing sensation at the time of injury, and the athlete may feel or hear a "pop." Palpable tenderness and spasm will be noted in the involved muscle, and a defect may also be palpable with third-degree strains. Swelling, ecchymosis, and pain with passive stretch and active contraction will be consistent with the degree of injury.

It is important to note that a number of other conditions can refer pain to the groin and mimic the signs and symptoms of muscular strain. Other causes of groin pain, listed in table 10.1, should be considered in evaluation of this area.

## CHRONIC AND OVERUSE SOFT TISSUE INJURIES

Because of the repetitive stresses placed on the hip and pelvis during locomotion and cutting and jumping maneuvers, chronic conditions caused by inflammation and muscle tightness are seen more often than acute injuries. Structural and

## Table 10.1 Potential Causes of Groin Pain

| Condition |
| --- |
| Muscle strain |
| Infection and inflammation of lymph nodes |
| Inguinal and femoral hernias |
| Kidney stone |
| Legg-Calvé-Perthes disease |
| Referred pain from lumbar region |
| Sacroiliac joint dysfunction |
| Stress fracture of the femoral neck |
| Synovitis of the hip joint capsule |
| Trochanteric and iliopsoas bursitis |
| Apophysitis (young athletes) |
| Epiphyseal injuries (young athletes) |

functional abnormalities at the hip can have a significant impact on the entire lower extremity.

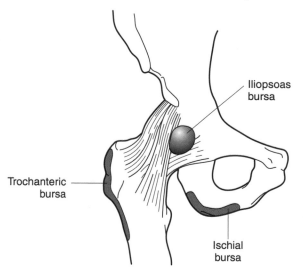

**I Figure 10.4** Location of the iliopsoas, trochanteric, and ischial bursae.

### Bursitis and Snapping Hip Syndrome

Although numerous bursae surround the hip and pelvis, chronic bursitis usually involves the trochanteric, iliopsoas, or ischial bursae (figure 10.4).

### Trochanteric Bursitis

The trochanteric bursa sits between the iliotibial (IT) band and the greater trochanter. Tightness in the IT band, repetitive insult to the lateral hip, excessive Q-angle, hip anteversion, leg length discrepancy (long leg), and running on a slanted street (downhill side) may cause abnormal friction and irritation of the bursa between these structures. The athlete will complain of pain or deep aching in the lateral hip, palpable tenderness, and crepitus over the greater trochanter. Swelling and redness may be present if the bursa is acutely inflamed. The athlete may also complain of pain radiating down the lateral leg and a "snapping" sensation when the IT band travels over the greater trochanter and inflamed bursa during hip flexion and extension.

### Iliopsoas Bursitis

Iliopsoas bursitis most often results from overuse activities. The athlete will complain of pain in the anterior groin with hip flexion. Because the bursa is deep to the adductor muscles, it is difficult to evaluate and palpate for tenderness. Because of the difficulty in palpating the specific structures, iliopsoas bursitis is often mistaken for a muscular strain. In chronic bursitis, snapping in the groin may also occur as the iliopsoas passes over the lesser trochanter and inflamed bursa.

**Ischial Bursitis**

The ischial bursa, which lies over the ischial tuberosity, may become painful and inflamed with excessive friction. As the ischial tuberosities bear the weight in sitting, repetitive hip flexion and extension of one leg and then the other can lead to bursal irritation. The athlete will complain of pain with sitting, palpable tenderness over the ischial tuberosity, and pain with passive hip flexion and active/resistive hip extension. Ischial bursitis is often difficult to differentiate from proximal hamstring tendinitis.

### Piriformis Syndrome

The piriformis muscle is an external hip rotator that originates on the pelvis and passes through the greater sciatic foramen to its attachment on the posterior superior aspect of the greater trochanter of the femur. Anatomically, the sciatic nerve usually passes underneath the piriformis as it exits the greater sciatic foramen. However, in ~12% of the population, the sciatic nerve splits and the fibular portion passes through the piriformis muscle (figure 10.5). Trigger points, tightness, or spasming in the piriformis can result from overuse or repetitive activities, causing buttock pain and symptoms of sciatic nerve irritation. Muscle spasm and tightness can compress the sciatic nerve, resulting in referred pain and tingling down the posterior thigh. Other signs and symptoms include pain and limited range of motion with hip internal rotation and palpable tenderness deep to the gluteals.

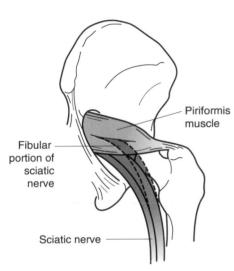

**Figure 10.5** In the majority of the population, the sciatic nerve passes underneath the piriformis, but in ~12% of the population the sciatic nerve splits, and its fibular portion passes through the piriformis with the tibial portion still passing underneath.

## TRAUMATIC FRACTURES

While traumatic hip and pelvic fractures commonly result from motor vehicle accidents and from falls in persons who are elderly, they occur rarely in the healthy athlete as a result of sport activity. While some such fractures are quite obvious, others are not; some may mimic a muscle strain. Fractures are more common in adolescents, and all hip and pelvis pain resulting from traumatic mechanisms should be carefully evaluated in young athletes.

### Hip and Pelvic Fractures

Hip fractures, which most frequently occur through the femoral neck, typically result from a direct blow to the lateral hip. Acetabular fractures may occur in conjunction with a hip dislocation or from a hard landing on a single leg (e.g., hurdling) that drives the femoral head into the acetabulum. Pelvic fractures are probably the least common; but when they do occur, they typically result from high-impact or crush-type mechanisms as seen in sports such as auto racing, skiing, or horseback riding.

Signs and symptoms will include immediate pain, swelling, and loss of function. With hip fractures and dislocations, the injury is usually quite obvious, as the involved leg will appear shortened and will be externally (fracture) or internally (dislocation) rotated. For less obvious fractures, if the athlete is able to move the hip and lower extremity at all, she will most certainly be unable or unwilling to bear weight. Pelvic fractures due to crush injuries can be life threatening, as there may be considerable hemorrhage. The athlete with a suspected traumatic fracture should be evaluated and continually monitored for shock.

### Avulsion Fractures

Avulsion fractures, more common in sport than in other physical activities, result from a violent contraction or tractioning of the attaching muscle. Kicking hard against

The athlete with a suspected traumatic fracture of the hip or pelvis should be closely evaluated and continually monitored for shock.

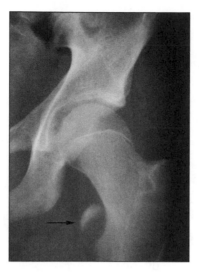

**Figure 10.6** Avulsion fracture of the lesser trochanter.

an immovable object or performing a quick, explosive movement can produce tremendous tractioning forces at the bony attachment and cause the tendon to pull away from the bone. Common sites for avulsion fractures are the anterior superior iliac spine (ASIS, sartorius), anterior inferior iliac spine (AIIS, rectus femoris), lesser trochanter (iliopsoas) (figure 10.6), and ischial tuberosity (hamstring). Avulsion fractures are more common in younger, skeletally immature athletes who have yet to obtain closure of the apophyseal joint than they are in adult athletes.

The athlete will complain of a sudden and sharp pain at the time of injury and may report hearing or feeling a snap or pop. Immediately after injury, the athlete will be unwilling to move the extremity. Tenderness will be observable along the bone, and a palpable defect in the myotendon unit near the attachment or a muscle bulging away from the attachment may also be evident. Swelling may be immediate or delayed.

## DEFECTS AND ABNORMALITIES SECONDARY TO REPETITIVE STRESS

Given the primary weight-bearing function of the hip and pelvis, the large mechanical forces transmitted through the bone and joint structures make these structures vulnerable to repetitive stress-type injuries. Injuries of this type occur most commonly in runners. Here as well, particular concerns arise with the pediatric athlete.

### Osteitis Pubis

Osteitis pubis is characterized by irritation and inflammation of the pubic symphysis resulting from overuse and repetitive stress of the adductor muscles at their insertion (figure 10.7). Most often seen in runners, osteitis pubis produces signs and symptoms of groin pain, palpable tenderness over the pubic symphysis and bone, adductor tightness, and pain with passive abduction and active adduction. Pain will increase with activity and be alleviated by rest.

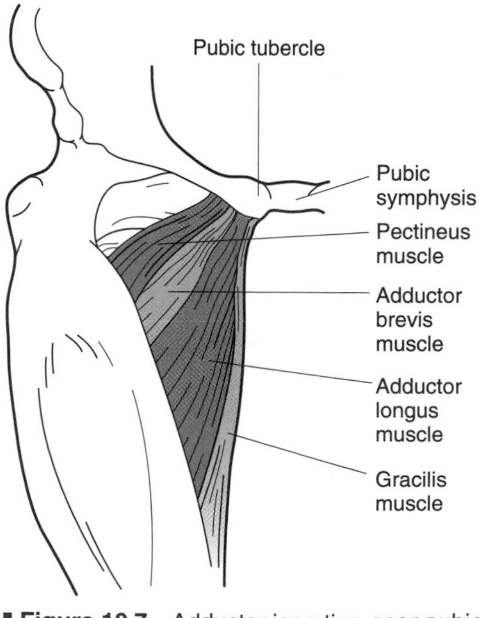

### Stress Fracture

Stress fractures of the femoral neck and pelvis occur most commonly in long-distance runners, particularly female runners. Athletes who have been inactive for long periods of time because of injury or who have recently and abruptly changed their training routine may also be at greater risk for stress injuries.

Stress fractures of the femoral neck result primarily from chronic and repetitive overload due to weight-bearing activities. Femoral neck stress fractures are more prevalent in athletes who have poor dietary habits, osteoporotic bone, leg length discrepancy, or other biomechanical abnormalities in the lower extremity that may impose abnormal stress on the bone. Signs and symptoms of femoral neck stress fracture include groin pain that may radiate out to the lateral hip or down the thigh. Initially, the athlete will complain of increased pain with weight-bearing

Pubic tubercle

Pubic symphysis

Pectineus muscle

Adductor brevis muscle

Adductor longus muscle

Gracilis muscle

**Figure 10.7** Adductor insertion near pubic symphysis.

activity that diminishes or disappears completely with rest, only to return once activity is resumed. Pain will become more constant if the offending activity and overstress continue. Palpable tenderness and pain with percussion to the greater trochanter may also be present.

The pubic ramus, which serves as the attachment site for the hip adductors, is also prone to stress fractures due to repetitive muscular stress. Endurance running activities are usually the primary cause. Signs and symptoms of a pubic stress fracture include pain in the groin radiating down the medial thigh and palpable tenderness along the bone. Initially, pain will increase with activity and lessen with rest; if stress continues, the pain will become more constant. Single-leg weight bearing, active/resistive adduction, or passive abduction may also reproduce pain.

### *Special Pediatric Concerns*

An athletic trainer who is accustomed to evaluating adult athletes may miss certain conditions in the pediatric athlete that are not typically seen in adults. These include apophysitis, epiphyseal fractures, slipped capital femoral epiphysis, and chronic synovitis. It is important to have a high index of suspicion for these injuries when you are evaluating the young athlete, as the injuries may have considerable consequences on later bone growth and development. Children or adolescents with groin pain lasting longer than a week should be referred to a physician.

### Apophysitis

Prior to ossification, the apophyseal joints are weaker than the myotendinous unit; they can become inflamed and can separate as a result of repetitive muscular contraction and stress. In some cases, a complete avulsion of the apophysis can occur following a forceful contraction of the attaching muscle. Often, apophysitis is mistaken for a muscle strain because it mimics many of the signs and symptoms of muscle strains in adults. Common sites for apophysitis are the insertions of the rectus femoris at the inferior iliac spine, the iliopsoas at the lesser trochanter, the adductors at the pubic ramus, and the proximal hamstring at the ischial tuberosity (figure 10.8). The young athlete will complain of pain and point tenderness near the myotendinous insertion. An enlarged bony prominence and crepitus may also be observable at the point of insertion. Pain will increase with passive stretch and active/resistive contraction of the attaching muscle. With complete avulsion, the athlete will complain of a pop and sharp pain in the hip or groin at the time of injury and may be unwilling to move the extremity. There may or may not be swelling in the area.

> **!** Children or adolescents with groin pain lasting longer than a week should be referred to a physician.

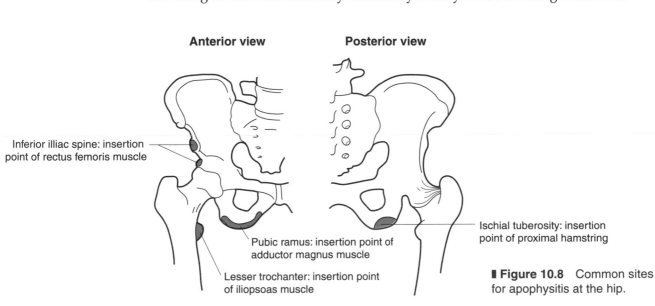

Anterior view    Posterior view

Inferior iliac spine: insertion point of rectus femoris muscle

Pubic ramus: insertion point of adductor magnus muscle

Lesser trochanter: insertion point of iliopsoas muscle

Ischial tuberosity: insertion point of proximal hamstring

▍**Figure 10.8**  Common sites for apophysitis at the hip.

### Epiphyseal Fractures

With traumatic forces at the hip, adolescents are more prone to fracture at the weaker epiphyseal plate than at the shaft of the bone. Epiphyseal fractures occur most commonly at the greater trochanter and capital femoral epiphysis. The fracture can be partial (separation) or complete (avulsion). With capital femoral epiphyseal fractures, the mechanism of injury and signs and symptoms are similar to those of a hip dislocation. The acute fracture may have been preceded by weakening and separation of the epiphysis over time. Athletes who present with a limp and complaints of intermitted groin pain that radiates down the medial thigh to the knee—with no recall of a specific injury—should be referred to a physician for further evaluation. Separation of the epiphysis can cause a secondary chronic synovitis.

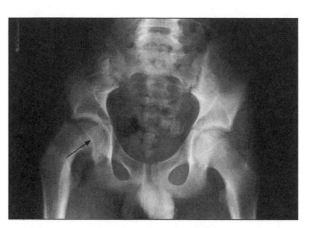

**▌Figure 10.9** Slipped capital femoral epiphysis on right (see arrow).

### Slipped Capital Femoral Epiphysis

A similar condition found in children and adolescents—which will also manifest itself as a limp and cause pain in the groin and thigh region—is a slipped capital femoral epiphysis. As the name implies, the capital femoral head has slipped or displaced at the epiphysis (figure 10.9). This injury results from progressive weakening of the epiphysis and not directly from athletic activity. Other signs and symptoms include decreased range of motion, particularly with internal rotation. Avascular necrosis and synovitis are frequent complications.

### Chronic Synovitis

Chronic synovitis is an inflammatory process at the hip joint that is characterized by chronic irritation and excess secretion of synovial fluid within the capsule. The excess synovial fluid can increase pressure within the joint capsule and occlude blood flow to the femoral head. Because of the depth of the joint capsule, this condition is very difficult to detect. Swelling will not be obvious, and pain may mimic that of a groin strain. Prolonged synovitis may lead to avascular necrosis of the femoral head.

## HIP DISLOCATION AND SUBLUXATION

Because of the relatively deep acetabular socket and numerous thick and strong supporting ligaments, the hip joint is one of the strongest and most stable joints in the body; therefore it takes tremendous forces to dislocate the hip. Most dislocations occur posteriorly with the hip and knee in a flexed position. A direct blow transmitted up the shaft of the femur, or less commonly an indirect internal rotational force with the foot firmly planted, can cause the femoral head to displace posteriorly to the acetabulum. Examples of common mechanisms include knee-to-dashboard contact during a traffic collision and landing hard on a flexed knee with the full weight directed through the long axis of the femur. In order for the hip to dislocate, significant stretching and tearing of the acetabular labrum and surrounding ligaments must occur.

Signs and symptoms include extreme pain, obvious deformity, and unwillingness to move the extremity. The leg will appear shortened and internally rotated. The athlete should be immobilized and immediately transported to emergency medical care via emergency medical services (EMS). Complications of hip dislocation include rupture of the artery to the head of the femur and avascular necrosis of the femoral head. With posterior dislocations, injury to the sciatic nerve may also result.

## NERVE AND VASCULAR INJURIES

Although nerve injury is uncommon at the hip and pelvis, the site most vulnerable to vascular compromise is the head of the femur. Avascular necrosis can occur in both children and adults as a result of either chronic inflammatory or traumatic injury mechanisms.

### Legg-Calvé-Perthes Disease

The condition known as Legg-Calvé-Perthes disease is characterized by avascular necrosis of the proximal femoral epiphysis. This is a chronic condition that develops slowly in children, more often in males than in females. For unknown reasons, vascularization to the epiphysis is diminished, causing degeneration and flattening of the femoral head articular cartilage. The child will complain of pain in the hip or groin that may radiate to the knee. Limping, decreased range of motion, and hip flexor tightness will also be noted. Again, any time a child or adolescent complains of hip or groin pain lasting more than one week, a physician should be consulted to rule out serious pathologies such as this.

### Avascular Necrosis of the Femoral Head

Nutrition and vascular supply to the femoral head is provided primarily by the artery to the femoral head that enters through the acetabulum. Avascular necrosis (osteochondritis dissecans) of the femoral head can occur when this artery is severed or is occluded for a prolonged period of time. This is a common complication following hip dislocations, fractures, or chronic synovitis and often necessitates a hip replacement.

## STRUCTURAL AND FUNCTIONAL ABNORMALITIES

Because of the weight-bearing function of the hip and pelvis, structural or functional abnormalities in this region can significantly alter biomechanical function in the lower extremity and may increase vulnerability to lower-extremity and back stress types of injuries. Therefore, understanding the abnormalities common in the hip will help you in your evaluation of chronic injuries in the lower extremity and trunk.

### Hip Anteversion and Retroversion

*Coxa valga is a condition in which the angle between the femoral shaft and neck is greater than 135°.*

Alterations in normal femoral angle can significantly affect biomechanics and muscle function in the lower extremity and influence Q-angle, genu varus/valgus, and patellar tracking. The normal alignment of the femur in relation to the hip and lower leg is determined by the degree of angulation of the femoral neck relative to the femoral shaft. The normal degree of angulation of the femoral head and neck is approximately 120-125° with a forward angulation of ~14-15° relative to the trochanters and distal femoral condyles (figure 10.10) (see next page). This angulation allows the head of the femur to be directed medially, superiorly, and slightly anteriorly to fit into the acetabulum. Coxa vara is a condition in which the degree of angulation is less than 120°, whereas coxa valga refers to an angle greater than 135°. In **hip anteversion**, excessive anterior angulation results in a toe-in gait (figure 10.11) (see next page). Hip anteversion will likely increase Q-angle and genu valgus at the knee. In **hip retroversion** there is a decreased anterior angle, producing a toe-out gait.

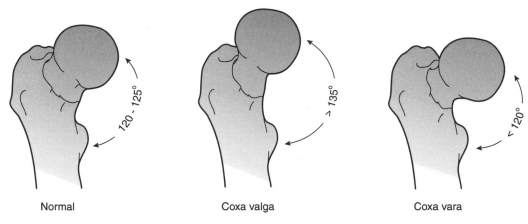

**Figure 10.10**    Normal angulation, coxa valga, and coxa vara of the hip.

### Leg Length Discrepancy and Pelvic Obliquity

Leg length discrepancies can be classified as true or apparent. A true leg length discrepancy is characterized by a bilateral difference in measurable length of the femur or tibial shaft. In the absence of a true length discrepancy, shortening on one leg may be caused by abnormalities in the hip and pelvis. This apparent leg length discrepancy may result from pelvic obliquity or a **hemipelvis**, in which one side of the pelvis is smaller than the other. Muscle tightness or sacroiliac dysfunction can also cause one leg to be drawn more superiorly than the other and can give the appearance of a leg length difference. Regardless of whether the difference is true or apparent, the asymmetry can cause pain and dysfunction in the hip, pelvis, or low back with weight-bearing activities. One should always assess leg length when an athlete reports with chronic hip, pelvic, or low back pain of unknown etiology.

### Gluteus Medius Weakness

Atrophy or weakness of the gluteus medius muscle will result in an inability to abduct the hip and maintain a level pelvis during gait. The ability to stand on one leg and maintain the opposite hip at the same level as the weight-bearing hip relies primarily on the function of the gluteus medius in the weight-bearing leg. The primary sign of gluteus medius weakness or dysfunction is a **gluteus medius lurch**, or **Trendelenburg gait**, a dropping of the non-weight-bearing hip during its swing-through phase (figure 10.12). These gait alterations can also result in increased hip, pelvis, and low back complaints.

**Figure 10.11**
Changes in lower extremity alignment secondary to hip anteversion.

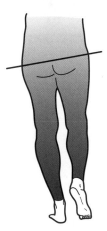
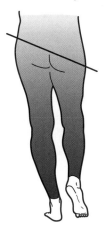

**Normal gait**

Negative Trendelenburg sign

**Abnormal gait**

Positive Trendelenburg sign

**Figure 10.12**
Trendelenburg gait.

# INJURY ASSESSMENT

The range of acute and chronic injuries of the hip and pelvis will require you to consider a number of factors when assessing injuries in this area. On the field, you could be faced with only a simple disabling contusion of the hip or a painful muscle strain, or on rare occasions you may encounter a traumatic hip dislocation requiring immediate medical assistance. In all cases, you must be able to quickly determine the nature of the injury in order to take the proper course of action without delay. Off the field, injuries of the hip and pelvis will not be as obvious as those on the field, as similar symptoms can represent multiple conditions, some of them quite serious. Therefore it is important that you acquire the assessment skills to be able to differentiate the possible causes of chronic pain and dysfunction and determine which may represent more serious underlying injury.

## ON-FIELD ASSESSMENT

In contrast to the knee and ankle, the hip joint is not often acutely injured in athletics; and severe acute hip injuries are rare. However, when an injury to this area does occur, it can be very debilitating. As with any on-field assessment, the athletic trainer must be able to quickly identify life- and limb-threatening conditions as well as recognize signs and symptoms of other serious injuries.

As you approach the athlete, survey the surroundings and note the athlete's injury response and body position. Your primary survey is consistent with surveying for all other joints in that you first assess for level of consciousness, airway, breathing, and circulation, and severe bleeding. If in the primary survey you note no life-threatening conditions, move on to your evaluation of the hip and pelvis.

### History

As always, gain a brief history from the athlete as to the mechanism of injury and the location, type, and severity of the symptoms. Remember that athletes often experience hip pain as inguinal or groin pain, whereas they more often feel lumbosacral pain in the buttocks and posterior thigh and possibly along the course of the sciatic nerve. Because of the close communication of the sacroiliac and hip joints with the sacral plexus and sciatic nerve, respectively, be sure to ask about any unusual sensations felt at the time of injury and currently, and find out whether there is any referred pain down the leg. Also check for other unusual sounds or sensations.

### Observation

With traumatic injuries, conduct a rapid visual check of skin color and moisture, pupil size, respiration, and pulse to assess for signs and symptoms indicating shock (see chapter 13).

Your initial observation should be for obvious and immediate signs of swelling, discoloration, and deformity. Observe bilaterally the position of the legs to see whether one leg appears shortened or internally or externally rotated. Whereas external rotation is more indicative of a fracture, internal rotation is more characteristic of a dislocation. Observe whether the athlete is willing to move the leg or hip, as well as the opposite limb. If you suspect a serious hip or pelvis injury, you should call EMS and observe the athlete for signs and symptoms of shock.

### Palpation

Palpation of the femoral pulse is performed in the femoral triangle where the femoral artery is most accessible. This artery is located midway between the adductor longus and sartorius just distal to the inguinal ligament. In the presence of severe trauma and suspected occlusion, you should palpate the artery for a pulse. Your palpation should also include a quick sensory test of the dermatomal distributions of the lumbosacral plexus if the athlete complains of pain wrapping around the pelvis or into the lower extremity (see neurological tests in the off-field assessment).

If no serious trauma or neurological symptoms are immediately observable, proceed with a brief but thorough palpation to assess for any tenderness, crepitus, or subtle deformities over the bony structures and muscular insertions as the athlete's pain and symptoms indicate. Palpate the anterior superior and inferior iliac spine, iliac crest, greater trochanter, posterior superior iliac spine (PSIS), ischial tuberosity, and sacroiliac joints. Be sure to include in your palpation the insertions of the sartorius on the ASIS, the rectus femoris on the AIIS, and the hamstring origin on the ischial tuberosity. If you do not note any bony tenderness, generally assess for tenderness or palpable defects in the adductor, abductor, and hip flexor muscle groups as needed to ascertain the extent of injury.

### Removal From the Field

If no fracture or dislocation is suspected, have the athlete perform slow, active range of motion of the lower extremities. If this does not cause a significant increase in pain, allow the athlete to sit and then stand. If the athlete tolerates these movements, assist him off the field. If, however, you have any doubt as to a potential fracture or dislocation, or if the athlete's pain is too severe to allow ambulation, you should have him transported on a stretcher to the sideline for a more thorough evaluation.

If you suspect a serious hip or pelvis injury, or the athlete is unable to ambulate under his own power or with assistance, do not hesitate to use passive transport to remove him from the field for a more thorough evaluation.

---

## Checklist for On-Field Assessment of the Hip, Pelvis, and Groin

### Primary Survey

✓ Survey surroundings.
✓ Obtain information from bystanders.
✓ Note position/response of athlete as you approach.
✓ Assess for level of consciousness, airway, breathing, circulation, severe bleeding.

### Secondary Survey

History

✓ Chief complaint
✓ Mechanism, location, and severity of pain
✓ Unusual sounds or sensations
✓ Any referred pain

### Observation

✓ Check for obvious and immediate signs of deformity, swelling, discoloration.
✓ Check for unusual positioning of the limb (shortened, rotated).
✓ Observe for any signs and symptoms of shock (wet, white, weak).

If deformity or evidence of severe trauma, notify EMS and monitor for signs and symptoms of shock.

### Palpation

✓ Check for bony tenderness, crepitus, or subtle deformities along the following:
  ✓ ASIS, AIIS, iliac crest, greater trochanter, PSIS, ischial tuberosity, sacroiliac joint
  ✓ Insertions for sartorius, rectus femoris, hamstring origin
  ✓ Check for palpable defects in the adductor, abductor, and hip flexor muscle groups.
  ✓ Compare bilaterally.

### Neurovascular Assessment

✓ Pulse (femoral)
✓ Sensory (L1-S2)
✓ Motor (L1-S2)

If evidence of possible fracture or significant injury, use passive transport to remove from field.

### Active Range of Motion

✓ For hip flexion, extension, abduction, adduction, internal and external rotation

If all tests are negative and athlete is able to complete active ROM, remove the athlete from field and assist as pain and symptoms dictate.

# SIDELINE ASSESSMENT

Before beginning the objective portion of the sideline assessment, the athletic trainer obtains a more detailed history of the injury from the athlete.

## History

From a more detailed history you gain information regarding the injury so that you can better determine its nature and severity. Ask further questions about the mechanism of the injury and the position of the limb when injury occurred. Determine whether the athlete was bearing weight at the time, and if so whether she was rotating on the weight-bearing leg. If the injury was a result of impact, ask her where on the body the impact occurred. Also note at this time any prior injuries to the hip and pelvis, as well as any previous injuries to the thigh or lower back that may be relevant.

## Observation

While obtaining the history, observe for signs of pain, the position of the injured hip and the way in which it is moved, and any difficulties or limitations with mobility and function. Observe how the athlete stands, sits, and moves from one position to another and how the hip is supported or guarded. If the athlete was able to ambulate off the field, note his ability to bear weight on the injured leg and his level of confidence in this regard. Check the area thoroughly for signs of discoloration and bruising, deformity, or swelling, especially over the bony prominences of the iliac crest and greater trochanter. Note any scars that would indicate previous injury or surgery.

## Palpation

Palpation around the hip area involves assessment of temperature, skin and soft tissue mobility, tenderness, defects, muscle spasm, swelling, and bony tenderness. The anterior, lateral, and medial hip can be palpated with the athlete supine; the posterior aspect is palpated with the athlete prone. If there is no table on the sideline, you can perform the palpation while the athlete is standing or lying on the ground, whichever he finds more comfortable.

### Supine

Bony palpation at the sideline is consistent with that during the on-field assessment. Starting with the iliac crests, palpate the rim of the iliac by following the crest anteriorly to the ASIS. Palpate the insertion of the abdominals and hip abductors along the iliac crest, a common site of contusions and strains. Follow the gluteus medius as it fans from the iliac crest to its insertion on the greater trochanter. A traumatic trochanteric bursitis will be tender to palpation off the superior aspect of the greater trochanter. Medial to and ~1 in. (2-3 cm) superior to the greater trochanter, you can palpate the inguinal ligament. You can palpate an inflamed psoas bursa beneath the midsection of the inguinal ligament. Medially and inferiorly to the inguinal ligament, the femoral triangle that is formed by the sartorius laterally, inguinal ligament superiorly, and adductor longus medially frames the femoral artery, femoral vein, and femoral nerve (figure 10.13). Deep palpation of

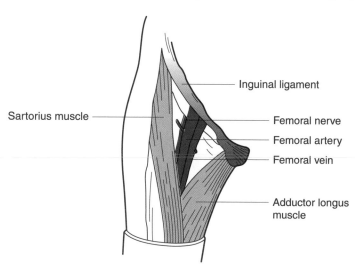

Sartorius muscle

Inguinal ligament

Femoral nerve

Femoral artery

Femoral vein

Adductor longus muscle

**▌Figure 10.13** The femoral triangle.

the hip joint is done indirectly, ~.5 in. (1-2 cm) distal to the inguinal ligament on the midpoint of a line between the greater trochanter and pubic tubercle. Although direct palpation of the joint is not possible, pain to deep palpation may be indicative of hip joint pathology. Palpate the pelvic tubercles by following the inguinal ligament medially. Pain to pressure on the tubercles may indicate pubic symphysis or sacroiliac pathology. Palpate the lateral (gluteus medius, tensor fascia), anterior (rectus femoris, sartorius), and medial (adductor group) thigh muscles to identify areas of tenderness, defects, spasm, swelling, and other pathology.

**Prone**

The iliac crests are identified and followed posteriorly to the PSIS, areas usually indicated by dimples in the lower back. Ischial tuberosities are located in the gluteal fold region with an upward and anterior palpation. Tenderness over this area may indicate an ischial bursitis or hamstring insertion pathology. Hip lateral rotators, especially the piriformis, are located from the greater trochanter in a superior and medial pattern toward the sacrum. The sciatic nerve lies midway between the ischial tuberosity and the greater trochanter as it exits from underneath the piriformis, and is best palpated in side-lying with the hip flexed. The sacral joints can be followed from the PSIS inferiorly and slightly medially. The sacrotuberous ligament is palpated between the ischial tuberosity and sacrum (figure 10.14). Unequal tension of these ligaments with right and left comparisons, accompanied by tenderness to palpation, may indicate either a ligamentous injury or sacroiliac dysfunction. You may note tenderness or spasm in these muscles. Also investigate the gluteal muscles and hamstrings for spasm, tenderness, and swelling.

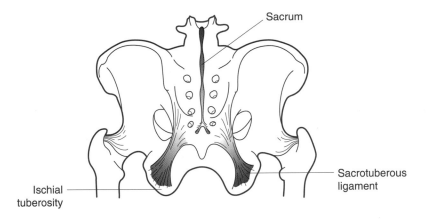

**▌Figure 10.14**   Location of the sacrotuberous ligament.

## *Range of Motion*

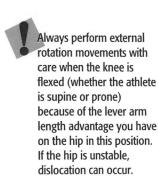

Always perform external rotation movements with care when the knee is flexed (whether the athlete is supine or prone) because of the lever arm length advantage you have on the hip in this position. If the hip is unstable, dislocation can occur.

Active and passive range of motion is assessed bilaterally in all hip motions while the athlete is lying down. After assessing active range of motion in supine and prone, perform passive range of motion, including overpressure, if active motion did not produce pain. Supine hip flexion should be performed both with the knee extended to include hamstring flexibility assessment and with the knee flexed to eliminate the influence of the hamstrings on hip movement (figure 10.15). The normal range of motion for hip flexion is ~115-125° with the knee flexed. Also assess hip abduction (~45-50°), hip adduction (~20-30°), and hip internal and external rotation (~45° each) with the hip flexed and extended before repositioning the athlete into prone to evaluate hip extension in both flexed and extended knee positions. You can also perform hip internal and external rotation with the athlete seated or prone, with the hip and

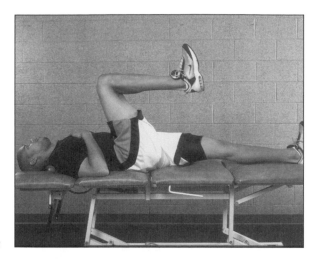 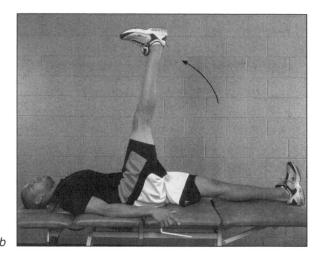

a                                                          b

■ **Figure 10.15** Active range of motion with the knee (a) flexed and (b) extended.

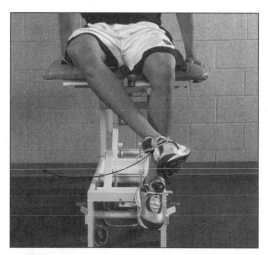

■ **Figure 10.16** Active range of motion for internal and external rotation of the knee while in a seated position.

knee flexed to 90° (figure 10.16). Always perform external rotation movements with care when the knee is flexed (whether supine or prone) because of the lever arm length advantage you have on the hip in this position. If the hip is unstable, dislocation can occur.

You can assess functional range of motion (and strength) in general by asking the athlete to perform a full squat. The athlete should be able to squat until the knees are fully flexed with the heels on the ground and the hamstrings in contact with the calf muscles. Observe for quality and quantity of movement. The athlete should not hesitate and should move through the motion smoothly, both in descending and in returning to standing. The hips should remain level and the buttocks should move under the athlete, not backward—which would indicate a compensatory movement to avoid pain. You can perform other quick checks of functional motion with the athlete in sitting by having the athlete cross her legs (hip flexion and adduction), with the lateral malleolus of one leg on the opposite knee (hip flexion, abduction, and external rotation).

### Strength

During strength assessment of hip flexion and extension, watch for hip rotation or abduction substitution.

Strength assessment is also performed bilaterally with the athlete in a lying position and in standing. On the table (or ground), position the athlete with the limb working against gravity for each muscle to be tested. In supine, resist the hip flexors manually with the knee extended (rectus femoris) and with the knee flexed (hip flexors). When the knee is extended, provide resistance either above the knee or just distal to it, with the hip at approximately 45° flexion. When the knee is flexed, provide resistance just proximal to the knee, with the hip at about 90° of flexion. Your choice of hand placement will depend on the athlete's hip flexor strength, your ability to resist the athlete, and the athlete's history of knee injury. Be careful to watch for hip rotation or abduction substitutions of this motion.

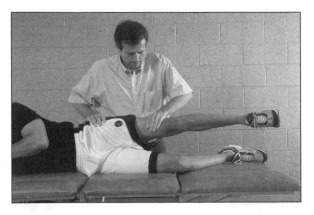

**▮ Figure 10.17**   Side-lying hip abduction strength assessment.

During strength assessment of hip abduction, watch for muscle substitution as indicated by the athlete's flexing or externally rotating the hip.

Resist hip abduction with the athlete in side-lying, the uninvolved leg on the bottom. Position the hip in midrange abduction and apply resistance (figure 10.17) either proximal or distal to the knee. Make sure that the athlete maintains the hip in pure abduction and does not flex it forward or externally rotate it when you apply manual resistance.

Hip extension strength is assessed with the athlete in prone. Perform the test with the hip in about 10° of extension with the knee flexed (gluteals only) and with the knee extended (gluteals and hamstrings) (figure 10.18, a-b). With the knee in extension, you can apply manual resistance either proximal or distal to the knee; when the knee is flexed, always apply resistance just proximal to the knee. For an accurate test result, ensure that the athlete does not try to compensate for weak hip extensors by rotating or abducting the hip during testing.

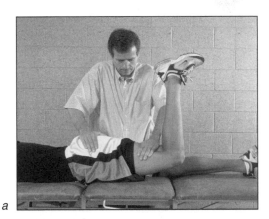
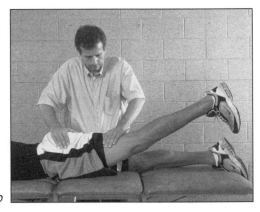

*a*   *b*

**▮ Figure 10.18**   Prone hip extension strength with (a) knee flexed to eliminate hamstrings, and (b) with the knee extended.

Comparisons are always made with the uninvolved leg to determine what strength is "normal" for the athlete. Always test the uninvolved hip first so the athlete knows what to expect on the injured side and will be less apprehensive and more willing to produce a maximal effort.

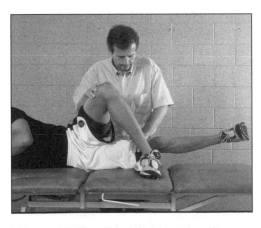

**▮ Figure 10.19**   Side-lying hip adduction.

Hip adduction is tested with the athlete in side-lying with the involved hip on the bottom. (If the athlete's hip is too tender for this position, you can perform the test in supine, but you must take this nongravity position into account when estimating the strength of these muscles.) With the athlete in side-lying, place the uninvolved leg in a figure-4 position with the hip and knee flexed and the foot flat on the floor in front of the knee of the involved leg. Then ask the athlete to lift the bottom leg upward, and apply manual resistance to the inner thigh proximal or distal to the knee (figure 10.19).

### Neurological and Circulatory Tests

Unless the athlete reports referred pain into the lower extremity below the hip, it is not necessary to perform neurological tests during the sideline assessment. These tests will be discussed in connection with the off-field assessment.

### Special Tests

As with most body segments, special tests are used to identify or rule out injuries unique to the hip and pelvis. Tests should be performed on both extremities for comparison between the right and left. The special tests typically used to define acute injuries will be described here. The section on the off-field assessment will cover tests used to identify nonacute injuries.

## Hip Pathology

### Hip Dislocation

Although an x-ray is the ultimate evaluation tool to determine hip dislocation, acute dislocations are not usually difficult to identify. The leg is often positioned in adduction and internal rotation. The greater trochanter is prominent, and the athlete reports severe pain, especially if she attempts to move the leg.

*Coxa vara is a condition in which the angle between the femoral shaft and neck is less than 120°.*

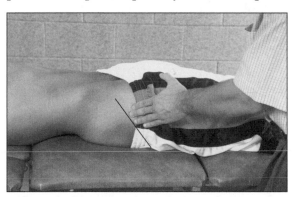

Congenital dislocations are more difficult to determine. One common test for these uses **Nelaton's line**, which is a line from the ischial tuberosity to the ipsilateral ASIS (figure 10.20). The test is positive when the greater trochanter is palpated above this line. This test can also be used to determine coxa vara.

**▮ Figure 10.20**  Palpation of the greater trochanter above Nelaton's line.

### Femoral Nerve Traction Test

This test assesses femoral nerve pathology that may emanate from the lumbosacral nerve roots (L2-4), causing pain in the groin and hip that radiates into the anterior thigh. The athlete lies on the unaffected side with the lower hip and knee flexed for stability and the top hip and knee placed in extension (figure 10.21). While the hip is maintained in about 15° extension, the knee is passively moved into flexion. The head should be maintained in slight flexion throughout the test. A positive sign is present if the athlete complains of pain, numbness, or tingling in the anterior thigh. The thigh should remain in slight abduction during the test so that the outcome is not a positive Ober's test (see off-field assessment special tests). The athlete's history and symptoms will help you determine whether the positive sign is related to femoral nerve or IT band pathology.

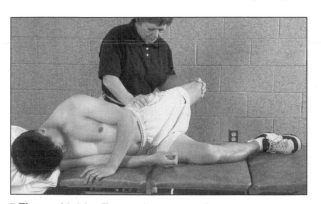

**▮ Figure 10.21**  Femoral nerve traction test.

### Stress Fracture Test

The stress fracture test, or **fulcrum test**, assesses for the possibility of a femoral neck stress fracture. With the athlete in a relaxed sitting position on the end of a table or bench, place your forearm under his thigh (figure 10.22). With the other hand, apply a downward pressure to the proximal knee. The test is positive if the athlete reports pain with the maneuver. Confirmation of a stress fracture requires a bone scan, so a positive finding warrants physician referral.

### Pelvis Pathology

Because of its complexity, along with the presence of multiple joints in multiple planes, the pelvis lends itself to several assessment procedures. There are many tests that can be used to identify sacroiliac pathology. This section will present only some of those that may be appropriate for acute injury assessment, including pelvic compression and pelvic distraction tests.

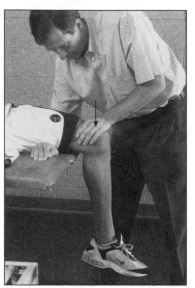

**∎ Figure 10.22**   Stress fracture test.

### Gaenslen's Test

Gaenslen's test is a general assessment that will indicate either a sacroiliac or hip pathology or an L4 nerve lesion. With the athlete in side-lying and the leg flexed at the hip and knee so that the knee is against the chest, stabilize the pelvis while extending the top leg (figure 10.23). Pain in the sacroiliac region is considered a positive sign. (Note: Although not as feasible for a sideline assessment, an alternative position for this test is with the athlete in supine, with both knees drawn up to the chest and one buttock off the edge of the table. The leg is slowly extended off the table. As before, pain in the sacroiliac region is a positive sign.)

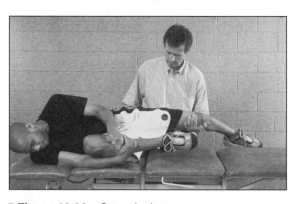

**∎ Figure 10.23**   Gaenslen's test.

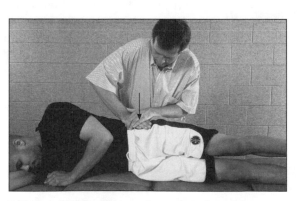

**∎ Figure 10.24**   Iliac crest compression test.

### Iliac Crest Compression Test

This test is used to stress the posterior sacroiliac ligaments. Place the athlete in a side-lying position with the involved side on top. Place your hands over the proximal iliac crest, and apply a downward force (figure 10.24). Pain in the sacroiliac joints is a positive sign for sacral joint irritation or sprain.

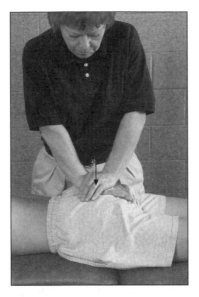

**Figure 10.25** Sacral apex compression test.

## Sacral Apex Compression Test

This test places a rotational stress on the sacroiliac joints. With the athlete prone, place the bases of both your hands over the sacral apex (figure 10.25) and apply pressure over the apex. Pain in the sacroiliac joints is a positive sign for this test as well.

## Anterior Distraction Test

This test, also known as the "**gapping test**," stresses the anterior sacroiliac ligaments. With the athlete supine, cross your arms so that your hands are on the athlete's opposite ASIS (figure 10.26). Apply a downward and outward pressure to each ASIS simultaneously. A positive sign occurs if the athlete reports posterior gluteal or leg pain. If the athlete complains of pain over the ASIS, you may use a pad between the ASIS and your hand.

## Posterior Distraction Test

The posterior distraction test, also known as **Hibbs' test**, evaluates the integrity of the posterior sacroiliac ligaments. Once cleared of any hip pathology, the athlete is positioned prone. With the pelvis stabilized, flex the knee to 90° and medially rotate the hip to its end point while palpating the sacroiliac joint on the same side (figure 10.27). The test is positive if palpation over the sacroiliac joint reveals greater laxity or movement on the involved side than on the uninvolved side.

### *Functional Tests*

If you judge that the athlete's signs and symptoms are relatively minor, perform a functional assessment to ensure that hip and pelvis pain will not return or be

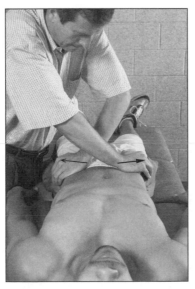

**Figure 10.26** Anterior distraction test.

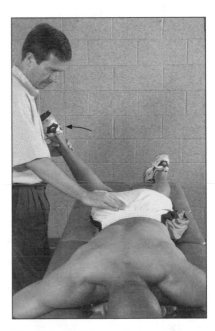

**Figure 10.27** Posterior distraction test.

reproduced when the athlete resumes activity. The lower-extremity functional tests described for the ankle (chapter 8) are appropriate here—tailored, of course, to the athlete's sport demands.

## OFF-FIELD ASSESSMENT

As with other segments, if the athlete is first seen in the health care facility, many times the injury will be in a postacute or chronic stage, and adequate evaluation will require additional assessment tools. Here the off-field assessment procedure is presented in chronological order; for elements that are the same as for the sideline assessment, readers are referred back to that section of the chapter.

### History

The history obtained from the athlete off the field includes the same elements as for the sideline assessment. You will ask additional questions to obtain a clear and accurate injury profile and to determine the stage of the injury (acute, postacute, or chronic/overuse)—and, if the injury is chronic, how the pain profile has changed over time. Ask questions to determine the time of injury or symptom onset, any change in pain or symptoms throughout the day, aggravating and easing factors, injury response to training, and level of irritability.

### Observation

When the athlete enters the facility, observe for gait deviations (stride and cadence), stance abnormalities, inequality of weight distribution side to side, and difficulties moving from standing to sitting or transferring onto and off the table. Observe for any hesitancy or guarding of the hip when the athlete is moving or transferring to a different position. Note how the trunk rotates and the hips move as the athlete walks. Observe the stance for its width, for knee angulation (Q-angle, genu valgus), and for the position of the feet. Standing in a toe-out position may indicate hip retroversion, whereas a toe-in stance and accentuated genu valgus may indicate hip anteversion. Check for obvious signs of a leg length discrepancy by comparing the levels of the greater trochanters and posterior knee creases. Check the levels of the ASIS and PSIS bilaterally. If the ASIS is lower and the PSIS is higher on one side, there may be an anterior rotation of the sacrum on that side. If both the ASIS and PSIS are elevated, an upslip of the pelvis on that side may be present.

In addition to posture, gait, and stance, observe the area of injury for signs of swelling, discoloration, or deformities. Also observe the erector spinae and gluteal muscle masses for equal tone and contour bilaterally, noticing any evidence of muscle atrophy or spasm.

### Differential Diagnosis

Since the low back, knee, and ankle may refer to the hip, differential diagnosis tests must be performed to rule out the possibility of referred pain from other body segments. Quick tests for differential diagnosis include standing lumbar range of motion in all planes with overpressure, squats, and active knee and ankle ranges of motion through each movement with overpressure. You can also use the lumbar quadrant position, extension, lateral flexion, and rotation to the same side with overpressure to eliminate the low back as a referral source of hip pain (figure 10.28). None of these quick tests except the squat should reproduce the athlete's pain. If any do, you should further evaluate the specific area as the possible source of pain before proceeding further in the hip evaluation.

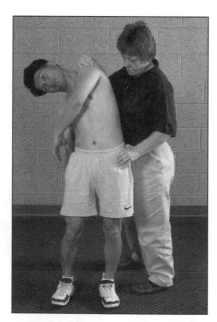

**▌Figure 10.28**  Lumbar quadrant position for clearing the low back as a source of hip pain.

## Checklist for Sideline Assessment of the Hip, Pelvis, and Groin

### History

Ask questions pertaining to the following:

✓ Chief complaint
✓ Mechanism of injury (contact vs. noncontact, rotational stress, weight bearing vs. non-weight bearing, etc.)
✓ Unusual sounds or sensations
✓ Type and location of pain or symptoms
✓ Previous injury
✓ Previous injury to opposite extremity for bilateral comparison

### Observation

✓ Check for swelling (local or general), deformity, and discoloration.
✓ Note positioning and any limitations in mobility or function.
✓ Check standing alignment: levels of greater trochanters, PSIS from behind, ASIS from front, equal weight bearing.
✓ Observe gait—normal versus abnormal.
✓ Inspect for muscular atrophy, tone, previous scars, and the like.
✓ Make bilateral comparison.

### Palpation

Palpate for pain, tenderness, and deformity over the following:

✓ ASIS, iliac crest including insertion of the abdominals and hip abductors, iliac tubercle, greater trochanter, trochanteric bursa
✓ Inguinal ligament, femoral triangle borders and contents, pelvic tubercles
✓ Abductor, hip flexor, and adductor muscle groups and insertions
✓ PSIS, ischial tuberosity, piriformis and sciatic nerve, sacroiliac joint, sacrotuberous ligament
✓ Gluteus maximus
✓ Hamstring (proximal and origin on ischial tuberosity)
✓ Perform bilateral comparison

### Range of Motion

✓ Perform active ROM for hip abduction, adduction, flexion (knee flexed and extended), extension (knee flexed and extended), internal and external rotation.
✓ Bilaterally compare and note any pain or restricted ROM.
✓ Perform passive ROM for the motions listed after each active test.
✓ Bilaterally compare and note any pain or restricted ROM.

### Strength Tests

✓ Perform manual resistance to motions listed for ROM (may follow each active/passive test).
✓ Check bilaterally and note any pain or weakness.

### Neurovascular Tests

✓ Sensory, motor, and reflex testing for lumbosacral plexus
✓ Femoral pulse

### Special Tests

✓ Test for hip pathology (femoral nerve traction test, stress fracture test)
✓ Test for pelvis pathology (Gaenslen's, iliac compression, sacral apex compression, posterior distraction)

### Functional Tests

### Range of Motion

As with the sideline assessment, you will evaluate hip range of motion in flexion with the knee flexed and extended, extension with the knee flexed and extended, internal and external rotation, and abduction and adduction. Evaluate hip flexion, abduction, adduction, and rotation with the athlete supine; assess hip extension and rotation with the athlete prone.

### Strength

Strength also is evaluated in the same manner as in the sideline assessment. Rather than performing the complete range of motion assessment followed by the complete strength assessment for all motions, you can perform range of motion for one motion and then immediately perform the strength assessment for the same motion. This will increase efficiency and prevent repetitive movements and unnecessary positioning of the athlete during the examination. It is important to utilize gravity when testing for strength grades 3, 4, and 5 and to eliminate gravity during tests for 1 and 2 grades. Use a buildup of resistance up to the maximum that the athlete can tolerate, noting any strength differences bilaterally.

### Neurological Tests

The hip and pelvis are surrounded by nerves of the lumbosacral plexus. Sensory and motor nerves from this plexus innervate the hip and pelvis regions. Figure 7.8 (chapter 7) demonstrates the dermatomal distributions, and figure 7.27 and table 2.2 (chapter 2) indicate the motor nerve distributions for this region.

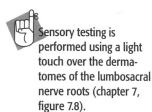

Sensory testing is performed using a light touch over the dermatomes of the lumbosacral nerve roots (chapter 7, figure 7.8).

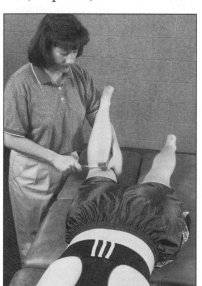

If you suspect neurological deficits, perform reflex testing on the patellar tendon and medial and lateral hamstrings tendons for L3-L4, L5-S1, and S1-S2, respectively. For each test, the muscle is placed in a midrange position, and the reflex hammer is tapped over the tendon. For the hamstring reflex, the athlete may be more comfortable, and the test may elicit a better response, if you place your thumb over the tendon and tap your thumb with the reflex hammer (figure 10.29).

**▌Figure 10.29**    Hamstring tendon reflex testing.

### Special Tests

This section presents special tests that identify nonacute pathology in the hip and sacrum region. Readers may refer back to the sideline assessment for descriptions of special tests for acute injury.

### Patrick Test

The Patrick test is also known as the **Faber (Flexion, Abduction, External Rotation) test** or **Jansen's test**. It is used to identify limited mobility of the hip, the possibility of iliopsoas spasm, or sacroiliac dysfunction. The athlete is supine with the involved leg flexed at the hip and knee so that the foot is crossed over the opposite knee (figure 10.30). Place one hand on the opposite ASIS to stabilize the pelvis and the other hand on the medial aspect of the knee of the involved leg. Passively move the leg into abduction, lowering the knee to the table. Mobility is normal and the response negative when the knee can be lowered so that the thigh is at least parallel to the opposite leg. The response is positive when the thigh remains elevated above the opposite leg.

**▌Figure 10.30**    Patrick test.

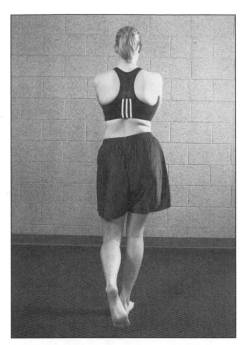

**▌Figure 10.31** A positive Trendelenburg test. Note: left hip has dropped indicating right gluteus medius weakness.

## Trendelenburg Test

This test assesses hip stability and abduction (gluteus medius) weakness. Have the athlete stand on one leg while you observe the non-weight-bearing hip (figure 10.31). With a normal response of the weight-bearing hip, there is a slight elevation of the non-weight-bearing hip. A positive sign occurs when the non-weight-bearing hip drops because of weakness of the weight-bearing hip abductors.

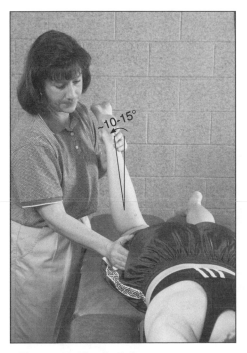

**▌Figure 10.32** Craig's test.

## Craig's Test

This test is used to identify retroversion and anteversion of the hip and is sometimes referred to as the **Ryder method** for retroversion and anteversion measurement. The athlete lies prone with his knees flexed to 90°. Palpate the greater trochanter and position the hip so that the greater trochanter lies parallel to the surface of the table (figure 10.32). The angle of the lower leg relative to the vertical is measured in this position. In the adult, a measurement of greater than 15° external rotation is considered hip anteversion. If the measurement is less than 8°, the hip is retroverted. An excessively anteverted hip will also be apparent with a toeing-in during standing, whereas a retroverted hip will produce a toeing-out.

### Leg Length Discrepancy

A difference in leg length can be a true discrepancy or an apparent limb shortening. To determine leg length discrepancy initially, have the athlete lie supine in a hook-lying position, and grasp her ankles with your thumbs on the medial malleoli (figure 10.33a). The athlete raises her hips and lowers them to the table. You will then passively extend the legs and compare the positions of the two medial malleoli (figure 10.33b). If the legs are unequal, you should proceed to determine whether the difference is true or apparent.

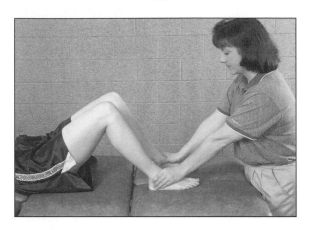

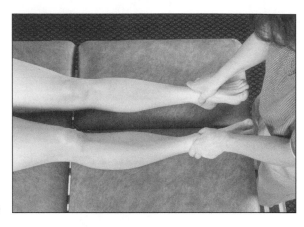

a                                                                                                b

■ **Figure 10.33**    Quick check for leg length discrepancy: (a) in hook-lying and (b) with legs extended.

A true leg length difference is present when the bones of the legs are not the same length. An apparent leg length difference is present as a result of soft tissue shortening, pelvic obliquity, spinal pathology, or other lower-extremity joint dysfunction.

A **true leg length discrepancy** measurement is made with the athlete supine and her legs fully extended. Place one end of a tape measure on her ASIS at its most prominent point. Place the other end on the medial or the lateral malleolus of the leg. (The likelihood of thigh girth influences on measurements is lower when the lateral malleolus is used.) Draw the tape tightly from the proximal to the distal point (figure 10.34). Identify a location just distal to the malleolus with your thumbnail pressed onto the tape measure at that point. You will need to be careful to use the same landmark location for left and right measures. Measurement differences greater than 0.6 in. (1.5) cm are considered abnormal.

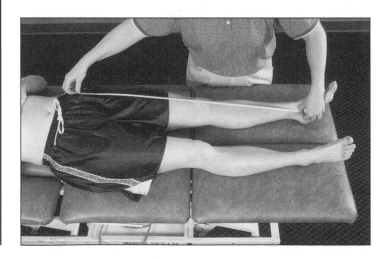

■ **Figure 10.34**    Measuring for true leg length discrepancy.

To measure **apparent leg length discrepancy**, have the athlete positioned in the same manner as for the true length measurement. Then take the measurement from the umbilicus to the left and right medial malleolus (figure 10.35). If there is a difference with the apparent test, but not the true test, the leg length discrepancy is due to factors (e.g., pelvic obliquity, hemipelvis) other than femoral and tibial leg length.

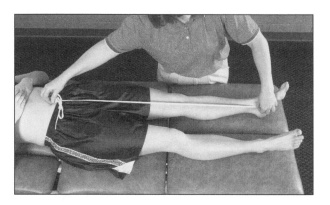

**▎Figure 10.35**   Measuring for apparent leg length discrepancy.

### Thomas Test

This test assesses the flexibility of the hip flexor muscles. The athlete lies supine and brings one knee up toward the chest, then pulls her knee to her chest to flatten her back to the table. A normal response is present when there is no change in the position of the extended leg. The test is positive if the extended leg becomes flexed so that the knee is raised off the table (figure 10.36). If the extended leg is pushed down, the hip flexor tightness may cause anterior rotation of the pelvis, and an increased lumbar lordosis will be noted. Abduction or external rotation of the leg can indicate tightness of the IT band.

### Rectus Femoris Contracture Test (Kendall Test)

This test, an extension of the Thomas test, can be performed as an assessment of both hip flexor and rectus femoris tightness. The athlete lies supine with her legs off the table up to midthigh level (figure 10.37). She flexes one knee to her chest and holds it in place with her arms. The knee over the edge of the table should remain flexed at 90°. A positive sign is present if the knee moves toward extension when the opposite knee is brought to the chest, indicating tightness in the rectus femoris.

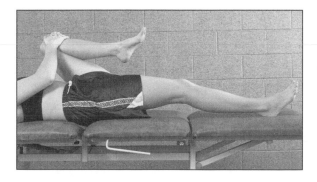

**▎Figure 10.36**   Thomas test.

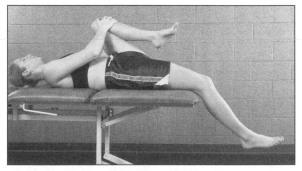

**▎Figure 10.37**   Rectus femoris contracture test (positive test shown).

## Ober's Test

Ober's test assesses tensor fascia lata and IT band tightness. With the athlete in side-lying and her bottom hip and knee flexed for stability, position her top leg in abduction and extension. The knee is kept extended throughout the test. Place one hand on the top pelvis, and support the top leg with your other hand (figure 10.38). Passively lower the leg into adduction. A positive sign occurs if the pelvis moves before the leg becomes adducted or if the leg remains in an abducted position. The test is also performed with the top knee flexed, although this is not advised; a greater stretch is placed on the IT band with the knee fully extended, whereas with the knee flexed the stretch is placed on the femoral nerve.

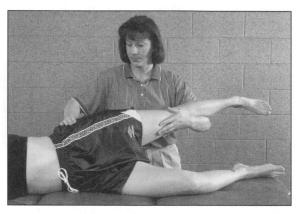

**Figure 10.38**   Ober's test.

## Piriformis Test

In addition to the sideline tests for assessing pathology in the pelvis, you can also use the piriformis test in the off-field evaluation. With the piriformis test you can check for tightness of the piriformis muscle (see earlier discussion of piriformis syndrome). With the athlete side-lying on the uninvolved leg, position his top leg with the knee flexed and the hip in 60° of flexion. Stabilize the pelvis and apply a downward pressure to the knee (figure 10.39). A positive sign is pain in the piriformis muscle. Sciatic pain with this test may indicate that the sciatic nerve runs through or is being compressed by the piriformis.

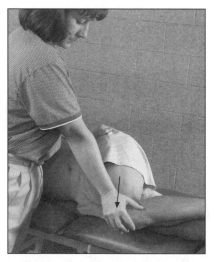

**Figure 10.39**   Piriformis test.

### Joint Mobility

The capsular pattern for the hip usually causes the greatest loss of motion in internal rotation; hip abduction and flexion will be the second most limited motions. External rotation will usually not be limited. Specific investigation of the hip joint to assess capsular tightness is warranted if this pattern of range of motion is present. You will need to compare right and left hips in order to determine abnormalities in hip joint mobility.

## Caudal Glide

The caudal glide (distraction) identifies gross hip joint mobility. The athlete lies supine with his hip in a loose-packed position, 30° flexion and abduction with slight external rotation. Grasp his thigh above the knee and apply a long-axis traction force by leaning backward (figure 10.40). Joint instability may be present if movement is excessive compared to that of the uninvolved joint or if you identify a telescoping of the joint during the distraction.

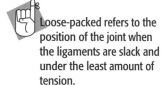

Loose-packed refers to the position of the joint when the ligaments are slack and under the least amount of tension.

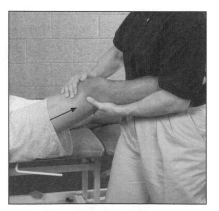

**Figure 10.40**   Caudal glide.

### Lateral Glide (Distraction)

The use of lateral distraction identifies general hypomobility of the hip joint. With the athlete lying supine, apply a mobilization belt around his proximal thigh and around your hips (figure 10.41). Place your near hand (nearest the athlete's head) over the greater trochanter to palpate for hip excursion while the far hand over the distal thigh prevents thigh abduction. Use your body weight to move the athlete's hip laterally. Compare with the uninvolved hip to identify abnormal mobility.

### Dorsal Femoral Glide

This maneuver is used to assess anterior-to-posterior joint mobility. The athlete lies supine with his hip flexed and adducted. Apply a downward force through the femur to move the head of the femur posteriorly (figure 10.42). Compare bilaterally and note any restriction.

### *Palpation*

Palpation of the hip and pelvis in the off-field assessment is the same as for assessment at the sideline. Palpation off the field takes place after all the other tests that have been described but prior to functional tests. By this time of the examination, you should have a reasonable suspicion of the tissue and specific segment involved and should focus your palpation on the appropriate areas.

### *Functional Tests*

The lower-extremity functional tests outlined for the ankle (chapter 8) are appropriate here as well. It is important to take into account the type of sport activity and to consider whether straight-plane running, rotational and cutting maneuvers, or single-leg jumping or landing maneuvers are inherent in the athlete's sport, and to perform functional testing accordingly.

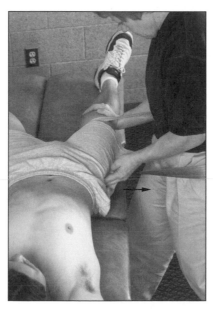

**▌Figure 10.41**  Lateral distraction of the hip joint (lateral glide).

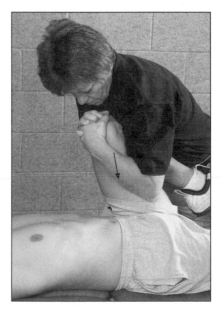

**▌Figure 10.42**  Dorsal femoral glide.

# Checklist for Off-Field Assessment of the Hip, Pelvis, and Groin

## History

Ask questions pertaining to the following:

- ✓ Chief complaint
- ✓ Mechanism of injury
- ✓ Unusual sounds or sensations
- ✓ Type and location of pain or symptoms
- ✓ Previous injury
- ✓ Previous injury to opposite extremity for bilateral comparison

If injury is chronic, ascertain:

- ✓ Duration of onset
- ✓ Level of irritability
- ✓ Aggravating and easing activities
- ✓ Training history

## Observation

- ✓ Check for visible facial expressions of pain.
- ✓ Check for swelling, deformity, abnormal contours, or discoloration.
- ✓ Observe for gait deviations, weight distribution, difficulties with movement.
- ✓ Observe overall stance, limb position, posture, and alignment (anterior, lateral, and posterior).
- ✓ Check muscle development and tone—areas of muscular spasm or atrophy.
- ✓ Bilaterally compare levels of ASIS, PSIS, greater trochanters, knee crease.

## Differential Diagnosis

- ✓ Clear lumbar spine, knee, and ankle.
- ✓ Assess active ROM—full squat.

## Range of Motion

- ✓ Perform active ROM for hip abduction, adduction, flexion (knee flexed and extended), extension (knee flexed and extended), internal and external rotation.
- ✓ Bilaterally compare and note any pain or restricted ROM.
- ✓ Perform passive ROM for the motions listed after each active test.
- ✓ Bilaterally compare and note any pain, restricted ROM, or difference in end feel.

## Strength Tests

- ✓ Perform manual resistance against same motions as for AROM.
- ✓ Check bilaterally and note any pain or weakness.

## Neurovascular Tests

- ✓ Sensory, motor, reflex of L1-S2
- ✓ Femoral pulse

## Special Tests

- ✓ Hip pathology (Patrick, Trendelenburg, Craig's, femoral nerve traction test, stress fracture test)
- ✓ Pelvis pathology (Gaenslen's, iliac compression, sacral apex compression, posterior distraction)
- ✓ Leg length discrepancy (true, apparent)
- ✓ Muscle restriction (Thomas, Kendall, Ober's, piriformis)

## Joint Mobility Assessment

- ✓ Caudal glide
- ✓ Lateral glide
- ✓ Dorsal femoral glide

## Palpation

Palpate for pain, tenderness, and deformity over the following:

- ✓ ASIS, iliac crest including insertion of the abdominals and hip abductors, iliac tubercle, greater trochanter, trochanteric bursa
- ✓ Inguinal ligament, femoral triangle borders and contents, pelvic tubercles
- ✓ Abductor, hip flexor, and adductor muscle groups and insertions
- ✓ PSIS, ischial tuberosity, piriformis and sciatic nerve, sacroiliac joint, sacrotuberous ligament
- ✓ Gluteus maximus
- ✓ Hamstring (proximal and origin on ischial tuberosity)

Perform bilateral comparison.

## Functional Tests

# SUMMARY

1. *Describe the etiology, signs and symptoms, and potential complications associated with acute and chronic injuries of the hip, pelvis, and groin commonly encountered in the physically active.*

   The hip and sacroiliac joints are among the strongest and most stable in the body. As such, they are able to withstand tremendous loads and incur fewer acute injuries than typically seen in the ankle and knee. The most common causes of acute injury are contusions, muscle strains (particularly in the groin), and sprains. Traumatic fractures and dislocations are rare, with stress fractures of the femoral neck and avulsion fractures being more common. Because of the repetitive stresses placed on the hip and pelvis during locomotion and cutting and jumping maneuvers, chronic conditions caused by inflammation and muscle tightness are seen more often.

2. *Identify conditions and concerns specific to the pediatric athlete.*

   Pain surrounding the hip and pelvis in children presents a different challenge for the athletic trainer who typically cares for physically active adults. Conditions specific to the pediatric athlete that one should consider or rule out in cases of hip and groin pain are apophysitis, epiphyseal fractures, slipped capital femoral epiphysis, and chronic synovitis. If these conditions are dismissed as a simple groin strain and proper treatment is not initiated, severe complications and permanent joint changes may result. Therefore when a pediatric athlete complains of groin or hip pain that lasts more than one week, it is important to refer the individual to a physician for follow-up and evaluation.

3. *Identify common structural and functional abnormalities of the hip and pelvis.*

   Structural and functional abnormalities at the hip can have a significant impact on the entire lower chain as well as on the lumbar spine. Abnormal angulation of the hip will result in hip anteversion or retroversion, causing changes in knee (Q-angle, genu valgus) and foot (toe-in, toe-out) alignment that in turn may predispose the lower extremity to stress-type injuries. Leg length differences, also common, can be the result of muscle or joint dysfunction (functional, apparent length difference) or can be a true difference in femoral and tibial length (structural). It is important to recognize and assess for these abnormalities with any chronic complaints in the knee, hip, or lumbar region.

4. *Perform an on-field assessment of the hip, pelvis, and groin, noting criteria for immediate medical referral and mode of transportation from the field.*

   Although the hip is not often acutely injured in sport, injuries to the hip can significantly impair an athlete's performance. On-field assessment requires the athletic trainer to have good observation and palpation skills and to be able to accurately and efficiently assess the athlete's injury severity, condition, and transport needs. Signs of obvious limb shortening or rotation of the leg should be noted, as they are indicative of a hip fracture or dislocation. If no obvious signs of trauma are present, the athletic trainer performs a quick palpation of the bony structures, muscular insertions, and major muscle groups for signs of tenderness and defects before having the athlete perform active range of motion and assisting him off the field.

5. *Perform a thorough and sequential sideline assessment of the hip, pelvis, and groin.*

   With the athlete on the sideline, one can make a more detailed assessment of the injury. Here the athletic trainer takes the time to obtain a more accurate history and to perform a complete assessment including palpation, range of motion, strength, neurological, and special tests. Special tests for this area during the sideline assessment may include tests that identify femoral neck stress fractures, sacroiliac sprain, and nerve pathology.

6. *Perform a thorough and sequential off-field assessment of the hip, pelvis, and groin, including differential diagnosis of referring back and lower-extremity pathologies.*

When an athlete presents in the athletic treatment facility, often the injury is chronic or postacute. Thus the assessment off the field is expanded to include special tests to evaluate the hip and pelvis for muscle shortening and/or weakness, sacroiliac joint dysfunction, structural and functional abnormalities, and joint restrictions. The evaluation also includes a differential diagnosis assessment to rule out any referring back and lower-extremity pathologies.

7. *Describe and differentiate potential causes and conditions of groin pain.*

Groin pain is a common complaint in people who perform running, sprinting, cutting, and rapid change-of-direction maneuvers. Although groin strains may be common, groin pain can also result from a variety of other pathologies including femoral neck stress fractures, inflamed lymph nodes, inguinal hernia, kidney stones, referred pain from the lumbar and sacroiliac regions, and chronic inflammatory conditions. It is essential to remember that groin pain in the adolescent may also indicate more serious hip joint pathologies. Therefore, when groin pain is present without a clear injury mechanism and when it persists for a significant period of time, one should have a high index of suspicion regarding these other conditions.

# REVIEW QUESTIONS

1. Why can contusions around the hip and pelvis be so painful and debilitating?

2. What are some of the common causes and signs and symptoms of trochanteric bursitis? What are some of the other common sites for chronic bursitis?

3. What are the common sites for avulsion fractures? Discuss the common mechanisms and the signs and symptoms associated with these injuries.

4. What is avascular necrosis? Discuss the cause of this condition and the types of injuries this complication may be associated with.

5. Describe the difference between true and apparent leg length discrepancy, and explain how you would differentiate between possible causes of a leg length difference in your evaluation. What potential problems are associated with a leg length difference?

6. When assessing active range of motion and strength for hip flexion and extension, why would it be important to test in both a straight-knee and a flexed-knee position?

7. What specific stress tests are used to evaluate the integrity of the sacroiliac ligaments?

8. Describe the special tests used to identify muscular restrictions around the hip and pelvis. Include the specific structure(s) that each test is designed to evaluate.

# CRITICAL THINKING QUESTIONS

1. Think back to the scenario at the beginning of the chapter. You have learned that, among other injuries, a femoral neck stress fracture, low back pathology, iliopsoas bursitis, and an adductor muscle strain can all refer pain to the groin area. Discuss how you would go about differentiating these four conditions in your assessment. Include in your discussion the special tests that you would use to identify or rule out each of these conditions.

2. You have an athlete complaining of sciatic-type pain down the posterior thigh and lateral lower leg. You have evaluated the athlete's lumbar spine and sacroiliac regions; there were no unusual findings, and you are unable to reproduce the athlete's pain with spinal motions. What muscular condition might you suspect as the cause of this sciatic pain, and how would your evaluation proceed? Considering the special tests learned in this chapter and in chapter 7, which special tests would you use to differentiate among possible causes of the nerve irritation?

3. A 25-year-old runner comes to you complaining of unilateral hip and back pain. As part of your assessment, you wish to rule out any functional or structural abnormalities that may be causing muscular balance or joint dysfunction. Considering the lower extremity as a whole (chapters 7-10), describe how you would assess for alignment abnormalities that may be contributing to this runner's lower back pain.

# CHAPTER ELEVEN

# Head
# and Face

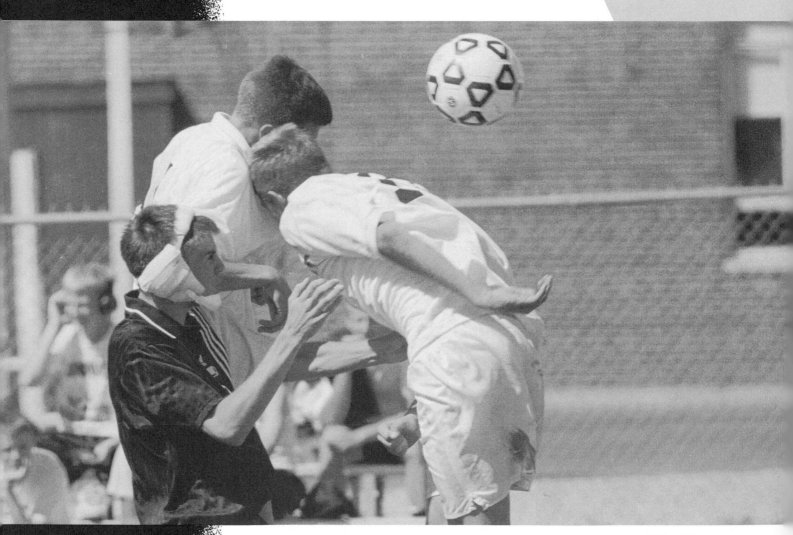

# OBJECTIVES

After completing this chapter, the reader will be able to do the following:

1. Describe the mechanisms, signs and symptoms, and potential complications associated with head and facial injuries commonly encountered in the physically active

2. Differentiate between signs and symptoms of concussion, skull fracture, and intracranial hemorrhage

3. Discuss the potential complications and delayed symptoms that may result from head trauma

4. Perform an on-field assessment of a potential head injury, keeping in mind the criteria for medical referral and mode of transportation from the field

5. Perform a thorough and sequential sideline assessment of a potential head injury, including special tests for cognition, balance, and coordination, keeping in mind the criteria for referral and follow-up evaluation

6. Perform a general assessment for facial injuries, including identification of differential signs and symptoms indicating associated head injury

7. Perform a complete neurological assessment of the cranial nerves

Amanda and Bart were as pumped up as the team was for the game that would decide whether they would make it to a bowl game this year. Late in the second quarter, Kevin, the second-string quarterback, came over to Amanda with concern about John, the first-string quarterback.

"I think something's wrong with John. . . . He seems confused out there and isn't running the plays I'm signaling in to him—I'll think that hit he took in the first quarter rang his bell."

"Thanks, Kevin, I'll take a look at him," Amanda said as she headed over toward John. "Hi, John, you doing okay?" Amanda could see by his eyes that John was a bit dazed.

"Huh? Uh, yeah . . . when is the first quarter going to be over, anyway?" John said, showing frustration.

Continuing her evaluation, Amanda found that John had a headache and was unable to recall what plays he had just run. The team physician agreed—it was clear that John had suffered a mild concussion. Amanda promptly went over to the coach and informed him that John would have to sit out for the rest of the half and that they would reevaluate him during halftime. The coach was not happy, but he understood; he cared about the safety of his players.

Amanda continued to check John every 15 minutes. About 30 minutes after the initial evaluation, she noticed that he was becoming more lethargic and less oriented to his surroundings and teammates. She also noted that he was more unsteady than before and that his grip strength was weaker on one side. She called the team physician over immediately and related her current findings. The ambulance was called and John was immediately taken to the emergency room, where it was found that he had a small subdural hematoma.

Amanda was glad she had continued to evaluate John even though his initial symptoms had appeared minor. She and Bart used the incident as a lesson for the student athletic trainers working the sideline, emphasizing the importance of repeated evaluations for athletes who suffer a head injury.

This chapter will address the recognition and assessment of injuries to the head and face and will equip you to thoroughly evaluate these injuries and to differentiate signs and symptoms that indicate a life-threatening condition. It is important to realize, though, that head and facial pain can be caused by medical conditions unrelated to sport activity. General medical conditions of the head, eyes, ears, nose, and mouth will be covered in chapter 13; you must keep these conditions in mind when an athlete complains of pain and symptoms in this region with no known injury mechanism.

The head is a complex anatomical structure that houses the brain and the sensory organs for sight, hearing, taste, and smell. Although athletes will frequently complain of head and facial pain, the causes can be quite varied and may sometimes indicate serious intracranial pathology. Therefore it is important that you understand the anatomical complexity and function of the structures in the head region in order to adequately assess the basis for injury and illness there. A complete anatomical discussion is beyond the scope of this chapter, which will deal instead with the more important structures of the nervous system as they relate clinically to specific injuries.

The bony structure of the head or skull, which provides protection for the brain and sensory organs, is divided into the cranium and facial bones. The cranium is composed of the frontal, occipital, ethmoid, sphenoid, and paired temporal and parietal bones. The facial skeleton includes the mandible and paired maxillae and nasal, zygomatic, lacrimal, and palatine bones. The only movable joint allowing appreciable range of motion is the temporomandibular joint, which is prone to both acute injury and chronic dysfunction. The bony skeleton is covered by the highly vascularized scalp, consisting of layers of skin and connective tissue. Because of this rich vascular supply, lacerations of the scalp and face will typically result in profuse bleeding.

Although the brain is well protected by the bony skeleton, it is not immune to injury with severe head trauma. The brain is covered by three layers, or **meninges**, that become clinically important when vascular disruption and bleeding occur between them. The **dura mater** is the outermost covering, consisting of a tough fibrous tissue that serves as the inner lining of the skull and provides protection to the brain. The middle meningeal artery, which is the largest of the meningeal arteries, passes through the **epidural space** between the temporal skull and dura mater. This artery is important in that it is often torn with skull fractures, resulting in significant bleeding and a rapid increase in intracranial pressure in the epidural space. Other vessels cross the dura mater, and their disruption with shearing forces can cause bleeding beneath the dura mater into the **subdural space**. The **arachnoid mater** is a delicate, transparent membrane that forms the intermediate covering of the brain. It is separated from the inner meningeal membrane, the **pia mater**, by the **subarachnoid space**, which contains cerebral spinal fluid.

Functional impairment with brain trauma will depend on the brain structures involved. The primary divisions of the brain itself include the cerebral hemispheres, brain stem, and cerebellum (figure 11.1). The two cerebral hemispheres, divided into four lobes (frontal, parietal, temporal, and occipital), function to control body movement, perception of sensation, and higher cerebral functions such as speech, learning, memory, and emotion. The two cerebral hemispheres are connected by the brain stem, which consists of the medulla oblongata and pons. The brain stem extends to the base of the skull and passes through the foramen magnum to become the spinal cord. The brain stem functions to transmit information between the cerebral hemispheres and the spinal cord and to control vital functions of respiration, heart rate, and blood pressure. On the posterior aspect of the pons and medulla is the cerebellum, occupying most of the posterior cranial fossa. Consisting of a midline portion and two lateral lobes, the cerebellum functions primarily to control motor functions that regulate posture, muscle tone, and coordination.

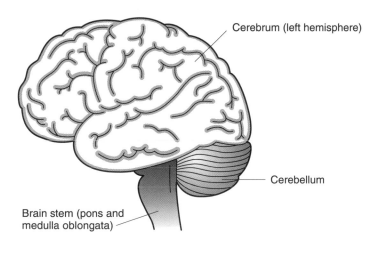

Cerebrum (left hemisphere)

Cerebellum

Brain stem (pons and medulla oblongata)

■ **Figure 11.1** Primary divisions of the brain.

Also emanating from the brain are 12 paired cranial nerves that are numbered from anterior to posterior according to their attachments to the brain (figure 11.2). The cranial nerves provide sensory and motor innervation for the head, neck, thorax, and abdomen (table 11.1). Their individual functions become important in the neurological assessment of head injuries to determine the location and extent of intracranial pressure or pathology.

# INJURIES TO THE HEAD AND FACE

Even with the use of protective equipment during sport activity, head and facial injuries occur frequently and can range widely from minor insults to serious, life-threatening conditions. It is essential for you to be well versed in the etiology and

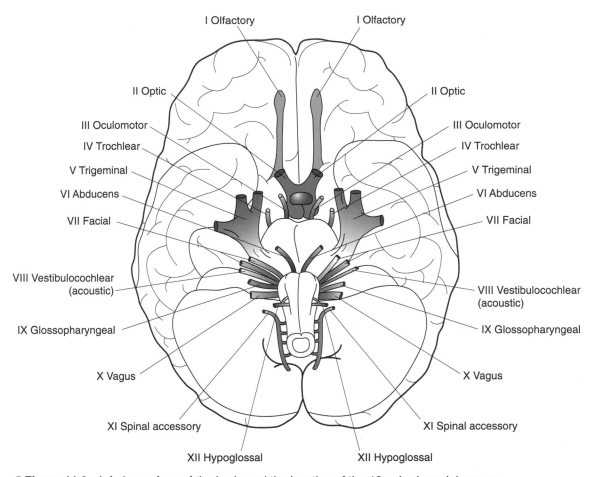

**Figure 11.2** Inferior surface of the brain and the location of the 12 paired cranial nerves.

| Table 11.1 | Function and Assessment of Cranial Nerves | |
|---|---|---|
| **Nerve** | **Name** | **Assessment** |
| I | Olfactory | Sense of smell |
| II | Optic | Peripheral vision, pupillary reflex to light |
| III | Oculomotor | Pupil size, pupillary reflex to light (consensual and direct reflex) |
| | | Raise eyelid |
| | | Eye movement (ability to look up and in) |
| IV | Trochlear | Eye movement (ability to look down and in toward nose) |
| V | Trigeminal | Clench teeth, side-to-side jaw movement |
| VI | Abducens | Lateral eye movement |
| VII | Facial | Wrinkle forehead, smile, frown |
| VIII | Vestibulocochlear (acoustic) | Tinnitus, hearing, equilibrium (Romberg test) |
| IX | Glossopharyngeal | Sense of taste, gag reflex |
| X | Vagus | Voice quality |
| XI | Spinal accessory | Shoulder shrug |
| XII | Hypoglossal | Stick tongue out, note any deviation to one side |

signs and symptoms of each of these conditions and to be able to quickly identify those symptoms that indicate a medical emergency and the need for immediate medical referral.

## HEAD INJURIES

Head injuries are common in athletics, representing the leading cause of death due to sport activity. Unfortunately, external signs resulting from head trauma have no bearing on the seriousness of brain injury. Even apparently mild head injuries have the potential to become life threatening, and you must be able to differentiate between the signs and symptoms of mild head injury or concussion and those indicating intercranial swelling or hemorrhage. Additionally, blows to the head can result in cervical injury. Therefore it is imperative to suspect a cervical injury in the unconscious athlete until you have proof to the contrary.

Head injury can result from either direct or indirect mechanisms. There are essentially two mechanisms of direct trauma, coup and contrecoup (figure 11.3). When the head is stationary and is struck by a moving object such as another player's helmet, a ball, or other sport implement, the brain will be traumatized at the location of impact. This is termed a **coup-type injury**. When the head is moving and makes contact with an immovable or more slowly moving object, the result is a deceleration or **contrecoup-type injury**. Using the head to tackle, falling and striking the head on the

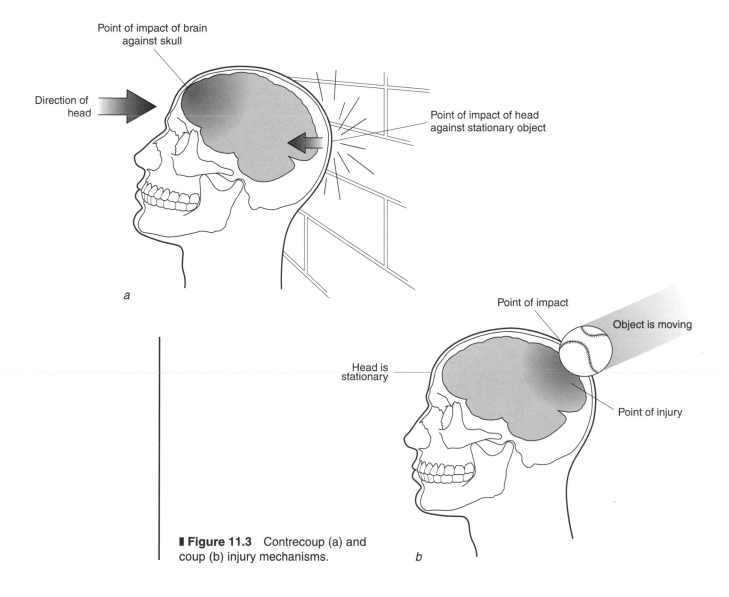

Point of impact of brain against skull

Direction of head

Point of impact of head against stationary object

a

Point of impact

Object is moving

Head is stationary

Point of injury

**▌Figure 11.3** Contrecoup (a) and coup (b) injury mechanisms.

b

*A **compression force** is a force that places direct pressure on a surface or soft tissue.*

*A **shear force** is a force that is directed parallel to a joint or soft tissue surface.*

*A **tensile force** is a force that tractions or pulls away from the surface.*

ground, and running into a goal post are examples of decelerating injuries that will cause the brain to "lag" in relation to the rapid deceleration of the head and to impact the side of the skull opposite the point of contact. Indirect mechanisms such as the transmission of forces through the spine and jaw, or whipping of the head with blows to the thorax with the neck muscles relaxed, can also cause head trauma. These mechanisms can produce three types of stresses to the brain tissues: compressive, shear, and tensile. Because of the protection provided by the skull and the cushioning of the cerebral spinal fluid, compression forces are usually well tolerated as force is dissipated by these structures. However, shearing forces that occur with movement of the brain within the skull are poorly tolerated (Cantu 1992).

Head injuries are typically classified into three categories:

- Mild head injury or concussion
- Intercranial hemorrhage
- Skull fractures

### Concussion

A **concussion**, caused by an agitation or shaking of the brain, is defined as a transient alteration in brain function without structural damage. Clinically, it is defined by the severity of injury. Multiple grading scales have been developed to classify the degree of injury based on either the duration of unconsciousness or the duration of posttraumatic amnesia. The system developed by Cantu (1992), presented in table 11.2, includes a practical and useful scale that considers both of these variables.

*Amnesia means loss of memory.*

Signs and symptoms include headache, dizziness, nausea, ringing in the ears (**tinnitus**), loss of consciousness, confusion, and amnesia. Signs and symptoms may vary considerably from one individual to another and according to injury severity. While it is often fairly easy to recognize second- and third-degree concussions, first-degree concussions may go unnoticed if the athlete does not report the symptoms. Often, mental confusion—of which the athlete will be unaware—is the only symptom, but it may be picked up by an astute teammate or coach who notices that the athlete is not with the game plan.

### Intracranial Hemorrhage

Although the skull provides good protection, it is also acts as an unyielding casing and pressure vise around the brain when intracranial swelling or hemorrhage occurs. When head trauma results in tissue edema or hemorrhage, pressure will build in the intracranial space, forcing the contents to shift down toward the only opening,

| Table 11.2   Cantu System for Classifying Severity of Concussion | | |
|---|---|---|
| **Grade** | **Loss of consciousness** | **Duration of posttraumatic amnesia** |
| Grade I (mild) | None | <30 min |
| Grade II (moderate) | <5 min | 30 min to <24 h |
| Grade III (severe) | ≥5 min | ≥24 h |

Reprinted, by permission, from R.C. Cantu, 1992, "Cerebral concussion in sport," *Sports Medicine* 14: 69.

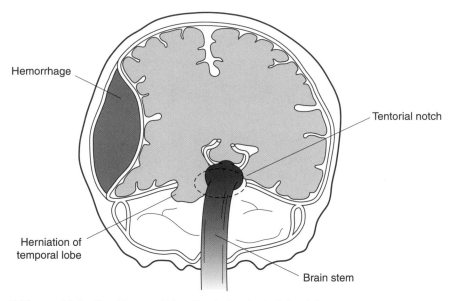

■ **Figure 11.4**  Swelling and bleeding in the tentorial notch.

the tentorial notch (figure 11.4). This will ultimately result in compression of the brain stem, the center for breathing, heart rate, and other life-sustaining functions. Unless pressure is relieved in a timely fashion, death will result.

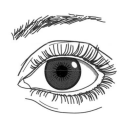

■ **Figure 11.5**  Unequal pupils indicating intracranial pressure.

A space-occupying hematoma will alter consciousness, vital signs, motor function, and pupillary function. Individuals with this injury will vary in their level of consciousness from fully awake, to drowsy or lethargic, to stuporous, to comatose. It will become increasingly difficult to arouse and awaken the person. Vital signs will indicate high blood pressure, decreased pulse rate, and changes in respiration. The most common observation is **Cheyne-Stokes respiration**, characterized by a rhythmic fluctuation between **hyperpnea** (rapid, deep breathing) and **apnea** (absence of breathing). Note that these altered vital signs are the opposite of those of shock, which are rapid shallow breathing, hypotension, and rapid pulse. Pupillary changes indicative of increasing intracranial pressure include pupil inequality (figure 11.5) and unresponsiveness to light. Motor deficits will range from weakness to paralysis. Unusual movements, such as a Babinski sign or decorticate or decerebrate posturing, are also indicative of severe brain damage. **Decorticate posturing** occurs with injury above the brain stem and is characterized by rigid extension of the legs and flexion of the arms, wrist, and hands in toward the chest (figure 11.6). **Decerebrate posturing**, a sign of upper brain stem injury, is a

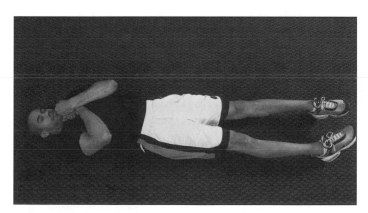

■ **Figure 11.6**  Decorticate posturing.

rigid extension of all four extremities, with the arms internally rotated and pronated (figure 11.7). A positive **Babinski sign**, or dorsiflexion of the great toe and splaying of the lesser toes with stroking of the plantar surface, is indicative of a lower brain stem injury.

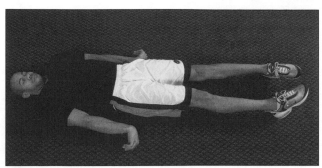

**Figure 11.7**    Decerebrate posturing.

It is important to note that these symptoms may not be observed immediately following injury but may be delayed for minutes, hours, or even days. However, once they appear, the athlete's condition can deteriorate quickly, resulting in death within minutes. Typically, the longer the period of consciousness or delay in symptoms following injury, the slower the hemorrhage and the progression of symptoms. Therefore, it is important to observe and monitor the athlete regularly for signs and symptoms of intracranial hemorrhage and to refer immediately when these are present.

In athletics, there are two primary types of intracranial hemorrhage—subdural and epidural hematomas:

Symptoms of intracranial hemorrhage may not appear immediately following injury and may occur at some delay. However, once symptoms do appear, the athlete's condition can deteriorate quickly and result in death if not immediately recognized.

Any athlete who loses consciousness, even for a brief period of time, should be closely examined and monitored following injury and throughout the next 24 h for signs and symptoms of intercranial hemorrhage.

• A **subdural hematoma**, or bleeding in the subdural space, is a medical emergency that is usually associated with severe closed head trauma and that has a high mortality rate (Cantu 1991). At the time of injury, the athlete is usually rendered unconscious and either will remain unconscious or will regain consciousness for a brief period of time before collapsing (Cantu 1991). Therefore, any athlete who loses consciousness, even for a brief period of time, should be closely examined and monitored following injury and throughout the next 24 h for signs and symptoms of intercranial hemorrhage.

• **Epidural hematomas** most often result from a skull fracture in the temporal region that tears the middle meningeal artery, resulting in a rapidly expanding hematoma. The direct trauma may or may not have been sufficient to cause brain trauma or loss of consciousness at the time of injury. Therefore, these injuries can be deceiving in that initially the symptoms may not be severe. However, after a brief period of consciousness, the athlete's condition will deteriorate rapidly, with death occurring within minutes if pressure is not relieved.

### Skull Fracture

Skull fractures result from direct impact; they are more common in sports utilizing a bat and ball, and in sports played on hard surfaces with the athlete not wearing a helmet, than in other types of sports. The fracture may be linear or hairline, resulting from a blunt force, or depressed, resulting from a more focused point of contact. The location of the fracture may be significant, as fractures that transverse a major artery may cause tearing of the vessel and an epidural hemorrhage. Other times, the fracture may aid in dissipating the force and lead to lesser brain trauma. Signs and symptoms of skull fracture include pain, palpable tenderness, swelling, discoloration, and possible depression. The overlying skin may or may not be lacerated. Discoloration around the eyes (**raccoon eyes**) and behind the ears (**Battle's sign**), and fluid draining from the nose (**rhinorrhea**) or ears (**otorrhea**), are additional signs indicative of a skull fracture. Loss of consciousness and other signs and symptoms of concussion may also be apparent.

### Second-Impact Syndrome

An athlete who returns to competition and sustains a second minor head trauma too soon after an initial head injury may be at risk for second-impact syndrome. **Second-**

**impact syndrome** is characterized by an autoregulatory dysfunction that causes rapid and fatal brain swelling. The athlete with previous and recent history of mild head injury who receives a blow to the head will initially exhibit signs and symptoms of a mild concussion. The second impact will usually not result in loss of consciousness, and the athlete will typically remain on her feet but may appear dazed (Cantu 1995). However, within minutes, she will collapse into a coma and show signs of cranial nerve and brain stem pressure. The mortality rate of second-impact syndrome is high, and therefore prevention is key.

Athletes who sustain even a mild head injury should be thoroughly examined and should be symptom free before returning to activity. Unfortunately, criteria for deciding when an athlete can safely return to competition are not well defined. In 1994 the National Athletic Trainers' Association Research and Education Foundation sponsored a summit on mild head injury in sports that brought together experts from neurosurgery, neuropsychology, rehabilitation, family practice, pediatrics, and athletic training to address this important issue. Research is ongoing to establish objective criteria for determining full recovery and safe return to activity following brain trauma.

### Post-Concussion Syndrome

Post-concussion syndrome can occur following mild head injury; the signs and symptoms are listed below. These symptoms may not always be easy to recognize and can persist for days, weeks, and even months after neurocognitive tests have returned to normal. Therefore, it is important to listen to and closely observe the athlete in the days following injury for subjective complaints that may relate to the head trauma.

## EYE INJURIES

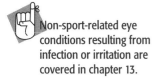 Non-sport-related eye conditions resulting from infection or irritation are covered in chapter 13.

Injuries to the eye, which most often result from direct contact, may involve either the corneal surface or internal structures of the eye. Eye injuries can be quite serious and may result in permanent damage if not recognized immediately or treated appropriately. All serious eye injuries should be immediately referred to an ophthalmologist for further evaluation and care.

### Periorbital Hematoma

A periorbital hematoma, or black eye, is caused by a direct blow and is characterized by discoloration and swelling of the orbital rim and cavity. Other signs and symptoms, including pain and vision impairment, may be present secondary to severe swelling of the eyelids. Although a periorbital hematoma is rarely serious and does

---

### Signs and Symptoms of Post-Concussion Syndrome

- Headache with exertion
- Dizziness
- Tinnitus
- Fatigue
- Irritability
- Frustration
- Difficulty in coping with daily stress
- Impaired memory or concentration

- Eating or sleeping disorders
- Behavioral changes
- Alcohol intolerance
- Decreased academic performance

*Source*: National Athletic Trainers' Association Research and Education Foundation. *Mild Brain Injury in Sports Summit Proceedings*. Washington DC, April 16-18, 1994.

not require medical referral, it is very important to thoroughly assess the eye itself for any associated trauma.

### Corneal Abrasion

A finger poke to the eye or a foreign body under the eyelid can scratch the outer surface of the cornea, resulting in a corneal abrasion. Abrasions can also occur when one attempts to remove a foreign body from the eye or removes a contact lens that has been in place too long. To prevent these types of abrasions, it is always better to flush the eye with saline, which should gently lift the foreign body off the corneal surface and out of the eye, than to try to remove the object manually.

Corneal abrasions are extremely painful. The athlete will often be unable to keep his eye open secondary to pain. The eye will appear red (**hyperemia**) and watery, and the athlete may complain of a gritty feeling—as if something were still in the eye even after the foreign body has been removed. Consequently visual acuity may be temporarily impaired. Fortunately, the eye heals quickly, and symptoms will diminish significantly over the first 24 h. Often the pain alone is sufficient to cause the athlete to seek medical attention.

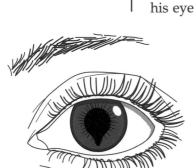

**▌Figure 11.8**   Corneal laceration and tear-shaped pupil.

### Corneal Laceration

Lacerations through the full thickness of the cornea are much less common than corneal abrasions but can occur when a sharp object, such as a fingernail, cuts the eye. The athlete will complain of acute pain and visual impairment. Distortion or disruption of the corneal surface will be observable, and the pupil may appear tear-shaped (figure 11.8). Athletes with a corneal laceration should be immediately referred to an ophthalmologist for further evaluation.

### Detached Retina

A sudden blow to the head or eye can cause the pigment layer of the retina to tear away or become detached from its neural layer on the inner, posterior surface of the eye. A detached retina is not readily apparent with visual observation, but symptoms indicating a possible detached retina include blurred vision, flashes, floating spots, or blind areas in one's field of vision. These symptoms may occur immediately after injury but may also be delayed for a time period from a few days to a few months. Suspicion of a detached retina warrants immediate referral.

### Hyphema

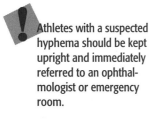

Athletes with a suspected hyphema should be kept upright and immediately referred to an ophthalmologist or emergency room.

Direct trauma to the eye can also result in a **hyphema**, or an accumulation of blood in the anterior chamber of the eye (figure 11.9). The chamber sits anterior to the iris and is normally filled with a clear, watery fluid (aqueous humor). Blood in the anterior chamber is readily apparent, as it will obscure the iris and pupil. The athlete will complain of impaired vision, pain, and a feeling of pressure in the eye. Hyphemas indicate a serious eye injury that can cause excessive pressure within the eye or can be associated with further underlying pathology. The athlete should be kept upright and immediately referred to an ophthalmologist or emergency room.

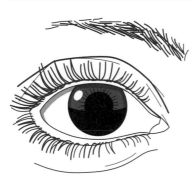

**▌Figure 11.9**   Blood in the anterior chamber (hyphema).

### Fractures

A fracture of the orbital floor, also known as a **blow-out fracture**, occurs as a result of a sudden increase in orbital pressure due to a direct blow to the eye. Blunt trauma such as being struck in the eye with a baseball or a racquet ball is a common mechanism. The pressure created by the blow will cause the thin, inferior wall of the orbit to fracture and displace inferiorly. Signs and symptoms include swelling, discoloration, and point tenderness along the inferior aspect of the eye. The injured eye may appear to sit lower than the uninjured one, and the athlete will be unable to look up because of entrapment of the inferior eye muscles at the fracture site (figure 11.10). The athlete will also complain of double vision (**diplopia**).

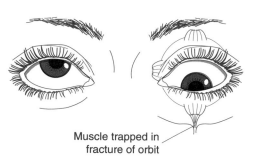

Muscle trapped in
fracture of orbit

**▌ Figure 11.10** Orbital blow-out fracture with the inability to look upward.

## EAR INJURIES

Injuries to the ear include lacerations and hematoma caused by blunt trauma to the side of the head. Chapter 13 covers ear conditions associated with illness and infection that athletes may experience but that are not a direct result of sport participation.

### Auricular Contusions and Cauliflower Ear (Auricular Hematoma)

The auricle, or external ear, comprises a single, elastic cartilage covered by a thin layer of skin that provides nutrition to the underlying cartilage. Contusions, friction, or repetitive trauma to the external ear can result in bleeding between the skin and cartilage. An observable hematoma (figure 11.11) will form, and the athlete will complain of considerable pain and tenderness. If the hematoma is left untreated and allowed to persist, separation of the cartilage from its nutritional supply will result in necrosis and degeneration of the cartilage. Permanent scarring and deformity resembling the cauliflower will also result.

### Lacerations

Lacerations of the ear, though uncommon, can result from a severe direct-impact or tensioning force. Athletes who wear earrings during sport participation are particularly at risk for lacerations of the earlobe, as the earring can get caught on a jersey and be violently pulled from the ear. Signs and symptoms include pain and bleeding. There may also be transient hearing loss if the laceration occurs secondary to direct impact, but hearing should return within minutes following injury.

General medical conditions of the nose and sinuses, covered in chapter 13, should be considered in the differential diagnosis when an athlete cannot recall a mechanism of injury.

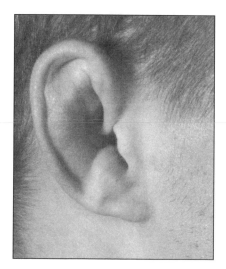

**▌ Figure 11.11** Cauliflower ear.

## NASAL INJURIES

Nasal injuries are the most common facial injury in sport. Nasal fractures are the most common facial fracture, and nosebleeds (epistaxis) frequently occur because of the rich blood supply in the nasal mucosa.

### Epistaxis

Although the majority of nosebleeds (epistaxis) result from direct trauma to the nose or face, some athletes can experience recurrent nosebleeds as a result of mucosal irritation, infection, exertion, or hypertension. The primary sign is mild to profuse bleeding from the nose. The athlete may also complain of pain and difficulty breathing secondary to swelling. Athletes with recurrent nosebleeds should be referred to a physician for further evaluation.

### Nasal Fracture

The prominence of the nose on the face and its thin bony structure increase its susceptibility to fracture. Common scenarios include contact with an opponent's elbow during a rebound and a softball bouncing up into the face from a "bad hop." The fracture may involve the bony bridge or the more distal movable cartilage. Bony displacement, usually lateral, is common. Signs and symptoms include pain, palpable tenderness, epistaxis (often profuse), probable deformity and crepitus, and immediate swelling. The nasal septum may also be damaged or severely deviated; this may restrict airflow through one of the nasal passages. Initially, breathing through the nose following a fracture is often difficult because of swelling. However, if an athlete continues to complain of restricted breathing once swelling subsides, deviations in the nasal septum should be ruled out. Athletes with suspected nasal fractures should also be evaluated for associated maxillary fractures and possible concussion and should be referred to a physician as appropriate.

### Deviated Septum

The nasal septum is a part bony and part cartilaginous structure that separates the nasal passageway into two narrow cavities. Minor deviations in the septum to one side or the other are common. However, severe deviations can occur as a consequence of congenital malformation or of direct trauma as already described. If the deviation is severe, it can restrict airflow, and the athlete will complain of difficulty with air exchange through one side of the nose. In this case, surgery may be necessary to repair the deviation.

## JAW AND MOUTH INJURIES

Direct contact and glancing blows to the face and chin can result in traumatic injury of other facial bones or the temporomandibular joint (TMJ). Chronic TMJ dysfunction may also occur in athletes and may be the source of other complaints of head and facial pain.

### Mandibular Fracture

Fractures to the mandible or jaw occur as a result of a direct blow, for example being struck by a ball or another player or making contact with the ground when falling.

*Malocclusion is an inability to approximate the upper and lower jaw/teeth in a normal bite.*

Often, two fractures will occur, one on either side of the jaw. The most common site of fracture is at the mandibular angle, near the socket of the third molar (Moore 1992) (figure 11.12). Fractures more proximal at the neck and coronoid process are usually associated with a dislocation. The athlete will complain of pain with jaw movement and will be palpably tender along the jaw line. Gentle tapping of the chin may also cause increased pain. Swelling, discoloration, malocclusion, bleeding around the teeth, and possible bony crepitus and deformity will also be noted.

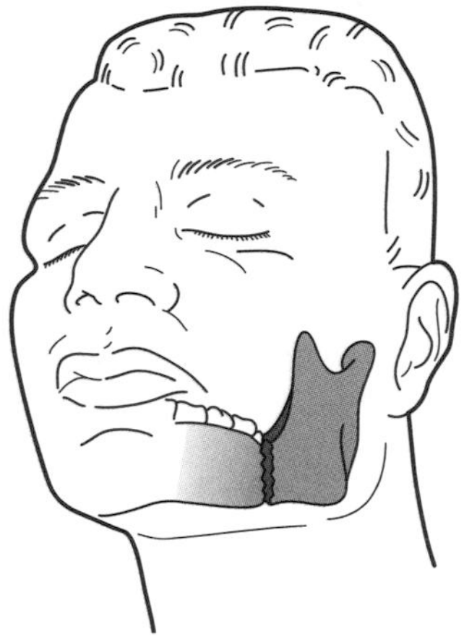

**Figure 11.12** Mandibular fracture at the mandibular angle near the socket of the 3rd molar.

### Maxilla Fracture

The maxilla comprises the bony surface between the mouth and the eyes. Blunt or direct trauma to the anterior face can cause fractures of the upper jaw and mouth. Signs and symptoms include pain, swelling, bleeding around the upper teeth, and discoloration below the eyes. The athlete will be tender to palpation and will complain of increased pain when biting down. Malocclusion, loose teeth, and crepitus may also be observable. Fractures to the maxillae may also occur concurrently with a nasal fracture, and epistaxis may result.

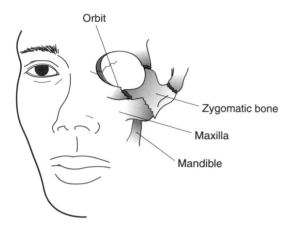

**Figure 11.13**  Zygomatic arch fracture.

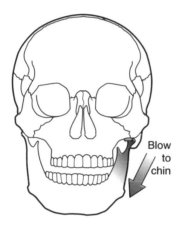

**Figure 11.14**  Malocclusion and lateral shift of the jaw.

### Zygomatic Arch Fractures

The inferolateral orbital rim is formed by the zygomatic or "cheek" bones. Zygomatic fractures are among the more common facial fractures and usually result from a direct blow to the cheek (figure 11.13). Signs and symptoms include pain, swelling, discoloration, and tenderness over the bony prominence. If the fracture is displaced, the cheek will appear flattened. Because the zygomatic bone forms part of the orbit, visual acuity and ocular alignment may also be affected.

### Temporomandibular Joint Dislocation

Dislocations of the TMJ usually occur anteriorly. As the mouth is opened, the proximal head of the mandible and articular disc glide forward (Moore 1992). A blow to the chin, or too much downward pressure on the lower jaw when the mouth is open, may cause the proximal heads of the mandible to dislocate. Simply opening the mouth too wide can also cause dislocation. Dislocation is usually bilateral, and the athlete will be unable to close her mouth. She will be in considerable pain, and deformity will be observable at the TMJ. A lateral blow or angular blow to the chin may also result in a unilateral dislocation or subluxation. In this case, there will be restricted range of motion and a malocclusion of the teeth (figure 11.14).

### Temporomandibular Joint Dysfunction

Temporomandibular joint dysfunction is characterized by chronic joint pain and crepitus that may also produce headaches and neck pain. Causes of TMJ dysfunction are direct trauma, arthritic conditions, poor approximation of the teeth when biting down, muscular tension, and grinding of the teeth at night. If the articular disc is displaced, clicking may also occur with opening or closing of the mouth or with chewing. If an athlete complains of chronic headaches or neck pain with no history of injury, the TMJ should be always be evaluated and included in the differential diagnosis assessment.

## DENTAL INJURY

Dental injuries related to athlete participation are discussed here; dental disease is discussed in chapter 13 within the context of general medical conditions.

The athlete may present a variety of dental complaints that may or may not be related to sport participation. Athletes will experience dental pain and injury secondary either to direct trauma to the mouth or to tooth disease resulting from poor hygiene.

Injuries to the teeth caused by direct trauma to the mouth are classified as fractures, intrusion, luxation, or extrusion.

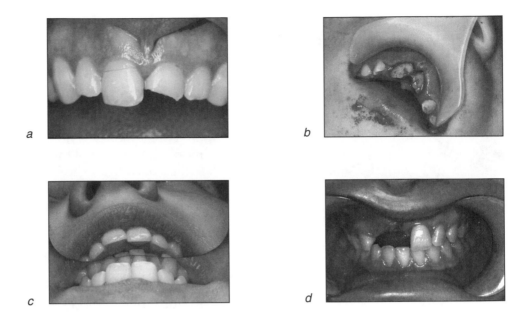

**Figure 11.15**    (a) Fracture, (b) intrusion, (c) luxation, and (d) extrusion (avulsion) of a tooth.

Tooth fractures may involve a simple "chipping" of the enamel or may extend into the dentin, pulp, or root (figure 11.15a). Involvement of only the enamel usually does not produce pain and is merely a cosmetic disruption, but fractures through the enamel into the structure of the tooth will cause considerable pain. In addition, the fracture may be visible, and there may also be bleeding around the gum secondary to trauma. Root fractures are not readily apparent, as the root is below the gum line and cannot be seen. However, the tooth will appear loose and crepitus may be present when one attempts to mobilize the tooth.

Traumatic forces to the mouth can also loosen a tooth in its **alveolar process** (tooth socket). An axial force applied to the tooth may cause an **intrusion**, in which the tooth is driven into the socket (figure 11.15b). Bleeding and tenderness of the tooth and gum will result, and the tooth will appear shorter than the adjacent teeth. The athletic trainer should not attempt to move the tooth if it is intruded.

If force is applied to the side of the tooth, the tooth may be displaced (luxation) or dislocated (figure 11.15c). The tooth will appear out of alignment or "crooked," and the gums may bleed. Dislocated teeth may also be partially extruded, or pulled from the socket. In this case, the tooth may appear higher or longer than the adjacent teeth. Complete **extrusions** will result in avulsion of the entire tooth from the socket (figure 11.15d). In cases of tooth extrusion or dislocation, the tooth can be gently returned to its normal position. In all cases, the athlete should be referred to a dentist for further evaluation.

It is also important to note that an abscess may form secondary to dental injuries. For this reason, athletes who sustain a fracture or displacement of a tooth should be instructed to report any increases in pain, sensitivity, or fever in the days following injury.

> ! Athletes who sustain a fracture or displacement of a tooth should be instructed to report any increases in pain, sensitivity, or fever in the days following injury that would indicate a secondary infection.

## ASSESSMENT OF HEAD INJURIES

A major blow to an athlete's head or chin should immediately arouse your suspicion of potential head injury. In evaluation of potential head injuries, your concern is not only whether the athlete exhibits any of the characteristic signs and symptoms, but also whether the signs and symptoms change or worsen over time. Your observation skills must be particularly keen in this assessment, as the behavior and response of the athlete will provide important clues to injury severity.

The assessment section of this chapter is divided into on-field and sideline assessment of head injury and sideline assessment of facial injuries. The on-field assessment of facial injuries is similar to that for head injury, as your primary concern on the field is the identification of life-threatening conditions and the need to rule out brain trauma. Off-field assessment for head and facial injuries is essentially the same as at the sideline; thus instead of off-field assessment guidelines, the discussion will present information on follow-up evaluation for head injuries. In fact, in any off-field or follow-up assessment, you should deliberately use the same evaluation techniques as in your on-field and sideline assessment so that you can compare your findings over time and determine whether the athlete's symptoms have improved or worsened.

## ON-FIELD ASSESSMENT

On-field assessment of a suspected head injury should begin with a primary survey to immediately determine level of consciousness and the presence of life-threatening conditions. Throughout the sideline assessment, you should closely monitor vital signs, level of consciousness, and signs and symptoms of intracranial hemorrhage.

### *Primary Survey*

As you approach the athlete, note the environment and surroundings and check for any potential hazards that may place the athlete at risk for further injury. Also note the position and any response of the athlete.

### Establish Level of Consciousness

The athlete with a head injury may range from conscious, coherent, and ambulatory to completely unconscious and unresponsive. Therefore your initial goal is to establish level of consciousness. Determine baseline level of consciousness by observing the athlete's eye opening and his motor and verbal response to a verbal command or a pain stimulus. Many use the Glasgow Coma Scale to objectively communicate an athlete's level of consciousness (table 11.3). If the athlete does not respond spontaneously or to verbal commands, use a pain stimulus to evoke a response or arouse him by applying supraorbital pressure just below the eyebrow, by rubbing your knuckle on his sternum, or by pinching the upper trapezius or inner aspect of his arm. The point system of the Glasgow Coma Scale, based on the athlete's response, provides both an initial assessment of level of consciousness and a means of monitoring changes in level of consciousness over time.

### Assess Vital Signs

If the athlete is moving and immediately speaks to you, you are assured that airway, breathing, and circulation are present. However, if she is unconscious, you should immediately assess vital signs. As with any unconscious athlete, a cervical spine injury should be suspected, and the head and neck should be immobilized throughout your evaluation process. If it is necessary to move the athlete to appropriately assess or care for her, you must follow cervical spine precautions. When establishing an airway, you should use a modified jaw thrust.

**Respirations** are evaluated for presence, rate, depth, and rhythm. Respiration is influenced by many parts of the brain and is a key vital sign that should be checked before anything else. Shock will produce rapid and shallow respirations; in contrast, intracranial hemorrhage will cause respirations to be slow and irregular. Cheyne-Stokes respirations, characterized by a rhythmic fluctuation between rapid, deep breathing (hypernea) and slow or absent breathing (apnea), may be observable.

Evaluate **pulse** for presence, strength, rate, and rhythm. A rapid pulse may be the result of the level of exercise just prior to injury, or it may be indicative of shock or increased pressure at the base of the brain. A decreased (less than 60 beats/min), bounding pulse is indicative of intercranial hemorrhage.

Any unconscious athlete with a suspected head injury should be treated as if he or she has a cervical spine injury until there is proof to the contrary. The head and neck should be stabilized throughout the evaluation process.

**Table 11.3   Glascow Coma Scale (Rate Best Response in Each Category)**

**Eye opening**

| | | |
|---|---|---|
| Spontaneous | 4 | |
| In response to voice | 3 | |
| In response to pain | 2 | |
| Does not open eyes | 1 | |
| | | Score _____ |

**Verbal response**

| | | |
|---|---|---|
| Oriented and easily converses | 5 | |
| Confused, but converses | 4 | |
| Inappropriate words | 3 | |
| Incomprehensible words | 2 | |
| No verbal response | 1 | |
| | | Score _____ |

**Motor response**

| | | |
|---|---|---|
| Obeys verbal commands | 6 | |
| Localized pain | 5 | |
| Withdraws from pain | 4 | |
| Abnormal flexion response (decorticate rigidity) | 3 | |
| Abnormal extension response (decerebrate rigidity) | 2 | |
| No response to pain | 1 | |
| | | Score _____ |

| | | |
|---|---|---|
| Total score | 15 | _____ |

You should also take blood pressure at this time. A rise in blood pressure (hypertension) will be noted with intracranial hemorrhage due to a compensatory response by the body to maintain blood flow through the brain as intracranial pressure increases. The blood pressure response to shock will be hypotension—opposite that for an intracranial hemorrhage.

**Other Immediate Observations**

As with any primary assessment, you should immediately observe and control for any severe bleeding and shock. As just mentioned, signs and symptoms of shock are essentially the opposite of those for an intracranial hemorrhage. Shock rarely develops from head injury alone and usually indicates that other trauma is also present.

Although you will evaluate pupillary reflexes and any evidence of lateralizing signs or unusual posturing (i.e., decorticate, decerebrate) in the secondary survey, your primary observation should also include these.

If the athlete remains unconscious or exhibits any positive signs, emergency medical services (EMS) should be summoned immediately. While waiting for EMS to respond, you will need to continually monitor vital signs and reevaluate every 5 min.

### *Secondary Survey*

If there is no immediate evidence of life-threatening injury, proceed with your secondary survey. In the on-field evaluation of a suspected head injury, the components of the secondary survey include history, observation, palpation, and neurological assessment.

### History

If the athlete is unconscious, ask bystanders what happened to get a sense of the mechanism of injury, as well as the direction and point of contact. If the athlete is conscious, ask him about the mechanism of injury and find out whether he recalls losing consciousness; also question him about the location, type, and severity of symptoms and any unusual sensations or feelings. Unusual sensations may include ringing in the ears (tinnitus), headache, or dizziness. Before moving the athlete, ask whether he has any cervical pain or radiating symptoms into the extremities. If he does, you should immobilize the head and neck, and your evaluation should include a cervical spine assessment.

Taking a history will not only help you determine the nature and severity of the symptoms; it will also provide an assessment of the athlete's orientation to time, person, and place. Although you will assess this more thoroughly on the sideline, the athlete's ability to articulate his symptoms and recall what happened or whether he lost consciousness will give you an initial assessment of brain function.

### Observation

Your on-field observation of the athlete should include a check for any immediate signs of skull fracture and brain trauma. Observe for any unusual body movements (posturing) or unusual behavior. Check for any unusual facial expressions such as drooling, drooping of one eyelid, or drooping of the corner of the mouth (lateralizing signs). Observe the athlete's level of consciousness and overall behavior. Does she appear alert and responsive, or is she restless, lethargic, or combative? Is she aware of her surroundings, or does she appear dazed and confused?

Your observation should also include an assessment of eye movement and responsiveness. Check the pupils for size, their equality left to right, and their reaction to light. Specifically, the pupils should be equal in size and should constrict when a beam of light is shone in the eye. Evaluate both direct (same eye) and consensual (contralateral eye) reflex. Also observe for unusual eye movements that would indicate cranial nerve pressure such as nystagmus (involuntary eye movement), lateral drift of one eye, or a downward and inward positioning of the eyes (cross-eye). If any of these signs are positive, you should assume serious brain injury and immediately summon EMS.

Also observe for swelling, deformity, discoloration, and bleeding or drainage from the nose or ears that would indicate a skull fracture. To determine whether drainage from the ears or nose contains cerebral spinal fluid, use a gauze to absorb some of the drainage. If cerebral spinal fluid is present, a yellowish halo will form around the area soaked with blood. Rhinorrhea (drainage from the nose) and raccoon eyes (discoloration around the eyes) may indicate a nasal fracture or a frontal skull fracture; Battle's sign (discoloration behind the ears) and otorrhea (drainage from the ears) may indicate a basilar skull fracture.

During your observation, continuously monitor the athlete's respirations and level of consciousness, being careful to note any changes from your earlier assessment. If any change in symptoms indicates a worsening in symptoms, rather than improvement, call EMS immediately.

If any change in symptoms indicates a worsening rather than improvement in the athlete's conditions, EMS should be summoned immediately.

If a depression or deformity is present on the skull, be very careful not to apply additional pressure to this area.

## Palpation

Carefully palpate the entire face and skull for tenderness, swelling, deformity, or depressions. If a depression or deformity is present on the skull, be very careful not to apply additional pressure to this area. With any deformities or depression, you should suspect a fracture. If the athlete is unconscious or incoherent, or is conscious and complains of cervical pain, you should also palpate the cervical spine for tenderness, swelling, and deformity.

## Neurological Tests

The need to perform neurological tests on the field will depend on your assessment thus far. If you are still unsure of the athlete's condition and his ability to ambulate off the field, you will perform a series of neurological tests.

A cranial nerve check will assess the integrity of each of the 12 cranial nerves. The name, function, and appropriate test for each cranial nerve are presented in table 11.1. If any one cranial nerve assessment produces a positive sign, you should suspect serious brain trauma and refer the athlete immediately.

A Babinski test can also be used to determine the presence of a brain lesion. Use a blunt object, such as the end of a reflex hammer or a pen, to stroke the plantar aspect of the foot from the heel, along the lateral aspect of the foot and across the ball of the foot. The test is positive if the great toe extends and there is splaying (abduction) of the other four toes. A normal response is flexion of the toes.

If you have not yet ruled out cervical spine injury, perform a cervical spine check for sensory and motor function. The procedures for the on-field assessment of cervical spine injuries are appropriate here (see chapter 3).

General **motor tests** are also used to assess for unilateral weakness and ability of the athlete to respond to commands. Ask the athlete to move all four extremities. Note any pain, unwillingness to move, unusual movements, or inappropriate responses. You can assess upper- and lower-extremity strength quickly with bilateral grip strength and resisted dorsiflexion/plantar flexion strength tests. Any positive tests are indicative of neurological pathology and mean that the athlete should be immobilized and passively transported for emergency medical care.

## Continuous Monitoring and Decision for Emergency Medical Referral

The condition of an athlete with a serious brain injury can quickly deteriorate, and death can occur within minutes. Therefore, it is imperative that you monitor vital signs and level of consciousness every 5 min until you have ruled out serious head trauma or are sure the athlete is stabilized or improving. Even then, the athlete should be reevaluated every 15-30 min. Because the individual's condition can deteriorate so quickly, if you have any doubt as to the severity of the head trauma you must not hesitate to seek emergency medical assistance. In addition to the positive signs already mentioned, any one of the following changes is reason for immediate referral:

- Decreasing level of consciousness (decreasing score on Glascow Coma Scale)
- Increase in blood pressure
- Decrease or irregularity in respirations
- Decrease or irregularity in pulse
- Unequal, dilated, or unreactive pupil(s)

## SIDELINE ASSESSMENT OF HEAD INJURY

Sideline assessment of a potential head injury serves as a follow-up to the on-field assessment, providing a more complete evaluation of neurological function. In some cases, your initial evaluation may take place on the sideline; for example, an athlete

# Checklist for On-Field Assessment of Head Injury

## Primary Survey

As you approach

✓ check surroundings and environment and gain history of event as necessary from bystanders if you did not witness.

When you reach the injured person, establish level of consciousness by checking

✓ eye opening,

✓ verbal response, and

✓ motor response.

If athlete is unconscious, immediately

✓ evaluate in the position found

✓ access vital signs by

   ✓ determining absence or presence of airway, breathing, and pulse (rate, rhythm, strength), and taking blood pressure.

✓ observe and control severe bleeding,

✓ observe for lateralizing signs and evidence of decorticate or decerebrate posturing,

✓ evaluate pupillary reflexes, and

✓ observe for shock (signs and symptoms opposite those of intracranial hemorrhage).

It is of utmost importance that you

✓ assume cervical spine injury until proven otherwise,

✓ summon EMS if you note any positive signs, and

✓ reassess vital signs every 5 min.

## Secondary Survey

✓ History

If athlete is conscious, ask questions pertaining to the following:

✓ Mechanism of injury

✓ Loss of consciousness

✓ Location, type, and severity of symptoms

✓ Unusual sensations (tinnitus, dizziness, headache, etc.)

✓ Complaints of cervical pain or any radiating symptoms into extremities

✓ Orientation to time, person, and place

## Observation

Observe for the following:

✓ Unusual body movements or behavior

✓ Unusual facial expressions (drooling, drooping of one eyelid or corner of mouth)

✓ Level of consciousness (alert, restless, lethargic)

✓ Pupils for size, equality, and reaction to light

✓ Unusual eye movements (nystagmus, cross-eye, or lateral drift)

✓ Otorrhea, rhinorrhea

✓ Swelling, deformity, bleeding, or discoloration (Battle's sign, raccoon eyes)

✓ Continued monitoring of respirations, level of consciousness

## Palpation

✓ Face and skull for tenderness, swelling, deformity, or depressions

✓ Pulse rate and intensity (Do this periodically.)

## Neurological Tests

✓ Babinski

✓ Cranial nerve check (table 11.1)

✓ Cervical spine check

✓ Active range of motion of all four extremities

✓ Grip strength and dorsiflexion strength

It is of utmost importance that you continue to monitor vital signs every 5 min, and refer immediately if changes in the following:

a. Level of consciousness (decrease)
b. Blood pressure (increase)
c. Pulse (decrease, irregular)
d. Respiration (decrease, irregular)
e. Pupils (unequal, dilated, unreactive)

If the athlete is stable and there are no signs of serious head injury, the athlete can be transported from the field with assistance as needed pending more thorough evaluation on the sideline.

may suffer a mild head injury that goes unnoticed until she comes to you complaining of a headache—or until you, the coach, or her teammates notice a change in her behavior or concentration. This scenario demonstrates the importance of constant alertness on the sidelines, particularly in contact sports, to signs and symptoms of unusual behavior in the athletes.

## History

The history obtained on the sideline is essentially the same as that on the field but includes further detail. You should repeat the questions you asked the athlete on the field to assess his memory before and after the injury event. Throughout the history portion of your evaluation, remember that you are also evaluating the athlete's cognitive function through his responses. You should also question the athlete about previous head injuries and concussions, including the date of the most recent episode.

In investigating the mechanism of injury, ask the athlete about the point of contact and the activity he was engaged in when the injury occurred. Asking him to describe the play the team was running will help you determine his memory function and the possible presence of **retrograde amnesia**. Also ask the athlete if he recalls losing consciousness, and if so, for how long. You can compare his recollection with your own observations or with those of other witnesses. If the athlete complains of unusual sensations such as tinnitus, dizziness, blurred vision, or headache, ask if these symptoms have improved or worsened since the injury occurred. A headache will almost always be present, and you should ask the athlete to describe the location and quality of the pain. Is the pain on the same side (coup mechanism) where the contact was made or on the opposite side (contrecoup mechanism)? Is the headache diffuse (concussion) or localized (skull contusion or fracture), or is it a pressure type of headache? If the athlete complains of an increasing pressure headache, intracranial edema and hemorrhage should be suspected and the athlete closely observed for associated signs and symptoms.

The history portion of the sideline evaluation should also include questions relating to the athlete's orientation to place, person, self, and time. To determine orientation to place, ask the athlete if he knows where he is or what he was doing at the time of injury. If the injury occurred during the game, does he know who the opposing team is and what the score is? To determine orientation to person, ask the athlete to identify you, a teammate, or a coach. Orientation to self is reflected in the athlete's response to his own name and his ability to tell you his age and birth date. Assess orientation to time by asking what month or day it is.

Once you have completed the history, you should have a better sense of the nature and severity of the injury, as well as an impression of the athlete's mental status in relation to memory and appropriateness of verbal response (confusion).

## Observation

If the athlete left the field under her own power, observe for any unsteadiness or imbalance. Once on the sideline, visually inspect again for signs of otorrhea, rhinorrhea, Battle's sign, or raccoon eyes. Note any swelling, discoloration, deformity, or bleeding from the scalp that you may have overlooked before. Look for bilateral symmetry of all facial structures and contours. Continue to observe for unusual body posturing, movement, or behavior. Note any signs such as nausea, vomiting, yawning, or unilateral weakness. If you are familiar with the athlete's normal behavior, note any changes in attitude or behavior. Examples of unusual behavior include confusion, lethargy, restlessness, and aggressiveness—or the athlete may appear argumentative or may repeat the same questions again and again. Observe facial expressions for evidence of drooping of the eyelid or of the corner of the mouth. Check appearance of the pupils bilaterally for size (dilation), equality, and shape. If any of these symptoms were present on the field, are they worse now, the same, or improved?

As in the on-field assessment, you should closely observe the athlete's eyes for unusual movements and reaction to light. To observe eye movement further, ask the athlete to track your finger. Observe the movements of her eyes as they follow your finger superiorly, inferiorly, and left to right. Note any difficulty in tracking, sluggishness, deviation from midline, or nystagmus.

Your observational assessment should continue throughout the entire evaluation process, including continuous monitoring of respirations for depth, rate, and rhythm.

### Palpation

Palpation, which is the same as for the on-field assessment, involves careful palpation of the skull and facial bones for evidence of trauma. You should also monitor pulse rate, strength, and rhythm periodically throughout the assessment.

### Neurological Tests

Neurological tests at the sideline are the same as on the field. Depending on the athlete's condition, you may perform them here for the first time or as follow-up to your on-field assessment to note any change in the athlete's condition. You will also use other special tests during the sideline assessment to evaluate neurological function in relation to cognition, balance, and coordination.

### Special Tests

Special tests, used to assess brain function, are classified as (1) cognitive tests for memory and concentration and (2) tests of balance and coordination.

### Cognitive Tests

Neuropsychological tests have been used routinely to determine cognitive function in relation to immediate memory, delayed memory, and concentration. It is important to note that according to some research, athletes with mild head injury do not always display significantly poorer performance on neuropsychological tests than uninjured controls (Guskiewicz et al. 1997). Therefore, failure to note deficits during these cognitive tests does not definitely rule out neurological dysfunction, and you should consider the results in conjunction with the overall findings of your objective and subjective assessments. However, if you observe profound confusion or loss of memory, or if the athlete shows signs of deterioration, you should immediately refer him to a physician for further evaluation.

> **Failure to note deficits during cognitive tests does not rule out neurological dysfunction. Consider the results in conjunction with the overall findings of your objective and subjective assessments.**

#### Retrograde Amnesia Assessment

**Retrograde amnesia** is assessed through questions to determine the athlete's ability to remember events prior to the injury. Retrograde amnesia may range from not remembering the injury event to total loss of orientation to person, self, place, and time. Although any list of questions will work, it is helpful to develop a standard list that you will use routinely and that will allow you to compare the athlete's responses over time. Order the questions so that they deal first with the injury event and subsequently progress back in time to activities immediately before injury, then to earlier in the day, and then to the previous day. Questions can be repeated every 5-15 min following injury and then daily during the recovery process to indicate whether memory is improving or worsening. A positive sign for retrograde amnesia is any loss of memory, and severity is based on how far back the loss of memory extends.

#### Anterograde Amnesia Assessment (Five-Object Recall)

Assessment of **anterograde amnesia** concerns the athlete's immediate memory and ability to recall events that have occurred since the injury. A five-object recall test assesses for the presence of anterograde amnesia through verbal presentation of five unrelated objects (e.g., baby, dog, perfume, sunset, hammer). To assess immediate memory, instruct the athlete that you are going to test her memory, and read a list of words. When finished, ask the athlete to repeat back to you as many words as she can remember. Then have her perform the same task two more times, each time repeating as many words as she can remember. Note any incorrect response or missed word.

To assess delayed recall, wait 2 to 5 min and then ask the athlete if she remembers the list of words that you read a few minutes earlier. Record any missed or incorrect word. For either test, an incorrect response or an inability to remember the words is a positive sign.

### Digit Span Test

A digit span test can consist of a one- or two-part protocol to assess concentration and immediate memory recall. Tell the athlete that you are going to read him a series of numbers. When finished, ask him to repeat the series of digits in the same order (part one) and in reverse order (part two). Start with a string of three numbers and progress on successive trials to strings of four, five, and six numbers. If the athlete responds correctly on one string, proceed to the next string, which will include one more number. If he responds incorrectly, repeat the test using the same string length but a different set of numbers. Record the number of successful trials.

### Serial 7 Test

The Serial 7 test is used to assess concentration and analytical skills. The athlete is asked to count backward from 100 to 0 by sevens (i.e., 100, 93, 86, 79, etc.). Inability to perform this or other similar math skills is a positive sign.

### Balance and Coordination Tests

Balance and coordination tests evaluate brain function through the athlete's ability to maintain postural equilibrium. Although there are sophisticated computer devices for assessing postural control and coordination, the more common field tests available for the sideline assessment include the Romberg, modified Romberg, heel-to-toe walking, heel-to-knee, and finger-to-nose tests.

### Romberg Test

The traditional Romberg test identifies cerebellum dysfunction through assessment of balance and equilibrium. The athlete performs the test with feet together, eyes closed, and arms at his sides (figure 11.16). In this position, the athlete should be able to stand stationary with minimal postural sway. A positive sign is present if the athlete substantially sways or if he loses his balance.

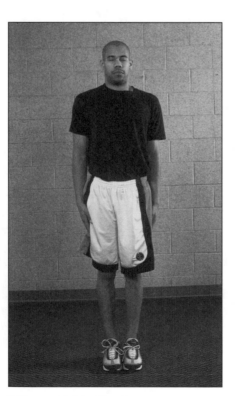

**I Figure 11.16**   Romberg test.

## Modified Romberg Test

Many variations of the Romberg test have been employed to assess postural equilibrium. A common modification has the athlete standing with legs shoulder-width apart, eyes closed, arms stretched out, and head tilted back (figure 11.17). You can make the test more challenging by having the athlete (1) stand in tandem (heel to toe), (2) lift one leg off the ground, and/or (3) touch his finger to his nose. A positive sign is excessive sway or loss of balance.

## Heel-to-Toe (Tandem) Walking

Having the athlete walk a straight line with a heel-to-toe gait is another way to assess balance and equilibrium (figure 11.18). Inability to walk a straight line, unsteadiness, or loss of balance is considered a positive test.

## Heel-to-Knee Test

If the athlete is supine, you can determine coordination by having him touch the heel of one foot to the opposite knee (figure 11.19). The test is performed first with eyes open and then with eyes closed. You can repeat the test by having the athlete alternate movement between the right and left side at increasing speed. A positive sign is any difference in movement side to side or an inability to perform the task smoothly and efficiently.

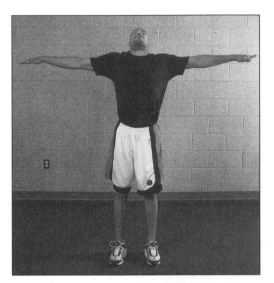

■ **Figure 11.17** Modified Romberg test.

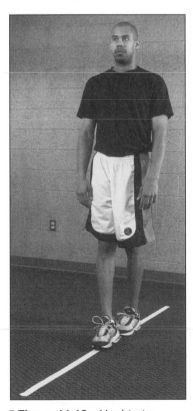

■ **Figure 11.18** Heel-to-toe (tandem) walking.

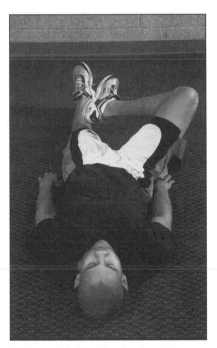

■ **Figure 11.19** Supine heel-to-knee test.

### Finger-to-Nose Tests

To assess upper-extremity coordination, have the athlete stand with arms outstretched and eyes open. Then ask him to alternately touch his nose with his left and right index finger, first with eyes open and then with eyes closed (figure 11.20). You can make the test more challenging by having the athlete alternatively touch his nose and then your finger as you move your finger from one position to another in front of him. Then compare the results of the test bilaterally; coordination difficulty or a side-to-side difference is a positive sign.

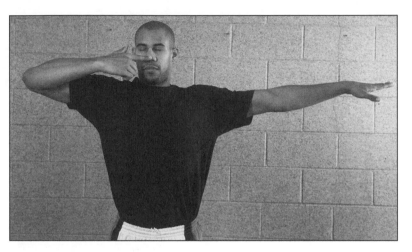

**Figure 11.20**    Finger-to-nose test.

### Repeated Testing and Decisions on Referral

Vital signs, pupillary response, and level of consciousness should be reevaluated every 15-30 min if the athlete is stable, and every 5 min if the athlete is unstable, until serious head injury is ruled out. It is essential that you be able to differentiate the signs and symptoms of a concussion from those of an expanding intracranial lesion, as the latter indicates a life-threatening medical emergency and makes immediate referral imperative. When your evaluation shows only signs and symptoms of a concussion, your decision regarding referral will depend on the degree of injury. Any athlete who exhibits signs and symptoms of a first-degree concussion for longer than 5 min should be removed from activity for the remainder of the day and closely watched for increasing signs and symptoms. Any athlete exhibiting signs and symptoms of a second- or third-degree concussion should be removed from activity and referred to a physician for further evaluation regardless of duration or improvement of symptoms.

## FOLLOW-UP (OFF-FIELD) ASSESSMENT OF HEAD INJURY

Follow-up assessment of mild head trauma during the first 24-48 h after injury should include home instructions for the athlete and his roommate or a family member to watch for signs and symptoms that would indicate a worsening condition. It is useful to have a prepared take-home instruction sheet that you can give to the person who will be staying with the athlete over the next 24-48 h following injury (see page 370). Even in mild cases that would appear to warrant little concern about serious brain injury, you should provide this information as a precaution, as signs of intercranial hemorrhage may be delayed or may progress slowly.

As already mentioned, your off-field assessment of head injuries should be the same as the sideline assessment. Repeated testing is fundamental to the assessment

## Checklist for Sideline Assessment of Head Injury

### History

✓ Previous head injuries

✓ Mechanism of injury and activity at time of injury

✓ Chief complaint

✓ Unusual sensations (tinnitus, dizziness, blurred vision, headache, unsteadiness)

✓ Location, type, and quality of pain (including headache symptoms)

✓ Loss of consciousness

✓ Orientation to place, person, self, and time

Throughout history, assess memory, appropriateness and quality of verbal response.

### Observation

✓ Visually inspect for the following:

   ✓ Otorrhea, rhinorrhea, Battle's sign, raccoon eyes (skull fracture)

   ✓ Halo effect for cerebral spinal fluid

   ✓ Swelling, deformity, discoloration, or bleeding of skull, scalp, or face

   ✓ Bilateral symmetry of facial structures

✓ Observe for the following:

   ✓ Unusual body posturing (decerebrate, decorticate)

   ✓ Unusual movement (vomiting, seizures, yawning, unilateral weakness)

   ✓ Unusual behavior (violent, combative, argumentative, repeating questions, confused)

   ✓ Unusual facial expressions (drooping of eyelid or corner of mouth)

   ✓ Level of consciousness (alertness, restlessness, lethargy)

   ✓ Pupil appearance (size, shape, equality)

   ✓ Pupil reaction to light (consensual and direct light reflex)

   ✓ Unusual eye movement (nystagmus, tracking difficulty, deviation from midline)

✓ Continued observation of vital signs (respiration depth, rate, and rhythm)

### Palpation

✓ Skull and face for point tenderness, swelling, deformity, depression:

   ✓ Compare bilaterally.

✓ Continued monitoring of pulse rate

### Neurological Tests

✓ Cranial nerve check

✓ Bilateral grip strength

### Special Tests

✓ Cognitive tests

   ✓ Memory

   ✓ Retrograde assessment (memory of events prior to injury)

   ✓ Anterograde assessment (five-object immediate and delayed recall)

   ✓ Concentration (Serial 7)

✓ Balance and coordination

   ✓ Romberg test

   ✓ Finger-to-nose test

   ✓ Heel-to-toe walking

Repeat testing every 15-30 min if stable, every 5 min if unstable, until serious head injury is ruled out, for the following:

✓ Vital signs

✓ Pupils

✓ Level of consciousness

### Functional Tests

✓ Performed only in cases in which athlete is otherwise symptom free under resting conditions

---

of head injury in order to determine whether symptoms are worsening, staying the same, or improving. Therefore it is helpful to have a standardized assessment protocol that allows clear documentation of your assessment and subsequent findings; this will enable you or another health professional to make objective comparisons over time. One such assessment instrument is the Standardized Assessment of Concussion (SAC) (McCrea et al. 1997) (see page 371). The SAC includes assessment of orientation, immediate memory, concentration, and delayed recall, and can be used for both sideline and follow-up evaluation. A check is placed by each correct answer; the checks are then added and totaled for each section and for the complete

## Take-Home Instructions for Head Injury

There are times when signs and symptoms of serious head injury may be delayed following injury. Therefore it is important that you observe the athlete frequently over the next 24-48 h for any changes in his or her condition or behavior. Call your athletic trainer or team physician if you have any questions, and seek medical attention immediately if you note any of the following signs and symptoms.

- A severe headache that increases in intensity and pressure
- Vomiting more than two to three times
- Any evidence of seizures or unusual body movements
- Unilateral weakness or inability to move one or both arms and legs

- Changes in facial expressions
- Changes in behavior such as increased irritability, agitation, or restlessness
- Increased mental confusion or loss of memory
- Increased lethargy, decreased level of consciousness, or difficulty in awakening
- Unusual eye movements or changes in size or position of one or both pupils
- Breathing rate that decreases below 12 breaths per minute or becomes irregular
- Pulse that decreases below 60 beats per minute or becomes irregular

> **!** Exertional maneuvers should never be used in the assessment of head injuries when the athlete is clearly dazed or is already exhibiting signs and symptoms.

assessment. Exertional maneuvers, also included in the assessment, are used only during follow-up assessment when the athlete is ready to begin simulating sport participation. Exertional maneuvers should never be used when the athlete is clearly dazed or is already exhibiting signs and symptoms.

The SAC is not intended as a stand-alone concussion assessment method or return-to-play measure. Rather, it provides a standardized, quantifiable measure of neurocognitive abnormalities that complements other aspects of the concussion assessment. Dr. Jeffrey Barth of the University of Virginia adds neurological questions to the checklist (see below):

### Functional Tests

Functional tests will enable you to assess whether the signs and symptoms of head injury have cleared and to establish the athlete's readiness to return to activity. Often, the athlete's symptoms (e.g., headache) will dissipate under resting conditions but will reappear when exercise is introduced. The SAC test initially provides for this functional assessment by using exertional maneuvers of jumping jacks, pushups, and crunches before cognitive and neurological testing. If symptoms are clear with these simple exercises, the athlete can perform activities more specific to his sport in progressively increased intensity and duration.

## Neurological Questions

| Neurological Part A | | Neurological Part B | |
|---|---|---|---|
| Vomiting present | Yes ____ | Nausea (since head injury) | Yes ____ |
| Dizziness present | Yes ____ | Headache (since head injury) | Yes ____ |
| Normal pupil reaction to light | No ____ | | |
| Normal eye tracking | No ____ | | |
| Equal pupil size | No ____ | | |
| Finger to nose 5 × | No ____ | | |
| Heel to toe 10 steps | No ____ | | |

# STANDARDIZED ASSESSMENT OF CONCUSSION (SAC)

## 1. ORIENTATION

Month: _____ 0  1

Date: _____ 0  1

Day of week: _____ 0  1

Year: _____ 0  1

Time (within 1 hr): _____ 0  1

Orientation total score _____ /  5

## 2. IMMEDIATE MEMORY

(All 3 trials are completed regardless of score on trial 1 and 2; total score equals sum across all 3 trials.)

| List | Trial 1 | Trial 2 | Trial 3 |
|------|---------|---------|---------|
| Word 1 | 0  1 | 0  1 | 0  1 |
| Word 2 | 0  1 | 0  1 | 0  1 |
| Word 3 | 0  1 | 0  1 | 0  1 |
| Word 4 | 0  1 | 0  1 | 0  1 |
| Word 5 | 0  1 | 0  1 | 0  1 |
| Total | 0  1 | 0  1 | 0  1 |

Immediate memory total score _____ /  15

(Note: Subject is not informed of delayed recall testing of memory.)

## NEUROLOGICAL SCREENING:

Loss of consciousness: (occurrence, duration)

Pre- and posttraumatic amnesia: (recollection of events pre- and post-injury)

Strength:

Sensation:

Coordination:

## 3. CONCENTRATION

*Digits backward.* (If correct, go to next string length. If incorrect, read trial 2. Stop after incorrect on both trials.)

| | | | |
|---|---|---|---|
| 4-9-3 | 6-2-9 _____ | 0 | 1 |
| 3-8-1-4 | 3-2-7-9 _____ | 0 | 1 |
| 6-2-9-7-1 | 1-5-2-8-6 _____ | 0 | 1 |
| 7-1-8-4-6-2 | 5-3-9-1-4-8 _____ | 0 | 1 |

*Months in reverse order.* (entire sequence correct for 1 point)

Dec-Nov-Oct-Sept-Aug-July
June-May-Apr-Mar-Feb-Jan) _____ 0   1

Concentration total score _____ /  5

## EXERTIONAL MANEUVERS

(when appropriate)

5 jumping jacks          5 push-ups

5 sit-ups                     5 knee-bends

## 4. DELAYED RECALL

| | | |
|---|---|---|
| Word 1 | 0 | 1 |
| Word 2 | 0 | 1 |
| Word 3 | 0 | 1 |
| Word 4 | 0 | 1 |
| Word 5 | 0 | 1· |

Delayed recall total score _____ /  5

## SUMMARY OF TOTAL SCORES:

Orientation _____ /  5

Immediate memory _____ /  15

Concentration_____ /  5

Delayed recall _____ /  5

Overall total score _____ /  30

Reprinted, by permission, from Michael McCrea.

### Criteria for Return to Play

The decision for return to play should be based on the subjective and objective findings of your follow-up assessment and should always be made in concert with the team physician. All symptoms should have completely cleared during both rest and exercise. The length of rest time mandated before return to activity, once the athlete is symptom free, will be dependent on the nature and severity of the injury, the duration of lingering symptoms, and the number of previous head injuries. Unfortunately, current guidelines for return to play lack sufficient scientific data and are based primarily on the athlete's subjective complaints. Researchers are currently attempting to identify more objective criteria of injury recovery through cognitive and balance testing (Guskiewicz et al. 1997). Until these data are available, it is important that you exercise caution and err on the conservative side if you have any doubt about an athlete's readiness to return. Any athlete who exhibits signs and symptoms of a concussion greater than first degree should be evaluated and cleared by a physician before being allowed to return to play. This is particularly true in athletes who have suffered a previous head injury.

## SIDELINE ASSESSMENT OF FACIAL INJURIES

The goal in the sideline assessment of facial injuries is to determine the structure involved and the nature and severity of the injury. Whereas examination of the face will be presented here as a single, generic assessment, your actual assessment will be more specifically tailored on the basis of the athlete's complaint and your observations. Whenever an athlete sustains significant trauma to the face (i.e., nasal, maxillary, or mandible fracture), you should also maintain a high suspicion of associated head injury and should rule this out during your injury assessment.

### History

History should include the typical questions addressing the mechanism of injury; the location, type, and quality of pain; unusual sounds or sensations; and previous injury. Since bleeding from the ears or nose and discoloration around the eyes and behind the ears can also result from skull fractures, it is important to determine the mechanism and the point of contact to the head or face. When you suspect eye or head trauma, you should also question the athlete about visual disturbances such as visual impairment, blurred vision, blind spots or decreased peripheral vision, flashes or floating spots (retinal detachment), and double vision (blow-out fracture). Also ask whether the athlete has any complaints of loss of hearing, headache, dizziness, or tinnitus.

### Observation

Throughout your observation, you should also be checking for any signs and symptoms of head injury, including those that relate to level of consciousness, body movements or posturing, and respirations.

Visually inspect bilaterally for signs of swelling, discoloration, flattening, or deformity of facial structures. Observation of facial structures should be performed in three planes: from in front of the athlete (frontal), from the side (lateral), and from a position above the head (superior) to allow you to see down the nose. Facial structures including the forehead, cheeks, orbits, and jaw angles should be symmetrical; and the chin and nasal bones should be midline. Observe for any bleeding from the nose (nasal or maxillary fracture) or around the teeth (tooth, maxilla, or mandibular fracture). Note the position of the eyes bilaterally for symmetry and midline position. An eye that exhibits a downward gaze or sits lower than the other may be indicative of an orbital blow-out fracture. You should also closely inspect the eyes for any change in size or shape of the pupil and evidence of hyperemia or hyphema. When observing the mouth and jaw, note the position and alignment of the teeth, the position of the jaw, and any malocclusion during approximation of the upper and lower teeth. Inspect the ear and auditory canal for signs of infection, swelling, discoloration, and hematoma formation. Throughout your observation, you should also be looking for any signs and symptoms of head injury, including those relating to level of consciousness, body movements or posturing, and respirations.

### Palpation

Wear gloves when palpating mouth structures.

Carefully palpate the soft tissue and bony structures of the face and head for signs of swelling, deformity, crepitus, depression, and point tenderness. The entire surface of the skull should routinely be palpated for areas of swelling and/or depressions. Palpate the forehead, orbital rims, zygomatic arches, maxilla, nasal bones, and mandible bilaterally for tenderness, contour, and crepitus. Palpate the TMJ in the external ear canal while the athlete opens and closes his mouth, noting any clicking, locking, or tenderness with movement (figure 11.21). Then palpate the teeth for looseness and fracture. All palpations should be performed bilaterally.

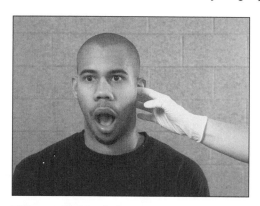

**I Figure 11.21**   Palpation of the temporomandibular joint.

### Special Tests

Special tests of the facial bones are limited; they include primarily the assessment of fractures and general assessment of vision (eye), smell and breathing (nose), and hearing (ears).

#### Bite Test

To assess for malocclusion or pain caused by fracture or dislocation, have athlete bite down on a tongue blade (figure 11.22). Positive signs include pain, weakness, and malocclusion of the jaw and teeth with biting.

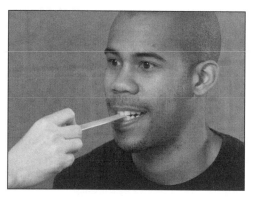

**I Figure 11.22**   Bite test.

#### Maxillary Fracture Test

Gentle mobilization of the upper jaw while the forehead is stabilized can help you identify a possible maxillary fracture (figure 11.23). Positive signs include pain, mobility, and crepitus.

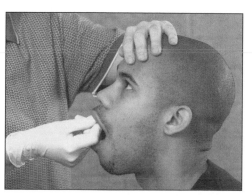

**I Figure 11.23**   Mobilization of maxillae for possible fracture.

## Percussion or Vibration Tests

Percussion or vibration applied to any bone can help you determine the presence of a fracture. Percussion/vibration tests include application of a tuning fork or a gentle tapping of the orbit, cheekbone, or mandible away from the area of tenderness. A positive sign occurs when the athlete feels pain at the site of injury.

## Vision

A simple 20/20 eye chart can be used to assess visual acuity following injury to the eye. Any athlete showing loss of visual acuity or evidence of blurred or double vision should be immediately referred to an ophthalmologist for further evaluation.

## Smell and Breathing

Loss of smell or difficulty in breathing can occur with epistaxis and nasal fractures, but smell and breathing should return to normal once bleeding and swelling subside. Loss of smell can also result from injury to the first cranial nerve (olfactory) and may be evidence of brain trauma. To assess for the presence of smell, have the athlete close her eyes and describe or identify a particular scent that you wave under the nose.

## Hearing

Transient hearing loss is not uncommon with blows to the head or ear, but hearing should return to normal shortly following injury. Loss of hearing may indicate rupture of the tympanic membrane, infection, swelling, or impacted cerumen. You can assess diminished or loss of hearing bilaterally by (1) rubbing two fingers together or (2) snapping your fingers beside the athlete's ear. Athletes with lost or diminished hearing in one ear may turn their head while you are talking in an effort to align the good ear with the direction of the sound. Whenever loss of hearing persists or is profound, you should refer the athlete to a physician for further evaluation.

### Range of Motion

Active range of motion for jaw and eye movement should be assessed when appropriate. Active range of motion for the jaw should include opening and closing of the mouth and side-to-side movement (figure 11.24, a-b). Normal range of motion for opening the mouth is approximately two to three finger widths. Note any pain, decreased range, or difficulty with movement. Side-to-side movement should be equal bilaterally.

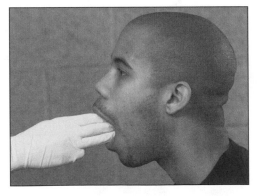
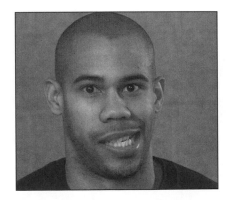

a                b

▮ **Figure 11.24** Active range of motion with (a) mouth opening of approximately 2-3 finger widths and (b) movement of the jaw side to side.

For active eye movement, ask the athlete to track your finger superiorly, inferiorly, and side to side. Compare eye movement bilaterally and note any restriction or difficulty with tracking. The two eyes should move together and should track your finger with smoothness and ease.

### Neurological Tests

Neurological assessment of the cranial nerves is performed when head injury is suspected or when loss of hearing, taste, or smell is noted. The assessment is the same as that for evaluation of head injury (see also table 11.1).

### Functional Tests

You may want to perform functional tests for further assessment of the extent of the athlete's injury and for determining safe return to participation. Pain with biting and chewing may indicate temporomandibular dysfunction or maxilla, mandible, or tooth pathology. Assessment of visual and auditory acuity during sport activity will help you determine whether the athlete's senses are sufficient to allow safe resumption of activity. Examples of functional tests for vision and hearing are having the athlete catch a ball, shoot a basket, or respond to a command from across the field or when she is distracted. You can also assess vestibular function through functional balance tests.

---

## Checklist for Sideline Assessment of Facial Injuries

### History
✓ Mechanism of injury
✓ Unusual sounds or sensations
✓ Location, type, and quality of pain
✓ Previous injury
✓ Complaints of impaired, blurred, or double vision
✓ Complaints of headache, dizziness, tinnitus (evidence of associated concussion)
✓ Complaints of loss of hearing

### Observation
✓ Swelling, deformity, flattening, or discoloration of facial structures
✓ Symmetry of facial structures
✓ Bleeding from nose or around teeth
✓ Position of eyes bilaterally
✓ Eyes for size and shape of pupil, corneal surface, hyphema, hyperemia
✓ Jaw position, malocclusion
✓ Position and alignment of teeth
✓ External ear and auditory canal
✓ Signs and symptoms of head injury (particularly with blows to the jaw)
✓ Bilateral check

### Palpation
Check for swelling, depressions, deformity, crepitus, and point tenderness:

✓ Forehead, orbital rim, zygomatic arch, maxilla, nasal bones, mandible
✓ Temporomandibular joint (clicking, locking, tenderness with movement)
✓ Soft tissue cartilage of the external ear
✓ Teeth for looseness, fracture
✓ Bilateral check

### Special Tests
✓ Assessment of smell
✓ Assessment of breathing (nasal passageway)
✓ Assessment of hearing
✓ Bite test

### Range of Motion
✓ Opening and closing of mouth (two to three finger widths)
✓ Side-to-side movement of jaw
✓ Eye movement (compare bilaterally and note restriction of movement)

### Neurological
✓ Sensory for smell, taste, or hearing (may indicate symptoms of head injury).
✓ Perform cranial nerve check if you have any suspicion of associated head injury.

# SUMMARY

1. *Describe the mechanisms, signs and symptoms, and potential complications associated with head and facial injuries commonly encountered in the physically active.*

   Even with the use of protective equipment during sport activity, head and facial injuries occur commonly and can range widely from minor insults to serious, life-threatening conditions. Head injuries, which can result from both direct and indirect mechanisms, represent the leading cause of death due to sport participation. Facial injuries typically result from direct insult and most commonly take the form of contusions, fractures, and lacerations. Although the majority of the injuries the athletic trainer encounters may not be life threatening, it is necessary to treat any injury resulting in neurological or sensory organ deficits as a medical emergency and to refer the athlete immediately to a physician for further evaluation.

2. *Differentiate between signs and symptoms of concussion, skull fracture, and intracranial hemorrhage.*

   Head injuries are typically classified into three categories: concussion, intracranial hemorrhage, and skull fractures. It is imperative that you be able to differentiate between the signs and symptoms of these different types of head injuries. A concussion will typically result in signs and symptoms of a diffuse headache, dizziness, nausea, and tinnitus and may produce confusion, amnesia, and loss of consciousness. Intracranial hemorrhage leading to swelling and pressure on the brain will cause characteristic changes in vital signs, motor function, and pupillary function. Skull fractures may or may not result in intracranial hemorrhage; these are identified by palpable tenderness and possible bony deformity as well as by the presence of discharge and/or discoloration of the eyes, ears, and nose.

3. *Discuss the potential complications and delayed symptoms that may result from head trauma.*

   Prompt recognition of neurological complications or evidence of increasing intracranial pressure is paramount to any evaluation following head trauma. Symptoms of intracranial hemorrhage may not be observable immediately after injury but may be delayed for minutes, hours, or even days. However, once symptoms of serious brain injury appear, the condition of the athlete can quickly deteriorate. Any time an athlete's symptoms worsen over time or neurological deficits are present, the athlete should be immediately referred for emergency medical care. Because the athlete's condition can deteriorate so quickly, an athletic trainer who has any doubt as to the severity of the head trauma must not hesitate to seek emergency medical assistance.

4. *Perform an on-field assessment of a potential head injury, keeping in mind the criteria for medical referral and mode of transportation from the field.*

   The athlete with a head injury may range from conscious, coherent, and ambulatory to completely unconscious and unresponsive. The on-field assessment of a suspected head injury begins with a primary survey to immediately determine level of consciousness and the presence of life-threatening conditions. In athletes who are unconscious, a cervical spine injury should also be suspected until there is proof to the contrary. The athletic trainer obtains a history from the athlete or from bystanders who witnessed the injury to determine the mechanism and nature of the injury. The observation includes assessment for unusual body movements, facial reactions, and pupillary responses, as well as a visual check for signs of swelling, deformity, discoloration, or drainage from the nose or ears. The skull and facial bones are then palpated for evidence of fracture, and pulse is monitored for changes in rate or strength. Neurological tests are performed to assess cranial nerve and motor function. Throughout the assessment the athletic trainer should closely monitor vital signs, level of consciousness, and signs and symptoms of intracranial hemorrhage.

5. *Perform a thorough and sequential sideline assessment of a potential head injury, including special tests for cognition, balance, and coordination, keeping in mind the criteria for referral and follow-up evaluation.*

   The sideline assessment is similar to the on-field assessment but includes a more complete history and neurological evaluation. The history is helpful for determining not only the mechanism and nature of injury, but also the athlete's level of consciousness and orientation. Special tests evaluate any loss of cognitive function such as memory, concentration, or analytical skills or any loss of equilibrium or balance. Assessment of head injury at the sideline is unique in that here it is imperative to repeatedly monitor vital signs and level of consciousness until serious head trauma has been ruled out or until it is clear that the athlete is stabilized or improving. This assessment uses the same history questions and the same protocol as on the field to aid in determining whether symptoms are improving or worsening over time and to allow more effective follow-up.

6. *Perform a general assessment for facial injuries, including identification of differential signs and symptoms indicating associated head injury.*

   The goal in the sideline assessment of facial injuries is to determine the structure involved, the nature of the injury, and its severity. If the structures of the ears or eyes are involved, the history should include questions regarding any difficulty with vision and hearing. The athletic trainer observes for any change, asymmetry, deformity, swelling, or discoloration of the facial structures and palpates all structures for tenderness, crepitus, and deformity. There are very few special tests for this region, with most used primarily as a functional assessment of the sensory organs. Movement of the jaw and eyes should also be evaluated, if these structures are involved, for any restriction or difficulty with movement. Whenever an athlete sustains significant trauma to the face (i.e., nasal, maxillary, or mandible fracture), it is important to maintain a high suspicion of associated head injury and to rule this out during the injury assessment.

7. *Perform a complete neurological assessment of the cranial nerves.*

   A cranial nerve check assesses the integrity of each of the 12 cranial nerves. It is important for the athletic trainer to memorize the functional test for each cranial nerve and include these tests in the neurological assessment of the head and face. Any time a positive sign is present with any one cranial nerve assessment, serious brain trauma should be suspected and the athlete referred immediately. Neurological evaluation of the trigeminal and facial nerves should also be included in assessment of facial trauma, as these nerves are sometimes traumatized or injured.

# REVIEW QUESTIONS

1. What are the two primary mechanisms of head injury? What types of stresses do these mechanisms place on the brain tissues, and which are least and best tolerated?

2. What are the two primary types of intracranial hemorrhage, and what structures are commonly involved in each? What changes in vital signs would indicate an expanding lesion?

3. What are the general classifications and signs and symptoms of concussion? How are these signs and symptoms different from those of an intracranial hemorrhage, and which ones indicate a medical emergency?

4. What are the signs and symptoms of a corneal abrasion, and how would you differentiate this condition from a corneal laceration?

5. Describe the difference between hyperemia and hyphema. Which of these conditions represents a medical emergency?

6. How are level of consciousness and orientation determined in an evaluation? Describe the evaluation procedure, and list the questions you would ask to determine an athlete's orientation to his or her surroundings.

7. Pupillary position, size, and responses are important in the evaluation of head and eye injuries. What would be considered abnormal in your observations of size, shape, and responsiveness, and what conditions might these abnormalities indicate?

8. Describe the common fractures of the facial bones and their general signs and symptoms. What special tests can be performed to help identify the presence of a fracture?

# CRITICAL THINKING QUESTIONS

1. An athlete sustains a blunt trauma to the eye and is in considerable pain. Discuss the various structures and conditions that may be associated with this mechanism. Which conditions and symptoms would warrant immediate medical referral, and how you would differentiate between minor and eye-threatening conditions in your evaluation?

2. While providing a history on the sideline, an athlete reports that this is the second concussion he has had in the past month. How might this information impact your (1) injury assessment and (2) your follow-up evaluation and return-to-play criteria?

3. An athlete receives a hard blow to the chin and complains of jaw pain and an inability to completely close her mouth. She also is complaining of a severe headache and dizziness. How would your evaluation proceed?

# CITED REFERENCES

Cantu, R.C. 1991. Minor head injuries in sports. In *Sports and the adolescent*, ed P.G. Dyment, 141-154. Philadelphia, Hanley & Belfus, Inc.

Cantu, R.C. 1992. Cerebral concussion in sport: Management and prevention. *Sports Medicine* 14: 64-74.

Cantu, R.C. and R. Voy. 1995. Second impact syndrome. *Phys Sports Med* 23: 27-34.

Guskiewicz, K.M., Riemann, B.L., Perrin, D.H. and L.M. Nashner. 1997. Alternative approaches to the assessment of mild head injury in athletes. *Med Sci Sports Exerc* 29: S213-221.

McCrea, M., Kelly, J.P., Kluge, J., Ackley, B., and C. Randoph. 1997. Standardized assessment of concussion in football players. *Neurology* 48(3): 586-588.

Moore, K.L. 1992. *Clinically oriented anatomy*. Baltimore: Williams and Wilkins.

National Athletic Trainers' Association Research and Education Foundation. 1994. *Mild brain injury in sports summit proceedings*, Washington, DC, April 16-18. National Athletic Trainers' Association.

## ADDITIONAL RESOURCE

Hillman, S.K. 2000. *Introduction to athletic training*. Champaign, IL: Human Kinetics.

# CHAPTER TWELVE

# Thorax and Abdomen

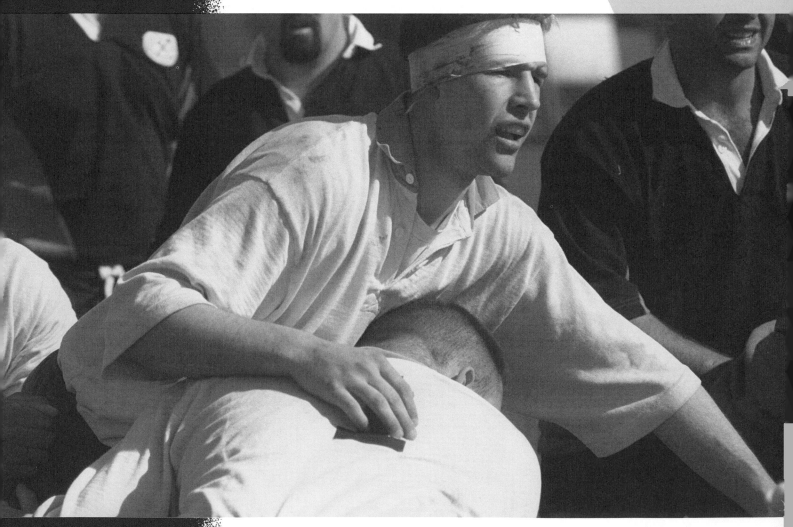

# OBJECTIVES

After completing this chapter, the reader will be able to do the following:

1. Describe the common mechanisms, signs and symptoms, and potential complications associated with injuries to the thorax commonly encountered in the physically active

2. Describe the common mechanisms, signs and symptoms, and potential complications associated with injuries to the abdomen commonly encountered in the physically active

3. Differentiate pathologies and signs and symptoms between cardiac contusion, tamponade, and concussion

4. Appreciate the potential for life-threatening injury resulting from direct and indirect trauma to the thorax and abdomen

5. Perform an on-field assessment of the thorax and abdomen, indicating criteria for immediate medical referral or continued observation

6. Perform an off-field assessment of the thorax and abdomen, indicating considerations for differential diagnosis

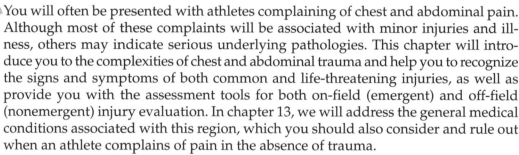

Jeremy was in his third year of lacrosse at Tucker University. As he was going for the ball during practice, a hard collision with a teammate sent him sprawling, and he landed hard on his back. Sharon, the athletic trainer who was covering practice, saw the collision and started to go over to check him; but then Jeremy got up and appeared to be okay.

"I'm okay," Jeremy yelled over to Sharon with a grimace on his face as he slowly trotted over to the rest of the team to continue practice. Even so, Sharon kept an eye on him. It was no more than 5 minutes later that Jeremy came over to see her. "Sharon, I don't feel so good."

Sharon noticed that Jeremy appeared a bit pale and clammy. "Tell me exactly what happened and where your pain is."

"I collided with John going for the ball and he hit me hard, right in the stomach, and knocked me flat. Now I feel kind of weak and nauseated. . . . My stomach hurts, too."

Sharon continued to question Jeremy as she inspected his abdominal region for signs of swelling or discoloration. "Are you having pain anywhere else?"

"Yeah, my left shoulder kind of hurts too." Sharon became concerned; she checked Jeremy's vital signs and found that his respirations were rapid and shallow and his pulse was fast. His blood pressure was about 90/50. It appeared that Jeremy was going into shock, and his symptoms indicated a potential spleen injury. Sharon immediately called 911 for emergency transport to the local hospital. As she waited for EMS to arrive, his symptoms continued to worsen, and his abdomen became rigid. She hoped EMS would get there soon. . . .

You will often be presented with athletes complaining of chest and abdominal pain. Although most of these complaints will be associated with minor injuries and illness, others may indicate serious underlying pathologies. This chapter will introduce you to the complexities of chest and abdominal trauma and help you to recognize the signs and symptoms of both common and life-threatening injuries, as well as provide you with the assessment tools for both on-field (emergent) and off-field (nonemergent) injury evaluation. In chapter 13, we will address the general medical conditions associated with this region, which you should also consider and rule out when an athlete complains of pain in the absence of trauma.

To understand and properly evaluate chest and abdominal injuries, you must first have an appreciation for the anatomical orientation and physiological function of the organs and structures of the thorax and abdomen. Although this chapter will present anatomical orientation where appropriate within the context of various pathologies, you are encouraged to review the general anatomy and physiology of this region before proceeding.

# INJURIES TO THE THORAX AND ABDOMEN

Injuries to the thorax and abdomen can result from a variety of mechanisms. Injury can occur as a consequence of violent muscle contractions and can even occur spontaneously without evidence of direct trauma. Blunt trauma or direct insult is the most common mechanism, and the one that presents the greatest concern for serious injury. Although the internal organs of the thorax and abdomen are well protected, they are vulnerable to injury during sport. Internal injuries often result from a hard fall; a helmet to the chest, lower back, or abdomen; or impact from a baseball, softball, or other sport implement. Because of the potential for life-threatening complications connected with these injuries, you should maintain a high suspicion of underlying pathology throughout your evaluation any time an athlete sustains a significant blow to the chest or abdomen.

# THORAX

Injuries to the chest wall and organs of the thoracic cavity can result from direct insult or violent muscle contractions; they also may occur spontaneously as a consequence of intense exercise. The most common injuries resulting from these mechanism are contusion, strains, sprains, and fractures of the chest wall. However, these same mechanisms can also traumatize the heart and lungs or cause internal bleeding—all effects that can have life-threatening consequences.

## Contusions

Because of the superficial nature of the anterior and lateral chest wall, rib and sternal contusions are common in contact sports in which chest protection is not worn or is inadequate. Signs and symptoms include localized pain, swelling, discoloration, periosteal irritation, and point tenderness. Deep inspiration may also result in pain if there is injury or irritation of the adjacent intercostal muscles or costochondral joints. Although severe contusions may be difficult to distinguish from a fracture, contusions will typically not display signs of bony crepitus or pain with indirect compression of the chest wall.

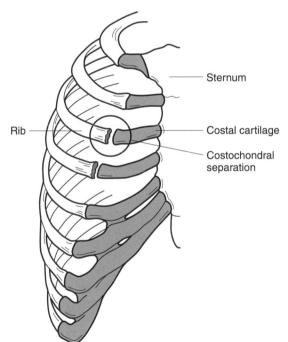

Rib — 
Sternum — 
Costal cartilage — 
Costochondral separation — 

**I Figure 12.1** Costochondral separation.

## Sprains

Sprains or separation of the costochondral joint can result secondary to anteriorly directed trauma to the sternum or lateral compression of the chest wall. Bouncing the barbell off the chest during bench press can also cause costochondral injury. Injury can range in severity from a mild sprain or irritation to separation and complete dislocation (figure 12.1). The athlete will complain of pain and point tenderness at the costochondral junction. With separation or dislocation, he will also complain of increased pain with deep inspiration, of crepitus or clicking, and of increased prominence of the joint. Swelling and discoloration may also be observable.

## Costochondritis

Chronic irritation and inflammation of the costochondral junction (**costochondritis**) can occur following acute, traumatic injury or as a result of chronic stress or repetitive activities such as coughing, rowing, or weight lifting. The athlete may have no history of trauma but will complain of a gradual onset of anterior chest wall pain and tenderness over the affected joint. Crepitus and mild inflammation may also be present. Rest, ice, and anti-inflammatory medication will typically resolve symptoms within a few weeks.

## Traumatic Fractures and Dislocations

Traumatic fractures can result from either a direct blow, indirect compression of the chest wall, or muscular tension. Rib fractures are much more common than sternal fractures. Because of the trauma associated with fractures of the thorax, you must be keenly aware of underlying pathology and potential resultant complications, particularly if the direction of force leads to compression of the chest wall or causes the fracture to displace inwardly.

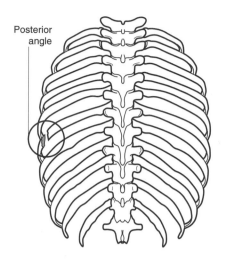

**Figure 12.2** Rib fracture at the posterior angle.

*Cyanosis is a bluish or purplish discoloration of the skin due to deficient oxygenation of the blood.*

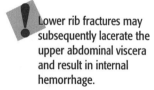

Lower rib fractures may subsequently lacerate the upper abdominal viscera and result in internal hemorrhage.

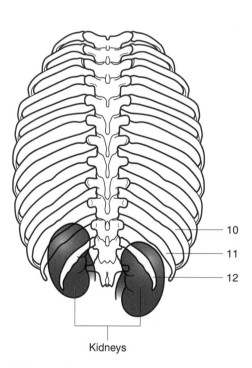

**Figure 12.3** Anatomical orientation of the left kidney to the posterior margin of the rib cage.

## Ribs

While the 1st through 4th ribs are well protected by the shoulder girdle and the 10th through 12th ribs are more mobile, the rigidly fixed 5th through 9th ribs are most prone to fracture. Fractures most commonly occur at the weaker, posterior angle (figure 12.2). Signs and symptoms include localized pain, point tenderness, swelling, discoloration, crepitus, and muscle guarding. Pain will increase with indirect chest wall compression, with deep inspiration, and with coughing, sneezing, laughing, or jarring. Because of increased pain with deep inspiration, the athlete will often present with rapid, shallow breathing to avoid pain. She may also rotate her trunk and lean toward the injured side to prevent muscle tensioning and pain.

Severe trauma can cause a **flail chest injury**, characterized by multiple fractures of three or more adjacent ribs. Fractures resulting from direct trauma are often more serious, as the fragment is more likely to be driven into the thoracic or abdominal cavity, leading to secondary visceral injury. For instance, when you suspect a lower posterior rib fracture, you should also be suspicious of potential kidney trauma (figure 12.3). Signs and symptoms associated with secondary lung injury include chest pain, difficulty breathing, cyanosis, and shock (see sections on pneumothorax and hemothorax). Therefore it is imperative to look beyond the suspected rib fracture and to monitor the athlete carefully for signs and symptoms of internal injury.

Nontraumatic or stress fractures of the rib also occur commonly in athletes, secondary to a violent twisting or muscle contraction frequently associated with violent coughing, overhead throwing, a golf swing, or rowing activities. As with traumatic fractures, the athlete will complain of localized pain and tenderness and increased pain with deep inspiration and trunk movement. Displacement is uncommon with a stress-type injury, and underlying injury is rarely a concern.

Although the first rib is well protected, nontraumatic fractures of this rib have also been documented in sport, secondary to falling on an outstretched or hyperabducted arm or a sudden, violent contraction of the scalenus anterior muscle (Fruh 1993). Signs and symptoms include sharp pain in the anterior triangle of the neck and palpable tenderness of the surrounding musculature (trapezius and scalenes). The athlete may also complain of radiating pain into the shoulder or scapula region, as well as possible neurological symptoms with secondary irritation or injury to the brachial plexus.

## Sternum

Fractures of the sternum are rare in contact sports, more often occurring secondary to high-velocity impact of the chest with the steering wheel in motor vehicle accidents. However, sternal fractures can result from a severe, direct blow to the anterior chest (e.g., when another player's helmet or a sport implement, such as a baseball, hits the chest at high velocities). The athlete will likely complain of a loss of breath immediately following injury because of the impact, as well as pain with deep inspiration. Examination will reveal localized pain, tenderness, ecchymosis, swelling, and possible deformity. Because of the severity of the blow necessary to cause a fracture, there is always a concern for underlying pleural (hemothorax, pneumothorax) or cardiac (contusion, tamponade) injury, or both, particularly if the sternum is displaced posteriorly. If underlying pathology is present, the athlete may also exhibit signs and symptoms of respiratory or circulatory distress. However, it is important to note that these signs and symptoms may not be present initially and can be delayed. Therefore any time an athlete receives a significant blow to the chest, he should be thoroughly evaluated and monitored carefully for signs of shock and respiratory and cardiac dysfunction following injury.

### Internal Injuries

Internal injuries in the thoracic region are quite serious and often life threatening. The thoracic cavity is divided into three sections or spaces: two separate pleural cavities housing the left and right lungs, and the mediastinum, which houses the heart, thoracic parts of the great vessels, the trachea, the left and right bronchi, and other important structures (figure 12.4). Although the thoracic cavity is well protected circumferentially by the sternum, ribs, and vertebral column, both blunt and penetrating trauma can injure these vital structures and compromise pulmonary or circulatory function or both. It is imperative that the athletic trainer be able to recognize the signs and symptoms of the following conditions and ensure immediate medical referral as appropriate.

### Pneumothorax

Surrounding each lung is a pleural sac. Its outer wall, the **parietal pleura**, adheres to the external wall of the pleural cavity. The inner layer, the **visceral pleura**, adheres to the surface of the lung. Between these two layers is a **serous fluid** that reduces friction and allows the two layers to move freely on one another as the lungs inflate and

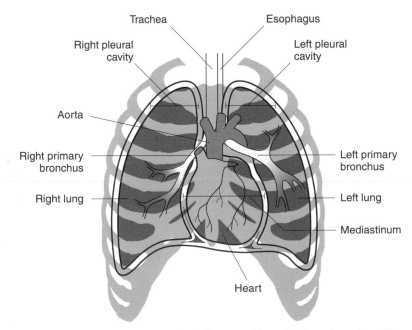

■ **Figure 12.4** Thoracic cavity and skeletal rib cage. Note the two pleural cavities and the structures of the mediastinum.

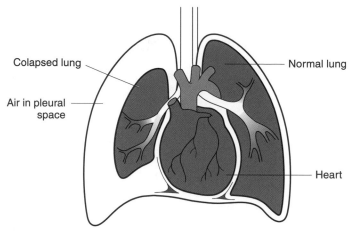

**Figure 12.5** Pneumothorax.

collapse with normal breathing. A pneumothorax occurs when air is allowed to enter this cavity, causing the lung to separate from the chest wall and reducing its volume (i.e., **lung collapse**).

A pneumothorax can be caused by traumatic injury or can occur spontaneously in the absence of trauma. A penetrating injury such as a rib fracture can rupture or lacerate lung tissue and allow inspired air to escape into the pleural space (figure 12.5). A hard blow to the chest with the glottis closed can result in rupture of the alveoli, or a **blow-out injury** More common in sport, however, is a spontaneous pneumothorax; this most often occurs in young, healthy athletes with no history of trauma, and may follow an intense bout of activity that causes small ruptures in the outer surface of the lung tissue. Signs and symptoms associated with a simple pneumothorax include upper chest pain, **dyspnea** (difficulty breathing) or shortness of breath, light-headedness, and decreased breath sounds with auscultation. If compromise is severe, the athlete may also be cyanotic. Athletes with a suspected pneumothorax should be immediately referred for emergency medical care.

Severe, life-threatening complications can arise if the air in the pleural cavity continues to increase, progressing to a tension pneumothorax. With a **tension pneumothorax**, the increasing pressure caused by the trapped air will cause the mediastinum to shift away from the injured side, compressing the heart and healthy lung and compromising their function (figure 12.6). Fatal hypoxia and acidosis will occur due to compression of the vena cava, decreased cardiac filling and output, and severely compromised lung volume. Signs and symptoms of a tension pneumothorax include acute respiratory distress, distended neck veins, circulatory compromise, tracheal deviation, decreased breath sounds, and severe restlessness and agitation. The athlete must be referred for immediate emergency medical care.

*Auscultation is a method of listening to internal sounds of the chest and abdomen with a stethoscope.*

*Hypoxia is a lack of oxygen.*

*Acidosis is an excess accumulation of acid in the body caused by cardiorespiratory compromise.*

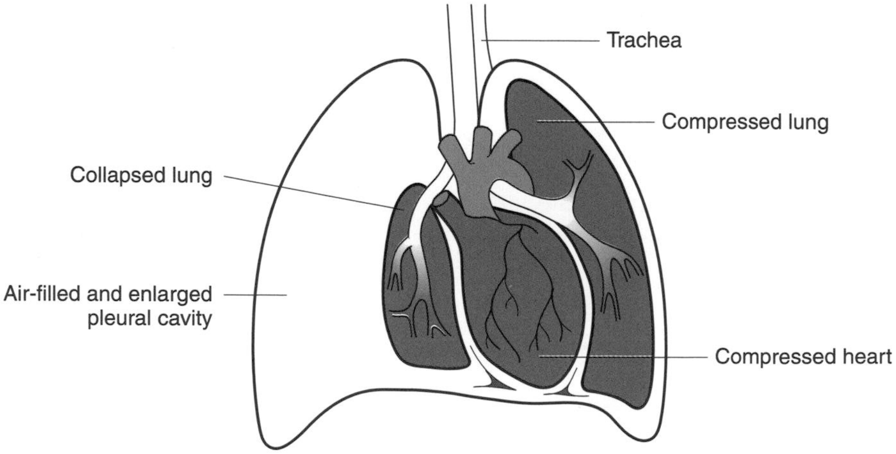

**Figure 12.6** Tension pneumothorax and shift of the mediastinum with compression of the heart and healthy lung.

*Hypovolemic shock is caused by internal hemorrhage resulting in decreased blood volume.*

Any blunt trauma to the chest should raise a high level of suspicion for underlying internal injury, and the athlete should be referred for immediate medical care in the presence of any symptoms of cardiorespiratory distress.

When an athlete collapses following blunt trauma to the chest, the athletic trainer should immediately assess for airway, breathing, and circulation and should summon emergency medical services.

## Hemothorax
Traumatic chest injuries, such as laceration of the lung tissue or an intercostal artery secondary to a penetrating rib fracture, can result in a hemothorax in which blood, rather than air, fills the pleural space. Signs and symptoms of a hemothorax include lung collapse and reduced or absent breath sounds on the involved side, severe chest pain, dyspnea, cyanosis, hypotension, and the coughing up of frothy blood. If bleeding is severe, hypovolemic shock, shift of the mediastinum, and collapse of the uninvolved lung may also result.

## Cardiac Contusion
Blunt trauma to the chest that causes compression of the heart between the sternum and the spine can result in a contusion to the heart muscle. High-velocity impact such as that of a baseball, hockey puck, lacrosse ball, or softball on the chest is a common mechanism in sport. Signs and symptoms of cardiac contusion include chest pain, neck vein distension, possible rhythm disturbance (**arrhythmia**), muffled heart tones, and changes on electrocardiogram indicating muscle injury. Signs and symptoms associated with shock and respiratory and cardiac distress may also be present, but these can vary considerably according to severity. Severe and life-threatening complications can result if the impact is sufficient to cause ventricular, coronary artery, or intraventricular septum rupture. Again, any blunt trauma to the chest should raise a high level of suspicion of underlying internal injury, and the athlete should be referred for immediate medical care.

## Cardiac Tamponade
Blunt trauma to the chest can also cause **cardiac tamponade**, or hemorrhage within the enclosed and inelastic pericardial cavity, if trauma is sufficient to rupture the myocardium or coronary artery. Fortunately, this occurs rarely in sport; but since the cause is often a penetrating injury such as a stab wound, this injury could potentially occur in sports such as javelin or fencing. Cardiac tamponade is characterized by compression of the heart and pulmonary veins, which prevents venous return to the heart. Signs and symptoms include neck vein distension due to the backup of venous flow, shock, hypotension, cyanosis, severe chest pain, and difficulty breathing. Cardiac tamponade is clearly life threatening and warrants immediate emergency medical care.

## Cardiac Concussion (Commotio Cordis)
A condition that has aroused considerable interest in recent years is cardiac concussion. Cardiac concussion, or commotio cordis, is characterized by immediate cardiac arrest and sudden death following a localized blunt, but seemingly inconsequential, blow to the chest (near the region of the heart) during sport activity (Maron et al. 1995). Many cases have been documented in which a blow to the chest from a sport implement—insufficient to cause structural injury to the sternum, ribs, or underlying heart—has resulted in immediate collapse (or collapse within seconds) and sudden death in young athletes with no previous history or evidence of heart abnormality or disease (Curfman 1998; Haq 1998; Maron et al. 1995). The most common offending projectiles are baseballs, softballs, and hockey pucks (Curfman 1998); but cardiac concussion has also resulted following impact from a lacrosse ball, cricket ball, helmet to the chest, hockey stick, body check in ice hockey, and karate kick (Haq 1998; Maron et al. 1995). Although the precise mechanisms for cardiac arrest from cardiac concussion are still uncertain, the primary cause is thought to be a premature beat precipitated by the impact, which in turn elicits ventricular fibrillation (Maron et al. 1995). Unfortunately, in most cases, resuscitation attempts have failed and death usually results. When an athlete collapses following blunt trauma to the chest, the athletic trainer should immediately assess for airway, breathing, and circulation and should summon emergency medical services (EMS).

# ABDOMEN

Traumatic injuries to the abdominal region include soft tissue injuries of the abdominal muscles, genitalia, and internal organs. While the thoracic cavity is protected by the skeletal rib cage, the abdomen is protected primarily by soft tissue structures. Thus contusions and muscular strains are the more common injuries in this region. Although these injuries are usually minor, they can cause considerable pain and disability if they are acute. Internal injuries, particularly to the solid organs, are also a concern with mechanisms of blunt trauma and most often involve the spleen and kidney. If internal hemorrhage results, the injury becomes life threatening if not immediately recognized and managed appropriately.

## *Contusion*

As with any other structure left unprotected during sport activity, the abdomen is prone to contusions secondary to direct contact. External abdominal structures most vulnerable to contusions include the abdominal muscles, the solar plexus, and the external genitalia.

### Abdominal Muscles

The abdominal muscles, which provide the chief protection to the abdominal cavity, are often exposed to direct trauma during sport activity. Severe muscular contusions are rare, since the underlying abdominal contents are soft and have sufficient "give" to dissipate blunt forces. Even so, injury to the muscle can result from direct trauma and gives rise to the typical signs of localized pain, swelling, tenderness, and ecchymosis. It is important to realize that blunt trauma of sufficient magnitude can also contuse the underlying abdominal viscera. Therefore, any time an athlete presents with a history of direct or blunt abdominal trauma, you should complete a thorough evaluation to rule out any signs and symptoms of visceral trauma prior to return to activity.

### Solar Plexus

A direct blow to the abdomen over the solar (celiac) plexus can cause momentary paralysis of the diaphragm and an inability to breathe. This syndrome, often referred to as "getting the wind knocked out of you," commonly results from the impact of a knee or helmet to the abdomen or from falling on a ball. This is a relatively minor condition typically requiring no treatment or referral; but it can produce considerable anxiety in the athlete, as she will be unable to breathe for a brief period of time. Signs and symptoms include abdominal pain, fear, anxiety, and difficulty breathing. The symptoms should dissipate quickly and normal breathing should resume without the need for medical intervention or treatment. By immediately recognizing the signs and symptoms of a blow to the solar plexus, the athletic trainer can assist in calming and reassuring the athlete until normal breathing resumes.

### Testicular Trauma

Testicular trauma or scrotal contusion is relatively common among physically active males, resulting from a direct blow to the external genitalia such as getting kicked or kneed in the groin. This injury can cause considerable pain, spasm, ecchymosis, and swelling. The athlete may also complain of nausea, and may vomit or faint if pain is severe. Except with severe contusions, the symptoms are usually short-lived and are often relieved when the athlete is placed supine and his knees are brought toward the chest. The athlete is typically able to return to activity after a few minutes. However, swelling and mild pain may linger for a few days. A **hydrocele** (swelling due to the accumulation of fluid within the tunica vaginalis, which is the membrane surrounding the testicle) or **hematocele** (rapid accumula-

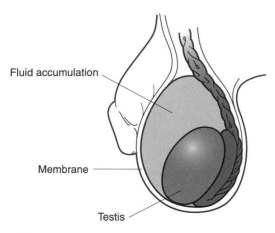

Fluid accumulation

Membrane

Testis

**∎ Figure 12.7** Testicular hydrocele. A hematocele may appear the same from the outside, but the fluid involved is blood rather than serous fluid.

tion of blood) may also form following trauma (figure 12.7). The athlete should be referred for medical evaluation whenever severe swelling is present, or when pain persists or symptoms worsen rather than improve. It is always wise to have the athlete examine the testicle following injury to check for any change in its appearance or position.

A potential complication of testicular trauma is torsion of the spermatic cord, in which the trauma causes the testicle to rotate in the scrotum. Torsion can also occur spontaneously in young males in the absence of trauma (see chapter 13, page 443). Signs and symptoms of testicular torsion include immediate or gradual onset of groin pain, heaviness in the scrotum, and change in the normal position or appearance of the testicle. This condition constitutes a medical emergency and requires immediate referral, as blood flow to the testicle will be compromised.

## Strains

The abdominal muscles function to stabilize, flex, and rotate the trunk during sport activity as well as to restrain the abdominal contents. Sudden muscle contractions or overstretch can strain these muscles and cause considerable disability because of their postural function. Strains and weakness in the lower abdominal region can also result in a herniation of the small intestines through the abdominal wall.

### Abdominal Muscles

Strain of the abdominal muscles (rectus abdominis, internal and external obliques) can result from a violent muscle contraction or trunk twisting movement. Chronic or repetitive overuse can also cause muscular strain. Signs and symptoms include pain, muscle spasm, and palpable tenderness. Swelling and discoloration may or may not be present. As with all muscle strains, the athlete will complain of increased pain with muscle contraction or with passive stretching of the involved muscle. Because the abdominal muscles are postural muscles and are involved in virtually every trunk movement, abdominal strains can be particularly bothersome to the athlete and slow to heal. Often, complete rest is necessary.

### Side Stitch

A side stitch or side ache is characterized by a sharp pain and/or spasm along the lateral abdominal wall, typically on the right side. This transient pain occurs most often with intense running activities and is more common early in the season. Although the exact cause is unknown, the side stitch is typically associated with muscle ischemia and poor conditioning, but has also been attributed to intestinal gas or to consumption of a large meal just prior to activity. The pain will often quickly subside with a reduction in activity or with deep, steady breathing. Stretching away from the side of pain or raising the arm overhead will also relieve symptoms. Once the pain dissipates, the athlete is usually able to return to activity without further problems.

### Hernia

A hernia is characterized by the protrusion of the small intestine through a weakened area in the anterior abdominal wall. The two most common sites of herniation are through the femoral ring and the inguinal region. Hernias can be congenital or acquired. Acquired hernias occur in sport when the already weakened area of the abdominal wall is further strained through lifting or other strenuous athletics-related activities. Herniation can also result from intense lifting, pushing, or coughing or from straining during defecation.

• **Femoral Hernia.** Anatomically, the femoral ring is an opening at the superior end of the femoral canal through which the femoral artery, vein, and lymphatic vessels pass into the lower extremity. The canal is widest at the femoral ring. With a **femoral hernia**, the abdominal viscera (usually small intestine) protrudes through the femoral ring and into the femoral canal (figure 12.8) (Moore 1992). It becomes visible or palpable just inferior to the inguinal ligament. It presents as a bulge or mass in the femoral triangle, inferolateral to the pubic tubercle and medial to the femoral vein. The mass may or may not be painful, but the athlete will typically complain of discomfort. Because of the rigid and defined boundaries of the femoral ring, strangulation of a femoral hernia is a concern. Strangulation occurs when the herniated contents become compressed and blood flow is compromised. If a strangulating hernia is left untreated, tissue necrosis will occur. Femoral hernias are more commonly seen in females because females typically have a wider femoral ring than males.

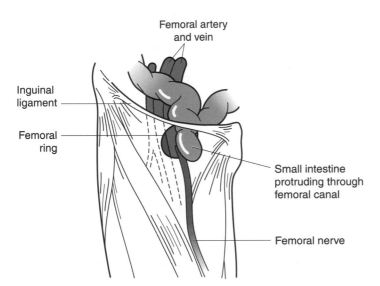

■ **Figure 12.8** Femoral hernia.

• **Inguinal Hernia. Inguinal hernias,** in which protrusion occurs through the inguinal canal, are commonly seen in males. The spermatic cord passes through the inguinal canal, which runs obliquely along the anterior inferior abdominal wall. The abdominal musculature provides much of the protection to the inguinal canal. There are two types of inguinal hernia, direct and indirect; the indirect type is the more common (75% of the cases) (Moore 1992). A direct hernia usually results from weakening of the anterior abdominal wall and protrudes anteriorly through the inferior portion of the inguinal (Hesselbach's) triangle. An indirect hernia will enter through the deep inguinal ring, inguinal canal, and superficial inguinal ring (figure 12.9). An indirect inguinal hernia will present as a mass in the inguinal region and may extend into the scrotum. The athlete may or may not complain of pain or tenderness in the region, depending on the extent of herniation. Having the athlete cough or bear down during palpation of the region will cause the herniation to further protrude momentarily due to an increase in intra-abdominal pressure. If the herniation does not retract and remains distended, strangulation of the herniated contents can occur secondary to restriction by the inguinal ring or twisting of the intestine. A strangulated hernia will cause severe pain and represents a medical emergency.

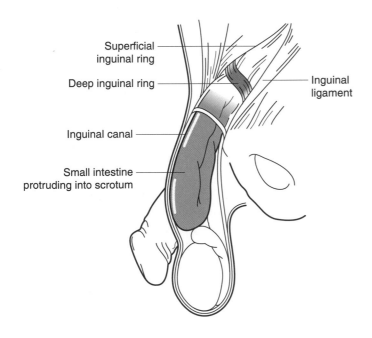

■ **Figure 12.9** Inguinal hernia.

### Internal Injuries

The abdominal cavity contains both hollow and solid organs that can be injured during sport activity. The hollow organs, which materials can pass through, include the stomach, large and small intestines, ureters, and bladder (figure 12.10a). The solid organs include the liver, spleen, pancreas, and kidneys (figure 12.10, a-b); because of their rich blood supply, injury to these organs can cause considerable hemorrhage. Injuries to the hollow organs are less common than injuries to the solid visceral organs, because of the hollow organs' ability to give and the solid organs' rigidity when trauma is directed at the abdomen. When an athlete presents with a history of severe blunt trauma to the abdomen, you should have a high index of suspicion of internal injury or hemorrhage. Therefore it is imperative for you to be able to recognize the signs and symptoms associated with internal injury and hemorrhage. When you suspect internal trauma, you should immediately refer the athlete for a thorough medical evaluation.

It is important that you keep in mind the location and orientation of the gastrointestinal organs in the abdominal cavity when considering what structures may be involved in various mechanisms of injury—particularly with regard to the location and direction of impact. To aid in identification and reporting of symptoms and

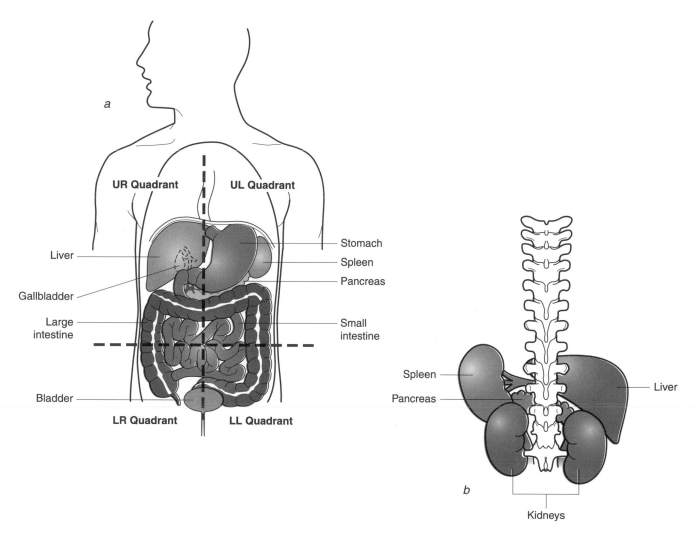

∎ **Figure 12.10** The gastrointestinal organs of the abdominal cavity from an (a) anterior and (b) posterior view. In (a), note the four quadrants of the abdominal cavity.

problems in the abdominal region, the abdominal cavity is divided into four quadrants, by imaginary transverse and horizontal lines that bisect the umbilicus, into the right and left upper and lower quadrants (figure 12.10a). However, it is important to remember that injuries to structures in one quadrant may cause pain or symptoms in another quadrant or may even refer symptoms to other body regions. Therefore you need to know not only the locations of these structures, but also their referral patterns (see table 12.1 later in this chapter).

### Bladder Rupture

The most common cause of a ruptured bladder is a direct blow to the abdomen with the bladder fully distended. This is rare in athletics simply because participating with a full bladder is too uncomfortable for most athletes. Athletes can easily prevent bladder ruptures by emptying the bladder prior to any athletic activity. The bladder can also be injured secondary to fracture of the pelvis. Signs and symptoms of a bladder rupture include a history of a direct blow or severe trauma to the abdomen, complaints of lower abdominal pain, and palpable tenderness and abdominal rigidity. Hematuria will be present, and the athlete will have difficulty with urination.

### Kidney Contusion

*Hematuria is blood in the urine.*

In contact sports, kidney contusions can occur secondary to a severe blow to the lower back. The kidneys sit on either side of the vertebral column between the levels of T12 through L3 (see figure 12.10b). The primary signs and symptoms of kidney trauma include deep aching in the lower back and flank region and possible muscle guarding. The pain may also wrap around anteriorly to the lower abdomen. Severe contusions can result in nausea, vomiting, and possible shock. Hematuria is a hallmark sign of kidney trauma but may or may not be visible to the naked eye and may require a urinalysis for identification. It is important to ask the athlete to check her urine for a change in color. Athletes with a suspected kidney contusion should be removed from activity and referred immediately to determine the extent of injury.

### Splenic Rupture

Rupture of the spleen can be a rapidly progressive injury that, if not recognized early, can lead to internal hemorrhage and possible death. In fact, splenic rupture is the most common cause of death due to abdominal trauma in sport. The spleen sits in the upper left quadrant and is protected by the 9th through 11th ribs (see figure 12.10a). It functions as a reservoir of red blood cells and produces antibodies and lymphocytes to fight illness and infection. The spleen is most vulnerable to injury after a systemic illness, such as mononucleosis, that causes the organ to become enlarged. Injury to the spleen can result from a direct blow to the left upper abdominal quadrant or a hard fall. The athlete will complain of left upper quadrant and flank pain and perhaps of nausea and vomiting. He will exhibit signs and symptoms of shock including a "wet" (cold, clammy skin), "white" (pale), and "weak" (weak, rapid pulse) appearance. Other signs and symptoms of hemorrhage include abdominal rigidity and rebound tenderness. If bleeding causes pressure or irritation of the diaphragm, a **Kehr's sign** will also be present, characterized by pain radiating into the left shoulder and partially down the arm. Athletes exhibiting any of these signs should be referred immediately. Removal of the spleen is often indicated.

A concern with splenic ruptures is that they can be deceiving and not readily apparent. The spleen can splint itself for a period of time, and hemorrhage can be delayed for hours, days, or even weeks after injury, with a subsequent lesser or inconsequential blow activating the hemorrhage. Therefore, it is imperative that an athlete who sustains blunt trauma to the abdomen be thoroughly evaluated following injury; she should also be instructed to watch for signs and symptoms of delayed hemorrhage and to seek medical attention immediately if they appear. Because of the increased risk of splenic rupture when the organ is enlarged, athletes with mononucleosis who are involved in contact, jarring, or running types of sports are restricted from these activities until the spleen has returned to its normal size. This may be difficult for the athletes to understand, as their symptoms of illness often clear before the spleen recovers.

# ASSESSMENT OF THE THORAX AND ABDOMEN

Assessment of the thorax and abdomen is rather complex in that symptoms of underlying pathology may not appear immediately, masking the seriousness of the situation. The ability to recognize signs and symptoms of internal injury and/or cardiorespiratory compromise can mean the difference between life and death, and often it is necessary to perform repeated assessments over time. Since the vast majority of injuries in this region will be acute or traumatic, and since the sideline and off-field assessments for this region are essentially the same, assessment of the thorax and abdomen will be divided here into on-field and off-field evaluations. The major difference between these assessments is their primary focus on emergent (on-field) versus nonemergent (off-field) conditions.

## ON-FIELD ASSESSMENT

Covering a soccer game, you see an athlete get kicked accidentally in the groin and go down on the field. Or consider the pitcher who goes down after sustaining a blow to the anterior chest from a line drive, or a football player who receives a blow to the left lower back from an opponent's helmet. Your goal in the on-field assessment is to initially assess for vital signs and life-threatening conditions, and then to gain an initial impression of the nature and severity of the injury. From this thorough but efficient evaluation, you can make the appropriate determination for medical referral and mode of transportation from the field.

### *Primary Survey*

As you approach the athlete, be observant of the surroundings, as well as the position and response of the athlete, which may provide important clues to the nature and extent of the injury. Is he lying still, or is he clutching his chest or abdomen?

Your first goal is to establish whether the athlete is conscious. Obviously, if he is doubled over in pain or is thrashing about, you will know this before you arrive at his side. If he is not moving, immediately assess for the presence of airway, breathing, and circulation. If he is breathing and has a pulse, check next for evidence of severe bleeding or trauma.

When an athlete sustains blunt trauma to the thorax and abdomen, there is always a chance of internal injury. Therefore, early in your assessment you should assess vital signs for evidence of cardiorespiratory distress, internal bleeding, and shock. Although symptoms of these conditions may not appear immediately, this assessment will provide a baseline for later comparison. How thoroughly you assess vital signs on the field will depend on the athlete's condition.

### Pulse

If the athlete has been exercising, her pulse will obviously be higher than normal and you will consider this in your interpretation. A normal pulse rate under resting conditions will be 60-80 beats/min. In well-trained runner, a lower pulse may also be normal. A rapid and weak pulse in an athlete is an indication of internal injury, shock, or both. The carotid artery at the neck is the best location for this assessment. Also note rhythm for evidence of arrhythmias, which may indicate a cardiac contusion or other cardiac trauma.

### Respirations

Respiratory distress will be obvious on observation. Normal respirations should fall between 12 and 24/min. Again, this value is likely to be higher after exercise. Dyspnea, or difficulty breathing, may be due to airway obstruction, chest wall injury, lung collapse, or chest compression. Deep quick (labored) respirations are also indicative of respiratory compromise (e.g., asthma ); and rapid and shallow respirations are characteristic of rib fractures, shock, and internal injury. In cases of abdominal trauma, the athlete will purposely limit his depth of respirations to movement of the upper chest to avoid movement in the abdominal region; this is one reason for rapid and shallow respirations. Respiration rates below 10/min or above 24/min are considered abnormal. Any signs of dyspnea demand prompt medical referral.

### Blood Pressure

Blood pressure will also provide an indication of shock and internal injury. A normal blood pressure should fall between 100 and 120 systolic and 70 and 80 diastolic. A blood pressure that falls below 100/60 may be indicative of shock or internal hemorrhage.

## Secondary Survey

Once you are assured that the athlete's vital signs are stable, proceed with your secondary survey. Again, because the severity of the condition may not be immediately evident, you will need to reassess vital signs periodically following significant trauma.

### History

If you did not do so as you approached, ask the athlete or bystanders, or both, about the mechanism of injury. If the mechanism was blunt trauma, try to determine the location, direction, and severity of the impact. Identify the athlete's chief complaint and the location, type, and quality of her pain or symptoms. Does she have any chest or abdominal pain? Is she nauseated? Is she having any difficulty breathing? Does the pain increase on inspiration? All these are relevant questions at this time. Keep in mind the orientation of the underlying structures, and remember that pain from the abdominal viscera may refer to other areas. For example, if the athlete complains of upper left quadrant pain and left shoulder pain, you should suspect a ruptured spleen. Chest pain and difficulty breathing are complaints consistent with a pneumothorax or hemothorax. Flank or groin pain is characteristic of kidney trauma, and pain in the upper right quadrant may indicate injury to the liver. Any time you suspect organ trauma, you should refer the athlete immediately.

### Observation

Continue to observe the overall response of the athlete for signs of pain, respiratory or cardiac distress, and signs of shock. Note his position and willingness to move. Is he lying still to avoid movement, or is he doubled over, or restless and agitated? Pain or avoidance of movement may indicate internal abdominal injury or peritoneal irritation. Abdominal pain and cramping will cause the athlete to double over; an athlete in respiratory distress will often be restless and agitated. Note the athlete's skin coloration. Immediately following exercise, the face should be flushed. A pale and moist appearance (wet and white) is indicative of shock and internal injury. Note the color of the skin around the lips and fingernails; a bluish tint (cyanosis) is indicative of respiratory compromise and inadequate oxygenation. Screen the chest and abdomen for signs of swelling, discoloration, lacerations, deformity, or asymmetry. Note the position of the trachea and check whether it is in midline or shifted to one side (tension pneumothorax). Observe the neck veins for distension (cardiac contusion, tension pneumothorax). Note any areas of discoloration at the site of trauma that may give you a sense of the severity or area of the impact. Consider whether the pain is near the site of impact or away from it; this may provide additional clues to the nature of the injury or the structure involved. Visually inspect the chest during respirations for complete expansion and for equal rise and fall on the two sides. If the athlete has multiple rib fractures and a flail chest, the movement of the fractured ribs will be the opposite of what you would expect during inspiration and expiration. Observe the abdomen for signs of guarding (pain, spasm) or distension (blood or fluid accumulation). If the athlete sustained significant trauma to the groin region, check the testicles for normal size and shape. Nausea and vomiting may also be observable; these signs are common with abdominal and groin trauma. If the athlete is coughing up blood (hemoptysis), there may be damage to the lung or bronchial passageway. Throughout your observation you should continue to monitor respirations and repeat vital signs as necessary, particularly if the athlete appears unstable.

## Palpation

Once you have determined the mechanism of injury and the athlete's chief complaint and have completed your observation, you should have a better sense of the location and nature of the injury. You will then proceed with palpation to quickly assess the potential structures that may be involved.

### Chest Wall

The chest wall is palpated for tenderness, swelling, deformity, crepitus, and asymmetry. Bony landmarks include the clavicle, sternum, xiphoid process, costochondral cartilage, thoracic vertebrae, scapula, and each rib (anterior, lateral, and posterior aspects). Also palpate the soft tissue for tenderness or defects in the pectoralis major and minor; intercostals on the anterior chest wall; serratus anterior and intercostals on the lateral chest wall; and the latissimus dorsi, erector spinae, and scapular muscles on the posterior chest wall. The inability to reproduce the athlete's chest pain by palpation of the superficial structures of the chest wall is an indication of internal pathologies.

### Abdomen

The abdomen is palpated for tenderness, distension, guarding, and rebound tenderness. It is best to palpate the abdomen with the athlete supine and her knees slightly flexed to relax the abdominal muscles. Begin with gentle palpation, with your fingers flat and together, starting at the umbilicus and then moving into each quadrant toward the costal, lateral, and iliac margins. Note any pain, tenderness, or defects of the abdominal musculature or their origins. If the abdomen in general is tender and distended, you should suspect internal bleeding and refer the athlete immediately. Also note any muscle guarding (spasm) or rigidity. Guarding is characterized by voluntary muscle spasm to protect injury of the abdominal wall and its contents. Rigidity, or a boardlike feeling that does not decrease when the muscles are relaxed, is indicative of internal bleeding. Rebound tenderness indicates irritation or inflammation of the peritoneum. Rebound tenderness is observed when the abdominal wall is depressed and then released. This will stretch the peritoneum and cause pain when the stretch/tissue pressure is released.

| Pulse |
|---|

The pulse should be periodically monitored via palpation for rate, rhythm, and strength. Note any change and continue to monitor for presence of arrhythmia or a rapid and weak pulse.

**Special Tests**

There are no special on-field tests for this region; your impression will be based primarily on the mechanism of the injury, the athlete's vital signs, and the observed signs and symptoms. If all signs are negative, the athlete can be removed from the field for further evaluation on the sideline.

**When to Refer**

Severe abdominal or chest trauma is uncommon in athletics; but you always should be prepared to evaluate and rule out such conditions, particularly when the athlete sustains blunt trauma to the flank, chest, or abdomen. To review, the cardinal signs of internal injury and shock include the following:

- Decreased blood pressure
- Rapid and weak pulse
- Wet, white, and weak appearance
- Rapid and shallow respirations

When any of these signs are noted, the athlete should be referred immediately for emergency medical attention. Other signs and symptoms that warrant immediate medical referral include any signs of respiratory distress (dyspnea); abnormal vital signs; cardiac arrhythmia; abdominal tenderness, rigidity, or distension; or any other signs that may indicate severe trauma. Remember, many of these signs and symptoms may not be observable immediately and may occur at some delay; therefore it is necessary to reassess the athlete periodically for any change in vital signs or symptoms. If all of the signs just listed are negative, the athlete can leave the field for continued monitoring on the sidelines.

## SIDELINE OR OFF-FIELD ASSESSMENT

The goal of your off-field assessment is to determine the SINS of the injury: **S**tage, **I**rritability, **N**ature, and **S**everity.

Not all injuries of the thorax and abdomen are immediately emergent, and some may be reported postacutely. Therefore your goal in the off-field assessment is to establish the SINS of the injury, to differentiate between other possible causes of the athlete's pain, and to rule out any latent underlying pathology that may manifest at some delay following the injury.

### History

All aspects of the history portion of the on-field assessment are applicable here. Since you may have not witnessed the injury or the athlete may be reporting it at some delay, other questions will also be relevant. Explore the mechanism of the injury and determine whether it was one of contact or noncontact. If noncontact, did the injury result from a sudden twist or muscle contraction that would indicate a soft tissue or muscle injury? For a contact injury, try to determine as closely as possible the location and area of impact, as well as the direction and intensity of the force. As the athlete describes the location, type, and quality of pain, is the location of pain consistent with the site of injury, or is it at some remote site, indicating secondary indirect trauma or referred symptoms?

Also explore other complaints at this time. If the injury is postacute, ask about the onset and duration of symptoms and any change in symptoms since the initial injury. Find out what activities increase or decrease symptoms, and establish the

## Checklist for On-Field Assessment of the Abdomen and Thorax

### Primary Survey

Observe surroundings and position and response of athlete as you approach.

✓ Establish level of consciousness.

✓ Check airway, breathing, circulation.

✓ Check for signs of severe bleeding, evidence of severe trauma.

✓ Check vital signs.

  ✓ Check pulse (rate, rhythm, strength).

  ✓ Check respirations (dyspnea, rate, depth).

  ✓ Take blood pressure.

### Secondary Survey

✓ History

✓ Ask athlete or bystanders about mechanism of injury:

  ✓ Location, direction, and severity of impact if blunt trauma

✓ Chief complaint

✓ Location, type, and quality of pain

✓ Presence and location of referred pain

✓ Difficulty breathing

✓ Feelings of nausea

### Observation

✓ Response and position of athlete, willingness to move

✓ Signs of respiratory or cardiac distress (dyspnea, cyanosis, neck vein distension, tracheal shift)

✓ Signs of shock (wet, white, weak)

✓ Skin coloration

✓ Signs of swelling, discoloration, lacerations, deformity, or asymmetry (superficial screen)

✓ Expansion and equal rise of the chest wall

✓ Abdomen for signs of guarding, rigidity, or distension

✓ Genitalia for swelling and abnormal appearance

✓ Continued monitoring of vital signs

### Palpation

✓ Chest wall for tenderness, swelling, deformity, crepitus, asymmetry

  ✓ Bony landmarks: clavicle, sternum, xiphoid process, costochondral cartilage, thoracic vertebrae, scapula, and ribs (anterior, lateral, and posterior)

  ✓ Soft tissue: pectoralis major and minor, intercostals, serratus anterior, erector spinae, scapular muscles

  ✓ Absence of palpable signs may indicate internal injury.

✓ Abdomen in all four quadrants for the following:

  ✓ Soft tissue tenderness or muscle guarding

  ✓ Rigidity and distension

  ✓ Rebound tenderness

✓ Continued monitoring of pulse

### Special Tests (None)

When to refer:

✓ Decreased blood pressure

✓ Rapid and weak pulse

✓ Wet, white, weak appearance

✓ Rapid and shallow respirations

✓ Dyspnea or cyanosis

✓ Cardiac arrhythmia

✓ Abdominal tenderness, rigidity, or distension

✓ Any abnormal vital signs

pain pattern. Has the athlete suffered any episodes of nausea, vomiting, or difficulty breathing? A sharp, sticking chest pain with inspiration is often associated with pleural irritation. If the injury was to the flank or abdominal region, ask the athlete whether he has noticed any blood in his urine; if he has not paid attention to this, have him check the next time he voids. And rather than looking only for the presence of blood, ask also about any changes in urine color. Bleeding is not always frank, and the athlete may miss a sign if he is looking only for a red coloration of the urine. Finally, does the athlete with chest wall or rib pain complain of increased pain with deep inspiration, coughing, or sneezing? If so, there may be an intercostal muscle strain, abdominal strain, or rib fracture, depending on the location of injury.

Gaining a history of previous injury and overall general health is also important at this time. Other general medical conditions unrelated to sport activity may also

General medical conditions of the cardiorespiratory and gastrointestinal systems can also refer pain to the thorax and abdomen. Whenever pain is present with no known mechanism of injury, these conditions must be considered and ruled out (see chapter 13).

cause pain or symptoms in the thorax or abdominal region. Therefore it is important to rule out factors such as asthma, upper respiratory illness, or gastrointestinal conditions that may be the source of the athlete's complaints (see chapter 13).

## Observation

Your inspection of the athlete will be consistent with that described for the on-field assessment and should include observation for abnormal respirations, skin color, abdominal guarding, athlete response, and signs of external trauma. With postacute injuries, swelling and discoloration will likely be more pronounced than they would normally be immediately following injury. Whether the athlete walks over to you on the sidelines or seeks your assistance in the athletic training room, note her position and posture. An athlete who is having difficulty breathing may be bent forward, with her hands resting on her knees; to relieve muscle strain and stretch, an athlete will often lean to the side of injury. This, as well as guarding or splinting of the arm or chest to protect the rib cage, may indicate a rib fracture. If the athlete is able to urinate and you suspect kidney trauma, inspect the urine yourself for presence of hematuria.

## Palpation

On the sideline or off the field you will palpate the chest wall and abdomen as described for the on-field evaluation. Place the athlete in a comfortable position (usually supine with knees and hips flexed) for maximal athlete relaxation and optimal palpation. Note areas of tenderness and consider both superficial and internal structures that may be involved. In addition to superficial palpation of the abdomen, you may also proceed with deeper organ palpation to assess for any pain or enlargement of the spleen, liver, or kidney. Deeper palpation of the abdomen takes practice and requires a sound knowledge of anatomical orientation of the abdominal viscera. Although direct palpation of these structures is difficult, it can be done (Munger and Baird 1980). To palpate near the liver, firmly place the digits of one hand under the right costal margin and have the athlete take a deep breath (figure 12.11). This will cause the diaphragm to descend and the lower right tip of the liver to move into the palpating hand. Lifting the right flank with your free hand will also improve the chance of liver palpation. To palpate the spleen, lift the left flank with your nondominant hand; with your other hand flat, depress the palpating digits just below and anterior to the 11th and 12th ribs and ask the athlete to take a deep breath (figure 12.12). A normal, healthy spleen will not be palpable. You can pal-

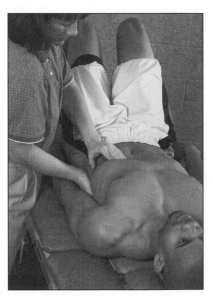

**■ Figure 12.12** Palpation technique for the spleen.

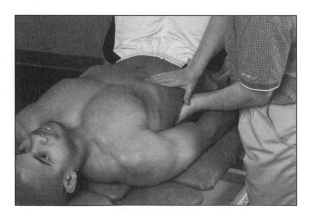

**■ Figure 12.11** Palpation technique for the liver.

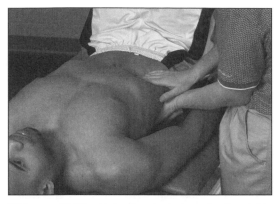

■ **Figure 12.13**    Palpation technique for the right kidney.

To help relax the athlete, begin your palpation away from the site of injury and slowly progress to the area of pain.

pate the right kidney by raising the flank with your free hand in order to move the kidney anteriorly toward your palpating hand on the anterior abdominal wall (figure 12.13).

If the athlete sustained severe testicular trauma that has not eased following injury, palpate or have the athlete palpate bilaterally for signs of swelling, tenderness, masses, change in consistency, or asymmetries. If there are any abnormalities, immediately refer the athlete to a physician for further evaluation.

## Special Tests

Very few special tests are available for identifying pathologies in the thorax or abdominal region. The primary tests used are compression tests for rib fractures and auscultation for abnormal heart, bowel, and lung sounds.

### Rib Compression (Spring) Tests

To assess for fractures of the lateral ribs, compress the chest wall by placing your hands on the anterior and posterior chest wall and squeezing them together (figure 12.14). This compression will cause tensioning of the lateral ribs. Pain or crepitus is a positive sign for fracture. You can use the same compression test for anterior or posterior rib fractures or for costochondral separation by applying a lateral compression stress with your hands placed on the lateral sides of the chest wall (figure 12.15). As before, pain or crepitus is a positive sign.

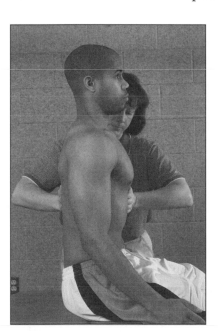

■ **Figure 12.14**    Anterior to posterior rib compression test.

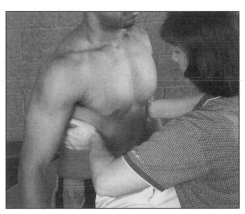

■ **Figure 12.15**    Lateral rib compression test.

*Rales are a crackling, popping, or bubbling sound heard with auscultation of the lungs.*

*Rhonchi are a loud whooshing sound heard with auscultation of the lungs, indicating air rushing over mucus in the bronchi.*

*Wheezing is a high-pitched whistling sound heard with auscultation, commonly noted with bronchial restriction in association with asthma.*

## Auscultation

Observation of heart, lung, and bowel sounds through auscultation may also be appropriate at this time and will provide further information about cardiopulmonary function or abdominal injury (figure 12.16). You will need training and practice in the use of auscultation techniques to be able to discern abnormal sounds such as decreased bowel sounds, decreased breath sounds, muffled heart tones, and arrhythmias. To listen to the abdomen, place the stethoscope over each quadrant. Gurgling and bubbling sounds are normal and will vary in intensity according to the time of day and the time the athlete had his last meal. Decreased or absent bowel sounds are indicative of internal injury or other serious underlying pathology and warrant immediate referral for further medical evaluation. Evaluate breath sounds over the thoracic surface while the athlete inhales and exhales. Check for decreased breath sounds that may indicate a pneumothorax. Other abnormal sounds include rales, rhonchi, or wheezing that may indicate other non-traumatic pulmonary conditions. Auscultation of the heart may reveal muffled or soft, faint heart tones, which are indicative of cardiac tamponade. You may also hear arrhythmias following cardiac contusion.

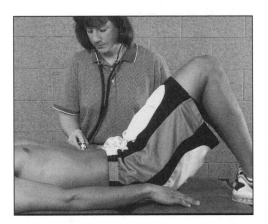

∎ **Figure 12.16** Auscultation of the abdomen with a stethoscope.

### Range of Motion

If you suspect muscular involvement or strain, perform active range of motion to assess for the presence of pain, guarding, or restricted motion with active muscle contraction. Motions to test include trunk flexion (abdominal crunch), rotation, lateral flexion, and hyperextension for assessment of the trunk and abdominal muscles (see chapter 7), as well as upper-extremity motions as indicated for assessment of the chest wall muscles (see chapter 4).

### Strength

Evaluate strength of the trunk and abdominal and chest wall muscles by resisting the same motions as tested for active range of motion. Please see chapters 4 and 7 for descriptions of these tests.

### Neurological Assessment

Neurological assessment in the abdominal and thoracic region is primarily sensory. It is common for thoracic nerve irritation to refer pain to the chest and abdomen. Figure 12.17 illustrates the dermatomes for each thoracic nerve root. Because of their overlapping patterns, it may be difficult to identify the specific nerve root involved; but if you note any abnormal sensations or pain that wraps around the thoracic region or abdomen, refer the athlete to a physician for further evaluation.

Neurological assessment of the thorax and abdomen also includes identifying referred pain patterns. A thorough knowledge of the pain referral patterns of the abdominal and thoracic viscera is essential to an accurate interpretation of the athlete's complaints. Common referral patterns for these structures are listed in table 12.1.

### Functional Assessment

You should assess functional performance only if all tests are negative and within the context of a decision about the athlete's readiness and ability to return to activity.

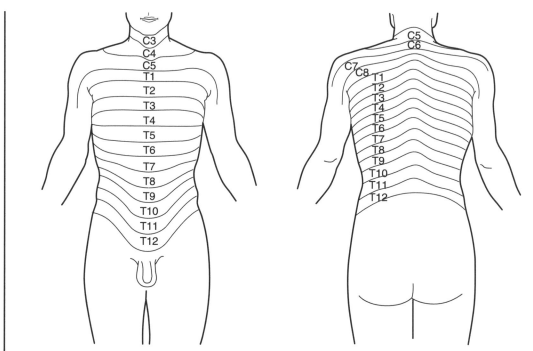

**Figure 12.17** Cutaneous dermatome patterns for thoracic nerve roots over the abdominal and thorax region.

| Table 12.1 Common Pain Referral Patterns of the Abdominal and Thoracic Viscera | |
| --- | --- |
| **Visceral organ** | **Area/pattern of referral** |
| Heart | Midsternal/epigastric, midback, left shoulder, and inner arm |
| Lung | Supraclavicular and neck regions |
| Liver | Upper right quadrant |
| Gallbladder | Upper right quadrant, right shoulder blade |
| Kidney | Flank into lower lumbar and groin area on same side |
| Spleen | Upper left quadrant, left shoulder |
| Stomach | Mid-thoracic region |
| Intestines | Umbilical region |
| Bladder | Lower, deep pelvic region |

This assessment may include aerobic exercise to ensure normal heart and lung function, and active sport-related movements to assess normal, pain-free muscular function. You should reassess signs and symptoms associated with the injury during and after the activity, noting any return of symptoms.

### Follow-Up Assessment

As has been mentioned throughout this chapter, signs and symptoms of internal injuries may not manifest themselves until hours or even days following injury. Therefore, ongoing or follow-up assessment and care of an athlete who has sustained blunt trauma should include frequent evaluation and instructions to the athlete about the signs and symptoms to watch for.

# Checklist for Off-Field Assessment of the Abdomen and Thorax

## History

✓ Ask athlete or bystanders about mechanism of injury:

 ✓ Contact versus noncontact mechanism

 ✓ Location, direction, and severity of impact if blunt trauma

✓ Chief complaint

✓ Onset, duration, and change in symptoms if injury postacute

 ✓ Activities that increase or decrease symptoms

✓ Location, type, and quality of pain

✓ Presence and location of referred pain

✓ Pain with coughing, sneezing, or deep inspiration

✓ Complaints of nausea, vomiting, difficulty breathing

✓ Presence of hematuria

✓ Previous injury history

✓ General medical health and history

## Observation

✓ Response, position, and posture of athlete

✓ Breathing pattern (dyspnea; respirations for rate, rhythm, and depth; chest wall expansion)

✓ Signs of cardiac distress (neck vein distension, tracheal shift)

✓ Skin coloration and moisture (cyanosis, white and wet)

✓ Abdomen for signs of guarding, rigidity, or distension

✓ Genitalia for swelling or abnormal appearance

✓ Blood in urine (hematuria) or sputum (hemoptysis)

✓ Signs of swelling, discoloration, lacerations, deformity, or asymmetry (superficial screen)

✓ Vital signs

 ✓ Respirations for rate, rhythm, and depth

 ✓ Blood pressure

 ✓ Signs of internal hemorrhage or shock

## Palpation

✓ Chest wall for tenderness, swelling, deformity, crepitus, asymmetry

✓ Bony landmarks: clavicle, sternum, xiphoid process, costochondral cartilage, thoracic vertebrae, scapula, and ribs (anterior, lateral, and posterior)

✓ Soft tissue: pectoralis major and minor, intercostals, serratus anterior, erector spinae, scapular muscles

✓ Abdomen and genitalia

 ✓ Soft tissue tenderness or muscle guarding

 ✓ Rigidity and distension

 ✓ Rebound tenderness

 ✓ Deep organ palpation (spleen, kidney, liver)

 ✓ Testicles for swelling tenderness, masses, abnormalities

✓ Pulse

## Special Tests

✓ Rib compression tests

✓ Auscultation of heart, lungs, and bowel

## Range of Motion

✓ Perform active ROM for trunk motions

✓ Perform active ROM for shoulder and scapular motions for muscles of the chest wall.

✓ Note difference bilaterally.

## Strength

✓ Perform resistance to same motions as in active ROM.

✓ Note weakness or difference bilaterally.

## Neurological

✓ Sensory of thoracic dermatomes

✓ Visceral referral patterns

## Functional Assessment

✓ Cardiorespiratory

✓ Musculoskeletal

## Follow-Up Assessment

✓ Instruct athlete about signs and symptoms to watch for.

✓ Perform periodic reevaluation for emerging signs and symptoms of internal injury.

# SUMMARY

1. *Describe the common mechanisms, signs and symptoms, and potential complications associated with injuries to the thorax commonly encountered in the physically active.*

   Injuries to the chest wall and structures in the thoracic cavity can result from direct insult or violent muscle contractions or may occur spontaneously as a result of intense exercise. The most common such injuries are contusion, strains, sprains, and fractures of the chest wall. However, these same mechanisms can also traumatize the heart and lungs or result in internal bleeding, which can have life-threatening consequences. Therefore it is essential for the athletic trainer to identify signs and symptoms of cardiorespiratory distress and to be able to differentiate those that indicate a medical emergency and the need for immediate medical referral.

2. *Describe the common mechanisms, signs and symptoms, and potential complications associated with injuries to the abdomen commonly encountered in the physically active.*

   Traumatic injuries to the abdominal region include soft tissue injuries of the abdominal muscles, genitalia, and internal viscera. While the thoracic cavity is well protected by the skeletal rib cage, the abdomen is protected primarily by the surrounding muscular wall. Consequently, contusions and muscular strains are the more common injuries in this region. Although these injuries are usually minor, when acute they can cause considerable pain and disability. Internal injuries, particularly to the solid organs, are also a concern with mechanisms of blunt trauma; these injuries most often involve the spleen and kidney. If internal hemorrhage results, the injury becomes life threatening if not immediately recognized and managed appropriately.

3. *Differentiate pathologies and signs and symptoms between cardiac contusion, tamponade, and concussion.*

   Blunt trauma to the anterior chest can cause injury to the heart. Cardiac contusion can result when the heart is compressed between the sternum and the spine. Cardiac tamponade is characterized by hemorrhage in the pericardial cavity, causing compression and compromise of the heart and pulmonary veins. Cardiac concussion, more common in adolescents, most often results from a blunt but seemingly inconsequential blow over the region of the heart. Each of these conditions represents a medical emergency; cardiac concussion often results in cardiac arrest and death. Any time an athlete receives blunt trauma to the anterior chest near the heart, cardiac injury should be suspected and vital signs immediately assessed.

4. *Appreciate the potential for life-threatening injury resulting from direct and indirect trauma to the thorax and abdomen.*

   The abdominal cavity contains both solid and hollow organs that can sustain injury during sport activity. When an athlete presents with a history of severe blunt trauma to the abdomen, the athletic trainer should have a high index of suspicion for internal injury or hemorrhage. Therefore it is imperative to be able to recognize the signs and symptoms associated with internal hemorrhage and shock. Suspicion of internal trauma warrants immediate referral of the athlete for a thorough medical evaluation.

5. *Perform an on-field assessment of the thorax and abdomen, indicating criteria for immediate medical referral or continued observation.*

   Severe abdominal or chest trauma is uncommon in athletics, but the athletic trainer should always be prepared to evaluate and rule out such conditions, particularly when the athlete sustains blunt trauma to the flank, chest, or abdomen. Therefore the goal in the on-field assessment is to initially assess for vital signs and life-threatening conditions, and then to gain an initial impression of the nature and severity of the injury. From this thorough but efficient evaluation one can make the appropriate determination for medical referral and mode of transportation from the field. If all of these signs are negative, the athlete can leave the field for continued monitoring on the sidelines. It is important to remember that many of these signs and symptoms may not be observable immediately and may occur at some delay; therefore, it is necessary to reassess periodically for any change in vital signs or symptoms. The ability to recognize signs and symptoms of internal injury and/or cardiorespiratory compromise can literally mean the difference between life and death, and these conditions often require repeated assessment over time.

6. *Perform an off-field assessment of the thorax and abdomen, indicating considerations for differential diagnosis.*

   Most injuries of the thorax and abdomen are not immediately emergent, and some may be reported postacutely. Therefore the goal in the off-field assessment is to establish the SINS of the injury, to differentiate between other possible causes of the athlete's pain (including general medical conditions), and to rule out any latent underlying pathology that may manifest at some delay following the injury.

# REVIEW QUESTIONS

1. Describe the common fractures of the chest wall. When would a suspected fracture cause you to be concerned about the potential for underlying pathology?

2. Describe the differences between a pneumothorax, a spontaneous pneumothorax, and a tension pneumothorax. How do their signs and symptoms differ, and which condition represents an immediate life-threatening injury?

3. What is commotio cordis? Describe the etiology and signs and symptoms of this condition and identify the populations most susceptible to this injury.

4. Testicular trauma is relatively common among physically active males. How would you differentiate between a minor and a serious injury?

5. What is a hernia, and what types of hernias are commonly seen in males versus females? What signs and symptoms would indicate these conditions?

6. What are the signs and symptoms of a kidney contusion?

7. As part of the primary survey, you are asked to take an athlete's vital signs. What vitals would you assess, and what are the cardinal signs and symptoms of internal hemorrhage?

8. From what you have learned in this chapter, list as many signs and symptoms as you can that would indicate immediate medical referral.

# CRITICAL THINKING QUESTIONS

1. During football practice you see an athlete receive a blow to the anterior abdomen. He is having difficulty catching his breath and is quite panicked. What condition(s) might you suspect, and how would you proceed in your evaluation to rule out serious pathology?

2. An athlete comes over to you on the sideline complaining of difficulty breathing and does not recall any specific trauma. Describe your evaluation of this athlete, including pertinent history questions and your objective assessment.

3. A wrestler is taken down hard on the mat, with his opponent landing on top of him. He complains of pain in his lateral chest wall and increased pain with inspiration. You suspect a rib fracture. To confirm your suspicions, how would your evaluation proceed from history through special tests?

# CITED REFERENCES

Curfman, G.D. 1998. Fatal impact—concussion of the heart [Editorial]. *N Eng J Med* 338(25):1841-1843.

Fruh, J.M. 1993. Fracture of the first rib in a collegiate soccer player. *J Sport Rehab* 2(3):196-199.

Haq, C.L. 1998. Sudden death due to low energy chest wall impact (commotio cordis) [Correspondence]. *N Eng J Med* 339(19):1398-1399.

Maron, B.J., Poliac, L.C., Kaplan, J.A., and Mueller, F.O. 1995. Blunt impact to the chest leading to sudden death from cardiac arrest during sport activities. *N Eng J Med* 333(6):337-342.

Moore, K.L. 1992. *Clinically oriented anatomy*. 3d ed. Baltimore: Williams & Wilkins.

Munger, B.L., and Baird, I.L. 1980. *Anatomy-Px: A practical introduction to anatomical correlates of the physical examination*. Baltimore: Williams & Wilkins.

# CHAPTER THIRTEEN

# Recognition and Referral of General Medical Conditions

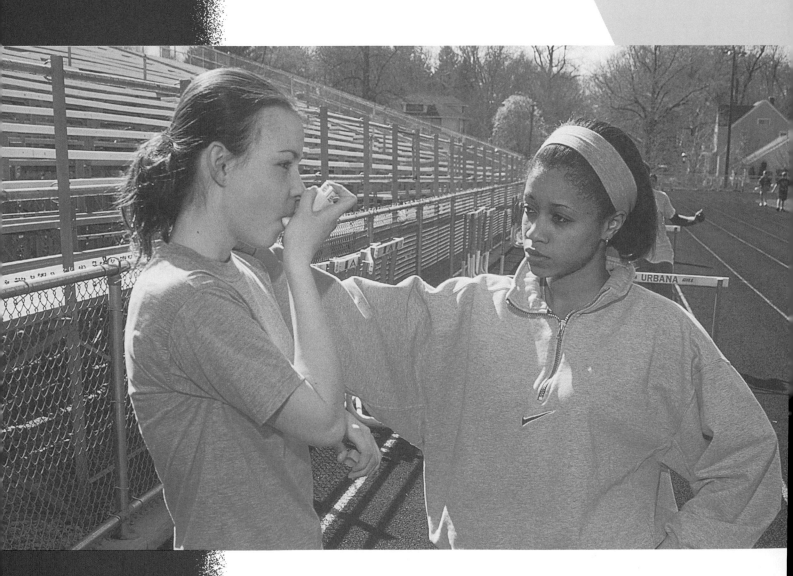

# OBJECTIVES

After finishing this chapter, the reader will be able to do the following:

1. Describe the signs and symptoms of a variety of medical conditions that may be encountered in the physically active

2. Appreciate the complications that may result from many of these conditions if not recognized and if left untreated

3. Determine which medical conditions require immediate, emergency medical referral and which require referral to a physician for diagnosis and treatment

4. Be able to perform an on-field assessment of an athlete who is unconscious and the etiology of the condition is unknown

Chelsea was an outgoing varsity lacrosse player. She always gave 100% and worked hard in practice. That is why it didn't take long for the coach to notice that something was wrong and to summon Patty, the athletic trainer, from the nearby athletic training room.

As Patty approached, she noticed that Chelsea seemed disoriented and didn't seem to be focused on any one thing. "Chelsea, are you feeling all right?" Patty asked, even though it was apparent she was not. Chelsea did not respond; she seemed agitated and confused, and was pacing. Patty remembered that Chelsea had revealed in her preparticipation examination that she had insulin-dependent diabetes. Patty smelled Chelsea's breath but didn't notice any odor. When taking Chelsea's pulse, she noted that it was rapid and weak and that her skin was pale and clammy. From her symptoms, it was likely that Chelsea was hypoglycemic and was going into insulin shock. Knowing Chelsea's condition, Patty was glad now that she had put a glucose packet in the field athletic training kit. Chelsea was not very cooperative, but allowed Patty to place the glucose under her tongue. Within minutes, Chelsea was acting more like herself.

"Do you know what happened?" Patty asked Chelsea.

"No, I don't really remember anything. I was practicing fine and then all of the sudden I got weak and light-headed. I thought maybe I needed some sugar, but I thought I could wait until after practice. I'm glad you knew what to do. . . . Thanks, Patty!"

When caring for the physically active, you may encounter a variety of general medical conditions and disabilities that are not directly related to physical activity but that can affect performance or overall health. Many of these conditions are of short duration and are accompanied by only minor signs and symptoms or disabilities. However, some can have severe, life-threatening consequences or can result in permanent disability if not recognized and treated appropriately. Other conditions represent permanent and preexisting disease states that require you to be aware of the athlete's history, as complications may arise during sport activity.

Although the majority of the conditions discussed in this chapter are beyond the scope of your ability to care for the athlete, you must be able to recognize their signs and symptoms in order to make the appropriate medical referral and ensure proper care for the athlete. When individuals participating in physical activity exhibit such signs and symptoms, it may be necessary to provide immediate first aid or emergency care; but referral to a physician is your ultimate responsibility. In many cases, you will not see the outward manifestations of these conditions but will learn of the problem from the concerned athlete. Because of the close relationship that develops through daily interaction, it is not uncommon for athletes upon recognizing symptoms to first confide in the athletic trainer rather than a physician. This is especially true in the case of more sensitive or potentially embarrassing symptoms when the athlete is unsure of what they signify or what to do about them.

This chapter will cover the general medical conditions you are most likely to see, according to body systems as presented in *Athletic Training Educational Competencies* (National Athletic Trainers' Association 1999). In some cases, the order has been slightly altered to enhance your comprehension and your understanding of related conditions. Since the goal of this chapter is primarily recognition, the discussion does not address specific assessment procedures for each condition; such assessment is usually the responsibility of the physician and requires diagnostic tests.

You will also find in this chapter the assessment procedures for evaluating an athlete who is unconscious and the cause is unknown. As this text has shown throughout, a variety of injuries and illnesses can result in a loss of consciousness. You will at times come upon an athlete who has become unconscious and you and other by-standers will not know the cause. This chapter includes a systematic assessment procedure that is not specifically related to any body region or medical condition to provide you with a strategic approach to this scenario.

# THE SKIN

Skin reactions, rashes, and lesions can result from a variety of conditions and agents. Most skin conditions are not life threatening, although they can be a nuisance and can linger if not treated soon after onset. Some can be treated with across-the-counter medications, but it is advisable for you to know your state's laws governing distribution of medications and also for you to obtain a confirmed diagnosis from a physician before administering any medication.

Some dermatological conditions are contagious and others are not. Those that are contagious must be carefully controlled to prevent their spreading. The athletic trainer must know which conditions are contagious and which are not.

The best treatment for any dermatological condition is prevention. Encouraging athletes to shower, wash hands, and seek prompt medical treatment at the onset of any condition can keep most dermatological conditions to a minimum.

For organizational purposes, skin conditions are classified in this chapter as either infectious, inflammatory, environmental exposures, or other.

## SKIN INFECTIONS

Localized skin infections can result from bacterial, viral, fungal, or parasitic agents.

### *Bacterial Infections*

Bacterial infections are typically of staphylococcal origin. These conditions are usually characterized by pustules, and the hair follicle is often the site of infection.

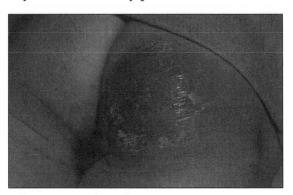

**❚ Figure 13.1**  Skin abscess.

#### Abscess

An abscess, which can occur in many different sites and can be either acute or chronic, is a localized infection that appears as a collection of pus (figure 13.1). Local tissue destruction and edema are common signs and symptoms. Acute abscesses are usually in a localized area of pain and increased warmth, demonstrating typical signs of inflammation. A chronic abscess is usually not as painful and is encapsulated by fibrous tissue.

#### Acne Vulgaris

Although acne vulgaris is commonly seen in adolescents, it can also occur as an adult-onset condition. It is the result of a heredity disorder of the hair follicles and oil glands that results in blackheads, cysts, and pustules (figure 13.2). Most cases exhibit acne lesions of varying depths on the face, neck, chest, shoulders, and back. Some people engaging in

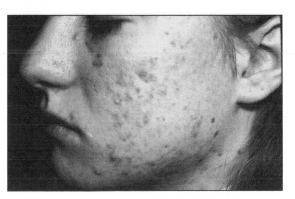

**❚ Figure 13.2**  Acne vulgaris.

physical activity may experience a flare-up of this condition as a probable result of increased perspiration and oil production during activity.

The dermatologist commonly has several options for treating acne vulgaris. Oral or topical antibacterial agents, topical antimicrobial agents, topical drying agents, and astringents to remove skin oils are commonly used. Oral antibiotics are not used with preadolescents or pregnant women because of the pigmentation changes they can produce in the permanent teeth of both preteens and fetuses.

### Carbuncle

*To **debride** means to clear a wound of infectious or foreign substances in an effort to promote healing and restore healthy tissue.*

A carbuncle, or boil, is a staphylococcus-based infection that affects several contiguous hair follicles connected by sinuses that are formed as the infection advances. Commonly located on the back of the neck, carbuncles occur most frequently in men. Signs include fever, a pus-filled lesion, and local pain. The skin surrounding the boil will be red and inflamed, with a hard, pus-filled core at the center (figure 13.3). This condition should be referred to the dermatologist, who can debride the area and prescribe antibiotics.

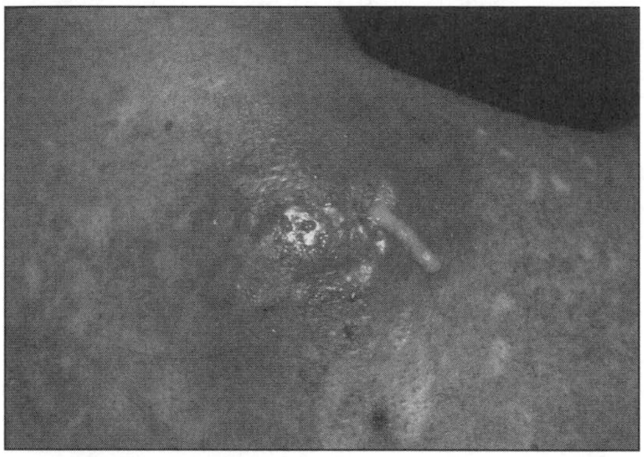

**Figure 13.3** Carbuncle.

### Cellulitis

Cellulitis is an inflammation of soft tissue or connective tissue. It usually involves skin and subcutaneous tissue and has a tendency to spread. Any infecting organism is capable of causing a cellulitis, but the most frequent cause is streptococci or staphylococci bacteria that affect an area of reduced resistance following injury or other trauma. Cellulitis is characterized by a general redness of the skin, swelling, pain, and warmth of varying proportions directly related to the severity of the condition (figure 13.4).

Physician referral is necessary so that proper antibiotic therapy can be instituted. Additional treatment may include rest and heat or moist dressings as prescribed by the physician.

### Folliculitis

Folliculitis, usually staphylococcal in origin, is an inflammation of the hair follicle. It frequently occurs in men with curly beards (pseudofolliculitis barbae) when the hair reenters the skin and causes a localized inflammation; however, it can occur in any hair follicle or body region. The inflammatory site becomes a pustule and displays signs of inflammation: redness, localized swelling, and tenderness (figure 13.5).

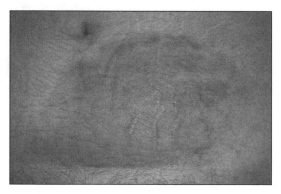

**Figure 13.4** Cellulitis.

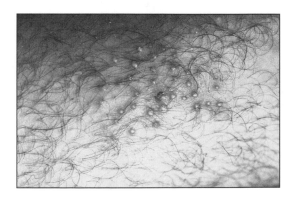

**Figure 13.5** Folliculitis.

The treatment is to dry the pustule with astringents or other agents used with acne vulgaris. When the folliculitis is prominent, the physician prescribes oral antibiotics. Scrubbing the face with an abrasive pad to prevent ingrown hair is a common method of prevention.

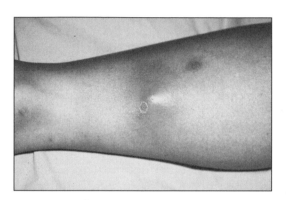

**I Figure 13.6**   Furuncle—boil at the hair follicle.

### Furunculosis

The common name for a furuncle is a **boil**—a localized infection of a hair follicle (figure 13.6). The common source of infection is staphylococcus bacteria. The local area is red, edematous, and tender. Since staphylococcal infections are highly contagious, the athlete must refrain from sport participation until the infection has healed.

Treatment includes moist hot packs and 10% topical benzoyl peroxide; the physician may order oral antibiotics. Prevention includes use of soap and good hygiene in regular showering.

### Impetigo

Impetigo, a contagious bacterial infection caused by either staphylococci or streptococci, is highly contagious in young children. It begins as pustules that go on to rupture and crust over (figure 13.7). These most commonly occur on the face and head but can spread to other areas.

Treatment includes referral to a physician for antibiotic medication. Use of soap and water for proper cleansing, followed by astringents or alcohol solutions to dry the lesions, is also advised.

### *Viral Infections*

Some skin infections are viral in origin; these include molluscum contagiosum, herpes simplex and zoster, and verruca plantaris and vulgaris.

### Molluscum Contagiosum

*A **papule** is a small raised bump on the skin that may or may not be painful.*

Molluscum contagiosum, a virally caused contagious infection of the skin, is characterized by small, round, flesh-colored papular lesions that occur most commonly on the face, trunk, axilla, perineum, and thigh (figure 13.8). You may see only a few papules, or there may be many. Athletes in contact sports are frequent transmitters of this disease.

Physician referral is necessary for treatment with prescribed medications.

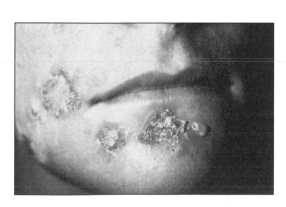

**I Figure 13.7**   Impetigo.

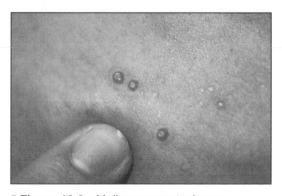

**I Figure 13.8**   Molluscum contagiosum.

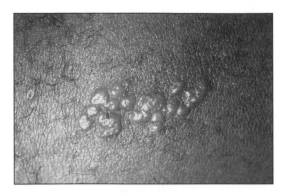

■ **Figure 13.9** Herpes simplex I.

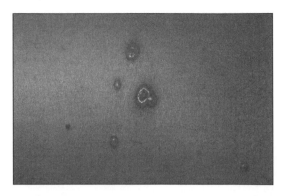

■ **Figure 13.10** Herpes zoster (chickenpox).

### Herpes Simplex

Herpes simplex infections are contagious viral infections caused by herpes virus I and II. They are characterized by an eruption of groups of vesicles (figure 13.9) and have a tendency to become reactivated and reappear with stress or fever. Herpes virus I that occurs on the lips or around the nose is also called a fever blister or cold sore. Herpes virus II occurs on the genitalia.

Acyclovir, an antiviral drug for herpes viruses, is available topically, orally, and by intravenous administration. Topical agents to dry the vesicles can also encourage the healing process. Prevention is the most effective means of control. Good hand-washing practices and use of gloves when one is applying medication to the sore will help reduce the spread. Direct contact with the sore should be avoided.

### Herpes Zoster

Herpes zoster is associated with two diseases, one that occurs in childhood and one that occurs in adulthood. The childhood version is known as chickenpox (**varicella**) and the adulthood version as shingles (zoster).

*A macule is a nonraised patch of skin with altered color.*

*Malaise is a vague, general feeling of illness and fatigue.*

• **Chickenpox** is characterized by skin lesions that begin as macules and progress to fluid-filled vesicles before they become crusty and scabbed (figure 13.10). The vesicles occur most often on the trunk, but in severe cases can spread to the face and extremities. The incubation period is two to three weeks. Fever and malaise can precede the appearance of macules. The older the individual is, the more intense the fever and malaise symptoms. Treatment is symptomatic, aimed at reducing fever and relieving itching. Care should be taken to avoid scratching the eruptions to prevent infection and later scarring. Hand washing and bathing are encouraged to minimize the risk of spreading the disease and causing an infection. The varicella vaccine used to protect against severe chickenpox has been available since March 1995. Routine vaccination of children at 12-18 months of age is recommended. Many states require vaccination prior to entry into the public school system. Immunity to further episodes of chickenpox occurs with one contraction of the disease.

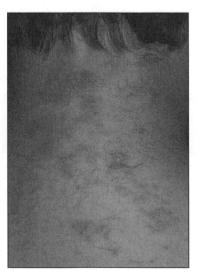

■ **Figure 13.11** Shingles.

• **Shingles** is a viral infection that affects the posterior nerve roots and dorsal ganglion in individuals usually over the age of 50. It is characterized by pain and vesicles that erupt along the inflamed nerve's cutaneous distribution on one side of the body (figure 13.11). In rare instances, vesicle eruption can be preceded for three to four days by flu-like symptoms of fever, malaise, chills, and/or headache. The vesicles become dry and scabbed after several days and then no longer contain the virus. Pain along the nerve's pathway as a result of nerve damage from the virus—post-herpetic neuralgia—is the most common complication; this can be severe and prolonged, lasting in some cases for months or years. Most commonly, the areas affected are the regions of trigeminal nerve and thoracic ganglia distribution. A primary complication of shingles is bacterial infections that can add to superficial tissue destruction and scarring.

Physician referral is recommended; however, there is no known effective treatment for herpes zoster. The drug of choice is acyclovir for treatment of shingles to reduce healing time, new vesicle formation, and pain duration. Symptomatic relief can occur with application of topical lotions or powders. Analgesics can be effective in pain relief.

### Verruca Plantaris

Verruca plantaris is commonly referred to as a plantar wart (figure 13.12). Caused by a virus, it results in hypertrophy and thickening of the epidermis layers. It occurs on the bottom of the foot and is flattened because of the pressure of weight bearing. The thickening can cause pressure and discomfort. These warts can occur as individual lesions or can cluster in groups called **mosaic warts**.

Most across-the-counter medications are ineffective in resolving plantar warts. In-season treatment includes symptomatic relief with protective or relief pads. In the off-season, referral to a physician for plantar wart removal is most effective, although there is no assurance that plantar warts will not return.

### Verruca Vulgaris

Verruca vulgaris is a common wart caused by a papilloma virus (figure 13.13). These warts occur in areas of frequent trauma or infection such as the hands, elbows, knees, face, and scalp. Distinctive in their appearance, they show sharp demarcation and some elevation, have either an irregular or a round border, are firm, and vary in color from light gray to near black.

These warts will sometimes spontaneously regress, but they can also be excised by a physician.

### *Fungal Infections*

Fungal conditions are generally referred to as tinea or ringworm infections. Specific names typically reflect their location.

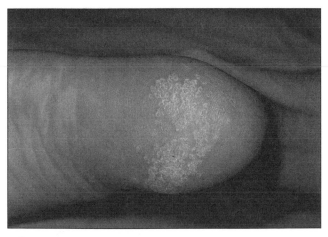

**▌Figure 13.12**   Plantar wart.

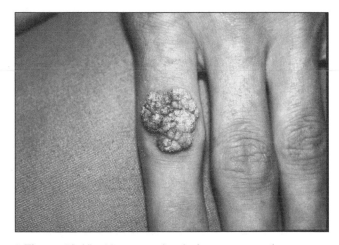

**▌Figure 13.13**   Verruca vulgaris (common wart).

## Ringworm

Although ringworm is one of many fungal diseases of the skin (tinea infection), the term is commonly used for a fungus that affects the scalp, trunk, and upper extremi-

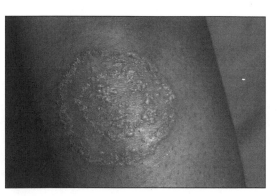

**Figure 13.14** Tinea corporis (ringworm).

ties. It is also known as **tinea corporis**. The lesion is a well-defined ringlike eruption that has red or brown plaques with a raised border and may itch or burn (figure 13.14). The lesion can be dry and scaly, moist, or crusted. It is spread by direct contact with the person who has the fungus or through indirect contact with items such as combs, clothing, and towels.

Topical antifungal medications, across-the-counter and prescription doses, are the most common form of treatment. Good hand-washing tech-

nique helps reduce transmission of the fungus, and sharing items such as combs, towels, and clothing should be discouraged.

## Tinea Capitis

This highly contagious ringworm infection, typically seen in children, affects the scalp (figure 13.15). The lesions are scaly, grayish patches in which the hair becomes dull, broken, and thin. The area affected can include either small ringed patches or much of the scalp.

Referral to a physician for necessary topical medication must be part of the treatment program, since tinea capitis does not spontaneously resolve.

## Tinea Cruris

Tinea cruris ("**jock itch**") is fungal infection that affects the groin (figure 13.16). It has the characteristic ringworm appearance and can cause itching, redness, scaling, and cracking. Prevention, which is the best method of treatment, includes using good showering and drying techniques, wearing clean cotton clothing, and avoiding clothes made of synthetic materials such as nylon. Antifungal medications are available in across-the-counter and prescription doses for treatment of tinea cruris. Not sharing towels and clothing are also good prevention habits that will limit spread of the fungus.

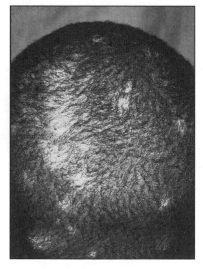

**Figure 13.15** Tinea capitus (ringworm of the scalp).

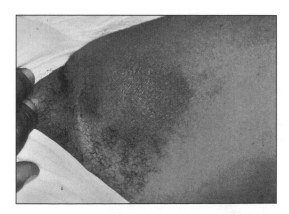

**Figure 13.16** Tinea cruris (jock itch).

### Tinea Pedis

Tinea pedis (athlete's foot) is fungal infection that affects the feet (figure 13.17). The skin can appear red, scaly, and cracking and is often itchy. The prevention and treatment course for tinea pedis is the same as for other ringworm infections. Cleansing and drying the feet properly, wearing clean socks, and avoiding walking barefoot are appropriate prevention steps.

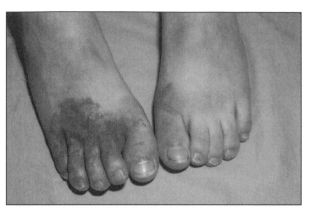

**I Figure 13.17** Tinea pedis (athlete's foot).

### Tinea Versicolor

Tinea versicolor is a noncontagious ringworm infection that affects the horny layers of the skin and hair follicles (figure 13.18). A yeast fungal infection, it appears first as a salmon-colored, then as a scaly, patch of skin that does not pigment. Usually found on the trunk, it will appear as either a white or a brown patch of skin.

## Parasitic Infestations

Parasitic infestations of lice and itch mites can result in infection and irritation of the skin. These infections are typically found in the hair of the scalp and pubic regions.

### Pediculosis

Pediculosis is an infection of the skin caused by lice (figure 13.19). The body region that is affected is indicated by the name: **pediculosis capitis** is caused by the head louse, **pediculosis corporis** by the body louse, and **pediculosis pubis** by the crab louse. Lice of this third type infest hairs of the genital region; infestation is commonly referred to as "crabs." The most prevalent symptom is severe itching. Louse eggs, called nits, can be seen attached to the hair shaft close to the root, as well as on clothing. Secondary bacterial infections from scratching can occur. Direct contact is the means of transmission from one individual to another. Treatment includes physician referral for medication to eradicate the parasite. Thorough laundering of clothing and bed linen will also be necessary.

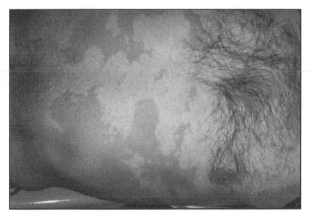

**I Figure 13.18** Tinea versicolor.

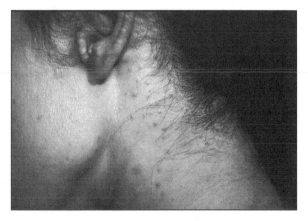

**I Figure 13.19** Pediculosis capitis.

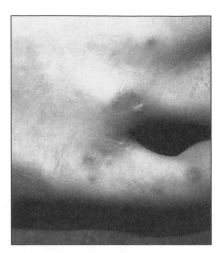

**Figure 13.20** Scabies.

### Scabies

Scabies is caused by the itch mite. The impregnated female mite burrows into the skin and deposits her eggs in the tunnel. The larvae hatch and accumulate around hair follicles. The typical signs and symptoms include the appearance of elevated burrows on the skin and itching. The most common sites are the interdigital spaces of the hands, axilla, trunk, and genital regions (figure 13.20).

Treatment includes prescribed medicated shampoo with gamma benzine hexachloride for the whole body, with repeated applications as necessary; laundering of clothing and bed linens; and prophylactic treatment of team members and others in contact with the individual.

## INFLAMMATORY CONDITIONS

General inflammatory conditions of the skin include dermatitis, eczema, and psoriasis.

*Erythema is redness of the skin.*

*Vesiculations are small ruptures or blistering of the skin.*

### Dermatitis

Dermatitis is simply defined as an inflammation of the skin. Contact dermatitis, the most common dermatitis condition, is a delayed reaction to direct contact with an allergen (figure 13.21). It is characterized by erythema, edema, itching, and vesiculations of varying degrees. The first step in treatment is removal of the offending substance. Physician referral for medications such as adrenocortical steroid ointments is recommended.

### Eczema

Eczema is the generic term used to describe chronic dermatitis. It is characterized by scaling, erythematous, edematous, papular, vesicular, crusty skin and is often accompanied by itching and burning (figure 13.22). As with other dermatitis, removal of the irritant is key to treatment. Treatment of the lesions depends upon their stage. Moist lesions are treated with drying agents, while crusting and scaling lesions are treated with petrolatum or hydrophilic ointments.

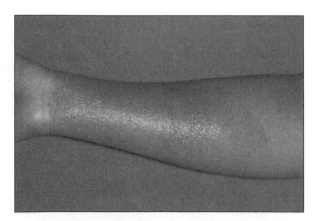

**Figure 13.21** Contact dermatitis.

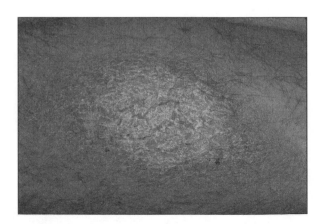

**Figure 13.22** Eczema.

### Psoriasis

Psoriasis is a usually chronic condition of unknown etiology that exhibits characteristic eruptions on the extensor surfaces of the extremities, especially the elbows, knees, back, and scalp (figure 13.23). The eruptions are circumscribed, erythematous papules covered with silvery scales. The frequency and duration of their recurrences and remissions vary. Treatment includes referral to a physician for medical care. Medications are usually prescribed to treat the signs and symptoms of psoriasis, but there is no effective treatment for prevention or remission.

## ENVIRONMENTAL EXPOSURES

Skin lesions can be also caused by environmental conditions such as allergens and by overexposure to heat and cold. The common terms for these conditions are hives, frostbite, and sunburn.

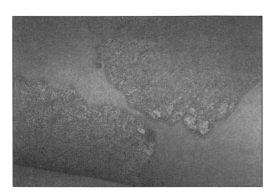

**▌ Figure 13.23**    Psoriasis.

*A **wheal** is a reaction of the skin surface characterized by an elevation of a patch of skin that is smooth and red in appearance.*

*__Histamine__ and __kinins__ are chemical substances found in the body that, when released, cause dilation and increased permeability of blood vessels.*

*__Eosinophils__ are leukocytes or other granulocytes that are released secondary to an allergen or a parasitic infection.*

*__Serum__ is a watery fluid.*

### Hives

Hives, or **urticaria**, is a dermal hypersensitivity reaction to an allergen. Common allergens include any substance to which one's exposure causes an abnormal reaction, such as insect bites, foods, dust, mold, or certain medications. A wheal formation that occurs on the skin can range from small red dots to large, raised, reddened areas (figure 13.24). Edema and erythema, resulting from release of histamine and kinins, are accompanied by wheal formation caused by exuded serum, eosinophils, and other white blood cells and local distension of blood and lymph vessels.

Most people who have hypersensitivity reactions are aware of them and know the steps to take after exposure. When first-time reactions occur, the individual should be referred to the physician. Hives will subside within one day to two weeks, depending on the severity of the reaction. Symptomatic relief of itching can be obtained with use of antihistamine medications and antipruritic topical agents. Of course, removal from the allergen is strongly recommended.

### Frostbite

Frostbite is a potentially serious condition of local tissue destruction consequent to exposure to cold, resulting in freezing of the superficial and possibly deeper tissue layers. It can range from mild to severe. Mild cases display erythema, itching, numbness, and mild pain. If exposure to cold continues, the skin can become pale, waxy, and firm to the touch. There may be some swelling with pain, numbness, or burning that can continue for several weeks. Severe cases are characterized initially by paresthesia and painless blisters and ultimately lead to tissue destruction and gangrene (figure 13.25).

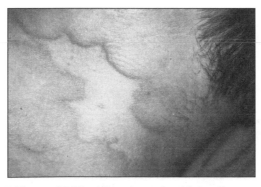

**▌ Figure 13.24**    Hives in a wheal formation.

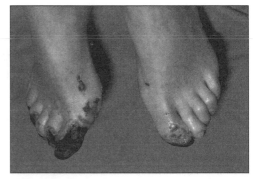

**▌ Figure 13.25**    Severe frostbite.

Initial treatment includes warming the tissue in warm water below 40.6° C (105° F). Rubbing the skin should be avoided. People with signs of frostbite should be immediately referred to a physician.

### Sunburn

Sunburn, a common skin condition caused by overexposure to the sun's ultraviolet rays, is characterized by redness, pain or burning sensation, itching, and increased heat of the skin. Blisters may also be present with more severe sunburns, resulting in peeling of the damaged skin layer a few days later. When the sunburn is severe and occurs over a large portion of the body, there may also be fever and general malaise. This is a condition that can and should be prevented with habitual use of sunscreen, as repetitive damage to the skin can lead to skin cancer. Individuals with fair skin are particularly susceptible, but this is not to say that dark-skinned individuals are immune. All athletes engaged in outdoor activities, regardless of season, should protect their skin by using sunscreen.

## OTHER LESIONS

Other lesions involving the dermis can result in buildup of tissue or fluid due to mechanical friction or glandular occlusion. These conditions include blisters, calluses, and sebaceous cysts.

### Blisters

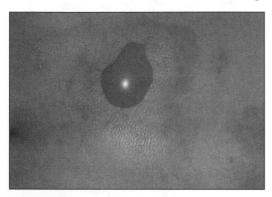

**I Figure 13.26**  Blister.

A blister is a separation of the skin's dermis and epidermis layers caused by a heat buildup from friction. Fluid, either serous or blood, fills the area (figure 13.26). The preferred method of treatment is to protect the area with a sterile bandage. If the blister breaks, the area should be cleansed using sterile technique; an antiseptic ointment should be applied and secured with a sterile dressing. Large or infected blisters should be referred to the physician for lancing and debridement.

Prevention is the best method of treatment. Athletes should wear properly fitted shoes with adequate sock protection, should break in shoes before wearing them for athletic participation, and should keep calluses well trimmed.

### Calluses

Calluses are the result of excessive friction. Skin builds up in an area of high friction as a means of self-protection (figure 13.27). Calluses typically form in the feet and hands over areas of high friction, stress, and bony prominences. As a callus forms, the skin becomes thicker and less flexible and elastic, moving as a larger-than-normal unit and becoming more susceptible to tears. Calluses should be kept trimmed and manageable, but should not be completely removed so as to leave sufficient protection of more sensitive skin layers. Prevention steps include wearing two pairs of socks, including a thin cotton sock next to the skin, or gloves on the hands. Use of lanolin or oils to keep the skin moist and soft can also help.

If the callus should tear, it is treated as any other open wound. Protection from infection is crucial. The wound should be cleansed, protected with an antiseptic or antibiotic ointment, and covered with a sterile dressing.

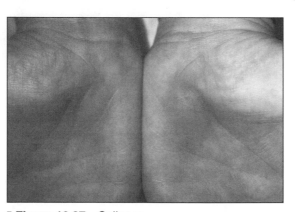

**I Figure 13.27**  Calluses.

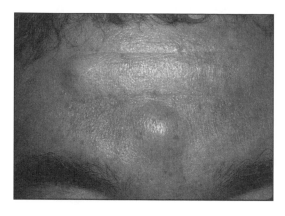

■ **Figure 13.28**    Sebaceous cyst.

### Sebaceous Cysts

A sebaceous cyst is a benign cystic tumor of the skin that develops because of occlusion of a sebaceous gland in the dermis. It is a firm, round, movable, and nontender mass that most commonly develops on the scalp, face, back, or scrotum (figure 13.28). Discomfort will be present if the cyst is infected.

Treatment includes physician referral for excision of the cyst sac. If the cyst is small, the physician may puncture the cyst to drain it rather than excise it.

## EYES, EARS, AND MOUTH

Irritation and infection in the eyes, ears, and mouth are common complaints in the physically active. These conditions can cause considerable pain, hampering performance until they are resolved. Most are caused by bacterial or viral infections.

## EYE CONDITIONS

Redness and irritation of either or both eyes, which can be quite painful, can result from infection, the presence of foreign bodies, or allergens. Two common eye conditions are conjunctivitis and sties.

### Conjunctivitis

**Conjunctivitis**, or "pinkeye," is an irritation and inflammation of the outer surface of the eye or inner eyelid. It can be caused by allergies or infection (viral or bacterial) or by direct contact (e.g., contact with an airborne substance, hand contact). While allergic conjunctivitis typically involves both eyes, viral or bacterial conjunctivitis usually begins in one eye but may spread to the other. The athlete will complain of pain, itching, and burning or a scratchy sensation in the eye; and the eye will appear red and swollen. Sensitivity to light (**photophobia**), blurred vision, and a yellowish discharge from the eye may also be noted secondary to the irritation and infection. Viral conjunctivitis, which frequently accompanies an upper respiratory infection, is quite contagious and can easily spread to the unaffected eye or to teammates. It is imperative that the athlete, as much as possible, avoids touching the eye and immediately washes her hands after having done so in order to avoid spreading the infection. Treatment includes removal of the irritant, eye washes, and referral to a physician for an ophthalmic solution.

### Sties

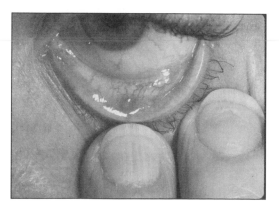

■ **Figure 13.29**    Sty.

The glands and hair follicles of the eyelid can also become irritated and swollen as a consequence of infection or obstruction. A **sty** is an infection or obstruction of a ciliary gland of the eyelid. **Chalazia**, or cysts of the sebaceous glands, may also form. Both result in focal redness and swelling that gradually appears as a small nodule or "bump" along the margin of the eyelid (figure 13.29). A painful pustule may develop over subsequent days. Pain and general eye discomfort will be the primary complaint.

## EAR CONDITIONS

Earaches can be caused by a variety of conditions. Pain can be referred from the jaw or teeth but is most often caused by inflammation in the external auditory canal. These conditions can be quite painful and can result in a temporary loss of hearing due to inflammation.

> Neither you nor the athlete should attempt to remove excessive wax buildup with a cotton swab; this is contraindicated, as it could cause further impaction and discomfort.

### Impacted Cerumen

Excessive wax buildup in the external auditory canal can lead to loss of hearing, tinnitus, and feelings of pressure or pain within the ear. On observation, the accumulation of wax will be visible in the ear canal. While the temptation may be to remove the wax with a cotton swab, this is contraindicated, as it could cause further impaction and discomfort. The athlete should be referred to a physician and the ear flushed with warm water for gentle removal.

### Otitis Externa (Swimmer's Ear)

Bacterial infections from water accumulation in the swimmer's ear are a common cause of inflammation in the external ear canal. Inappropriate or aggressive use of a cotton swab can also irritate the external canal. Signs and symptoms of otitis externa include pain, itching or burning, and possible drainage from the ear. The external ear may be tender to palpation, and pulling on the earlobe will increase pain. The athlete should be referred to a physician for the appropriate medication.

### Otitis Media

Otitis media is characterized by inflammation or infection of the tympanic cavity or middle ear. Within this cavity are the auditory ossicles (malleus, incus, and stapes) as well as tympanic muscles and nerves. Infections of the middle ear and tympanic membrane (eardrum) can be extremely painful. Signs and symptoms include severe earache, swollen and red eardrum, fever, dizziness (**vertigo**), tinnitus, and possible hearing loss. Middle ear infections are often associated with viral upper respiratory infections. The pain alone typically drives the athlete to a physician for evaluation and treatment. Persons with suspected otitis media should always consult a physician before flying.

## DENTAL AND GUM DISEASE

Frequently athletes neglect dental hygiene and may suffer from tooth and gum conditions or disease. When signs and symptoms of tooth or gum disease appear, the athlete should be referred to a dentist for evaluation and dental care.

### Gingivitis

**Gingivitis** is an inflammation of the gum that results from the presence of bacteria in and around the gums caused by food deposits and inadequate brushing or flossing. Brushing the teeth too aggressively or in a lateral versus up-and-down motion can also cause gum irritation. The gums will appear red and swollen, and the athlete will complain of pain and bleeding when brushing the teeth. If hygiene does not improve, gingivitis can progress to periodontitis (**pyorrhea**).

### Periodontitis

**Periodontitis**, a more serious condition caused by bacteria, results in loss of alveolar bone and recession of the gum line. Signs and symptoms include pain and bleeding with brushing, tooth sensitivity to cold and hot drinks or foods, red and swollen gums, breath odor, and possible loosening of the teeth.

### Dental Caries

Tooth pain may result from **dental caries** (cavities) or abscess. Dental caries are caused by decay and degeneration of the tooth enamel, allowing exposure, irritation, and infection of the tooth's pulp. The athlete may complain of a toothache and sensitivity with chewing or with drinking hot and cold fluids. If the infection passes through the root of the tooth into the periodontal tissues, an **abscess** may form in the adjacent gum. Signs and symptoms include a severe, unrelenting toothache that may radiate into the sinus, jaw, or ear depending on the location of the infected tooth. Pain will worsen when the person drinks hot or cold fluids. The gum will likely be swollen and red, and the tooth may be tender and loose when mobilized. A fever may also be present.

# RESPIRATORY SYSTEM

Irritation and infection (viral and bacterial) can occur throughout the respiratory system and passageways. Upper respiratory conditions are common and may affect the nose, throat, tonsils, and sinuses. A less frequent but more serious condition is infection of the lower respiratory system (bronchi and lungs). Other respiratory conditions not associated with infection include allergic rhinitis, asthma, hay fever, and hyperventilation. It is important that you be able to recognize and differentiate those conditions that can result in serious respiratory compromise, as they can be life threatening if the athlete does not receive timely and appropriate treatment.

## UPPER RESPIRATORY CONDITIONS

An upper respiratory infection (URI) is any infection that affects any portion of the upper respiratory system (conducting pathway) including the tonsils, nose, throat, sinuses, and neck lymph nodes. As previously noted, middle ear infections can also be associated with URIs. Upper respiratory infections can be viral or bacterial in origin. The common cold, flu, sinusitis, laryngitis, pharyngitis, and tonsillitis are examples of these conditions. Specific signs and symptoms and treatment procedures will vary according to the specific area involved and the cause of the infection. If a URI affects one area, the athletic trainer must be aware that other aspects of the upper respiratory system can become involved and must watch closely for changes in signs and symptoms. Referral to a physician is indicated if any URI does not appear to take a normal course or follow a normal duration. Additionally, referral to a physician may also be indicated for medication administration to relieve annoying symptoms.

Often the athlete will continue to work or engage in physical activity despite symptoms. Although the signs and symptoms associated with these conditions are relatively minor and may have a limited effect on performance, adequate rest is essential for quick resolution. Moreover, whenever a high fever accompanies these conditions, the athlete should be removed from participation until fever is reduced. Any athlete with a fever over 100° F should not be allowed to participate until the fever has gone down or a physician has given clearance. Athletes with high fevers who engage in activities that further increase core temperature may be at risk for febrile seizures.

Athletes with high fevers (>100° F) who engage in activities that further increase core temperature are at risk for febrile seizures.

### Systemic Infections

General URI conditions are multisymptomatic, as they typically affect both the nose and throat and may also involve the eyes and ears.

## Common Cold

Common colds are viral infections that affect the upper respiratory system and are sometimes referred to as rhinoviruses. The incubation time is short, 18 to 48 h, with the onset typically heralded by a scratchy throat, sneezing, nasal discharge, and general malaise. Fever can sometimes accompany a cold, especially in children. Congestion headache, reduced smell and taste sensations, nasal congestion, cough, and general achiness are frequent complaints. Symptoms usually run their course in 4-10 days, but additional factors such as sinusitis, bronchitis, or tonsillitis can extend their duration.

Treatment is symptomatic relief with the use of antipyretics, antihistamines, decongestants, and analgesics. Since a cold is caused by a virus, antibiotics are not recommended as treatment unless it is apparent that a bacterial infection accompanies the cold. Increased fluid intake and rest are an important part of the treatment.

*Antipyretics are fever-reducing agents.*

*Analgesics are pain-reducing agents.*

## Influenza

Influenza, or flu, is a highly contagious viral infection that affects the body in general and the upper respiratory system. Symptoms include fever, chills, general weakness, fatigue, body aches and pains, and inflammation of the upper respiratory system with moderate signs and symptoms of sore throat and cough. Mild cases last about two to three days, whereas more severe cases last for four to five days with residual symptoms of weakness and fatigue persisting for up to a few weeks. Treatment is for relief of symptoms, since there is no medication at present for viral infections. Bed rest is recommended until after the temperature has returned to normal; increase in fluid intake is strongly recommended, and medications for relief of pain and temperature can help make the individual more comfortable. Additional complications such as sinusitis, ear infection, and staphylococcus-based infections can occur; these require antibacterial therapy. Careful monitoring of symptoms and physician referral are therefore recommended.

### Nose and Throat

Signs and symptoms of URIs may also appear more localized, involving primarily the nose or throat.

## Rhinitis

Acute inflammation or infection of the nasal passageways, usually virus or allergy based, results in annoying nasal mucosa discharge. Obstructed breathing (congestion) can occur with excessive mucosal discharge and swelling of the nasal passages. A runny nose and sneezing are often the first signs of a URI. Medications are used primarily to control the mucosal discharge and decrease congestions.

## Sinusitis

Inflammation of the nasal and facial sinuses can result from either viral or bacterial exposure but is also commonly associated with predisposing conditions such as chronic rhinitis, obstructive drainage, allergy exposure, general debilitation, dental abscess, or exposure to extreme temperature and humidity. Those with a previous history of sinus infections seem to be more susceptible to repeat episodes with future URIs. Periorbital pain and edema, frontal headaches, nasal congestion, tenderness to pressure over the sinuses, fever, and general malaise are frequent complaints. Physician referral for symptomatic relief with the use of antipyretics, decongestants, or analgesics is advisable. Sinus irrigation may be necessary in lingering cases. Antibiotics are used for those cases that are bacterial based or that develop secondary bacterial infections. It is important, particularly with sinus infections, that an athlete who is on antibiotics follow the physician's directions and take the medication until it is completely gone. Because of the closed sinus spaces, sinus infections are slow to clear, and if not completely resolved, the infection will return.

*Dysphagia is pain with swallowing.*

## Pharyngitis

Inflammation of the pharynx can result from either a viral or a bacterial infection and is often an extension of sinusitis, tonsillitis, or adenoid infection. A burning or dry throat is commonly accompanied by chills, fever, hoarseness, and dysphagia. Treatment includes rest, fluid intake, and medication for symptomatic relief. Antibiotics are used for bacterial-based infections.

## Laryngitis

Acute inflammation of the larynx is usually a secondary result of a common cold, sinusitis, pharyngitis, or tonsillitis. A tickling sensation or rawness in the throat with a frequent need to clear the throat is often accompanied by a change in the voice, hoarseness, or loss of voice. If edema of the larynx is present, the person may have difficulty breathing (dyspnea).

Treatment includes bed rest, ingestion of fluids, and resting the voice; antibiotic medication may be indicated if the condition is bacterial in origin. Steam inhalation and cough or anesthetic lozenges can also encourage symptomatic relief.

*Adenoiditis is an inflammation of the glandular lymph tissue at the back of the pharynx.*

## Tonsillitis

Although acute inflammation of the tonsils is often the result of a bacterial infection, chronic tonsillitis is frequently related to predisposing factors such as a common cold or adenoiditis. Acute tonsillitis presents with signs and symptoms of chills, fever, malaise, headaches, body aches, and severe pain in the throat with difficulty swallowing. Symptoms of chronic tonsillitis, on the other hand, include a sore throat, mild fever, and nasal discharge. In either case, the tonsils will be red and edematous, and a whitish pus may be observable at the back of the throat. Acute tonsillitis is treated with antibiotics and symptomatic relief. Chronic tonsillitis may be best treated with a tonsillectomy.

# BRONCHIAL AND LUNG INFECTIONS

Infections of the bronchials and lungs are more serious than URIs. Although bronchitis can be caused by both infectious and irritating agents, pneumonia represents a very serious lung infection that requires immediate medical referral and treatment.

## *Bronchitis*

Inflammation of the bronchial tree, which can be either acute or chronic, can result from either an infection or a reaction to an irritating agent. Acute bronchitis is associated with a URI such as a common cold or other viral infection of the nasopharynx, throat, or upper bronchial tree. It may also be associated with a secondary bacterial infection. While acute bronchitis can affect children or adults, chronic bronchitis occurs commonly in adults and is the result of chronic diffuse obstructive pulmonary diseases such as emphysema or pulmonary fibrosis. Cigarette smokers frequently have chronic bronchitis.

Symptoms of acute bronchitis are those of most URIs, including nasal mucous discharge, malaise, slight fever, general achiness, and sore throat. A cough is usually dry and nonproductive in the first few days but becomes productive with a mucoid secretion in later stages. A hissing or crackling (rales) may be heard with auscultation (see chapter 12). A lingering cough may continue for weeks after other symptoms have subsided.

*An **expectorant** is a drug used to increase flow and decrease the viscosity of mucus in the respiratory passageway.*

Physician referral is advisable to ensure proper treatment of possible complications and the administration of appropriate medications. If systemic symptoms are present, the athlete should be placed on bed rest until the fever is gone. Fluid ingestion is encouraged. Symptomatic relief can be offered with administration of a variety of drugs including antipyretic, analgesic, expectorant, and bronchodilator medications.

### Pneumonia

Pneumonia is an infection of the alveolar spaces that is usually bacterial based but can be viral. Bacterial infections are grouped as pneumococcal and include Group A hemolytic streptococcus and Types 1 and 2 staphylococci. Pneumonia is frequently preceded by a URI in an athlete. Other factors that influence pneumonia onset in adults include alcoholism, malnutrition, debilitation (being bedridden), aspiration, coma, or bronchial tumor.

*Tachypnea refers to the presence of rapid respirations.*

*Tachycardia means rapid pulse.*

Pneumococcal pneumonia is the most common form of pneumonia. Pneumococci enter the lungs via the respiratory passages and lodge in the alveoli, where an inflammatory process is initiated. The edema formation serves as a rich culture medium within which the pneumococci proliferate; they spread to other alveoli and lobes. Signs and symptoms include fever, chest pain, tachycardia, difficulty breathing (dyspnea), respiratory distress (tachypnea), and a nonproductive hacking cough advancing to a cough with sputum (mucus) that is pinkish in the early stages and later changes to a rusty color. The rusty color is a hallmark sign of pneumococcal pneumonia, as is an expiratory grunt. Rales can be heard with a stethoscope in the affected lobe. As the infection progresses, the alveoli become fluid filled, severely limiting gas exchange. Therefore, it is imperative that the person receive treatment as soon as any of these symptoms appear.

Treatment includes bed rest, fluids, oxygen administration, and medications including antibiotics, analgesics, and antipyretics. Many cases require hospitalization.

## OTHER RESPIRATORY CONDITIONS

Not all respiratory conditions are infectious in origin. Both chronic and acute respiratory conditions can be caused or exacerbated by allergens in the environment or can be induced by exercise or stress. These include hay fever, asthma, and hyperventilation.

### Hay Fever

Hay fever is an allergic rhinitis that occurs seasonally because of the individual's reaction to airborne pollens. Depending on the allergy, the person may be most susceptible in the spring, summer, or fall. A profuse watery nasal discharge is accompanied by itching of the eyes, nose, and mouth. Sneezing is common, along with conjunctivitis, frontal headaches with increased sinus pressure, and irritated nasal mucous membranes.

*Sympathomimetic refers to a group of medications that mimic the actions of the sympathetic nervous system to cause vasoconstriction and open respiratory passageways.*

Treatment is to remove the allergen if the reaction is allergy based. Medications may be prescribed to minimize irritating symptoms; these may include antihistamines in nose drop, inhalant, or oral form; decongestants; and sympathomimetic oral medications. Sometimes, if allergies are severe, it is necessary to provide surgical or chemical treatments to alter discharge ability or nasal sensitivity.

### Asthma

Asthma, a respiratory condition characterized by paroxysms of dyspnea, coughing, and wheezing, has been seen in increasing frequency over the past few years. Millions of Americans experience asthma; many deaths occur each year due to complications when the condition is left untreated. Asthma is usually triggered by an environmental irritant, allergen, medication, or exercise that causes a reactive narrowing of the trachea, bronchi, and bronchioles. The result is a widespread, reversible narrowing of the airways (bronchospasm). An improper exchange of oxygen and metabolic wastes (mucus) results as the airway is narrowed, and breathing becomes more labor intensive with an increase in airflow resistance. Resulting signs and symptoms of an acute, severe asthma attack include spasmodic coughing, chest pain and tightness, wheezing, high pulse and respiratory rate, retraction of the neck muscles on inhalation, restlessness and agitation, and possible fainting. The athlete will usually be positioned upright and be leaning forward with his hands on his knees, laboring to breathe. If the attack is severe and little or no air is being moved, wheezing may be absent.

Although **exercise-induced asthma** is being seen in increasing frequency, its cause is essentially unknown. Exercise-induced asthma can occur in young adult athletes who have no other history of asthma. The signs and symptoms, often more subtle, may consist of only a repetitive cough and/or slight wheezing either during intense exercise or after activity.

*Anticholinergic refers to medication used to block the action of the neurotransmitter, acetylcholine, to relax smooth muscle.*

When providing immediate care for an athlete with asthma, it is important that you maintain a calm, reassuring attitude in an effort to relax the person, who undoubtedly will be anxious and panicky. If asthma is part of an allergic response, the allergen should be avoided whenever possible. A variety of medications are effective in treating asthma, whether exercise induced or pathogenically related. Usually, the athletes you encounter will have a previous history of asthma and will be well versed in the use of their medications. Bronchial dilators and bronchial smooth muscle relaxers (anticholinergics) are the primary medications used. Anti-inflammatories and corticosteroids are also commonly prescribed. Although medication can be dispensed in inhaled, oral, or intravenous form, the inhaler is the most common mode of delivery, with the inhalant self-administered. People who do not respond to their inhaler medication should be taken to a physician without delay. Table 13.1 lists the common drug therapies used for bronchial asthma. It is important that you become familiar with these medications, actions, and side effects, as you will encounter this condition often and may need to help athletes obtain their medication when an attack occurs.

## HYPERVENTILATION

*Respiratory alkalosis is a deficiency of carbonic acid in the blood caused by excessive elimination of $CO_2$. It is also referred to as "metabolic alkalosis."*

Hyperventilation is characterized by a breathing rate and/or depth in excess of that required to eliminate carbon dioxide ($CO_2$). Usually transient, it typically results from factors such as metabolic disturbances, panic, or fear and may occur in unconditioned athletes during exercise. An athlete who is hyperventilating will breathe off too much carbon dioxide, which will result in respiratory alkalosis. This causes symptoms of numbness or tingling around the mouth and in the hands and feet, as well as

| Table 13.1 | Common Drug Therapies for Bronchial Asthma | |
| --- | --- | --- |
| **Drug type** | **Examples** | **Action** |
| Anticholinergic | Ipratropium bromide (e.g., Atrovent) | Bronchodilation by relaxing smooth muscle |
| Beta agonist | Albuterol (e.g., Proventil, Ventolin), isoetharine metaproteronol (e.g., Alupent, Metaprel), terbutaline (e.g., Brethine) | Dilates bronchial tubes |
| Corticosteroid | Beclomethasone (e.g., Anti-Beclomethasone), Prednisone | Fights inflammation and prevents narrowing of airways |
| Mast cell inhibitor | Sodium cromoglycate | Inhibits release of chemical mediators of inflammation |
| Methylxanthine | Theophylline, triamcinolone (e.g., Azmacort) | Dilates bronchial tubes; increases diaphragmatic contractility; stimulates respiratory center |

light-headedness. A sharp, stabbing chest pain is also a frequent complaint, causing people to panic further because they think they may be having a heart attack. Breathing into a paper bag to take carbon dioxide back in has been effectively used to rapidly reverse the condition. However, this technique is no longer recommended, as overcompensation (hypoxia) may ensue if the individual continues to breathe excess $CO_2$ for too long (Caroline 1995). Therefore, the best course of action is to simply calm and reassure the athlete in an effort to restore normal respiration rate and depth. When assessing an athlete who appears to be hyperventilating, you should monitor the rate and depth of respirations and rule out other pathological conditions that may also produce rapid respirations (see chapter 12).

# CARDIOVASCULAR SYSTEM

Cardiovascular conditions are often serious; they may involve either the heart itself or the peripheral vascular system. Blood pressure and volume are closely monitored and maintained throughout the body via a balance of sympathetic and parasympathetic nervous system control. However, illness, injury, and chronic disease states may alter or compromise cardiovascular function. You will need to understand and recognize the following cardiovascular conditions so that you can provide appropriate medical referral and care.

## HYPERTENSION

*Neurogenic means originating in or controlled by the nervous system.*

**High blood pressure** is the common term for **hypertension**, which involves an elevated systolic and/or diastolic blood pressure and is associated with generalized arteriolar vasoconstriction. High blood pressure is considered to be present when pressure is consistently over 140/90 mmHg at rest. Heredity can play a predisposing role in its onset. Other determining factors include renal, adrenal, and neurogenic pathologies. Hypertension generally affects adults in the early 30s. In the early stages, there is no change in cardiac output, pulse rate, or blood volume because of a concomitant increase in arterial blood pressure. In fact, the only symptom for many years may be an elevated blood pressure. Lesser symptoms can occur, including periodic fatigue, dizziness, headaches, weakness, and insomnia. Over time, cardiac hypertrophy and changes in electrocardiogram readings are common. Hypertension is a major contributor to renal dysfunction, angina pectoris (chest pain), myocardial infarction (heart attack), cardiovascular accidents, congestive heart failure, stroke, and retinal changes.

Prevention includes a variety of lifestyle changes such as a diet low in fat and high in complex carbohydrates, regular exercise, weight control, and control of stress influences. The individual needs to avoid excessive use of hypertension-producing substances such as coffee, tea, tobacco, salt, and alcohol. Goals of treatment with prescribed medication include reduction of blood pressure to within normal limits.

Many factors such as exercise, anxiety and tension, illness, or pain can temporarily increase blood pressure. Therefore, a single reading is not usually sufficient to determine the condition, particularly when taken under conditions that are less than resting and relaxed. It is often helpful to take an athlete's blood pressure over consecutive days and to have the person quiet and relaxed for at least the previous 5 min. You should document these recordings and provide the documentation to the physician when you refer the athlete; this is valuable information that will aid in the diagnosis. Athletes with mild hypertension should be examined by a physician prior to athletic participation.

## HYPERTROPHIC CARDIOMYOPATHY

Hypertrophic cardiomyopathy is a serious disease of the myocardium (heart muscle), resulting in enlargement of the muscle cells of the ventricular septum and left ventricular walls. It is also referred to as **asymmetrical hypertrophy**, idiopathic hypertrophic subaortic stenosis, and muscular subaortic stenosis. Although the specific etiology is unknown, many believe that it occurs because a mutation of the genetic code for components of the heart muscle's cross-bridges causes changes in the important chemomechanical transduction of impulses through the heart. The enlarged left ventricular wall has more stiffness than normal, causing a backflow of blood to the atrium and lungs and reduced blood flow to the body. Although many patients have no symptoms, others experience symptoms such as shortness of breath, chest pain, and dizziness. Shortness of breath (dyspnea) occurs because of the backflow of circulation from the left ventricle to the pulmonary circulation. Angina (chest pain) occurs because of the inadequate flow of oxygenated blood to the heart muscle. Dizziness and fainting symptoms (**syncope**) occur because of reduced blood flow to the brain.

The disease, often undetected, has a wide range of effects. Some individuals have no symptoms and lead a normal life, never realizing they have hypertrophic cardiomyopathy. Others develop progressive symptoms that limit their activity level. In extreme cases, the condition can result in sudden death during physical activity in otherwise healthy athletes who do not suspect that they have it. While this condition points to the importance of a cardiovascular screen in the preparticipation physical exam, it may not always be identified. Therefore, any time you observe or are aware of signs and symptoms associated with cardiovascular compromise or distress, immediately refer the individual to a physician before allowing further participation.

If you are working with a physically active person who is not a competitive athlete and has hypertrophic cardiomyopathy, first consult with the person's physician to find out what level of activity he or she may safely maintain. Treatment includes proper diet and good personal health habits. The person with this condition should avoid isometrics as well as all forms of strenuous exercise. Moderate exercise such as walking or biking is advised. The person should avoid dehydration and also avoid hot tubs and saunas that increase heart rate and blood pressure and encourage dehydration. Beta blockers and calcium channel blockers are common drugs of choice to relax the heart muscle and maintain good heart rhythm in those diagnosed with hypertrophic cardiomyopathy.

## HYPOTENSION

Hypotension is a subnormal (low) blood pressure. The most common type is **orthostatic hypotension**, in which the blood pressure drops when the individual suddenly moves to a standing position. Orthostatic hypotension is defined as a decrease of at least 20 mm Hg in systolic blood pressure upon movement from a supine to a standing position. It can be caused by cardiac pump failure, diminished blood volume available within the vascular system, venous pooling, medication, and neurogenic pathologies. The condition is transient, but produces a brief period of light-headedness, dizziness, weakness, or nausea. Persistent episodes, or episodes that result in syncope, should be evaluated by the physician for underlying causes prior to continued participation.

Treatment includes steps to relieve causative factors such as changing position slowly, avoiding alcohol, avoiding hot showers or baths, increasing salt intake to

*Sympathomimetics are drugs that stimulate the sympathetic nervous system to cause vasoconstriction of the blood vessels and increase blood pressure.*

*Hematocrit is the ratio of red blood cells to total blood volume.*

*Vasomotor refers to smooth muscle control of blood vessel size.*

*A nociceptor is a pain receptor.*

increase intravascular blood volume, and taking medications. Medications usually include over-the-counter sympathomimetics or prescription-dose sympathetic agonists to increase blood pressure; fludrocortisone to promote renal sodium reabsorption and arteriole sensitivity to norepinephrine; or erythropoietin to restore normal hematocrit.

# MIGRAINE HEADACHE

Migraines are recurring vascular headaches of a sudden onset with associated gastrointestinal and visual disturbances. The exact cause is unknown, but it is believed that migraines may be related to allergies, stress, hormonal imbalance, toxins, or vasomotor disturbances. There is often a family history. It is believed that the migraine process starts with head pain that results from **extracranial** vasoconstriction in the scalp and dura. Vasoconstriction in **intracranial** circulation also takes place, resulting in reduced oxygen to the brain to cause neurogenic symptoms such as vision changes and speech difficulty. A reactive vasodilatation to meet the brain's oxygen needs affects the neck and scalp arteries, triggering a release of prostaglandins and other chemicals that produce inflammation, swelling, and increased pain sensitivity. Stimulation of nociceptors resulting from scalp artery dilation causes the throbbing pain.

Migraines are divided into two types, classic and common. Classic migraine attacks are preceded 10 to 30 min earlier by an aura that produces neurological symptoms. The person may experience visual disturbances such as seeing flashing lights, sometimes with a temporary loss of vision. Photophobia is common. Common symptoms of classic migraines are speech difficulty; tingling of the face or hands; weakness on one side of the body; and an intense throbbing pain that starts on one side of the head around the temple, forehead, eye, ear, and jaw and advances to the other side. Classic migraines last for one to two days whereas common migraine symptoms last for three to four days.

Common migraines, which are more prevalent, do not have an aura preceding onset. The standard symptom, photophobia, is often accompanied by other symptoms including throbbing around the eye, nausea, vomiting, mood changes, and severe headache.

Physician referral for analgesic medications administered orally, rectally, or intravenously may be necessary. If analgesic medication can be administered early enough, full migraine symptoms can sometimes be avoided. Fluid ingestion, rest in a darkened room, and relief of stress can help to minimize symptoms.

## SHOCK

Shock is a state of circulatory collapse in which the cardiovascular system does not provide enough circulating blood to the body. Shock occurs for one of three reasons:

1. The heart is damaged and ineffective in pumping blood (cardiogenic shock).
2. Blood volume is lost so that there is an insufficient quantity to flow through the system (hypovolemic shock, anaphylactic shock, and septic shock).
3. The blood vessels dilate so that there is ineffective perfusion of fluid through the system (neurogenic shock).

Shock can occur with any injury; the athletic trainer must be aware of the possibility of shock, know the symptoms of shock, and take efficient and effective steps in the proper treatment of shock when it occurs.

**Cardiogenic shock** occurs when the heart fails or works very ineffectively; common causes include myocardial infarction, viral myocarditis, valvular heart disease,

*Viral myocarditis is inflammation of the heart muscle caused by a viral infection.*

and other myocardial inflammatory diseases. **Hypovolemic shock** occurs as the result of a decreased volume of blood available in the circulatory system. This is secondary to loss of blood because of bleeding, internal organ injuries, or fractures. **Metabolic shock** occurs when the blood volume is reduced secondary to loss of body fluid as a consequence of illness that causes diarrhea, excessive urination, or vomiting. When there is damage to the spinal cord and the nerves that innervate smooth muscle, **neurogenic shock** results as the blood vessels lose their tone and dilate; although there is no fluid loss, the amount of fluid available for circulation throughout the system is not sufficient for the system to continue functioning (i.e., the size of the container is significantly increased in relation to the volume of fluid it contains, and the fluid is no longer sufficient to maintain blood pressure and adequate circulation).

**Psychogenic shock** is a transient condition that occurs when a person faints; a sudden involuntary nervous system reaction causes vasodilation and pooling of blood in the peripheral blood vessels. Reduced blood flow to the brain leads to fainting. Since the condition is transient, circulation is soon restored to normal. **Anaphylactic shock** is a hypersensitivity reaction to an allergen. As part of the allergic reaction, the blood vessels dilate to cause a decreased volume of circulating blood. There can also be some leaking of fluid out of vessel walls (increased permeability) that will add to the reduced blood volume available for circulation. **Septic shock** results in severe dilation of the blood vessels and reduces circulating blood volume in response to bacterial infections. The bacterial infection also damages blood vessels, causing loss of blood volume through vessel walls.

Signs and symptoms of shock are progressive and can eventually lead to loss of consciousness and even death if left untreated. Early signs include cold, wet skin; profuse sweating; paleness that can change to cyanosis in later stages; shallow, rapid, labored, or irregular breathing; weak, rapid pulse; nausea or vomiting; anxiety or restlessness; dull, lusterless eyes; dilated pupils; and gradually falling blood pressure. Once blood pressure signs are evident, the individual is well into shock development.

The shock victim should be taken immediately to an emergency care facility. Prior to and during transport, an adequate airway should be maintained, and bleeding should be controlled with compression and elevation. Proper splinting of fractures to minimize bleeding, maintaining body temperature, keeping the athlete comfortable, allowing nothing to eat or drink, and continual monitoring of vital signs are also important. Shock is an emergency situation and must be attended to with efficiency, calm, and appropriate care.

For additional information on the care and treatment of shock, refer to *Introduction to Athletic Training* (Hillman 2000), chapter 8.

## Summary of Signs and Symptoms Associated With Shock

1. Restlessness
2. Anxiety
3. Thirst
4. Nausea and vomiting
5. Cold, clammy, and pale skin (wet, white)
6. Weak, rapid pulse
7. Shallow and rapid respirations
8. Decreased level of consciousness (confusion, dizziness)
9. Decreased blood pressure
10. Dilated pupils

*Vasovagal refers to a reflex dilation of blood vessels and a pooling of blood in the extremities.*

## SYNCOPE

Syncope (or fainting) is a sudden, temporary loss of consciousness most commonly resulting from either a physiological or an emotional stress that causes a vasovagal reaction. This most often occurs in standing or with sudden changes in position (i.e., sudden sit to stand). It can also happen as a result of reduction in blood volume produced by heavy sweating, violent coughing spells that rapidly change blood pressure, heart or lung disorders, side effects of medications, seizures, or any condition that results in inadequate glucose or oxygen supply to the brain.

Syncope is a transient incident that results from a sudden increase in vasodilation of peripheral blood vessels without a concomitant increase in cardiac output. These events cause a reduced blood flow to the brain and consequently fainting. Preceding symptoms include a sudden change in position, weakness, cold sweat, nausea, abdominal discomfort, dimming vision, and a roaring sound in the ears (Caroline 1995). Once the person is supine (horizontal), the blood flow to the brain is restored, and consciousness quickly returns. Although there are few residual effects, one must take care to evaluate for any possible injury consequent to any fall during fainting. It is important to recognize that a syncopal episode can be caused by a variety of factors, some cardiac in origin. Fainting should never be dismissed or considered a normal response, and the athlete should be referred to a physician to determine the underlying cause for the episode.

> Syncope can result from a variety of factors, some cardiac in origin. Fainting should never be dismissed or considered a normal response, and the athlete should be referred to a physician to determine the underlying cause for the episode.

# ENDOCRINE SYSTEM

Sometimes an athlete under your care has an endocrine disorder that necessitates daily medication and continual monitoring. Pancreatic (diabetes) and thyroid dysfunction are the most common conditions that you will encounter. Although they do not prevent an athlete from participating, complications may arise during or apart from exercise as a result of these conditions. It is important that you understand these conditions and be able to recognize signs of complications in order to provide emergency assistance to the athlete when needed. It is important to note that endocrine complications can occur in athletes with both good and poor disease management. A complication, in and of itself, is not an indication of poor disease management; it may convey that there is a problem temporarily, something that is totally unplanned, like a developing cold virus, infection, or may be an indication that the treatment or medication regimen needs to be adjusted. Knowing the history of the athletes under your care and the medications that they take will help you provide optimal care.

## DIABETES MELLITUS

Diabetes mellitus is an autoimmune disorder that causes a deficiency in glucose metabolism. Insulin, a peptide hormone responsible for glucose utilization, is either not secreted by the islets of Langerhans in the pancreas, or is prevented from being utilized in the body. Diabetes mellitus occurs as one of two types, insulin-dependent diabetes mellitus (IDDM) or type I diabetes, and non-insulin-dependent diabetes mellitus (NIDDM) or type II diabetes. Insulin-dependent diabetes mellitus usually occurs in children and in non-obese adults, whereas NIDDM most often occurs in obese adults. Insulin-dependent diabetes is the result of insufficient insulin production in the pancreas. Individuals with NIDDM have an insulin-producing pancreas, but the body's sensitivity to the insulin hormone is significantly diminished. In both types of diabetes, glucose, rather than being metabolized by target tissue, remains in the bloodstream where it is partially filtered through the kidneys. Prolonged blood glucose elevation eventually damages organs and tissues and can lead to blindness, kidney failure, recurring infections, and cardiovascular insufficiency that can in turn cause cardiac complications, neuropathy, and extremity amputation.

### *Signs, Symptoms, and Control*

Several early signs and symptoms of diabetes are most prevalent in IDDM; signs and symptoms in NIDDM are slower to progress and can remain subtle and unnoticed for extended periods of time, even months. Frequent urination, a hallmark sign, occurs because glucose excretion draws with it large amounts of water. Rather than using glucose, the body utilizes other sources of energy, primarily fats. When fats are metabolized, acetones and ketones are generated as waste products that cause a change in the blood's pH (ketoacidosis). In an attempt to restore normal pH, the body increases its elimination of carbon dioxide through deep expirations. Acetones are expired, producing a characteristic odor on the breath usually described as sweet or fruity or sometimes like fingernail polish remover. Rapid weight loss occurs as the body excretes glucose and uses fat stores for metabolism. Excessive thirst and dry skin are present because of the dehydration from frequent urination. Fatigue and weakness occur; and in the absence of treatment, shock and a diabetic coma ensue.

*A **bolus** is the rapid administration of an injectable medication.*

Early diagnosis and control with diet, exercise, and medication are key to proper diabetes management. Normal blood glucose levels range between 70 and 120 mg/dl. The person with diabetes should attempt to maintain as nearly normal levels as possible to minimize side effects of diabetes. Medication for IDDM requires from one to several daily subcutaneous insulin injections. Insulin pumps are also available that allow insulin to be administered continuously as well as provide multiple boluses of insulin as needed through a soft catheter implanted beneath the skin in the subcutaneous layer. Individuals with NIDDM typically control blood glucose levels through diet, oral medication, or both. Diet and exercise are important components of good diabetes control for both type I and type II groups.

### *Glycemic Reactions*

If a person with diabetes has too much insulin in the body, the blood glucose levels will drop below normal and a **hypoglycemic** reaction will occur. If there is too little insulin, glucose levels are elevated above normal levels, and the body becomes **hyperglycemic**. The athletic trainer must be aware of the differences in the signs and symptoms between these two conditions, since the treatments are opposite (see table 13.2).

#### Hypoglycemia (Insulin Shock)

**Hypoglycemia**, or **insulin shock**, can be life threatening. The symptoms, which are nonspecific, include sweating, trembling, fatigue and weakness, light-headedness, irritability, headache, intoxication-like behavior, apprehension, mental confusion, and—in advanced stages—convulsions and coma. Memory loss, lack of coordination, and slurred speech may also be noted. Since activity lowers blood glucose levels, athletes with diabetes should be monitored closely during times of unexpected increased activity and during early-season workouts when diet, insulin, and activity balances may not yet be established.

If the athlete in insulin shock is unable to swallow, do not attempt to force liquids or foods; instead, immediate transportation to an emergency care facility for intravenous glucose administration is necessary to avoid possible brain damage or death.

If you have an athlete with diabetes on one of your teams, maintain a supply of glucose tablets (available from drug stores) or other sugar substance in the athletic training kit, or have quick and easy access to fruit juice, sweetened soft drinks, or food during practice and games and while on the road.

Many athletes who have had diabetes for some time understand the disease and take precautionary measures to minimize the risk of hypoglycemic reactions. There are times, however, when unanticipated schedule changes or altered activity levels may precipitate a hypoglycemic reaction. The athletic trainer should keep a supply of glucose tablets or glucose packets, designed for hypoglycemic episodes, in the athletic training kit, or have quick and easy access to sweetened drinks or foods. If candy is the only sweet substance available, hard candy with a high sugar content should be ingested, not chocolate-based, which has a high fat content. Administration of candy, fruit juice, sugar-sweetened soft drinks, sugar, or other glucose-containing substances should be immediate upon observation of changes in the athlete's behavior. If the athlete is unable to swallow, do not attempt to force liquids or foods; instead, call EMS for immediate medical care

## Table 13.2　Comparisons of Hypoglycemia and Hyperglycemia Signs and Symptoms

| | Hypoglycemia | Hyperglycemia |
| --- | --- | --- |
| Onset | Rapid onset, occurring within minutes | Slow onset, occurring over a span of hours and even days |
| Neurological changes | Irritability, mental confusion, dizziness, bizarre behavior, slurred speech, memory loss, headache, dilated pupils; in severe cases, seizures and coma | Lethargy |
| Skin | Cold, clammy; profuse sweating | Warm and dry |
| Muscular changes | Weakness, fatigue, muscle tremors, incoordination, ataxic gait | Weakness and fatigue |
| Cardiorespiratory changes | Weak, rapid pulse | Rapid pulse (tachycardia) |
| | No odor on breath | Deep, rapid breathing (Kussmaul respirations) and characteristic odor of acetones on breath |
| Genitourinary/gastro-intestinal changes | None | Nausea and vomiting, excessive urination, excessive thirst, excessive eating |

and transportation to an emergency care facility for intravenous glucose administration to avoid possible brain damage or death.

Hypoglycemic reactions are minimized when the athlete's diabetes is well controlled. A snack about 30 min prior to exercise will help reduce insulin reactions. If activity is prolonged, the athlete should ingest about 10 g of carbohydrates every 30 min. Routine exercise programs allow the athlete to anticipate the necessary balance between exercise, food, and insulin, providing an optimal condition for good control of blood glucose levels.

### Hyperglycemia (Diabetic Coma)

In its advanced stages, hyperglycemia is referred to as **hyperglycemic shock**, or **diabetic coma**. This condition develops over a period of days as the individual's blood glucose levels rise. Failure to take insulin, severe illness or infection, or poor dietary control can be precipitating factors that disrupt glucose levels and lead to this condition. The symptoms include those mentioned earlier as onset symptoms. You will smell the characteristic odor of acetones (the "fruity/sweet" smell) on the individual's breath, and the person will be lethargic. When you suspect hyperglycemia, you should refer the athlete to a physician. Most athletes who are in good control do not suffer hyperglycemic shock. However, illness—particularly flu-like symptoms that result in fever, dehydration, and loss of appetite—presents special concerns for athletes with diabetes in terms of glucose regulation. Therefore, when athletes with diabetes become ill, you should routinely refer them to a physician for proper management and care.

### Differential Diagnosis and Immediate Care

It is sometimes difficult to distinguish between the symptoms of hyperglycemia and hypoglycemia. Lethargy, listlessness, and confusion can occur with either condition. If you are unsure which condition the athlete has, you should assume she is hy-

If you are unsure whether the athlete is suffering from hypoglycemia versus hyperglycemia, administer sugar. If the athlete does not start to respond within 2 or 3 min after receiving sugar, candy, or sweetened beverages, you should suspect hyperglycemia.

poglycemic and administer glucose tablets or sugar. If the athlete is hypoglycemic, she needs sugar immediately; but if she is hyperglycemic, additional ingestion of glucose tablets or sugar will not significantly advance the condition. If the condition is a hypoglycemic reaction, the athlete should respond to the treatment within a few minutes, but if it is hyperglycemic, her condition will not change. If she does not start to respond within 2 or 3 min following administration of sugar, candy, or sweetened beverages, you should suspect hyperglycemia. The athlete should be transported to an emergency care facility for immediate treatment.

## HYPERTHYROIDISM

*Hyperkinesis is an abnormal increase in movement or purposeless muscle movement.*

*Goiter is an enlargement of the thyroid gland visible as a swelling in the front of the neck.*

Hyperthyroidism can develop during times of emotional or physical stress. It is an autoimmune condition in which an excessive amount of thyroid hormone is present in the body. This leads to an increase in the body's metabolic activity to cause weight loss regardless of any increased food intake. With an increase in metabolic activity comes a concomitant increase in body temperature; so the individual does not tolerate hot environments, suffers from excessive sweating, and must significantly increase fluid intake. Increased sympathetic activity results in an increased heart rate, tremor, and protrusion of the eyeballs. Impaired muscle function and weight loss contribute to muscle weakness. Increased appetite and hyperkinesis are usually present. Other frequent manifestations of hyperthyroidism are goiters, bursitis, and systolic hypertension. If a goiter is present, the individual may have difficulty breathing or swallowing.

*Ablation is surgical removal.*

Treatment is ablation of the thyroid tissue with surgery or radiation, or control of thyroid levels with medication. Antithyroid drugs bring the hyperthyroidism under control within eight weeks, but continued intake of medication is often necessary for a year or longer. Radiation with iodine is a common treatment but carries a risk that hypothyroidism will develop or repeated treatments may be necessary. Surgical removal of the thyroid has a 90% cure rate, but surgical risks include nerve damage and hypothyroidism.

## HYPOTHYROIDISM

Hypothyroidism may result from an iodine deficiency but can also occur following radiation exposure or from hypothalamic or pituitary damage. Many of the symptoms are the opposite of those seen with hyperthyroidism. Since thyroid hormones regulate the rate at which the body utilizes calories for energy expenditure, hypothyroidism causes a reduction in body metabolism and weight gain even without any change in caloric intake. Additional effects are a loss of appetite, intolerance to cold, decreased sweating, reduced heart rate, constipation, coarse and dry hair, premature graying in young adults, thick and dry skin, swollen eyelids, numbness and tingling in the hands, lethargy, slowness of movement, and sleepiness. In the very young, the condition is known as **cretinism**; growth is stunted, hair growth is sparse, reproductive organs are improperly developed, and mental retardation occurs. If hypothyroidism is left untreated, more profound symptoms can occur including enlargement of the heart, psychiatric disorders, dyspnea, slowed mental processing, inability to maintain normal body temperature, and loss of consciousness. Several years of untreated hypothyroidism leads to **myxedema**, a condition marked by drowsiness, cold body temperature, and possible coma.

Treatment is provided with regular administration of synthetic thyroid hormone medication to deliver normal thyroxin levels throughout the body. Although most symptoms of hypothyroidism disappear after a week of medication, the person must continue daily medication throughout life. Correct dosage administration is critical, since too much thyroxin can promote coronary artery disease and osteoporosis.

*A **duodenal ulcer** is a disruption in the mucosal membrane of the duodenum (first part of the small intestine).*

# PANCREATITIS

Pancreatitis, an inflammation of the pancreas, can be either acute or chronic. The most common cause is a partial obstruction of the pancreatic duct because of a penetrating duodenal ulcer, edema following surgery or abdominal trauma, peritonitis (chapter 12), or a systemic disease. An acute attack often follows a precipitating factor such as alcohol or opiate ingestion, or a large meal. The escaped pancreatic enzymes cause a severe reaction of the surrounding tissues. Symptoms include nausea, vomiting, and severe pain that can be crampy and dull or poorly defined. The pain can radiate to the back, substernum, or flanks. It is usually worse when the individual attempts to lie down. Constipation or diarrhea can be present, as can diminished bowel sounds and abdominal distension. Vascular collapse and death can ultimately occur. Most cases are mild, but severe cases have a high mortality rate. Physician referral is indicated any time there are reduced bowel sounds (see chapter 12). Suspected pancreatitis should be referred to the physician for diagnosis and treatment with antibiotics, analgesics, or surgery.

# GASTROINTESTINAL TRACT

Gastrointestinal complaints are among the most common medical conditions that you will encounter in physically active people. They can be caused by inflammation, viruses, bacteria, and diet. They are particularly troublesome, and often restrict participation secondary to the pain and discomfort created by the accompanying symptoms.

## APPENDICITIS

Inflammation of the appendix can occur in an athlete of any age. You must be aware of signs and symptoms, since immediate referral to a physician is necessary to avoid dangerous and life-threatening situations. Appendicitis can be acute or chronic but is triggered by a bacterial infection lodged within the appendix. A low-grade fever accompanies lower abdominal cramps or sharp pains that become more centralized over the right lower quadrant. Nausea and vomiting are also common. There will be muscle guarding and rigidity of the abdominal wall, pain, and rebound tenderness in the right lower quadrant and around the umbilicus.

Immediate physician referral is necessary for either administration of antibiotic medication or surgical intervention.

## COLITIS

Inflammation of the colon typically occurs during the second through fourth decades of life as a result of certain food hypersensitivities, bacterial or viral infections, psychogenic disorders, or an autoimmune process. The onset can be sudden but most often is slow and insidious, beginning with bowel urgency, abdominal cramps, or bloody mucus in the stools and progressing to looser stools, frequent bowel movements, and severe cramps. Fever, nausea, vomiting, and moderate malaise are common systemic symptoms. Lower abdominal tenderness is present.

*Glucocorticoid is an adrenal cortical hormone that is used primarily to protect against stress and to affect protein and carbohydrate metabolism (Taber 1997).*

Physician referral is recommended, and treatment often includes bed rest; fluid intake; change in diet; intravenous medication and supplements; medications such as anticholinergics (to reduce intestinal motility), antibacterial agents, and glucocorticoids; and stress management techniques.

## CONSTIPATION

Constipation can result from a variety of factors, including poor hydration, stress, poor diet, medications, and neurogenic disorders. Constipation is frequently asymptomatic but can cause cramps and general abdominal discomfort.

Prevention of constipation includes adequate hydration, achieved by drinking several glasses of water daily. It also includes a dietary reduction in simple carbohydrates and an increase in complex carbohydrates and fresh fruits and vegetables, as well as balance in the diet. Use of bulk laxatives can increase bulk within the colon and encourage regular bowel movements. Laxatives, suppositories, and enemas can relieve constipation, but it is generally not wise to take them on an ongoing basis.

## DIARRHEA

Diarrhea is characterized by loose, liquid, or frequent bowel movements. Diarrhea is usually short-term, but if it lasts for more than two weeks it is considered persistent or chronic. It is usually a symptom of other factors including ulcerative colitis, parasitic infections, bacterial infections, diverticulitis, irritable colon syndrome, malabsorption syndrome, gastroenteritis, medication reactions, food additives such as sorbitol or fructose, food allergies, travel with exposure to contaminated water or food, excessive use of laxatives, or stress and anxiety.

The key to managing diarrhea is identification of the cause to remove or reduce it rather than merely treating the symptoms. Proper medication to manage diarrhea can be prescribed once the underlying cause has been determined. Many across-the-counter antidiarrheal drugs such as Lomotil (diphenoxylate with atropine) or Pepto-Bismol are effective in managing acute diarrhea related to irregular or indiscriminate eating as often occurs on team road trips. Additional steps in the care of athletes with diarrhea include preventing dehydration, having the athlete avoid beverages containing caffeine or alcohol (since caffeine will promote diarrhea and alcohol will dehydrate the body), and having the athlete maintain good nutrition. Chronic diarrhea can be prevented with sensible steps such as drinking only clean or purified water, using proper food-handling techniques, and maintaining good hand-washing habits.

Individuals who have prolonged diarrhea (more than two to three days) should be referred to the physician for further evaluation and treatment. Not only can diarrhea be a sign of more serious conditions; when prolonged, it can cause dehydration and electrolyte imbalances that can lead to metabolic shock.

## ESOPHAGEAL REFLUX

Esophageal reflux occurs when the esophageal sphincter between the esophagus and stomach does not close completely. Acid from the stomach can enter the esophagus and cause what is commonly termed **heartburn**. The condition is aggravated when the individual lies recumbent. The person is encouraged to sleep in a semirecumbent position and to seek medical attention for medication to help reduce acid content in the esophagus. The greatest danger with esophageal reflux is the possibility that gastric acid will be aspirated into the trachea and cause pulmonary complications.

## GASTRITIS

*Antiemetics are drugs that control nausea and vomiting.*

Gastritis is an acute or chronic condition in which the mucous membrane of the stomach becomes irritated or inflamed. Acute gastritis can result from ingestion of abrasive substances such as alcohol, salicylates (e.g., aspirin), antibiotics, sulfur products, excessively acidic or spicy food, or allergenic foods. Acute gastritis is usually of short duration, subsiding within 24 to 48 h, and presents with symptoms of nausea, vomiting, headache, vertigo, sensation of fullness, malaise, and possible fever. Treatment includes abstention from solid foods, with ingestion of only clear liquids. Soft foods are gradually introduced and then a bland diet is consumed for at least two weeks. Antiemetics and analgesics are used for symptomatic relief as needed.

*Humoral refers to a bodily fluid or semifluid such as a hormone.*

Chronic gastritis is the consequence of a bacterial infection that stimulates a cellular and humoral response, resulting in irritation of the mucosa and possibly leading to ulcer disease. The bacteria are unique in that they thrive in an acidic environment. Treatment includes antibiotic therapy along with medication that reduces hydrochloric acid secretion to allow the bacteria to become more sensitive to the antibiotic medication.

## GASTROENTERITIS

Gastroenteritis is an inflammation of the stomach and intestine mucous membrane—an acute condition that people commonly refer to as food poisoning. The cause is ingestion of virus or bacteria or excessive intake of irritating substances such as alcohol, salicylates, cathartics, or heavy metals. The severity of the symptoms is directly related to the nature and dose of the irritant ingested. There is a sudden onset of nausea, as well as vomiting, malaise, abdominal cramps, and diarrhea. A fever is usually present if the condition is infection based. Gurgling bowel sounds can be heard with a stethoscope. Dehydration and electrolyte imbalances can occur with vomiting and diarrhea. Treatment includes intravenous therapy for restoration of electrolyte balances and hydration until vomiting has stopped. Medications for symptomatic relief are usually prescribed. Once the individual has started drinking fluids, gradual introduction of soft foods and a bland diet is the usual protocol.

## INDIGESTION

Indigestion is a nonspecific term that refers to either improper digestion or deficient absorption of food in the digestive tract. Also known as digestive upset, or **dyspepsia**, it can result from irregular eating, ingestion of foods to which the individual is unaccustomed or allergic, and anxiety or stress. Symptoms include stomach upset, nausea, or flatulence. Treatment commonly includes one of a large selection of across-the-counter medications for relief of symptoms, for example Pepto-Bismol, Tums, Rolaids, and Gaviscon. Avoidance of irritating foods and control of anxiety and stress are prevention steps advisable for individuals who experience regular episodes of indigestion.

## ULCERS

Ulcers involve a more severe form of gastritis and include an erosion of the mucous membrane of the stomach, duodenum, or lower esophagus. Ulcers can take the form of duodenal or gastric ulcers and are also referred to as peptic ulcer disease. They are thought to be caused primarily by the helicobacter pylori *(H. pylori)* bacterium. Prior to its discovery in 1982, ulcers were thought to be the result of ingestion of spicy foods, hyperacidity, or increased stress. The hallmark symptom is a gnawing or burning pain in the epigastrium. Pain occurs most often when the stomach is empty, can last from minutes to hours, and is relieved by eating or taking antacids. Bleeding can result from erosion of the stomach wall and will present as a coffee-colored emesis (vomitus) if the bleeding is slow, as a more distinct red if the bleeding is more rapid. Additional but less common symptoms can include nausea, heartburn, vomiting, weight loss, and diarrhea. Physician referral for antibiotic medication accompanied by medication to reduce stomach acid is the usual treatment protocol.

## IRRITABLE BOWEL SYNDROME

Irritable bowel syndrome is a noninflammatory, non-serious disorder that affects the large bowel. Failure of the large bowel to function smoothly is reflected in the accompanying symptoms. The cause is unknown, but the syndrome occurs more often in women than in men; symptoms are seen more often during menstruation and times of stress and are aggravated with ingestion of fats, chocolate, milk products, alcohol, and caffeine. A significant number of people with irritable bowel syndrome demonstrate signs of depression, anxiety, or other psychological problems. Symptoms include abdominal cramps with painful constipation or diarrhea. Although most often the condition involves constipation, influences such as bacteria, virus, toxins, or prolonged antibiotic use can cause diarrhea. Typically, bowel movements produce hard stools covered with mucus and may be interspersed with episodes of diarrhea. There may also be bloating and gas. Lower quadrant tenderness will be present with palpation.

Physician referral for differential diagnosis to rule out more serious conditions is advisable. Treatment includes resolving possible stress and anxiety issues. Encouragement and education regarding regular diet and eating habits with adequate fluid and fiber intake should also be part of the treatment protocol. Reduction in the use of laxatives should be encouraged. Antispasmodic drugs, fiber supplements, or stool softeners are commonly prescribed.

# EATING DISORDERS

The eating disorders known as anorexia and bulimia can be serious and life threatening. The athletic trainer must be aware of their signs and symptoms and report any suspected cases to the physician for care and treatment.

## ANOREXIA NERVOSA

Anorexia is a severe psychological disorder characterized by a self-induced food aversion and extreme weight loss. Although the condition can affect males, females are 10 times more often affected and usually experience amenorrhea as a side effect. Anorexia typically begins either in the preteen years or early in the teen years but may not manifest until later in the 30s or 40s; females from professional or managerial families are most often affected. Athletes involved in activities in which body image is important and small size is advantageous, such as gymnasts, dancers, divers, jockeys, wrestlers, and crew coxswains, are particularly vulnerable.

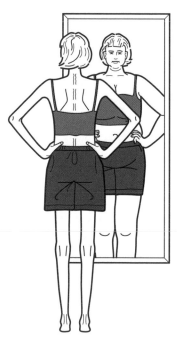

■ **Figure 13.30**   People with anorexia see themselves as overweight when they actually are severely underweight.

Anorexia may appear initially as normal dieting and as concern about weight loss but becomes an obsession to be thin. People with anorexia do not see themselves as thin, even when their appearance is emaciated and they are grossly underweight (figure 13.30). Food and caloric intake and expenditure become their central focus, with food often limited to 300-600 calories daily. They show a need and compulsion to exercise often and excessively. Signs and symptoms include weight loss greater than 25% of body weight, behavior directed toward weight loss, peculiar patterns of handling food, intense fear of gaining weight, disturbances in body image, and amenorrhea in women. Secondary symptoms include constipation, pale and dry skin, dry hair, low blood pressure, electrolyte imbalances, dehydration, subnormal temperature, broken sleep, reduced pulse rate, brittle bones, and slight edema around the ankles. The athlete may become withdrawn and may have difficulty concentrating or

## Primary and Secondary Signs and Symptoms of Anorexia Nervosa

**Primary Signs and Symptoms**
- Weight loss greater than 25% of body weight
- Behavior directed toward weight loss
- Peculiar patterns of handling food
- Intense fear of gaining weight
- Disturbances in body image
- Amenorrhea in women

**Secondary Symptoms**
- Constipation
- Pale and dry skin

- Dry hair
- Low blood pressure
- Electrolyte imbalances
- Dehydration
- Subnormal temperature
- Broken sleep
- Reduced pulse rate
- Brittle bones
- Slight edema around the ankles

thinking clearly. At meals with the team, the athlete may play with the food or move the food on the plate to give the impression of eating, may hide the food to feign eating, or may encourage others to eat more. In later stages, the person with anorexia, like someone who has bulimia, will resort to laxatives that can produce persistent abdominal pain, cause fingers to become edematous, and damage bowel muscles to further add to constipation. Severe and prolonged starvation efforts can result in dangerous electrolyte imbalance and dehydration that can become life threatening.

Treatment may include hospitalization for psychological counseling, progressive and closely monitored weight gain, and an effort to establish new eating habits. People with anorexia are frequently reluctant to admit that they have a problem. Since they do not view themselves as underweight, but overweight, changes in attitude and behavior are often difficult.

## BULIMIA NERVOSA

Individuals who have bulimia are of normal weight but use techniques such as vomiting and ingestion of diuretics and laxatives to prevent weight gain. Individuals who suffer from bulimia tend to be slightly older than those with anorexia. Like those with anorexia, they have an exaggerated fear of getting fat, but they do not attempt to lose weight, only maintain it. Episodes of uncontrolled binge eating followed by vomiting are frequent. People with bulimia are often perfectionistic and outgoing individuals who enjoy pleasing others. Because of frequent vomiting episodes, symptoms such as enlarged salivary glands around the throat become evident, and tooth enamel is dissolved by stomach acids. Calluses on the knuckles and sores at the corners of the mouth may also be present. Irregular heart rate, muscle weakness, kidney damage, and epileptic seizures are additional symptoms that can result from frequent vomiting and electrolyte disturbances. Because outward signs are minimal and subtle, bulimia is more difficult to detect than anorexia. However, at times these conditions are found in tandem, and weight loss is evident (**bulimarexia**).

The treatment uses the same protocol as for anorexia, but it can sometimes be easier for the person with bulimia to comply with treatment protocols. An individual who has bulimia often feels guilty and ashamed of her behavior, and the binge eating-vomiting behavior is time consuming and exhausting. Admitting to the problem may be a relief, but counseling and support with a change in lifestyle and environment are necessary for successful treatment.

## OBESITY

Although prevalent in society, obesity is not normally seen in the athletic population. The number of overweight youths has more than doubled in the United States in the past 30 years, and inactivity may be the primary reason. Almost half of those in the 12-to-21 age group, and more than one-third of high school students, do not participate in regular exercise. Sumo wrestlers, football players, and heavyweight wrestlers are the athletic groups that may exhibit obesity. Body weight over 20% of the desired weight is considered in the obese range. Weight over 40-50% above desired weight is considered morbidly obese and can be life threatening. Various methods of determining body fat mass relative to lean body mass are available; these are the best methods for defining desired body weight.

For more information on techniques for determining body fat mass, refer to *Introduction to Athletic Training* (Hillman 2000), chapter 4.

Nutritional counseling referral is advisable for individuals interested in lowering their body fat. A balanced diet combined with regular exercise is the most effective means of achieving weight loss, but this should be instituted under the guidance of a nutritional counselor or physician.

# SEXUALLY TRANSMITTED DISEASES AND DISEASES TRANSMITTED BY BODY FLUID

Sexually transmitted diseases are common today and represent very sensitive conditions both socially and medically. These conditions can raise considerable concern and stigma among teammates, and athletes are often reluctant to report their signs and symptoms. Because of the sensitive issues surrounding sexually transmitted diseases, you must be able to deal with the athlete with professionalism and confidence. Although these conditions may bring with them dangers of transmission to other athletes, confidentiality and education are of utmost importance.

## HUMAN IMMUNODEFICIENCY VIRUS AND ACQUIRED IMMUNODEFICIENCY SYNDROME

Human immunodeficiency virus (HIV) weakens the immune system by destroying lymphocytes (T cells), lessening the body's ability to defend itself against infections and malignancies that can be deadly. Human immunodeficiency virus advances through a progression of stages, beginning with transient infections and HIV, continuing to acquired immunodeficiency syndrome (AIDS)-related complex diseases, and leading to AIDS. Approximately 70% of those infected with HIV will develop AIDS within 10 years. Acquired immunodeficiency syndrome is actually a collection of life-threatening diseases that occur as the individual's immune system becomes progressively weaker and less resistant to infection and malignancies.

Normal T-cell count is 800-1300. An individual may remain in HIV status for several years before the disease advances to AIDS; AIDS is usually defined by a drop in the T-cell count below 200 as a result of HIV. At this point, the individual's health declines more rapidly.

HIV cannot be transmitted through casual contact, kissing, or touching; it is transmitted through unprotected sexual activity, intravenous drug use, breast-feeding from HIV-infected women, infection from contaminated needles, and less often through transfusion of blood products. The likelihood that transfusions will cause HIV infection has decreased greatly in recent years because of improved techniques for blood screening. Although HIV can infect any age group, the greatest number of cases are seen in the most sexually active age group, ages 24 to 44. While in the late 1990s approximately 80% of HIV cases were men and 20% were women, the incidence of new female cases is increasing at a faster rate than new male cases.

Although there is no cure for HIV, recent advances in medication combinations have improved the health and longevity of HIV patients. The medical "cocktails" include an expensive combination of a relatively new class of drugs called protease inhibitors taken throughout the day. These medications keep HIV in check and have reduced the death rate by 50%.

Athletes with HIV should notify the athletic trainer of the condition. Because of the persisting social stigma and often unfounded fears connected with HIV, the athletic trainer should respect patient confidentiality by not passing this information on. Standard sterile technique relating to care of open wounds and disposal of contaminated supplies should be maintained as with any other condition.

For more information on proper sterilizing techniques and contaminant disposal, refer to *Introduction to Athletic Training* (Hillman 2000), chapter 8.

# HEPATITIS

Hepatitis is an inflammation of the liver caused by either infectious or toxic substances. It is one of the most frequently reported infectious diseases in the United States, surpassed only by gonorrhea and chickenpox. There are five known types of hepatitis: A, B, C, D, and E. They are defined by the manner of transmission and the length of time the individual can remain a carrier. Hepatitis A and E are communicated from one person to another through fecal-oral transmission following food handling without proper hand washing, and can evolve into epidemic situations. Hepatitis B, C, and D are transmitted through blood, semen, and other bodily fluids. Hepatitis B is hardier than the HIV virus but is communicated in similar ways, such as the sharing of contaminated needles, unsafe sex, and transmission from mother to infant at birth. Hepatitis D thrives only in the presence of a hepatitis B infection. People can also contract hepatitis by eating the wrong kind of mushroom, ingesting alcohol excessively, eating raw shellfish from contaminated waters, taking too much Tylenol, and ingesting anything that causes liver inflammation.

Infectious hepatitis—hepatitis A—is most contagious before signs of jaundice appear. Hepatitis A is usually acute and without lasting effects on the liver. Hepatitis B produces more severe symptoms than either A or E, but does not carry as great a risk of causing chronic hepatitis as does hepatitis C. Although the progression is slow, occurring over 10 to 30 years, hepatitis C has the greatest chance of advancing to cirrhosis and liver failure.

Early symptoms of hepatitis include flu-like symptoms such as fever, fatigue, nausea, diarrhea, general achiness, and loss of appetite. Jaundice is a hallmark sign. Acute viral hepatitis usually disappears within 4 to 16 weeks without any treatment beyond adequate diet and rest. Chronic hepatitis can cause periodic health disturbances and lead to cirrhosis and occasionally to liver failure.

Antibody vaccines are available for hepatitis A and B. Individuals who are sexually active, health care workers with possible exposure to hepatitis (including certified athletic trainers), and intravenous drug users are all encouraged to obtain the hepatitis B vaccine. Parents of infants should also have their babies immunized against hepatitis B. Those traveling with teams overseas should have hepatitis vaccines before leaving the country. Athletes suspected of having hepatitis should be referred to a physician. Care of athletes with hepatitis requires use of sterile technique with open wounds and proper disposal of contaminated items.

## CHLAMYDIA

Chlamydia is the most common bacterial sexually transmitted disease in the United States. Because 75% of infected women and 50% of infected men do not show symptoms, the disease often goes untreated. Teenage girls and young women under the age of 25 have the highest incidence rate. When signs and symptoms are present, they may include painful urination (dysuria) and a pus discharge in males, or vaginal discharge, pelvic pain, and dysuria in females. Although chlamydia can be easily treated, when untreated it can lead to a number of severe problems including pelvic inflammatory disease, infertility, chronic pelvic pain, and tubal pregnancy with risk of death. Untreated chlamydia in males can result in urethral infection and swollen and tender testicles.

Prevention through education is the best means of treatment. Screening of men and women in the high-incidence age groups is also advocated. Antibiotic therapy under the guidance of a physician is the standard of care for those infected with the disease.

## GENITAL WARTS

*Urethritis is an inflammation of the urethra.*

*Purulent means containing or consisting of pus.*

*Epididymitis is an inflammation of the epididymis.*

*Endometritis is an inflammation of the endometrium of the uterus.*

Genital warts, or **condylomata acuminata**, are located in the perineum and perianal region. They are caused by the human papilloma virus (HPV), and it is estimated that 1 million new cases occur each year (Taber 1997). Genital warts are contracted through sexual contact, and the individual will typically have a history of unprotected sexual contact with an infected person or with multiple partners. These viral warts begin as tiny pink swellings and may coalesce to form a fibrous overgrowth covered with thickened epithelium. They may appear as single or as colonized warts with a cauliflower-like appearance and are usually not painful. To prevent their spread, the individual should abstain from sexual contact or use a condom during intercourse until healing is complete. In women, these warts may be associated with cervical cancer; thus it is important that the individual seek medical attention for further evaluation.

## GONORRHEA

*A chancre is a sore or ulcer.*

Gonorrhea is a bacterial infection, the infection rate of which is climbing rapidly. Females aged 15 to 19 have the highest rate of gonorrhea. Sexual intercourse is the chief means of transmission. Although symptoms are not always apparent, males can develop an acute urethritis with dysuria. Urinary frequency and urgency can also occur along with a yellow, purulent discharge. The lips of the urinary meatus can be red and swollen. Although 50% of females do not have symptoms, when symptoms are present they can include a purulent urethral discharge, a cervical discharge, or swollen **Bartholin glands**. In untreated cases, sterility, urethritis, prostatitis, and epididymitis may occur in males. Females may also become sterile and may develop endometritis and pelvic inflammatory disease. Either sex may develop gonococcal arthritis and conjunctivitis.

Sexual abstinence and proper condom application and consistent use are the best modes of prevention. Antibiotics are the drug of choice for treatment of gonorrhea.

## SYPHILIS

Syphilis is an acute venereal bacterial condition. The syphilis bacterium is transmitted during vaginal, rectal, or oral sex; it can also be transmitted through open wounds or through direct contact with bodily fluids or blood. If symptoms occur, they are usually seen as genital or anal lesions in the form of a chancre that starts as a papule and then ulcerates. Chancres can also appear, however, almost anywhere on the body, including the hands, eyelids, and mouth. As the chancre is fading, a rash in the form of either rough, "copper penny" spots on the palms of the hands and bottom of the feet, or small blotches or scales all over the body, can become visible. The rash can appear as a prickly heat rash, as slimy white patches in the mouth, or as chickenpox-like bumps— or may be hardly noticeable. The rash may be present for two to six weeks and spontaneously disappear. The groin lymph nodes may be enlarged. If left untreated, syphilis can progress to a secondary syphilis as the disease spreads through all tissues of the body and causes highly infectious generalized skin lesions and conjunctivitis, periostitis of the long bones, hepatitis, headaches, fatigue, weight loss, and nephritic (renal) syndrome. Late syphilis is indicated by nonspecific chronic inflammatory conditions that can affect cardiovascular and central nervous system functions.

Although prevention and education are the treatment of choice, antibiotic therapy is the standard of treatment for individuals who have contracted syphilis. One dose of penicillin usually effects a cure. Any unusual discharge, sores, or rashes—especially in the genitourinary and groin region—should be referred to a physician for diagnosis and treatment. Sterile technique is always the management technique of choice with transmissible diseases. An athletic trainer who has been bitten or scratched by someone with syphilis should contact a physician and obtain a prescription for antibiotic therapy.

# GENITOURINARY TRACT AND ORGANS

The genitourinary tract and organs include the kidneys, bladder, urinary tract, and the external genitalia. Gynecological conditions will be discussed separately in the next section.

## KIDNEY STONES

Kidney stones is the common term for **urinary calculi**. Found anywhere in the urinary system, including the kidney, ureter, bladder, or urethra, they are composed of urinary salts that are precipitated. They occur more often in middle-aged males than in any other group.

*Hematuria means blood in the urine.*

If kidney stones stay within the kidney, the individual may remain asymptomatic. If a stone moves from the kidney and obstructs the ureter, severe **renal colic** ensues as the smooth muscle of the ureter forcefully contracts to relieve the obstruction. The pain, which is extreme, may start in the back or flank and radiate across the abdomen into the groin, genitalia, and inner thigh. Nausea, vomiting, sweating, chills, urinary frequency or urgency, and shock may occur, as can microscopic hematuria.

The patient is transported to an emergency care facility for relief of symptoms. Renal colic is one of the most severe pains people can experience, so morphine or another powerful analgesic is commonly administered along with antispasmodic medications. Adequate fluid intake should be encouraged. Small stones eventually pass through the ureter and are discharged. Larger stones may require surgical intervention to relieve the obstruction. This can be performed with lasers for effective yet minimally invasive results.

## URETHRITIS

Urethritis, or inflammation of the urethra, is also known as a urinary tract infection (UTI) that is isolated to the urethra. This type of infection occurs more frequently in women than in men, and it is a poorly understood phenomenon. Symptoms, although not always present, may include urinary frequency and urgency, painful or burning urination, cloudy or even reddish urine if hematuria is present, general malaise, and lower abdominal pain. Men may experience a fullness of the rectum.

Antibacterial medications will usually resolve the problem within a couple of days, but antibiotics are taken for up to two weeks to assure a cure. Actions such as increasing fluid intake and decreasing smoking and ingestion of caffeine or alcohol may aid in reducing symptoms. Preventive steps include drinking plenty of fluids (especially water), not delaying urination, and avoiding feminine sprays and douches.

## URINARY TRACT INFECTION

As just discussed, urethritis is a form of UTI. A UTI is also present if the bacterial infection spreads to other segments of the urinary system. In advanced cases, the infection spreads to the bladder and ureter. When kidneys are affected, symptoms of urethritis as well as other symptoms such as back pain, fever, nausea, and vomiting can be present. Although the reason for a greater incidence of UTI in women than in men is unclear, there are several conjectures. Women who use a diaphragm are more likely to develop urinary infections than those who use other birth control methods. Sexual intercourse can trigger an infection for some women. The female's urethra is short and close to the vagina, as well as closer to the anus than in males, so the female's bladder may be easier for bacteria to access than the male's.

Antibacterial drugs are used to treat UTIs. As with urethritis, the medication is taken for about two weeks even though symptoms subside after a two-day administration. Prevention steps are the same as those listed for urethritis.

## SPERMATIC CORD TORSION

*Infarction is necrosis of a tissue or organ resulting from obstruction of the local circulation secondary to a clot or occlusion of the vessel.*

*The **cremaster muscle** is continuous with the internal oblique and functions to draw the testes to a more superior position in the scrotum.*

*The **cremasteric reflex** is a drawing up of the scrotal sac with ipsilateral stroking of the upper, inner thigh.*

Spermatic cord torsion, or testicular torsion, occurs when the testicle twists on the spermatic cord, leading to venous occlusion and engorgement followed by arterial ischemia, risking testicular infarction (figure 13.31). Torsion can also occur spontaneously in young males in the absence of trauma. Predisposing factors include anatomic abnormalities of the insertion of the tunica vaginalis or spermatic artery anomalies, a nonexistent or very long gubernaculum, a poorly placed or long epididymis, or an abnormal testicular position. Trauma to the scrotum followed by swelling or a vigorous cremaster contraction in combination with any predisposing factor can result in testicular torsion. There is a sudden or gradual onset of severe unilateral scrotal pain accompanied by scrotal swelling and sensation of heaviness, as well as nausea and vomiting. The involved testis is tender and firm and is elevated in comparison to the contralateral testis; edema is present with scrotal erythema, the cremasteric reflex is absent ipsilaterally, and scrotal elevation does not relieve the pain. This condition constitutes a medical emergency and requires immediate referral, as blood flow to the testicle will be compromised.

Manual detorsion of the testicle will provide pain relief. If necessary, the athlete can be instructed in self-administration of manual detorsion technique. Most torsions rotate inward and toward the midline, so manual detorsion must occur in the opposite direction, with a twisting outward and laterally away from the midline. This derotation may have to be repeated two or three times, depending on the athlete's pain symptoms. Manual detorsion has a 30-70% success rate. If the technique is successful, the athlete should still be referred to a physician for evaluation and follow-up care. If it is unsuccessful, emergency transportation to a hospital for surgical release is necessary to save the testis.

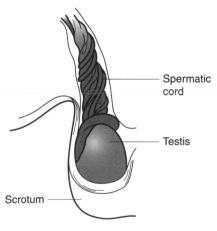

Spermatic cord

Testis

Scrotum

**▌Figure 13.31**   Spermatic cord torsion.

## HYDROCELE

A hydrocele is an accumulation of fluid around the testicle. Hydroceles are most common at birth and will usually resolve without assistance by 18 months of age with the closure of the processus vaginalis. Adult hydroceles result from direct trauma, infections, or radiotherapy. Symptoms include a sensation of heaviness and mild discomfort radiating into the inguinal region and sometimes into the back. Enlargement of the scrotal sac can occur in standing and decrease in recumbency, and scrotal consistency can range from soft to tense. There is commonly no pain.

Prior to treatment, a differential diagnostic assessment to rule out testicular torsion must be made. It is also necessary to determine the need for surgical release of the hydrocele. Adult hydroceles often require surgical intervention; thus physician referral is necessary in the presence of any changes in the size, shape, or consistency of the testicle.

## VARICOCELE

A varicocele is an enlargement of the internal spermatic veins that develops because of defective valves in the veins, allowing a backflow into the testicle (figure 13.32).

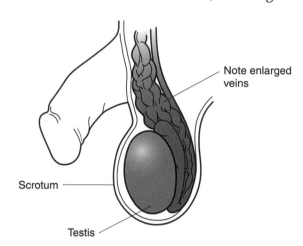
This can result in sterility. The left spermatic vein is more often affected than the right because the left vein enters the left renal vein at a right angle and can become compressed by the mesenteric artery at this site. Blood pooling with increased temperature and congestion can influence sperm production. Often the affected testicle is smaller than the other one, and when the individual is asked to bear down, blood backflow can be palpated.

Note enlarged veins

Scrotum

Testis

■ **Figure 13.32** Testicular varicocele.

If pain is present or the size difference between the testicles is significant, surgical repair is indicated. Surgery is usually successful and sperm count is restored in up to 70% of the patients.

# GYNECOLOGICAL DISORDERS

Elite athletes frequently experience gynecological disorders, as excessive or intense exercise can be a cause of menstrual dysfunction. Other conditions such as painful menses and vaginal infections or irritation can also cause discomfort and affect athletic performance. This section will also cover breast conditions.

## MENSTRUAL DYSFUNCTION

Female athletes may complain of a variety of menstrual dysfunctions, including pain, menstrual irregularity, or loss of menses.

### *Amenorrhea*

*Imperforate means lacking the usual or normal opening.*

Amenorrhea is the absence of a menstrual cycle. There are three types of amenorrhea: primary, secondary, and irregular. Primary amenorrhea is present when menstruation has not started by age 16. There are several causative factors, including an imperforate hymen, ovarian dysfunction, or hormonal imbalance. Secondary amenorrhea occurs when menstruation stops after at least one to three menstrual periods. Factors that can produce secondary amenorrhea include pregnancy, menopause, stress, weight change, breast-feeding, anemia, excessive exercise, ovarian cysts, and medications. Irregular amenorrhea is present either when periods occur inconsistently or when there are only a few annually; causes can be factors related to secondary amenorrhea. Female athletes most often experience secondary or irregular amenorrhea.

Amenorrhea is often associated with disordered eating, low body weight, and excessive exercise, not all of which need be pathological. The incidence of osteoporosis (bone loss) and of stress fractures is higher in amenorrheic women than in others. Physician referral is necessary to determine the cause of amenorrhea and appropriate treatment. Hormones, hormone stimulators, thyroxin, other medications, nutrition counseling, and other measures may be indicated depending on the results of an examination and laboratory tests.

### Oligomenorrhea

Oligomenorrhea is defined as an irregular menses, characterized by infrequent or light periods or both. Causes can include rapid weight loss, anorexia or bulimia, high levels of or significant changes in exercise, and some medications and illicit drug use. The athlete should be referred to a physician, who will determine the cause of the oligomenorrhea before selecting the most appropriate treatment. No treatment is required unless the cause is pathological, or unless the individual wishes to become pregnant or to maintain a balance of hormone levels.

### Dysmenorrhea

*Prostaglandins are fatty acids that perform a variety of hormone functions.*

Dysmenorrhea, also known as "menstrual cramps," includes pain during menstruation that is severe enough to interfere with normal activity. Additional symptoms can include nausea, vomiting, and severe abdominal pain. Women who have dysmenorrhea have an abnormally high concentration of prostaglandins in their menstrual fluid. Release of prostaglandin into the uterus stimulates the smooth muscle there to contract, limiting oxygen supply to the uterine wall by inhibiting blood supply. Once menstrual flow begins, the prostaglandin is discharged, causing symptoms to subside after the first few days of the period.

Across-the-counter analgesics and anti-inflammatories may provide adequate relief of pain. Hot baths and massage may also encourage muscle relaxation and increase circulation. Exercises may aid in abdominal muscle relaxation. In more severe cases, prescription-dose prostaglandin inhibitors may be necessary to relieve symptoms. Some women also find relief with contraceptives.

## PELVIC CONDITIONS

Pain or symptoms in the pelvic and vaginal regions are usually caused by yeast and bacterial infections. These conditions include vaginitis, candidiasis, and pelvic inflammatory disease.

### Vaginitis

**Vaginitis** is the medical term for vaginal infections. Of the number of organisms that can cause vaginitis, the most common are bacteria, yeast, and parasites. Bacteria cause a thin, milky white or gray discharge that has an unpleasant, foul, or musty odor, and perhaps discomfort or burning. Untreated conditions can lead to pelvic inflammatory disease, endometritis, cervicitis, and other obstetric complications. Treatment includes antibiotic medication. Yeast infections are discussed separately in the next section.

**Trichomoniasis** is a parasite that can cause a yellow-green-gray frothy or sticky discharge that sometimes has a fishy or foul odor. The condition can cause occasional itching and painful irritation. Difficulties with pregnancy can occur if the woman is infected during pregnancy. Prescription medication is necessary to treat this condition.

It is important to realize that vaginal infections are common among women and should be attended to when symptoms are first recognized. A correct diagnosis is crucial to an effective treatment outcome, and referral to an obstetrician for appropriate tests is necessary for an accurate diagnosis. Prevention plays a significant role in reducing the risk or spread of infection. Women can take several preventive steps. They should avoid douching, since it upsets the delicate pH balance and can increase the spread of organisms; other recommendations are to avoid tight clothing and to use cotton undergarments to help keep moisture (an environment in which many organisms thrive) to a minimum. Good hygiene will also help prevent the spread of organisms. Scented toilet paper, feminine deodorants, and harsh soaps can decrease even further the health of any irritated area. Safe sex practices will help to prevent sexually transmitted infections.

### Candidiasis

Candidiasis, or yeast infection, is actually caused by a fungus. Small numbers of this fungus are present normally in the vagina; but when the number increases, symptoms occur. The variety of causes include tight clothing, warm weather, stress, diabetes, pregnancy, obesity, and medications such as antibiotics, steroids, and birth control pills. Symptoms can include pain during sex, vaginal itching and burning, and a curdlike, white discharge. Candidiasis is not dangerous, and symptoms usually decrease with treatment.

Treatment includes across-the-counter antifungal medication inserted as vaginal suppositories, creams, or tablets. If the infection persists, a physician should be consulted to rule out other diseases and establish the cause. Preventive steps include wearing loose clothing and cotton underwear and avoiding douches unless instructed by a physician to use them.

### Pelvic Inflammatory Disease

Pelvic inflammatory disease (PID), also called **salpingitis**, is a serious complication of sexually transmitted diseases. It is a bacterial infection that attacks the female reproductive system, spreading from the vagina to the womb, fallopian tubes, and ovaries. It occurs as a result of an untreated bacterial infection of the vagina. Gonorrhea is a common preceding infection. In addition to sexual transmission, females can get PID from an intrauterine device. Symptoms may not always be present but include painful stomach cramps, bleeding, fever, chills, an upset stomach, and an odorous discharge. If untreated, the condition can lead to sterility and is in fact the major cause of sterility in young women. Women with PID have an increased risk of ectopic (tubal) pregnancy.

Prevention of PID includes monogamous relationships, use of condoms, or abstinence. Treatment includes use of antibiotic therapy to destroy the bacteria. Intrauterine devices should be removed before therapy is initiated. The woman's sexual partner should also be examined and treated if indicated to avoid episodes of reinfection.

## BREAST CONDITIONS

It is not uncommon for the breast to be tender prior to menstruation. Normal changes in the breast will affect both breasts simultaneously and symmetrically. However, there may be times that an athlete comes to you out of concern, complaining of changes in the appearance or feel of the tissue in one of her breasts. In the majority of these cases the changes are benign, but it is important that they be evaluated and malignancy (cancer) ruled out.

### *Benign Conditions*

Benign (noncancerous) conditions can be caused by fibrocystic changes and fibroadenomas. Because it is often difficult to differentiate between benign and malignant changes in breast tissue without diagnostic tests, all individuals (whether male or female) who note changes in their breast tissue should be referred to a physician for proper diagnosis.

### **Fibrocystic Changes**

Fibrocystic changes do not represent a disease state but rather a benign development of multiple fibrous lumps or small cysts caused by an overreaction of the breast to normal hormones produced during ovulation (Tetzlaf 1998). Fibrocystic changes are common in women between 20 and 50 years of age, affecting over 50% of all women. The fibrous lumps or cysts often become larger and more tender prior to menstruation. Coffee, tea, cola drinks, chocolate, and some diet and cold medications are thought to promote the growth of fibrocystic lumps (Tetzlaf 1998).

### **Fibroadenomas**

Fibroadenomas, which are benign tumors that occur most frequently in women between the ages of 18 and 35, are characterized by solid lumps of fibrous and glandular tissue. They account for nearly all breast tumors found in women under age 25 (Tetzlaf 1998). They are usually nontender, except possibly prior to menstruation, and are mobile when palpated.

### *Cancer*

Breast changes such as lumps, dimpling, or puckering of the skin and thickening or swelling in the breast that do not go away may be warning signs of breast cancer, warranting immediate referral to a physician for evaluation. Other signs and symptoms to be concerned about include skin irritation, distortion, retraction, and scaliness; and changes or tenderness in, or secretion from, the nipple. If the tumor is malignant and not detected and treated early, it will continue to grow and invade adjacent, healthy tissue. As with any cancer, if left unchecked it can spread to the nearby lymph nodes and travel through the lymph system and bloodstream to other parts of the body (**metastasis**).

### *Early Detection and Self Examination*

Breast cancer is second only to lung cancer as a cause of cancer-related deaths in women. Although the risk of breast cancer increases with age and may be higher in some women (see below), every female is at risk for breast cancer. In fact, 75% of women diagnosed with breast cancer have none of the associated risk factors other than being female or their age (Tetzlaf 1998). While breast cancer cannot be prevented, it can be effectively treated and cured if recognized early. Therefore, educating your athletes and encouraging breast self-examination (see page 448) in women 20 years and older may ultimately save a life.

## Risk Factors Associated With Breast Cancer

- Women as they get older, particularly for women over 50
- Women who have a personal or family history of breast cancer
- Women who have had a biopsy confirm atypical hyperplasia
- Women who menstruated early
- Women with late-onset menopause

- Women who have recently used oral contraceptives or postmenopausal estrogens
- Women who have never been pregnant or who had their first child at a late age
- Women of higher education and socioeconomic status
- Women who smoke

Data from American Cancer Society, 1999, *Facts and Figures*.

# Breast Self-Examination

A woman who thoroughly examines her breasts each month is likely to notice any changes that might signal the onset of cancer. The few minutes it takes to perform breast self-examination (BSE) may mean the difference between detecting a cancer when it is likely to be small and still confined to the breast and detecting a cancer that is relatively large and likely to have spread beyond the breast.

The purpose of BSE is to become familiar with how your breasts look and feel so you can readily recognize changes and report them immediately to your health care provider. You'll be watching for changes such as a lump or thickening, dimpling or puckering of the skin, or differences in size and shape.

If you're not clear on the following steps of BSE, ask your doctor.

**1.** Lie on your back with a pillow under your right shoulder. Place your right hand behind your head. Using the pads of the middle three fingers of your left hand, examine all of your right breast tissue—including tissue that extends into your armpit, up to your clavicle, and down to the bottom of your rib cage—by firmly massaging small areas in one of three patterns. Select the pattern that is most comfortable to you and use it consistently.

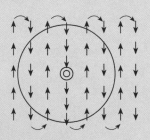 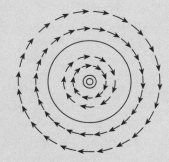 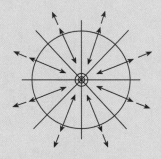

**2.** Examine your left breast, placing the pillow under your left shoulder, using the fingers of your right hand, and repeating the instructions for step one.

**3.** Repeat the examination of each breast, this time while standing with one arm behind your head. Many women find it helpful to do this part of the exam while they're in the shower because soapy hands move more easily over wet skin.

**4.** Stand in front of a mirror and note the texture and color of skin as well as the shape and contour of the breast.

**5.** Gently squeeze the nipple of each breast and report any discharge to your health care provider at once.

**6.** Conduct BSE each month. If you're menstruating, do it a few days after your period ends, when your breasts are less tender. Women who don't have regular periods should select a specific day of the month and do BSE on that same day each month.

# VIRAL SYNDROMES

Viral syndromes are systemic conditions caused by viral infections. They are often highly contagious and may have prolonged symptoms. Infection usually occurs well before signs and symptoms appear, with incubation periods of two weeks or more. Complications such as enlarged visceral organs and sterility may result from one or more of these conditions. Viral syndromes include mononucleosis, mumps, and measles. Chickenpox (herpes zoster), previously described in relation to skin conditions, is also classified as a viral syndrome.

## INFECTIOUS MONONUCLEOSIS

Most cases of infectious mononucleosis, or "mono," are caused by the **Epstein-Barr virus**, a member of the herpes group of viruses. This condition can affect any age group, but most cases are seen in the 15-to-30 age range. The disease is transmitted through direct contact with saliva of an infected person. A common means of transmission is sharing beverage containers or food utensils.

Incubation is two to seven weeks after contact, and symptoms can last a few days or several months. Most commonly, they disappear in one to three weeks. Symptoms are vague and include general malaise, headache, fatigue, chilliness, loss of appetite, and puffy eyelids. As the disease progresses, additional symptoms—swollen and tender lymph glands, sore throat, and fever—emerge. Tenderness and enlargement of the spleen, difficulty swallowing, and bleeding gums can also be present. Adults over the age of 30 who contract the disease can have a more severe episode and longer-lasting symptoms. Additional symptoms for this age group can include ruptured spleen, pericarditis, and liver involvement. If an athlete of any age competes while the spleen is enlarged, there is a chance of rupture; thus physical activities requiring contact or jostling are contraindicated.

Physician referral for a diagnosis should be made in suspected cases. A heterophil antibody blood test "monospot" confirms the diagnosis and eliminates other differential diagnoses. Treatment includes restricting vigorous activity until all symptoms have disappeared. Since an enlarged spleen is susceptible to injury, athletes should be restricted from weight lifting and competitive sport until recovery is complete. There is no specific medication for treatment of mononucleosis, but the athlete should maintain a well-balanced diet, prevent dehydration with adequate fluid intake, and take across-the-counter analgesics for symptomatic relief of headache and muscle aches. Antibiotics are not prescribed, since the disease is caused by a virus and will not respond to medication.

## MEASLES

Measles is a highly contagious viral infection (**rubeola**) transmitted through the air: breathing the same air as an infected person can cause an individual to contract measles. Because of its ease of transmission, epidemics—usually occurring in the spring in a two- to three-year cycle—are common. Incubation period is about 9 to 11 days, with about two weeks between exposure and the appearance of the measles rash. The time of infectivity begins two to four days before the rash appears and ends two to five days after it appears.

Symptoms include a fever as high as 105° F (40.6° C), rash, runny nose, photophobia, watery eyes, or hacking cough. Small, irregularly shaped spots with a red periphery and blue-white centers (Koplik spots) in the mouth appear one to two days before the rash and are hallmark signs of measles. The rash, which begins about three or four days after the other symptoms, takes the form of irregular papules around the hairline of the face and neck and rapidly spreads to the trunk and extremities. The rash fades in the same way, first in the face and neck and then through the rest of the body, usually completing its course in about six days. The disease takes about 10-14 days to run its course.

Complications such as croup, bronchitis, pneumonia, conjunctivitis, hepatitis, and encephalitis can occur with measles. Symptoms and complications are more severe in adults. A vaccine should be routinely administered to infants after 13 months of age. Public schools in most states require immunization prior to school admission. A vaccine either before or within three days after exposure to the disease will be effective in preventing illness. Vaccines made before 1979 may not be effective, so people who were vaccinated before 1980 should receive another measles vaccine if an outbreak occurs.

Vaccinations are not given to pregnant mothers or to individuals who have depressed immune systems. Persons who are allergic to eggs or neomycin are also in danger of severe reactions from the vaccine.

*Reye's syndrome is a rare, often fatal childhood disease that can cause damage to the brain and other vital organs. The incidence of Reye's syndrome has been linked to aspirin use in children.*

Individuals with measles can take across-the-counter medications to reduce the fever, but children should not take aspirin because of the risk of developing Reye's syndrome. Clear fluids are used to maintain good hydration and reduce the chance of lung infections. A cool-mist vaporizer may relieve cough symptoms. Rest in a darkened room and abstention from reading and watching television because of photophobia are advisable.

## MUMPS

Mumps is a highly contagious viral infection that affects the salivary glands, especially the parotid glands. It is spread through droplet infection or direct contact with saliva. Most cases are seen in children, ages 5 to 15, and occur with greatest frequency in the late winter and early spring. The incubation period is 14 to 28 days, after which symptoms appear. These include chillis, headache, malaise, swelling of salivary glands, and exquisite tenderness over the angle of the jaw where the salivary glands are located. Fever and sore throat with difficulty swallowing or chewing also occur and last for 24 to 72 h.

Complications associated with mumps most often affect individuals past puberty and can affect the testes or ovaries, resulting in sterility. Males may suffer from painful inflammation of the testicles, with up to 25% of these cases resulting in sterility. Other rare complications include facial nerve palsy and effects on the central nervous system, pancreas, kidneys, or breasts.

The mumps vaccine is usually provided in a single injection as part of the MMR (mumps, measles, rubella) immunization. When people do contract mumps, treatment is for relief of symptoms; it includes bed rest until the fever subsides, analgesics for pain, clear fluid intake to prevent dehydration, and a soft diet to minimize pain caused by chewing.

# NEUROLOGICAL DISORDERS

Neurological disorders represent a wide range of conditions of varying etiologies that have an ultimate effect on some aspect of the nervous system; some are acute and others are chronic. Each can result in significant complications if not recognized or properly treated.

## TETANUS

Tetanus is commonly called "lockjaw." Caused by the tetanus bacillus, it enters the body through an open wound that has been in contact with dirt or soil. The bacillus attaches to the local nerve, moves to the spinal cord, and becomes anchored to the motor nerves. It prevents normal synaptic inhibition, so a tetanic contraction of the muscles occurs. Most commonly, stiffness of the jaw and neck is produced, with stiffness of the extremities occurring less often. Headaches, fever, and convulsions can be early symptoms. As the disease progresses, facial, back, neck, and abdominal muscles become rigid. Additional complicating factors include sphincter rigidity, dysphagia, convulsions, cyanosis, or asphyxia; death can result. Any suspicion of tetanus infection in an athlete warrants immediate referral to a physician.

The best treatment is prevention with an updated tetanus toxoid immunization. A tetanus toxoid booster is currently effective for 5-10 years. Wound care should be addressed immediately using proper cleansing and sterile technique. If you are uncertain of the person's immunization status, you should refer the athlete to a physician and she should receive a tetanus toxoid booster as soon as possible following injury.

## EPILEPSY

Epilepsy is a chronic condition characterized by recurring seizures. Seizures are a spontaneous and involuntary neurological aberration caused by an unregulated and abnormal electrical brain activity; they can last from a few seconds to a few minutes. The many causes of epilepsy include head trauma, infectious diseases, metabolic disorders, tumors, congenital abnormalities, and drugs. Epilepsy can also be idiopathic in nature, without an identifiable cause, usually appearing from 5 to 20 years of age.

Although seizures are a sign of epilepsy, you should not assume that all seizures are epileptic. They can occur as one-time events resulting from traumatic incidents and other disorders such as extremely high fever, heatstroke, central nervous system trauma, and hyperventilation. Trauma can cause seizures at any age and may not become evident for up to two years following the injury. Infectious diseases such as bacterial meningitis or herpes encephalitis can also produce seizures. Other sources are premature birth or complications at the time of delivery, metabolic disorders including hypoglycemia or diabetes, drug or alcohol withdrawal, and brain tumors.

*Tonic refers to a sustained contraction of a muscle or muscle group.*

*Clonic refers to a rapid contraction and relaxation of a muscle or muscle group.*

The various types of seizures are classified as partial or focal seizures and generalized seizures. Focal or partial seizures affect only certain parts of the brain and usually involve only one part of the body, such as the face or arm, in a tonic-clonic activity. There is usually no loss of consciousness; other symptoms can include seeing flashes of light, pupil dilation, sweating, or tingling or jerking that can begin in one part of the body and advance to other segments. Focal seizures can progress rapidly to generalized convulsions.

Generalized seizures are of various types, but the most common are the petit mal and grand mal seizures. Although most people have no warning, some will experience an aura or feeling that precedes an episode seconds or minutes before its onset. Precipitating factors for seizures can include stress, missed meals and medications, lack of sleep, alcohol, or fever. Petit mal seizures are brief episodes of consciousness impairment that occur in childhood and are usually outgrown by the age

### Possible Etiologies of Adult Seizures

The cause of seizures in adults cannot always be determined, but you should consider the following possibilities:

1. Insufficient oxygen in blood
2. Intracranial pathology
   - Head injury or space-occupying lesion (e.g., brain tumor, subdural hemorrhage)
   - Stroke
3. High fever
4. Meningitis
5. Metabolic or chemical problems
   - Low blood sugar (hypoglycemia)
   - Exposure to toxins or drug overdose
   - Withdrawal from alcohol or drugs

of 20. The individual may appear to be daydreaming or staring off into space and be unaware that the episode has occurred once it is over. A grand mal seizure, also called a tonic-clonic seizure, occurs with a sudden loss of consciousness in which the person falls to the ground as the body's muscles enter a state of total tonic contractions. After about 1 min, the body goes into the clonic phase, during which the body jerks for 2 to 3 min. Breathing can become shallow during the tonic phase; during the clonic phase the individual may bite his tongue or lips or experience fecal and/or urinary incontinence. After the seizure, the person is very lethargic and may drift into sleep or experience additional seizures. There is usually no memory of the seizure, and the person may have postseizure symptoms of headache, drowsiness, nausea, muscle soreness, or disorientation, sometimes lasting several days.

First-aid treatment of epileptic seizures consists of protecting the individual from nearby hazards, loosening the clothing around the neck, removing eyeglasses, and protecting the head from injury. If you know the person has epilepsy or has a medical identification, you should turn her on her side to allow saliva to drain and ask if she wants to go to the hospital. If there is no history of seizure, or if the person is pregnant, has diabetes, or has been injured, take steps to obtain emergency transportation to an emergency care facility.

During a seizure, there are specific actions that should be avoided. Never restrain the individual; do not place objects in her mouth, since they may obstruct breathing; and do not move her unless there is a risk of injury. Do not offer liquids until she is completely awake.

Individuals with epilepsy should carry identification indicating their condition. If the individual is an athlete, the athletic trainer should be informed of the situation. High-risk sports such as football, skiing, and scuba diving are usually not recommended. Seizures can often be controlled with a combination of adequate rest, balanced diet, avoidance of stimulants, minimization of stress, and medication.

Treatment usually includes anticonvulsive medication for prevention of seizures. Many drugs are available, so the specific drugs selected will depend upon the type of seizure, the side effects of the drug, and the individual's health and age. It is common to try a number of drugs or combinations of drugs before finding the correct medication and dosage to bring the seizures under control. Some of the medications often used are Tegretol, Dilantin, phenobarbital, and Rivotril.

## REFLEX SYMPATHETIC DYSTROPHY

Reflex sympathetic dystrophy (RSD) is a multisystem, multisymptom disorder. Its effect on the sympathetic nervous system results in a multitude of symptoms and problems. It usually follows an injury and most frequently affects the hand in upper-extremity injuries or the foot in lower-extremity injuries. The etiology is unknown.

The primary symptom of RSD is severe, constant pain, usually a burning sensation that occurs in the involved extremity, especially distally. It is accompanied by pitting or non-pitting edema, bluish skin color, coolness of the distal extremity, and reduced motor function. The color and temperature changes are thought to occur because of increased sympathetic stimulation. This abnormal sympathetic stimulation causes vasospasm of the arterioles, tissue swelling secondary to capillary release of fibrin and plasma, stiffness secondary to tissue ischemia, and eventual soft tissue fibrosis.

Reflex sympathetic dystrophy can go through three stages of progression:

• **Stage I** lasts an average of three months and is characterized by the onset of severe, burning pain at the site of injury. This is accompanied by hyperesthesia, local edema, muscle spasm, limited mobility, and vasospasms that cause the skin to appear red, warm, and dry and then change to cyanotic, cold, and sweaty. In mild cases this stage may last only a few weeks and spontaneously resolve.

*Brawny edema is long-term leathery swelling of tissue.*

*Trophic refers to disordered or altered nutrition.*

*Ankylosed refers to fusion or fixation of a joint.*

*Dystrophy is a muscular disorder characterized by weakness and fibrosis.*

*Sympathectomy means removal of sympathetic nerves.*

• **Stage II,** lasting for three to six months, is marked by a more severe but diffuse pain than seen in stage I. Swelling spreads and changes to a brawny edema. Spotty osteoporosis can become evident on x-ray. Hair becomes scant, and nails become brittle and grooved. Atrophy is apparent at this stage.

• **Stage III** is apparent through noticeable and irreversible trophic changes. Atrophy continues; interphalangeal joints become stiff and eventually ankylosed, and contractures of flexor tendons become apparent. X-rays will reveal more diffuse and marked osteoporosis.

If the condition continues untreated, dystrophy and then atrophy occur with less chance of recovery. The key to treatment is early recognition and intervention while the condition is still reversible. Anti-inflammatory agents, beta blockers, analgesics, tricyclics, tranquilizers, and calcium channel blockers are all drugs that may relieve RSD symptoms. Nerve blocks performed as either intravenous regional blocks or sympathetic blocks are sometimes used to reduce sympathetic nerve stimulation to the area. Pain and edema control with desensitization activities and stiffness prevention are early treatment steps. Modalities for pain and edema control and active exercises to facilitate edema reduction and functional return are encouraged as tolerated. In extreme cases, sympathectomy or the implantation of stimulators or an infusion pump may be indicated.

## MENINGITIS

Meningitis is an infection of the cerebral spinal fluid that can be either bacterial or viral. It is sometimes referred to as spinal meningitis. Bacterial meningitis is usually more severe and can result in brain damage, hearing loss, or death. Viral meningitis is rarely as serious, with recovery occurring in about 7 to 10 days. Establishing the specific cause of meningitis is crucial to effective treatment.

Symptoms are similar for all meningitis and occur over several hours to a couple of days. They include headache, stiff neck, and high fever. Nausea, vomiting, confusion, photophobia, and drowsiness can also be present. Seizures can occur secondary to meningitis.

Viral meningitis is contagious, as are some forms of bacterial meningitis. Spread is through direct contact with respiratory and throat secretions such as saliva, sputum, or nasal mucus. Coughing, sneezing, and kissing are common means of transmission of bacterial meningitis.

Prevention is the best method to treat meningitis. Avoid contact with individuals who have meningitis; and if contact occurs, use thorough hand-washing techniques. There is no vaccine against viral meningitis, but there is a vaccine against some of the bacterial meningitis strains. Treatment for bacterial meningitis includes immediate referral to a physician for appropriate antibiotics for the specific bacterial strain, prevention of dehydration, maintenance of good nutrition, and rest. There is no effective medication for viral meningitis, which usually resolves on its own; but steps to relieve symptoms, prevent dehydration, and assure proper nutrition and rest should be followed.

## SYSTEMIC DISEASES

Other systemic diseases not previously covered in relation to viral, cardiovascular, or neurological conditions include those that affect the blood and joints. Previous chapters have dealt with arthritic conditions as they relate to specific body regions. The following sections cover iron-deficiency anemia, sickle cell anemia, and Lyme disease.

## IRON-DEFICIENCY ANEMIA

Anemia is characterized by a deficiency of red blood cells, hemoglobin, or total blood volume. Although there are various causes of anemia, iron-deficiency anemia occurs the most frequently. A deficiency of iron in the blood brings about a decrease in the quantity of red blood cells. Since red blood cells contain hemoglobin, the oxygen carrier of the blood, anemia reduces the body's ability to deliver oxygen to cells throughout the body.

Iron deficiency occurs as a result of insufficient iron quantities in the diet, reduced iron absorption ability of the body, blood loss, or lead poisoning. Anemia is seen more frequently in women than in men because of female blood loss during menstrual bleeding and because of the smaller stores of iron in women as compared to men.

A diet rich in iron can reduce the risk of anemia. Foods rich in iron include red meat, egg yolks, raisins, fish, legumes, and liver. Foods enriched with iron include flour, bread, and some cereals. Symptoms of iron-deficiency anemia include pale skin, fatigue, weakness, shortness of breath, low blood pressure, headache, decreased appetite, and irritability. Tests for hematocrit and hemoglobin blood levels are commonly used to identify iron-deficiency anemia.

Treatment of anemia begins with identifying the cause of the condition and then taking steps to eradicate it. Iron supplements are usually provided along with a diet rich in iron. In most cases, blood levels will return to normal after a two-month treatment course. Iron supplements are best absorbed on an empty stomach, but some individuals cannot tolerate the stomach upset that can occur. Since antacids and milk can interfere with iron absorption, they should not be ingested while taking iron supplements.

## SICKLE CELL ANEMIA

Sickle cell anemia is a genetic mutation of the red blood cells. Normal red blood cells are round, but sickle cells are sickle-shaped. The condition occurs most predominantly in blacks. About 1 in every 400 African-Americans is born with sickle cell anemia. The disease becomes apparent after the child's first year.

Signs and symptoms include pain in the chest, joints, back, and abdomen that can range from mild to severe; swelling in the feet and hands; jaundice; kidney failure; repetitive infections; or gallstones or strokes at an early age.

There is currently no medication for treatment of sickle cell anemia. Treatment is aimed at prevention of complications and symptomatic relief. Analgesics, oxygen, and fluid replacement are recommended during painful episodes. Since individuals with sickle cell anemia are prone to pneumonia, vaccinations against pneumonia should be provided. Diet supplementation of folic acid can be useful. Recent attempts to cure sickle cell anemia through chemotherapy and bone marrow transplant have been successful on a limited basis.

## LYME DISEASE

Lyme disease first became known in 1975 when a large number of children in and around the town of Lyme, Connecticut, were being diagnosed with juvenile rheumatoid arthritis. Investigations uncovered deer ticks infected with a bacterium that were responsible for the outbreak of arthritis.

Symptoms of the disease occur as a red rash in the form of a small red spot at first that expands over the next few days or weeks. The rash usually occurs at the site of the tick bite; it is often a red ring surrounding a clear central area and can range from a dime in size to an area that covers the entire back. Additional symptoms can include typical flu-like symptoms such as fever, headache, stiff neck, body aches, and fatigue. If the disease is not recognized and is left untreated, additional symptoms that can occur later may include arthritis with swollen and painful joints; Bell's palsy; numbness, pain, or weakness of the limbs with poor motor coordination; an irregular heartbeat that can precipitate dizziness or shortness of breath; and less common problems such as hepatitis or severe fatigue. Therefore, early recognition is key.

The best method of preventing Lyme disease is to avoid deer ticks. Most people become infected during the summer when ticks are most prevalent and people are outside in wooded areas and grasslands where ticks are present. Walking in the center of trails and wearing long-sleeved shirts and long pants will reduce tick exposure, and use of tick and insect repellents can also help. Treatment of Lyme disease includes the use of antibiotics such as doxycycline or amoxicillin. The sooner treatment is initiated, the better and quicker the recovery.

# ASSESSMENT OF THE UNCONSCIOUS ATHLETE

There will likely be times in your career that you will come upon an athlete who is unconscious and the etiology of the condition is unknown. Although unconsciousness may be the consequence of a traumatic injury as noted in previous chapters, it may also result from a variety of general medical conditions and drug interactions. Therefore your assessment of an athlete who is unconscious for no known reason should proceed systematically to assess for life-threatening conditions and to identify potential signs and symptoms that may indicate the cause for unconsciousness. Most of the assessment techniques you will use in this general assessment of the unconscious athlete have been described in previous chapters. Therefore, in this section you will read about the general framework and be referred back to appropriate chapter(s) for the details. As you proceed through the various components of this evaluation, consider the variety of conditions you have learned about throughout this text that may result in unconsciousness and produce a positive sign.

## PRIMARY SURVEY

Your first goal is to assess for unconsciousness and life-threatening conditions by evaluating vital signs and determining whether severe bleeding is present. Attempt to arouse the athlete by calling his name. Check airway, breathing, and circulation for presence of respirations and pulse. Remember that you do not know the cause for the athlete's unconsciousness, so until you have ruled out cervical spine injury you must proceed in your assessment using spinal precautions (chapter 3). If pulse or breathing is absent, call EMS and begin cardiopulmonary resuscitation. There is no need to continue the evaluation. If respirations and pulse are present, check immediately for signs of severe bleeding; and if these are present, control before proceeding further.

## SECONDARY SURVEY

In your secondary survey, your goal is to continue to assess for life-threatening conditions and to look for signs that may provide a clue to the cause of the athlete's unconsciousness. However, considering the number of conditions that may cause abnormal findings, the primary goal is not so much to determine the nature of the injury or illness as it is to identify positive signs so that you can make appropriate decisions on referral and immediate emergency or first-aid care. Your primary assessment tools include a history from bystanders, observation, and palpation techniques.

### History

Obviously, the athlete who is unconscious will not be able to give you any information. However, you may gain valuable information about the history of the event or the athlete from the environment and or bystanders or both. As you look at the surroundings, check for any evidence that would indicate a traumatic event. Information from bystanders can be very helpful and can yield important clues. Ask bystanders if they have any idea what might have caused the athlete to become unconscious. Did they witness an accident or event that would indicate trauma, or was there no apparent trauma or injury mechanism? Did they note whether the loss of consciousness was gradual or rapid in onset? Sudden onset is common with such conditions as syncopal episodes, concussion, and epilepsy, whereas a gradual onset is characteristic with increasing intracranial hemorrhage, shock, heat illness, and diabetic coma. Ask how long the athlete has been unconscious. If bystanders observed the athlete lose consciousness, try to determine the level of consciousness or the behavior of the athlete beforehand and the activity the athlete was engaging in. In other words, was she confused or disoriented, or did she seem to be fine just prior to becoming unconscious? Did she complain of any pain, illness, or other symptoms before losing consciousness? Pain in the abdomen may be a clue to internal hemorrhage, and chest pain may indicate pathology of cardiorespiratory origin.

Finally, do any bystanders know the athlete well enough to know aspects of her medical history that may have been a contributing factor? For instance, does the athlete have diabetes or epilepsy? Has she lost consciousness before, and if so, what was the cause of the previous episode? Friends may also know whether the athlete is taking any medications or is abusing drugs or alcohol. The more information you can gain from bystanders, the more precisely you may be able to define the athlete's condition and the more information you will be able to provide to emergency medical personnel when they arrive.

### Inspection

The aim of your visual inspection is to note any observable signs that would indicate a life-threatening condition, as well as clues to the type of trauma or illness. As you approached the athlete, you might have already observed the head, neck, and extremities for deformities or unusual position. Note any unusual body posturing (decorticate or decerebrate rigidity, chapter 11) that would indicate head trauma or brain injury. If the athlete appears relaxed and in normal position, this is usually a good sign. Note any evidence of seizure activity and take the appropriate actions to protect the athlete from further injury.

Although you have already checked for presence of breathing, recheck respirations for presence, rate, depth, and rhythm. Are the respirations rapid and shallow (shock, syncope), or slow, shallow, and/or irregular (i.e., head injury)? Note any signs of respiratory distress such as wheezing or difficulty with air exchange. Chapters 11 and 12, as well as earlier sections of this chapter, covered conditions that could alter respirations.

Inspect the skin for temperature, coloration, and moisture. Is the skin hot and dry, which could indicate heat-related illness? Or is it cool, pale, and clammy, which might indicate shock and internal hemorrhage? Is the athlete cyanotic around the lips and face? This could indicate inadequate oxygenation.

Next, check pupils for size, equality, and reaction to light (chapter 11). An athlete who has simply fainted will have equal and reactive pupils. Pupils that are equal and dilated may be indicative of a grand mal seizure or shock. Pinpoint pupils are indicative of drug overdose. Dilation, inequality, or lack of reactivity of one pupil is indicative of a space-occupying brain lesion.

Inspect the mouth for bleeding and evidence of an unusual odor. Remember, the hyperglycemic athlete will have a sweet, fruity breath odor (see discussion of diabetes in this chapter). An athlete who has suffered a seizure may have bitten her tongue, and bleeding may be observable.

Inspect head to toe for evidence of trauma. Inspect first around the head, scalp, and neck for any swelling, deformity, or discoloration that would indicate a skull fracture or head injury. Check the ears and nose for rhinorrhea and otorrhea (chapter 11). Inspect for swelling, deformity, or discoloration of the chest wall, trunk, or abdomen that may indicate a rib fracture or underlying internal pathology (chapter 12). Lastly, inspect for swelling, deformity, or discoloration of the extremities. Although injuries to the extremities usually in themselves do not cause loss of consciousness, these signs may indicate the severity of trauma and other conditions (i.e., shock and internal injuries) that may have resulted.

If this inspection reveals any positive signs, call EMS at once.

### Palpation

You will use palpation to confirm the presence and strength of palpable vital signs and to check for evidence of trauma through a head-to-toe screen. First palpate the pulse for presence, rate, and strength. Also take and record blood pressure at this time. Hypertension and bradycardia may indicate intracranial hemorrhage (chapter 11), whereas a rapid, weak pulse and low blood pressure are indicative of shock and internal hemorrhage (chapter 12). The pulse will also be fast and weak secondary to a variety of medical conditions previously noted in this chapter.

After assessing vital signs, perform a head-to-toe evaluation. Palpate the head, neck, and scalp for deformity, crepitus, depressions, or swelling. Palpate the chest, trunk, and extremities for signs of deformity (fracture and dislocation), crepitus (fracture), unusual contours, and swelling that would indicate trauma. Palpate the abdomen for distension and rigidity to discern evidence of internal injury.

### Level of Consciousness

Finally, assess the depth of level of unconsciousness if this was not determined earlier in your assessment. You should reassess this, as well as vital signs, constantly throughout the evaluation to monitor for worsening or improvement in the athlete's condition. Use the Glasgow Coma Scale described in chapter 11 (page 360) to determine whether the athlete is drowsy, stuporous, or comatose. The state is one of drowsiness if the athlete can be aroused with verbal stimuli; it is one of stupor if he can be aroused with painful stimuli such as a pinch to the trapezius or the inner arm or thigh. If the athlete responds to no stimulus, either verbal or painful, he is said to be comatose.

### When to Refer

No special or functional tests are used in the assessment of the unconscious athlete, unless the athlete regains consciousness and one has a better sense of the cause. Your history, observation, and palpation should give you sufficient information for determining the need to summon EMS and provide emergency first aid. In almost all cases of unconsciousness, the athlete should be referred to a physician for evaluation. Immediate emergency referral is warranted in any of the following situations:

- The athlete fails to regain consciousness within a few minutes.
- The cause for the unconsciousness cannot be determined, even if consciousness is regained.
- Any abnormal vital signs are present.
- Any signs of serious or life-threatening injury or illness are noted.

## Checklist for the Assessment of an Unconscious Athlete

As with any emergency situation, you should begin your assessment with a *primary survey:*

✓ Attempt to arouse athlete; call name.

✓ Check airway (cervical spine precautions).

✓ Check breathing (look, listen, feel).

✓ Check circulation.

✓ Check for severe bleeding.

If you are able to rule out the necessity for immediate EMS, you may proceed to your *secondary survey:*

### History

Try to obtain from bystanders or the surroundings as much information as possible about the following:

✓ The cause (trauma vs. no apparent trauma)

✓ Whether loss of consciousness was gradual or rapid in onset

✓ Duration of unconsciousness

✓ Level of consciousness or behavior prior to loss of consciousness

✓ Any complaints made by the athlete prior to losing consciousness

✓ Any medical history that might have contributed

### Inspection

✓ Note position of head, neck, and extremities for deformities.

✓ Note any unusual body posturing (decerebrate or decorticate rigidity).

✓ Note presence of seizure and take appropriate action to protect the athlete.

✓ Determine presence of and note any irregularities in rate, depth, and rhythm of respirations.

✓ Inspect skin for temperature, coloration, and moisture.

✓ Check pupils for size, equality, and reaction to light.

✓ Check mouth for bleeding (seizures) or unusual odors (diabetes).

✓ Inspect for swelling, deformity, or discoloration around the head, neck, or scalp.

> ✓ Inspect for otorrhea and rhinorrhea.

✓ Inspect for swelling, deformity, or discoloration of the chest wall, trunk, and abdomen.

✓ Inspect for swelling, deformity, or discoloration of the extremities.

### Palpation

✓ Determine presence, rate, and strength of pulse.

✓ Take and record blood pressure.

✓ Palpate head, neck, and scalp for deformity, crepitus, and swelling.

✓ Palpate chest, trunk, and extremities for deformity, crepitus, and swelling.

✓ Palpate abdomen for distension and muscle rigidity.

### Assess Level of Unconsciousness (Glasgow Coma Scale)

> ✓ Drowsiness (athlete is aroused by verbal stimuli)

> ✓ Stupor (athlete is aroused by painful stimuli: pinch trapezius or inner arm or thigh)

> ✓ Coma (no response to any stimulus, verbal or painful)

### Functional Tests

✓ None

### Refer when any of the following occurs:

✓ Athlete does not regain consciousness.

✓ Cause for unconsciousness cannot be determined even if consciousness is regained.

✓ Any abnormal vital signs are present.

✓ Any positive signs are noted on exam.

# SUMMARY

1. *Describe the signs and symptoms of a variety of medical conditions that may be encountered in the physically active.*

   This chapter has dealt with a large number of common and less common medical conditions. Some of those presented are prevalent in youngsters and some are more prevalent in adults. The conditions covered arise from a spectrum of sources ranging from viral or bacterial infections to genetic dispositions.

2. *Appreciate the complications that may result from many of these conditions if not recognized and if left untreated.*

Many of the conditions referred to in this chapter may present serious, even life-threatening complications if not recognized and managed appropriately. Cardiovascular and respiratory conditions, some sexually transmitted diseases, severe eating disorders, and endocrine disorders are all examples of conditions that one must recognize in order to prevent serious complications or death.

3. *Determine which medical conditions require immediate, emergency medical referral and which require referral to a physician for diagnosis and treatment.*

It is the responsibility of the certified athletic trainer to be aware of the signs and symptoms of serious conditions so that he or she can make proper medical referral. An awareness of these conditions can facilitate an early diagnosis, prevent complications, and advance an effective and efficient recovery.

4. *Be able to perform an on-field assessment of an athlete who is unconscious and the etiology of the condition is unknown.*

There will be times when an athlete loses consciousness and there will be no knowledge of the etiology of the condition. Assessment of the unconscious athlete in this situation is designed to identify immediate life-threatening emergencies through both primary and secondary surveys and to identify clues to the cause of the unconsciousness. The primary survey is consistent with primary surveys in other situations, and the goal is to identify the status of airway, breathing, and circulation and evidence of severe bleeding. The secondary survey includes a history from the bystanders and the surroundings, as well as assessment of vital signs and a head-to-toe evaluation through observation and palpation.

# REVIEW QUESTIONS

1. Describe the appearance and signs and symptoms of the following skin conditions:
   - Cellulitis
   - Carbuncle
   - Herpes simplex I
   - Verruca vulgaris
   - Ringworm
   - Tinea cruris
   - Pediculosis
   - Eczema

2. Name at least four conditions that may result in ear pain. What are their signs and symptoms, and when should an athlete be referred to a physician for treatment?

3. Describe the differential signs and symptoms of influenza and the common cold. Under what circumstances, in relation to these conditions, should an athlete not be allowed to practice?

4. What causes bronchitis? How would you differentiate this condition from pneumonia?

5. What are the signs and symptoms of an acute asthma attack? How would you manage this condition initially, and when would you refer the athlete for medical care?

6. What are the physiological reasons for shock? Describe the various types of shock and the characteristic signs and symptoms.

7. What causes a syncopal episode? When should an athlete who has fainted be referred for a medical evaluation?

8. Describe the difference between a diabetic coma and insulin shock. What are the characteristic signs and symptoms of each?

9. Discuss the gastrointestinal disorders commonly seen in the physically active. What signs and symptoms would warrant physician referral?

10. Why is it difficult to evaluate an athlete with suspected anorexia nervosa? What signs and symptoms would cause you to suspect this condition?

11. What causes amenorrhea? What other conditions are commonly associated with amenorrhea, and what concerns might you have for an athlete with amenorrhea?

12. How is mononucleosis different from other viral conditions? What are the potential complications of "mono," and what signs or symptoms contraindicate physical activity?

13. What is the difference between a focalized and a generalized seizure? What are potential causes for seizure activity?

# CRITICAL THINKING QUESTIONS

1. An athlete comes to you complaining of pain and burning with urination. What conditions might you suspect, and what questions might you ask the athlete to help determine the cause for these symptoms?

2. A thorough medical history obtained during the preparticipation physical examination at the beginning of the year can provide valuable information regarding previous medical conditions that may resurface or impact physical activity. If you were asked to design a health history questionnaire, what questions would you include?

3. You notice an athlete standing on the sidelines who is leaning forward and appears to be having difficulty breathing. As you approach her, you can see the panicked look on her face and can hear wheezing. What condition(s) might you suspect, and how would your assessment proceed? What questions might be particularly important to ask this athlete that may aid in her immediate care?

4. You learn that an athlete on your team has IDDM. What potential complications might you expect with this condition? What strategies would you use to prepare for these complications, and what signs and symptoms would you look for?

5. A wrestler comes to you complaining of a rash on his skin. You know that a number of skin lesions are infectious and contagious. How would you go about evaluating this athlete, and what conditions would prohibit continued activity?

6. An athlete complains of a "rash" in his groin area. You can tell he is embarrassed and uncomfortable telling you this, but he was concerned enough that he needed to talk to someone. How would you deal with this athlete, and how would your assessment proceed to determine the need for medical referral?

# CITED REFERENCES

Caroline, N.L. 1995. *Emergency care in the streets*. 5th ed. Boston: Little, Brown.

National Athletic Trainers' Association. 1999. *Athletic training educational competencies*. 3rd ed. Dallas: National Athletic Trainers' Association.

Taber, C.W. 1997. *Taber's cyclopedic medical dictionary*. 18th ed. Philadelphia: F.A. Davis Co.

Tetzlaf, J. 1998. *A guide to breast health care*. Chicago: Budlong Press Co.

# ADDITIONAL RESOURCE

Hillman, S.K. 2000. *Introduction to athletic training*. Champaign, IL: Human Kinetics.

# GLOSSARY

**ABCs:** Airway, Breathing, and Circulation.

**ablation:** Surgical removal.

**abrasion:** Broad scraping or shearing off of superficial skin layers.

**abscess:** Localized collection of pus on any body part, caused by bacterial infection.

**accessory motion:** Subtle gliding movement that occurs within and between the joint's inert structures. Usually accessed with joint mobility tests. Also known as joint play.

**acidosis:** Excess accumulation of acid in the blood caused by cardiorespiratory compromise.

**active ROM:** Voluntary movement of a joint through a range of motion without assistance.

**acute:** Of sudden onset and of short duration, typically resulting from a one-time event or mechanism.

**adenoiditis:** Inflammation of the glandular lymph tissue at the back of the pharynx.

**adhesive capsulitis:** When an inflamed capsule develops adhesions and subsequent contractures causing severe limitations in range of motion.

**alveolar process:** The part of the maxilla or mandible that contains the tooth socket.

**amenorrhea:** Absence or cessation of menses.

**amnesia:** Loss of memory.

**analgesic:** Pain-reducing agent.

**anaphylactic shock:** Shock that occurs as a hypersensitivity reaction to an allergen.

**anesthesia:** Absence of sensation.

**ankylosed:** Refers to fusion or fixation of a joint.

**annulus fibrosis:** Outer covering of the intervertebral disc that acts to withstand tension and prevent distortion of disc material.

**anterograde amnesia:** Loss of an athlete's immediate memory and ability to recall events that have occurred since the injury.

**anteversion:** Excessive anterior angulation of the femoral head resulting in a toe-in gait.

**anticholinergic:** Medication to block the action of the neurotransmitter acetylcholine to relax smooth muscle.

**antiemetic:** Drugs that control nausea and vomiting.

**antipyretic:** Fever-reducing agent.

**ape hand deformity:** Deformity characterized by extension of the thumb and alignment in the same plane as the fingers.

**apnea:** Absence of breathing.

**apophysitis:** Inflammation of a bony projection or outgrowth serving as a muscle attachment.

**apparent leg length discrepancy:** A measurement difference when taken from the umbilicus to the left and right medial malleolus.

**apprehension sign:** When a person reacts to or limits motion due to a fear or sensation of impending joint dislocation or stress.

**approximation:** To bring two structures near or in contact with one another.

**arachnoid mater:** A delicate, transparent membrane that forms the intermediate covering of the brain.

**arcade of Frohse:** A fibrous band located at the proximal edge of the supinator muscle near the edge of the extensor carpi radialis brevis and radial capitellar joint.

**arrhythmia:** Disturbance or irregularity in the rhythm of the heart.

**assessment:** A procedure through which an athletic trainer determines the severity, irritability, nature, and stage of an injury.

**asymmetrical hypertrophy:** Enlargement of the muscle of the ventricular septum and left ventricular walls. Also referred to as idiopathic hypertrophic subaortic stenosis.

**atrophy:** Wasting away or decrease in the size of a muscle or other tissue or organ.

**auscultation:** Listening for abdominal and thoracic sounds with a stethoscope.

**avascular necrosis:** Tissue death resulting from a lack of blood supply.

**avulsion:** Forceful tearing away of a part or structure such as bone, skin, or tendon.

**axonotmesis:** Partial disruption of a nerve.

**Babinski sign:** Dorsiflexion of the great toe and splaying of the lesser toes with stroking of the plantar surface, indicative of a lower brain stem injury.

**Bartholin glands:** Small mucous glands located on the lateral walls of the vagina near the vaginal opening.

**baseball finger:** Rupture of the extensor digitorum longus tendon from the distal phalanx. Also referred to as mallet finger.

**Battle's sign:** Discoloration behind the ears.

**benediction deformity:** Wasting of the hypothenar, dorsal interossei, and fourth and fifth lumbrical muscles resulting from ulnar nerve palsy. Also known as bishop's deformity.

**bilateral comparison:** Comparison of an injured side with an uninjured side.

**bishop's deformity:** Wasting of the hypothenar, dorsal interossei, and fourth and fifth lumbrical muscles resulting from ulnar nerve palsy. Also known as benediction deformity.

**blister:** Separation and accumulation of fluid or blood between superficial skin layers.

**blood pressure:** Tension exerted against the arterial walls when the heart is pumping (systolic) and when at rest (diastolic).

**blow-out fracture:** Fracture of the orbital floor occurring as a result of a sudden increase in orbital pressure from a direct blow to the eye.

**blow-out injury:** An injury occurring from a hard blow to the chest while the glottis is closed, which results in rupturing of the alveoli.

**boil:** Localized infection of skin, gland, or hair follicle. Also known as furuncle.

**bolus:** Rapid administration of an injectable medication.

**bone spur:** Bony outgrowth.

**Bouchard's nodes:** Nodules or bony enlargement of the proximal interphalangeal joints of the hand.

**boutonniere deformity:** Deformity characterized by flexion of the PIP joint and hyperextension of the DIP joint most often resulting from injury to the central slip of the extensor digitorum tendon at its insertion at the base of the middle phalanx.

**boxer's fracture:** A fracture specifically involving the neck of the fifth metatarsal.

**brawny edema:** Leathery hardening or thickening of tissue due to chronic inflammation.

**break test:** An efficient test for strength obtained by applying isometric resistance while the joint is in a neutral midrange position.

**Brudzinski test:** A test used to determine nerve root irritation, meningeal irritation, or dural irritation by flexing the hip.

**bulimarexia:** Eating disorder characterized by both anorexic and bulimic behaviors.

**burners:** Nerve injury (usually brachial plexus) with classic symptoms of immediate sharp, burning pain radiating down the distal extremity.

**bursa:** Synovial-filled membrane that lies between adjacent structures to limit friction and ease movement.

**bursitis:** Inflammation or swelling of a bursa.

**burst fracture:** Fracture of the C1 vertebra. Also known as a Jefferson fracture.

**calcaneal exostosis:** A condition characterized by excess calcium formation resulting in increased prominence of the posterior calcaneus, commonly referred to as pump bump.

**capsular pattern:** A pattern of limited joint motion that is unique to each joint, resulting from restriction in the joint capsule.

**capsular restriction:** A restriction in joint range of motion due to capsular adhesions or scarring.

**capsulitis:** Inflammation of the joint capsule.

**cardiac tamponade:** Hemorrhage within the enclosed and inelastic pericardial cavity.

**cardiogenic shock:** A condition characterized by inadequate blood flow and cardiovascular system collapse due to inadequate cardiac output.

**carpal tunnel syndrome:** A condition of the wrist and hand characterized by compression of the median nerve as it passes through the carpal tunnel.

**cauda equina:** The terminal portion of the spinal cord.

**cauda equina syndrome:** Compression of the terminal portion of the spinal cord usually caused by a central disc herniation resulting in bowel and bladder dysfunction.

**caudal:** Away from the head.

**cephalad:** Toward the head.

**cervical radiculitis:** Pain referred down the arm from cervical nerve root compression.

**chalazia:** A sebaceous cystlike tumor on the eyelid.

**chancre:** A sore or ulcer.

**Cheyne-Stokes respiration:** Breathing pattern characterized by a rhythmic fluctuation between hyperpnea and apnea.

**chronic:** A condition of gradual onset and of prolonged duration usually resulting from an accumulation of minor insults or repetitive stress.

**chronic instability:** Abnormal joint laxity due to permanent slackening of a joint ligament and/or capsule.

**clonus:** A very brisk and exaggerated reflex response.

**closed chain:** A segment where the distal end is fixed or in contact with the ground.

**closed wound:** An injury that does not involve disruption of the skin surface.

**comminuted:** To break into pieces or multiple fragments.

**comparable sign:** A positive response indicating either a reproduction of the athlete's symptoms or an alteration of the symptoms.

**compartment syndrome:** A significant rise in intracompartmental pressure caused by severe bleeding within a muscular compartment that can compromise neurovascular structures.

**compound dislocation:** An injury in which a displaced joint penetrates the skin surface so that the bone is exposed.

**compound fracture:** An injury in which a displaced fracture penetrates the skin surface so that the bone is exposed.

**compression:** To squeeze or press together.

**compression force:** Placing direct pressure on a surface or soft tissue.

**concussion:** A transient alteration in brain function without structural damage caused by an agitation or shaking of the brain.

**condylomata acuminata:** Genital warts.

**conjunctivitis:** An irritation and inflammation of the outer surface of the eye or inner eyelid, more commonly known as pinkeye.

**contrecoup-type injury:** An injury occurring when the moving head makes contact with an immovable or more slowly moving object. Also referred to as a deceleration injury.

**contusion:** The compression of soft tissue by a direct blow or impact sufficient to cause disruption or damage to the small capillaries in the tissue, commonly referred to as a bruise.

**costochondritis:** Inflammation of the costochondral junction.

**coup-type injury:** An injury in which the brain is traumatized at the location of impact when the head is stationary and is struck by a moving object.

**coxa valga:** Femoral neck angulation >135 degrees.

**coxa vara:** Femoral neck angulation <120 degrees.

**Cram test:** Another name for the bowstring test.

**cretinism:** Hyperthyroidism in the very young, resulting in stunted growth, sparse hair growth, improperly developed reproductive organs, and mental retardation.

**cubital tunnel syndrome:** A term that collectively describes ulnar neuropathy and compression at the elbow.

**cubital valgus:** Excessive valgus angulation of the extended elbow.

**cubital varus:** A decreased valgus angulation or actual varus angulation of the extended elbow. Also referred to as gunstock deformity.

**cyanosis:** A bluish or purplish discoloration of the skin due to deficient oxygenation of the blood.

**De Quervain's disease:** Tenosynovitis of the abductor pollicis longus and extensor pollicis brevis tendons and their sheaths on the radial side of the thumb.

**debride:** To clean a wound of infectious or foreign substances in an effort to promote healing and restore healthy tissue.

**decerebrate posturing:** A rigid extension of all four extremities with the arms internally rotated and pronated, which is a sign of upper brain stem injury.

**decorticate posturing:** A rigid extension of the legs and flexion of the arms, wrist, and hands toward the chest.

**deep tendon reflex:** An involuntary muscle contraction in response to a tendon tap.

**degenerative:** Chronic deterioration of a joint or tissue structure over time.

**dental caries:** Cavities.

**dermatome:** An area of skin innervated by a single spinal nerve root.

**diabetic coma:** Unconsciousness due to a lack of insulin. Also referred to as hyperglycemic shock.

**differential diagnosis:** An evaluation to rule out the involvement of other joints or regions as the cause for the symptoms.

**diplopia:** Double vision.

**dislocation:** Complete disassociation or displacement of one joint surface on another.

**distraction:** An assessment or mobilization technique where longitudinal force is applied to a joint to separate opposing joint structures.

**drop arm test:** A test that assesses the integrity of the rotator cuff.

**dura mater:** The outermost covering of the brain consisting of a tough fibrous tissue that serves as the inner lining of the skull and provides protection to the brain.

**dyspepsia:** Either improper digestion or deficient absorption of food in the digestive tract.

**dysphasia:** Pain with swallowing.

**dyspnea:** Difficulty breathing.

**dystrophy:** Muscular disorder characterized by weakness and fibrosis.

**ecchymosis:** Discoloration of tissue.

**embolism:** Obstruction of a blood vessel by a blood clot.

**end feel:** The quality of the feel or sensation felt by the evaluator when pressure is applied to the joint at the end of the range of motion.

**eosinophils:** Leukocytes or other granulocytes that are released secondary to an allergen or a parasitic infection.

**epicondylitis:** An overuse injury to the tendinous attachments of the flexor/pronator group at the medial epicondyle or the extensor/supinator group at the lateral epicondyle. Also referred to as "tennis elbow."

**epidural hematoma:** A tear in the middle meningeal artery resulting in a rapidly expanding hematoma in the epidural space.

**epidural space:** The space between the skull and dura mater.

**epiphysis:** A secondary ossification center or growth plate.

**Epstein-Barr virus:** A member of the herpes group of viruses, which is the source of most cases of infectious mononucleosis, or "mono."

**erythema:** Redness of the skin.

**evaluation:** The systematic process used to assess an athlete's or patient's condition.

**exercise-induced asthma:** Asthma that occurs during exercise.

**exostosis:** Excess calcium formation resulting in increased prominence of a bone surface.

**expectorant:** A drug used to increase flow and decrease the viscosity of mucus in the respiratory passageway.

**extension:** Movement that decreases the angle of a joint.

**extensor lag:** Inability to fully extend the knee during active motion, but full passive motion is present.

**extracranial:** Outside the skull.

**extrusion:** Avulsion or disassociation of a tooth from the tooth socket.

**Faber (Flexion, Abduction, External Rotation) test:** Also known as the Patrick test or Jansen's test.

**fasciculation:** Involuntary contraction of muscle fibers innervated by a single motor unit.

**fatigue:** A reduced capacity to do work.

**faun's beard:** A hairy patch overlying the lumbar spine, indicative of spina bifida occulta.

**femoral hernia:** A condition occurring when the abdominal viscera protrude through the femoral ring and into the femoral canal just inferior to the inguinal ligament.

**fibular:** Peroneal.

**fibularis:** Peroneus.

**first-degree:** An injury classification characterized by mild tissue disruption and disability.

**flail chest injury:** An injury characterized by multiple fractures of three or more adjacent ribs.

**flatfoot:** A condition caused by hypermobility resulting from increased ligament laxity and muscle weakness on the plantar surface of the foot. Also known as pes planus.

**flexibility:** The degree of pliability or adaptability of a muscle, tendon, or joint.

**flexion:** Movement that increases the angle of the joint.

**forearm splints:** Periostitis occurring in the forearm.

**forefoot:** Composed of the tarsometatarsal, intermetatarsal, metatarsophalangeal, and interphalangeal joints.

**Fowler test:** The relocation test used to assess anterior instability. Also known as the Jobe relocation test.

**fracture:** Disruption or break in the continuity of a bone.

**fulcrum test:** A test that assesses the possibility of a femoral stress fracture.

**functional deformity:** Deformity that does not involve permanent structural changes and typically results from mechanical dysfunction.

**furuncle:** An infection of the hair follicle. Also known as boil.

**gamekeeper's thumb:** Ulnar collateral ligament rupture of the first metacarpophalangeal joint. Also known as "skier's thumb."

**ganglion:** A cyst that is characterized by herniation of synovial fluid through the joint capsule or synovial sheath of a tendon. Also known as a synovial cyst.

**gapping test:** Stress test for the anterior sacroiliac ligaments.

**genu recurvatum:** Excessive knee hyperextension.

**genu valgus:** Lateral angulation of the tibia relative to the femur.

**genu varum:** Medial angulation of the tibia relative to the femur.

**gingivitis:** Inflammation of the gums that results from the presence of bacteria typically caused by food deposits and inadequate brushing or flossing.

**glide force:** A force applied to the joint where the distal surface is moved in a straight (transverse) plane on the proximal joint surface.

**gluteus medius lurch:** A drop of the non-weight-bearing pelvis and hip during its swing-through phase. Also known as Trendelenburg gait.

**goiter:** Enlargement of the thyroid gland.

**golfer's elbow:** Also known as medial epicondylitis.

**gunstock deformity:** A carrying angle less than the normal 5° or 15° valgus angulation. Also known as cubital varus.

**heartburn:** A condition in which the acid from the stomach enters the esophagus.

**Heberden's nodes:** Nodules or bony enlargement of the distal interphalangeal joints of the hand.

**heel spur:** A bony outgrowth on the anterior inferior surface of the calcaneus due to tractioning of the plantar fascia.

**hematocele:** Rapid blood accumulation within the membrane surrounding the testicle.

**hematuria:** Blood in the urine.

**hemipelvis:** A condition in which one side of the pelvis is smaller than the other.

**herniation:** Development of a protruding structure (e.g., vertebral disc) or organ (e.g., intestine) through its outer wall or cavity where it is contained.

**Hibbs' test:** A test of the posterior sacroiliac ligaments. Also known as the posterior distraction test.

**high blood pressure:** A condition involving an elevated systolic (>140mmHg) and/or diastolic (>90mmHg) blood pressure associated with generalized arteriolar vasoconstriction. Also known as hypertension.

**hindfoot:** Composed of the distal tibiofibular (syndesmosis), talocrural (tibia, fibula, and talus), and subtalar (talus, calcaneus, navicular) joints.

**hip anteversion:** Excessive anterior angulation of the femoral neck that results in a toe-in gait.

**hip pointer:** A contusion to the iliac crest.

**hip retroversion:** Decreased anterior angulation of the femoral neck producing a toe-out gait.

**histamine:** Chemical substance found in the blood that, when released, causes dilatation and increased permeability of blood vessels.

**hydrocele:** Fluid accumulation within the membrane surrounding the testicle.

**hyperemia:** Redness of the eye.

**hyperesthesia:** Heightened or increased sensitivity to sensory stimuli.

**hyperglycemic:** A condition that occurs if there is too little insulin and glucose levels are elevated above normal levels. Also known as high blood sugar.

**hyperglycemic shock:** Shock induced by a lack of insulin (abnormally high blood sugar). Also referred to as diabetic coma.

**hyperkinesis:** Abnormal increase in movement or purposeless muscle movement.

**hypermobility:** Excessive motions in one or more planes.

**hyperpnea:** Rapid, deep breathing.

**hypertension:** Elevated blood pressure, usually considered when pressure is greater than 140/90 mmHg.

**hypertrophy:** An increase in the size of a muscle or other tissue or organ.

**hyphema:** An accumulation of blood in the anterior chamber of the eye.

**hypoesthesia:** Diminished sensation.

**hypoglycemia:** Low blood sugar.

**hypovolemic shock:** A condition that occurs as the result of decreased blood volume in the circulatory system.

**hypoxia:** Lack of oxygen.

**imperforate:** Lacking the usual or normal opening.

**incision:** A full thickness cut in the skin by a sharp object or instrument, resulting in smooth, even wound edges.

**infarction:** Necrosis of tissue or organ from obstruction of local blood flow.

**inguinal hernia:** Protrusion of the small intestine through the inguinal canal or abdominal wall.

**instability:** Abnormal or excessive joint laxity or excursion.

**insulin shock:** Shock resulting from a severe hypoglycemic reaction resulting from an overdose of insulin.

**intra-articular:** Within the joint capsule.

**intracranial:** Within the skull or cranium.

**intrathecal:** Within the spinal canal.

**intrusion:** A condition in which the tooth is driven into the socket.

**ischemia:** Tissue anemia caused by a lack of blood flow to an area.

**Jansen's test:** A test used to identify limited mobility of the hip, also known as the Patrick test or Faber (Flexion, Abduction, External Rotation) test.

**jersey finger:** Rupture of the flexor digitorum longus tendon form the distal phalanx of the finger.

**Jobe relocation test:** Test used to assess anterior instability. Also known as the Fowler test.

**jock itch:** A fungal infection in the groin region. Also known as tinea cruris.

**joint mice:** Loose fragments within the joint.

**joint mobilization:** A passive evaluation of joint movement to assess the capsular structures of the joint.

**joint play:** Accessory motion.

**Jones' fracture:** A fracture of the base of the fifth metatarsal usually caused by tractioning of the peroneus brevis tendon.

**Kehr's sign:** A sign characterized by pain radiating into the left shoulder and partially down the arm, usually indicative of a spleen injury.

**Kernig test:** A test in which the neck is flexed to determine nerve root irritation, meningeal irritation, or dural irritation.

**kyphosis:** Excess posterior convexity of the thoracic spine.

**laceration:** Tearing of the skin resulting in jagged, uneven wound edges.

**Lachman-Trillat test:** Another name for the Lachman test. Also known as the Ritchie test or the Trillat test.

**Liségue's test:** Another name for the straight leg raise test.

**Little League elbow:** A valgus traction force injury of the medial elbow that may start out as an inflammatory response or apophysitis and progress to an avulsion of the apophysis if the repetitive stress continues.

**loose-packed position:** Positioning of the joint where the ligaments are at their resting length and under the least amount of tension.

**lordosis:** Excessive anterior convexity of the cervical and lumbar spine.

**lower motor neuron:** Peripheral motor nerves that originate in the spinal cord and innervate skeletal muscle.

**lung collapse:** A reduction in lung volume. Also know as a pneumothorax.

**luxation:** Complete disassociation of two joint surfaces. Also referred to as dislocation.

**macule:** A non-raised patch of skin with altered color.

**malaise:** A vague, general feeling of illness or fatigue.

**malingering:** Pretending to be injured.

**mallet finger:** Avulsion of the extensor digitorum longus from the distal phalanx. Also known as baseball finger.

**mallet finger test:** A common name for the extensor tendon avulsion test.

**malocclusion:** An inability to approximate the upper and lower jaw or teeth in a normal bite.

**manual muscle test:** A graded strength test performed by applying manual resistance to a segment to evaluate a particular muscle or muscle group.

**McIntosh test:** Also known as the lateral pivot shift maneuver.

**meninges:** The three layers that cover the brain and spinal cord.

**metabolic shock:** Cardiovascular collapse secondary to a loss of body fluid as a consequence of illness that causes diarrhea, excessive urination, or vomiting.

**metastasis:** The spread of malignant cells through the lymphatic system from one body part to another.

**metatarsalgia:** A general term used to describe metatarsal pain. Also used as a term for Morton's neuroma.

**midfoot:** Composed of the talocalcaneonavicular, cuneonavicular, intercuneiform, and calcaneocuboid joints.

**miserable malalignment syndrome:** Another name for patellofemoral pain syndrome.

**mosaic warts:** Warts clustered in groups.

**motor tests:** Tests used to assess neuromuscular integrity and muscle strength.

**muscle fasciculations:** Involuntary muscle contractions that occur secondary to injury or pain, involving only a few muscle fibers innervated by one motor unit.

**muscle spasm:** Involuntary muscle contraction involving the entire muscle, which occurs secondary to injury, fatigue, or pain.

**muscle tremors:** Involuntary muscle contractions involving several motor units, which occur secondary to injury or pain.

**myositis:** Inflammation of a muscle or its connective tissue.

**myositis ossificans:** A condition that occurs when the body's inflammatory response during absorption of a hematoma causes calcification or bony deposits to form in the muscle.

**myotome:** A muscle or muscle group that is innervated by a single nerve root.

**myxedema:** A condition that occurs secondary to chronic hypothyroidism marked by drowsiness, cold body temperature, and possible coma.

**Nelaton's line:** A line from the ischial tuberosity to the ipsilateral ASIS used to determine congenital hip dislocations.

**neuralgia:** Ache or pain along the distribution of a nerve.

**neurogenic shock:** A condition that occurs when there is damage to the spinal cord and the nerves that innervate smooth muscle, resulting in loss of vascular tone.

**neuroma:** Thickening of a nerve or "nerve tumor" secondary to chronic irritation and inflammation.

**neuropathy:** A general term to describe any pathological condition of the nerve.

**neuropraxia:** Transient or temporary loss in nerve function.

**neurotmesis:** Complete severance of a nerve.

**nociceptor:** Pain receptor.

**nursemaid's elbow:** Subluxation or dislocation of the radioulnar joint, where the radial head is pulled down into and becomes caught in the annular ligament.

**nystagmus:** Involuntary lateral oscillatory movement of the eyes.

**objective:** A sign or symptom that is perceptible to other persons or is measurable.

**observation:** A visual recording or assessment.

**open chain:** A segment where the distal end is not fixed or in contact with the ground.

**open wound:** An injury that involves a disruption in the continuity of the skin.

**orthostatic hypotension:** A condition in which the blood pressure drops when a person suddenly moves to a standing position.

**osteochondral:** Referring to bone (osteo) and cartilage (chondral).

**osteochondritis dissecans:** Avascular necrosis of a joint's articular surface.

**osteochondrosis:** Alterations and degenerative changes of the subchondral bone. Precursor to osteochondritis dissecans.

**osteophyte:** A bone spur or bony outgrowth.

**otorrhea:** Fluid draining from the ears.

**overpressure:** An application of pressure at the end of a joint's physiological motion to assess end feel and ligamentous integrity.

**overuse injury:** An injury due to repetitive microtrauma that often follows periods of inadequate rest or recovery, overactivity, or repetitive overloading of a structure.

**pallor:** Loss of skin coloration due to decreased blood flow.

**palpation:** A skilled evaluation using the sense of touch to identify soft tissue or bony abnormalities.

**papule:** A small raised bump on the skin that may or may not be painful.

**paresthesia:** Impaired or altered sensation such as a tingling, burning, or numbing.

**parietal pleura:** The outer wall of the pleural sac that adheres to the external wall of the pleural cavity.

**pars interarticularis:** The region of bone between the superior and inferior articular facets.

**passive ROM:** Movement of a joint through a range of motion by someone other than the person being assessed.

**pediculosis capitis:** A parasitic infection of the hair on the head, caused by the head louse.

**pediculosis corporis:** A parasitic infection of the body, caused by the body louse.

**pediculosis pubis:** A parasitic infection in the pubic region, caused by the crab louse.

**periodontitis:** Loss of alveolar bone and recession of the gum line due to bacteria. Also known as pyorrhea.

**periosteum:** The fibrous membrane covering the bone.

**periostitis:** Inflammation of the outer lining of the bone (periosteum).

**pes cavus:** An abnormally high or excessive arch.

**pes planus:** An abnormally low or absent arch. Also known as "flatfoot."

**photophobia:** Sensitivity to light.

**physiological motion:** The active motion of the joint that occurs in the planes of motion. Flexion, extension, adduction, abduction, and rotation are examples of physiological motions.

**pia mater:** The inner meningeal membrane of the brain.

**pitting edema:** Soft tissue swelling that results in skin depression after pressure is released.

**popliteal pressure test:** Another name for the bow-string test.

**Pott's fracture:** Avulsion fracture of the medial malleolus and shear fracture of the lateral malleolus.

**primary assessment/survey:** The initial evaluation aimed at the assessment of immediate life-threatening conditions.

**prolapse:** A bulge or weakening of a structure (e.g., disc bulge).

**pronation:** To rotate downward. In the foot, this represents a composite of three motions: eversion, dorsiflexion, and abduction in the open chain; in the closed chain, eversion, plantar flexion, and abduction, which occur at the joint. In the forearm, this represents turning the hand downward or posteriorly.

**proprioception:** Awareness of position or movement of the body or a body segment.

**prostaglandins:** Fatty acids that perform a variety of hormone functions.

**protrusion:** A condition of being thrust forward or projecting outward.

**psychogenic shock:** A transient condition of shock that results in fainting due to fear, anxiety, or emotional stress that causes a sudden involuntary nervous system reaction, vasodilation, and pooling of blood in the peripheral blood vessels.

**pulmonary embolism:** Obstruction of the pulmonary artery usually due to a thrombus (blood clot) in the lower extremity breaking loose.

**pulse:** A palpable and rhythmic throbbing or wave in the arteries caused by contractions of the heart.

**pump bump:** Increased prominence of the posterior calcaneal tuberosity. Also known as a calcaneal exostosis.

**puncture:** A small hole or wound caused by a sharp, penetrating object.

**purulent:** Containing or consisting of pus.

**pyorrhea:** Loss of alveolar bone and recession of the gum line as a result of bacteria. Also known as periodontitis.

**quadrant position:** Placement of a spinal segment in lateral flexion, extension, and rotation to the same side as the symptoms.

**raccoon eyes:** Discoloration around the eyes caused by skull fracture.

**radiculitis:** Referred pain secondary to nerve root compression.

**rales:** A crackling, popping, or bubbling sound heard with auscultation of the lungs.

**Reagan's test:** A test to assess lunate instability. Also known as the lunatotriquetral ballottement test.

**reflex:** An involuntary muscle contraction in response to a stimulus (e.g., tendon tap).

**renal colic:** Extreme pain that starts in the flank or back and radiates across the abdomen into the groin, genitalia, and inner thigh.

**respirations:** Rhythmic breathing or air exchange in and out of the lungs.

**respiratory alkalosis:** A deficiency of carbonic acid in the blood caused by excessive elimination of $CO_2$.

**retrograde amnesia:** Loss of memory and inability to recall events before the traumatic event.

**retroversion:** Decreased anterior angulation of the femoral neck resulting in a toe-out gait.

**rhinorrhea:** Fluid draining from the nose.

**rhonchi:** A loud whooshing sound heard with auscultation of the lungs, indicating mucus in the bronchi.

**Ritchie test:** Another name for the Lachman test. Also known as the Lachman-Trillat test or the Trillat test.

**rubeola:** A highly contagious viral infection. Also known as measles.

**Ryder method:** Test used to identify retroversion and anteversion of the hip. Also known as Craig's test.

**salpingitis:** A serious complication of sexually transmitted diseases in which a bacterial infection attacks the female reproductive system, spreading from the vagina to the womb, fallopian tubes, and ovaries. More commonly known as pelvic inflammatory disease (PID).

**scapular winging:** A protrusion of the vertebral border of the scapula away from the posterior chest wall as a result of serratus anterior muscle weakness.

**sciatica:** Referred pain down the lower extremity along the sciatic nerve distribution.

**scoliosis:** A lateral or "S" curvature of the spinal column.

**second-degree:** An injury classification used to describe moderate tissue disruption and disability.

**second-impact syndrome:** An autoregulatory dysfunction of the brain that causes rapid and fatal brain swelling, usually a result of a secondary brain insult that is often minor.

**septic shock:** A condition that results in severe dilation of the blood vessels and cardiovascular system collapse in response to bacterial infections.

**sequelae:** The progressive course of a pathological condition.

**sequestration:** Separation. Describes an advanced stage of disc herniation where the inner disc material becomes separated from the annulus fibrosis.

**serous fluid:** Watery fluid that moistens surface membranes.

**shear force:** A force that is directed parallel to a joint or soft tissue surface.

**shinsplints:** A general term used to describe pain and inflammation of the musculotendinous unit and/or periosteum along the anteromedial border of the tibia. Also known as medial tibial stress syndrome.

**shock:** A condition of inadequate peripheral blood flow, secondary to trauma, that results in cardiovascular collapse.

**sign:** Evidence of injury that is observed or can be objectively measured.

**silver fork deformity:** Dorsal displacement of the distal fragments of the radius and ulna in relation to their proximal shafts; characteristic deformity of a Colles's fracture.

**SINS:** Stage, Irritability, Nature, and Severity of an injury.

**skier's thumb:** Ulnar collateral ligament rupture of the first metacarpophalangeal joint. Also known as "gamekeeper's thumb."

**SOAP notes:** Documentation of **S**ubjective findings, **O**bjective findings, overall **A**ssessment, and subsequent **P**lan for the athlete based on an assessment.

**spasm:** Involuntary muscle contraction.

**Speed's test:** A test used to examine the integrity of the biceps tendon.

**spina bifida occulta:** A congenital malformation of the lumbar spine characterized by incomplete closure of the posterior lamina at birth.

**spinal stenosis:** A developmental or congenital narrowing of the spinal canal.

**spondylitis:** An inflammation of the facet joint and its surrounding capsule.

**spondylolisthesis:** A secondary condition to bilateral spondylolysis, characterized by a forward subluxation of the involved vertebrae in relation to the vertebrae directly below.

**spondylolysis:** A fracture of pars interarticularis located between the inferior and superior facets.

**spondylosis:** Degenerative changes of the vertebrae and disc.

**sprain:** Stretching or tearing of a ligament or capsular structure.

**Sprengel's deformity:** A deformity characterized by an underdeveloped scapula that sits high on the posterior chest wall, caused by a failure of the scapula to descend properly.

**Spurling's test:** Cervical compression with the neck in extension and rotation to the involved side.

**stability:** Maintenance of equilibrium or relationship of joint structures with an imposed force.

**Stener lesion:** A complication of ulnar collateral ligament injury of the thumb in which the adductor aponeurosis gets caught between the ruptured ends of the ligament and prevents healing.

**stenotic:** Marked or characterized by narrowing of a tunnel or canal.

**stingers:** Common name for brachial plexus injuries with the classic symptoms of immediate sharp, burning pain radiating down into the arm.

**stone bruise:** Heel contusion.

**strain:** Stretching or tearing of a muscle or tendon.

**stress test:** A method of applying force to a structure to evaluate its integrity.

**structural deformity:** Deformity characterized by permanent structural changes in the bone or joint, which are usually congenital.

**sty:** An infection or obstruction of a ciliary gland of the eyelid.

**subacute:** Interim between acute and chronic, usually referring to later stages of the inflammatory process.

**subarachnoid space:** Space between the arachnoid mater and the pia mater that contains cerebral spinal fluid.

**subdural hematoma:** Bleeding in the subdural space.

**subdural space:** Space between the arachnoid mater and the dura mater.

**subjective:** Information gained from a person's impression or perception; not readily observed.

**subluxation:** An incomplete disassociation of two joint surfaces.

**sulcus sign:** A depression in the skin below the acromion with distraction of the glenohumeral joint.

**supination:** To rotate upward. In the foot, this represents a composite of three motions: inversion, plantar flexion, and adduction of the foot in the open chain; inversion, dorsiflexion, and adduction in the closed chain, which occur at the joint. In the forearm, the motion represents turning the hand upward or anteriorly.

**swan-neck deformity:** A deformity caused by hyperextension at the PIP joint and hyperflexion at the DIP joint due to disruption of the volar plate and tensioning of the flexor tendons.

**sympathomimetic:** A group of medications that mimic the actions of the sympathetic nervous system to cause vasoconstriction and open respiratory passageways.

**symptom:** A subjective complaint or an abnormal sensation described by the patient that cannot be directly observed.

**syncope:** Fainting or temporary loss of consciousness caused by inadequate blood flow to the brain.

**synovial fluid:** Fluid secreted by the synovial membrane to provide joint lubrication.

**tachycardia:** Rapid pulse.

**tachypnea:** Presence of rapid respirations.

**talotibial exostosis:** Excess bone growth on the anterior dome of the talus or distal tibia.

**tendinitis** (tendonitis): Inflammation of a tendon.

**tennis elbow:** An overuse injury to the tendinous attachments of the flexor/pronator group at the medial epicondyle or the extensor/supinator group at the lateral epicondyle. Also known as epicondylitis.

**tenosynovitis:** Inflammation of the synovial sheath covering a tendon.

**tensile force:** Traction or pulling away of a structure.

**tension pneumothorax:** A condition in which lung collapse and increasing pressure in the pleural cavity causes the mediastinum to shift away from the injured side, compressing the heart and healthy lung and compromising their function.

**theater sign:** Anterior knee pain that is exacerbated by ambulation after prolonged sitting.

**third-degree:** Injury classification used to describe severe, complete tissue disruption and disability.

**thoracic outlet syndrome** (TOS): A clinical term that describes compression of the neurovascular structures as they exit through the thoracic outlet at the base of the neck.

**thrombus:** Blood clot.

**tibial varum:** Medial angulation or bowing of the tibia.

**tinea corporis:** A fungus that affects the scalp, trunk, and upper extremities. Also known as ringworm.

**Tinel's sign:** Pain or radiation of symptoms reproduced with percussion or "tapping" over a nerve.

**tinnitus:** Ringing in the ears.

**tonic:** Refers to a sustained contraction of muscle.

**torticollis:** A deformity characterized by a lateral curvature of the cervical spine.

**traction:** Application of a longitudinal force to a joint to separate the proximal from the distal portion.

**transient neuropraxia:** Temporary sensory changes such as burning, tingling, or numbness, and/or motor changes (weakness to temporary paralysis) in both the upper and lower extremities as a result of spinal cord compression.

**transverse:** Horizontal orientation or at a right angle to the long axis of a structure of body.

**tremor:** Involuntary contractions of multiple motor units.

**Trendelenburg gait:** A drop of the non-weight-bearing pelvis and hip during its swing-through phase. Also known as a gluteus medius lurch.

**trichomoniasis:** Parasitic infestation of the genus Trichomonas.

**trigger finger:** Tenosynovitis of the flexor tendon sheath, most commonly seen in the third and fourth digits, resulting from thickening or nodules in the synovial sheath.

**trigger point:** A focal, hyperirritable area in the muscle or fascia that results in referred symptoms of pain, particularly when pressure is applied.

**Trillat test:** Another name for the Lachman test. Also known as the Lachman-Trillat test or the Ritchie test.

**trophic:** Disordered or altered nutrition.

**true leg length discrepancy:** A measurement difference in left and right leg length when measured between the ASIS and the medial or the lateral malleolus.

**turf toe:** Sprain of the first metatarsophalangeal joint. Also known as great toe sprain.

**unhappy triad:** Combined injury to the anterior cruciate ligament, medial collateral ligament, and medial meniscus.

**upper motor neuron:** Motor nerves originating in the cerebral cortex that send stimuli from the brain to the motor nuclei of the spinal cord.

**urethritis:** Inflammation of the urethra.

**urinary calculi:** Kidney stones.

**urticaria:** Dermal hypersensitivity reaction to an allergen. More commonly known as hives.

**vaginitis:** Inflammation or infection of the vagina caused by microorganisms.

**valgus:** A medially directed force or angulation of the joint.

**valgus stress:** A medially directed force applied to the lateral aspect of a joint to cause gapping of the medial joint and test the integrity of the medial joint structures.

**valsalva maneuver:** A test in which the athlete holds his/her breath and bears down or similarly blows into a closed fist to increase intrathecal pressure. A positive sign indicates a herniated disc or other space-occupying lesion within the spinal canal.

**varicella:** The childhood version of herpes zoster. Also known as chickenpox.

**varus:** A laterally directed force or angulation of the joint.

**varus stress:** A laterally directed force applied to the medial aspect of a joint to cause gapping of the lateral joint and test the integrity of the lateral joint structures.

**vasomotor:** Smooth muscle control of blood vessel size.

**vasovagal:** Reflex dilation of blood vessels.

**vertigo:** Dizziness.

**vesiculations:** Small ruptures or blistering of the skin.

**viral myocarditis:** Inflammation of the heart muscle caused by a viral infection.

**visceral pleura:** The inner layer of the pleural sac that adheres to the surface of the lung.

**volar:** Palmar aspect of the wrist and hand.

**Volkmann's ischemic contracture:** Contracture deformity of the wrist and hand resulting from ischemic necrosis of the forearm muscles.

**wheal:** A reaction of the skin surface characterized by an elevation of a patch of skin that is smooth and red in appearance.

**wheezing:** A high-pitched whistling sound heard with auscultation, commonly noted with bronchial restriction in association with asthma.

**winging of the scapula:** Protrusion of the vertebral border of the scapula away from the posterior chest wall as a result of serratus anterior weakness.

**Yergason's test:** A test for assessing bicipital tendinitis.

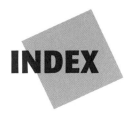

# INDEX

Note: The italicized *f* and *t* following page numbers refer to figures and tables, respectively.

# ABOUT THE AUTHORS

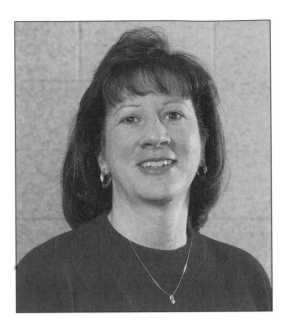

**Sandra J. Shultz**, PhD, ATC, CSCS, teaches and conducts clinical research in the Sports Medicine and Athletic Training Program at the University of Virginia. As a certified athletic trainer since 1984, she has a broad clinical perspective with experience at the collegiate, high school, and clinical settings, as well as Olympic and international levels.

Prior to coming to the University of Virginia, Dr. Shultz served as associate director of athletic training and rehabilitative services at the University of California at Los Angeles where two of her primary responsibilities were the direct health care of student athletes and the education of student athletic trainers.

She is a member of the National Athletic Trainers' Association (NATA), the American College of Sports Medicine, and the National Strength and Conditioning Association. She serves on the NATA Entry-Level Education Committee and the Appropriate Medical Coverage for Intercollegiate Athletics Task Force. She is actively involved in research related to sport injury risk and has received grant funding from the National Federation of State High School Associations and the NATA Research and Education Foundation.

Dr. Shultz attained a master's degree from the University of Arizona and a PhD from the University of Virginia. In her spare time, she enjoys running, traveling, and reading novels.

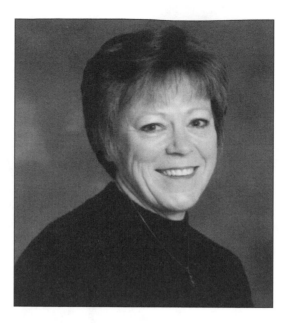

**Peggy A. Houglum**, MS, ATC, PT, has more than 28 years of experience in rehabilitation providing patient and athlete care since 1971. Her extensive background as a certified athletic trainer and physical therapist has provided her with a unique perspective regarding sports injury evaluations that make injury recognition and assessment techniques meaningful and appropriate.

Houglum has clinical experience with the United States Olympic Committee, the 1984 Olympics, the 1985 World University Games, and at universities and clinics.

A member of the National Athletic Trainers' Association and the Sports Section of the American Physical Therapy Association, Houglum received the NATA Most Distinguished Athletic Trainer Award in 1996. Currently chair of the NATA Continuing Education Committee, she also has served on the NATA Professional Education Committee, the NATA Education Council, and the NATA Clinical Education Committee.

Houglum attained her master's degree in athletic training from Indiana State University and is currently pursuing a PhD in Sports Medicine from the University of Virginia. She lives in Charlottesville, Virginia, and enjoys painting, cycling, and traveling in her spare time.

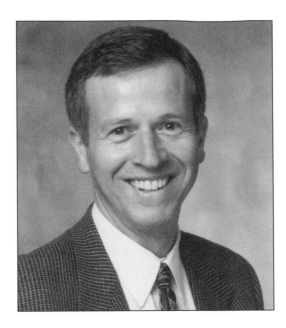

**David H. Perrin**, PhD, ATC, is the Joe Gieck Professor of Sports Medicine and the chair of the department of human services and curriculum director of graduate athletic training and sports medicine in the Curry School of Education at the University of Virginia.

Dr. Perrin is editor-in-chief of the *Journal of Athletic Training* and was the founding editor of the *Journal of Sport Rehabilitation*. He is author of *Isokinetic Exercise and Assessment* and *Athletic Taping and Bracing* and editor of *The Injured Athlete* (Third Edition).

For 13 years, Perrin served as a member of the NATA Professional Education Committee, helping to write the guidelines for accreditation of both undergraduate and graduate athletic training education programs.

Perrin's research interests include muscle performance, knee arthrometry, joint proprioception, and postural stability. His awards from the National Athletic Trainers' Association include the Sayers "Bud" Miller Distinguished Educator Award, the Most Distinguished Athletic Trainer Award, and the William G. Clancy, Jr., MD Medal for Distinguished Athletic Training Research. He is a fellow of the American College of Sports Medicine and a fellow of the American Academy of Kinesiology and Physical Education.

Dr. Perrin received his master's degree from Indiana State University and his PhD from the University of Pittsburgh. In his free time, he enjoys traveling, exercising, and vacationing at his lake cottage in Vermont.

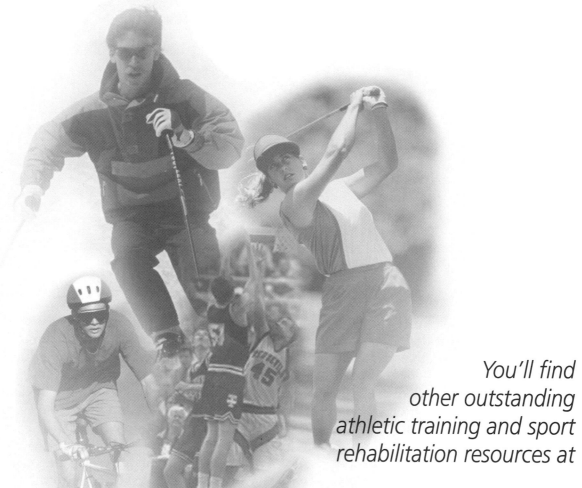

*You'll find
other outstanding
athletic training and sport
rehabilitation resources at*

# www.HumanKinetics.com

*In the U.S. call*

## 800-747-4457

Australia .................................... 08 8277 1555
Canada ................................... 1-800-465-7301
Europe ......................... +44 (0) 113 255 5665
New Zealand ............................... 09-523-3462

**HUMAN KINETICS**
*The Information Leader in Physical Activity*
P.O. Box 5076 • Champaign, IL 61825-5076 USA